Foot and Ankle Arthroscopy

Springer
New York
Berlin
Heidelberg
Hong Kong
London
Milan
Paris
Tokyo

Foot and Ankle Arthroscopy

James F. Guhl, M.D.
Medical College of Wisconsin
Milwaukee, Wisconsin

Melbourne D. Boynton, M.D.
Vermont Orthopaedic Clinic
Rutland, Vermont

J. Serge Parisien, M.D.
The Hospital for Joint Diseases and New York University
School of Medicine
New York, New York

Editors

With 429 Illustrations, 249 in Full Color

Springer

James F. Guhl
Emeritus Professor of Orthopaedic Surgery
Department of Orthopaedic Surgery
Medical College of Wisconsin
Milwaukee, Wisconsin 53226

Melbourne D. Boynton
Attending Orthopaedic Surgeon
Vermont Orthopaedic Clinic
Rutland, Vermont 05701

J. Serge Parisien
Chief of Arthroscopic Surgery
The Hospital for Joint Diseases
New York, NY 10128
and
Clinical Professor
Department of Orthopaedic Surgery
New York University School of Medicine
New York, NY 10016

Library of Congress Cataloging-in-Publication Data
Foot and ankle arthroscopy / editors, James F. Guhl, J. Serge Parisien, Melbourne D. Boynton.—3rd ed.
p. cm.
Includes bibliographical references and index.
ISBN 0-387-98511-5 (h/c : alk. paper)
1. Ankle—Endoscopic surgery. 2. Ankle—Examination. 3. Foot—Endoscopic surgery. 4. Foot—Examination. 5. Arthroscopy. I. Guhl, James F. II. Parisien, J. Serge. III. Boynton, Melbourne D.
[DNLM: 1. Ankle—pathology. 2. Ankle—surgery. 3. Ankle Joint—pathology. 4. Ankle joint—surgery. 5. Arthroscopy—methods. 6. Foot—pathology. 7. Foot—surgery. WE 880 F68605 2003]
RD562.A53 2003
617.5′84059—dc21 2002042728

Printed in Singapore.

9 8 7 6 5 4 3 2 1 SPIN 10675336

www.springer-ny.com

ISBN 0-387-98511-5 Printed on acid-free paper.

Springer-Verlag New York Berlin Heidelberg
A member of BertelsmannSpringer Science+Business Media GmbH

To Richard O'Connor
who taught me and who was my inspiration
in doing operative arthroscopy.

J.F.G.

To all physicians and their patients
who are pioneers in the exploration towards excellence
and the restoration of function.

M.D.B.

To my wife, May,
to my children, Christine, Dan, Ana, and Alex,
and to all my teachers, past and present.

J.S.P.

Preface

Thanks to the efforts and talents of the senior editor, James F. Guhl, M.D., ankle arthroscopy has established itself as an important tool in the armamentarium of the orthopedic surgeon and allied practitioner interested in the field of foot and ankle surgery.

In keeping with Dr. Guhl's philosophy, experienced surgeons have been invited to discuss various aspects of the management of foot and ankle disorders in order to present this book as a single-source reference regarding foot and ankle arthroscopy. Chapters pertaining to clinical examination, anatomy, and various arthroscopic techniques, including their indications, contraindications, and possible complications, are discussed with clarity, providing a wealth of useful, up-to-date information. New promising procedures are covered as well. The text also devotes a chapter to rehabilitation.

We express our deepest gratitude to all the contributors for a job well done. We also would like to thank the developmental editor, Merry Post, and the editorial staff of Springer-Verlag, Rob Albano and Sadie Forrester, for their invaluable assistance in the preparation and publication of this new edition.

James F. Guhl, M.D.
J. Serge Parisien, M.D.
Melbourne D. Boynton, M.D.
September 2003

Contents

Contributors

GREGORY R. APPLEGATE, M.D.
MRI Department
Valley Advanced Imaging Medical Group
6855 Noble Avenue
Van Nuys, CA 94105, USA
and
Assistant Clinical Professor
Department of Radiology
University of California, San Diego
San Diego, CA 92103, USA

STEPHEN L. BARRETT, D.P.M.
Director of Surgical Training
Institute for Peripheral Nerve Surgery
Baltimore, MD 21218, USA
and
25227 Borough Park Drive
Spring, TX 77380, USA

MELBOURNE D. BOYNTON, M.D.
Vermont Orthopaedic Cinic
Killington Medical Clinic
3 Albert Cree Drive
Rutland, VT 05701, USA

JOHN T. CAMPBELL, M.D.
Chief, Division of Foot and Ankle Surgery
Department of Orthopaedic Survery
Johns Hopkins University
Johns Hopkins Bayview Medical Center
4940 Eastern Avenue
Baltimore, MD 21224, USA

FREDERICK N. DAY III, D.P.M.
3339 Central Avenue, Suite F
Hot Springs, AK 71913, USA

WALTER A. DEL GALLO, M.D., P.A.
Calallen Orthopedics, LLP
Northwest Regional Hospital
14317 Northwest Boulevard, Suite A
Corpus Christi, TX 78140, USA

CHRISTOPHER W. DIGIOVANNI, M.D.
Department of Orthopaedic Surgery
Brown University School of Medicine
Rhode Island Hospital
593 Eddy Street
Providence, RI 02903, USA

MICHAEL F. DILLINGHAM, M.D.
Department of Orthopedic Surgery
Stanford University Medical Center
500 Arguello Street, Suite 100
Redwood City, CA 94063, USA

GARY S. FANTON, M.D.
Adjunct Clinical Assistant Professor
Department of Orthopedic Surgery
Stanford University Hospital
500 Arguello Street, Suite 100
Redwood City, CA 94063, USA

MICHAEL D. FELDMAN, M.D.
Department of Orthopedic Surgery
The Miriam Hospital
164 Summit Avenue
Providence, RI 02906, USA

RICHARD D. FERKEL, M.D.
Southern California Orthopedic Institute
6815 Noble Avenue
Van Nuys, CA 91405, USA

CAROL C. FREY, M.D.
Assistant Clinical Professor of Orthopedic Surgery
Department of Orthopedic Surgery
The David Geffen School of Medicine at UCLA
Los Angeles, CA 90095, USA
and
Orthopaedic Foot & Ankle Center
1200 Rosecrans Avenue, Suite 208
Manhattan Beach, CA 90266, USA

JAMES M. GLICK, M.D.
Clinical Professor
Department of Orthopaedic Surgery
University of California, San Francisco
1199 Bush Street, Suite 200
San Francisco, CA 94109, USA

JAMES F. GUHL, M.D.
Clinical Professor, Emeritus
Department of Orthopaedic Surgery
Medical College of Wisconsin
Milwaukee, WI 53226, USA

STEVEN L. HADDAD, M.D.
Assistant Professor of Clinical Orthopaedic Surgery
Northwestern University
Chicago, IL 60611, USA
and
Illinois Bone & Joint Institute
Glenview Medical Arts Building
2401 Ravine Way
Glenview, IL 60025, USA

LARS KONRADSEN, M.D.
Orthopedic Department
Gentofte Hospital
University of Copenhagen
DK-2900 Hellerup, Denmark

DR. RICHARD O. LUNDEEN, D.P.M.
Director, Podiatric Medical Information
Winona Memorial Hospital
3232 North Meridian Street
Indianapolis, IN 46208, USA

RICHARD J. MASON, M.D.
Attending Surgeon
Department of Orthopaedic Surgery
The Orthopedic Center
510 Idlewild Avenue
Easton, MD 21601, USA
and
Clinical Instructor
Department of Orthopaedic Surgery
Johns Hopkins University School of Medicine
Baltimore, MD 21205, USA

CRAIG D. MORGAN, M.D.
Morgan Kalman Clinic
2501 Silverside Road
Wilmington, DE 19810, USA

LAWRENCE OLOFF, D.P.M.
Staff, Stanford University Hospital
500 Arguello Street, Suite 100
Redwood City, Ca 94063, USA

J. SERGE PARISIEN, M.D.
Attending Orthopaedic Surgeon
Sport Medicine Service
Hospital for Joint Diseases
New York, NY 10003, USA
and
Clinical Professor
Department of Orthopaedic Surgery
New York University School of Medicine
New York, NY 10016, USA

PER RENSTROM, M.D., Ph.D.
Department of Orthopedics
Karolinska Hospital
Stockholm, 171 76 Sweden

MARC A. SAMSON, M.D.
Department of Orthopaedic Surgery
Good Samaritan Hospital
1245 Wilshire Boulevard, Second Floor
Los Angeles, CA 90017, USA

Lew C. Schon, M.D.
Director, Foot & Ankle Fellowship
Department of Orthopaedic Surgery
Union Memorial Hospital
3333 North Calvert Street
Baltimore, MD 21218, USA
and
Assistant Professor
Johns Hopkins University School of Medicine
Baltimore, MD 21205, USA

Neal C. Small, M.D. (Retired)
Associated Orthopaedics & Sports Medicine
4031 West Plano Parkway
Plano, TX 75093, USA

James P. Tasto, M.D.
Clinical Professor
Department of Orthopaedics
University of California, San Diego
San Diego, CA 92103, USA
and
San Diego Sports Medicine and Orthopaedics
6719 Alvarado Road, Suite 200
San Diego, CA 92120, USA

George Thabit III, M.D.
Department of Orthopedic Surgery
Stanford University Medical Center
500 Arguello Street, Suite 100
Redwood City, CA 94063, USA

C.N. van Dijk, Prof. Dr.
Department of Orthopedic Surgery
Academic Medical Center
University of Amsterdam
Room G4-219
P.O. Box 22660
1100-DD Amsterdam, The Netherlands

Carole S. Vetter, M.D.
Department of Orthopaedic Surgery
Medical College of Wisconsin
9200 West Wisconsin Avenue
Milwaukee, WI 53226, USA

CHAPTER 1

Gross and Arthroscopic Anatomy of the Foot

Carol C. Frey and Christopher W. DiGiovanni

The complex anatomy of the foot makes radiographic and arthroscopic examination difficult. On the other hand, advances in small-joint instrumentation and techniques have helped revolutionize the care of foot disorders. As arthroscopic technology develops, the surgeon is better able to treat pathology in the foot efficiently and in a less invasive way. Along with the advancements in technique, however, it is paramount that the surgeon understands the pertinent gross and arthroscopic anatomy of the foot. A better understanding of the difficult anatomy of the foot, and the hindfoot in particular, should greatly facilitate the performance of such surgery and proper recognition of abnormal pathology when it is present.

SUBTALAR JOINT

Gross Anatomy

The subtalar joint is divided into anterior and posterior sections by the sinus tarsi and tarsal canal (Fig. 1.1). The contents of the tarsal canal include the cervical ligament, talocalcaneal interosseous ligament, medial root of the inferior extensor retinaculum, fat pad, and blood vessels (Fig. 1.2).

The anterior portion of the subtalar joint, also known as the talocalcaneonavicular joint, includes its anterior and middle articulating facets. It also contains the talonavicular articulation and the spring ligament. The anterior subtalar joint is generally thought to be inaccessible to arthroscopic visualization owing to the thick interosseous ligament, which fills the tarsal canal. Because of this, the region normally has no connection with the posterior joint complex.

The posterior subtalar joint has a long axis located obliquely 40 degrees to the midline of the foot, facing laterally. It consists of the convex posterior facet of the calcaneus and the concave posterior facet of the talus. The capsule of the posterior subtalar joint is reinforced laterally by the cervical ligament and the calcaneofibular ligament, and it has a posterior pouch and a small lateral recess.

Arthroscopic Portals

Few studies in the literature have dealt with arthroscopy of the subtalar joint.[1–5] Parisien and Vangsness[1,2] described anterior and posterior portals; Frey et al.[3] described the middle portal; and Mekhail et al.[6] described the medial portal (Fig. 1.3).

The posterior portal is approached from the side. A trocar is inserted in an upward and slightly anterior manner approximately 2 cm posterior and just proximal to the tip of the lateral malleolus, making sure it is behind the lesser saphenous vein and sural nerve and anterior to the Achilles tendon.[7] In an anatomic study of portal placement and safety, the posterior portal was located an average of 25 mm (range 20–28 mm) posterior and 6 mm (range 0–10 mm) proximal to the tip of the fibula.[3] The poste-

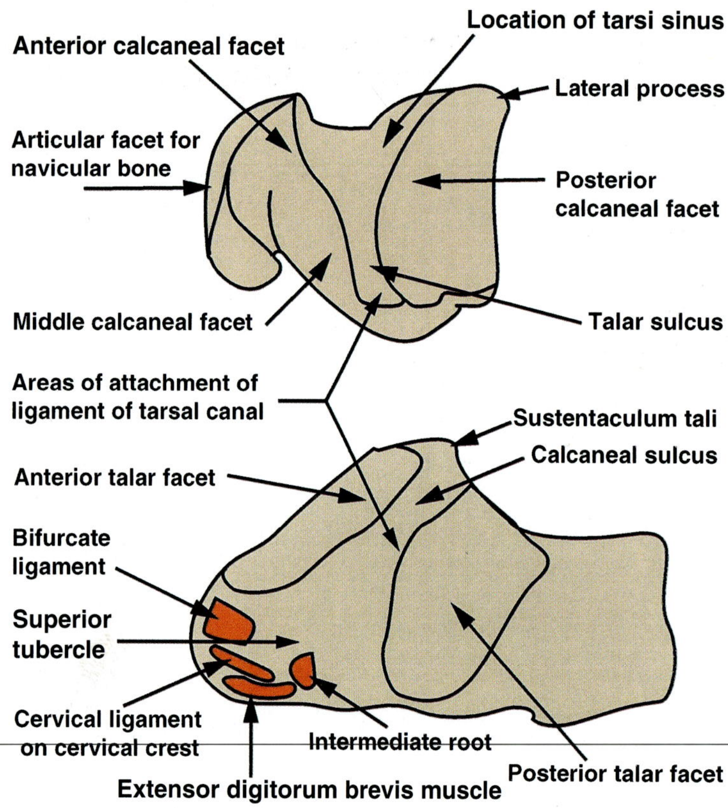

FIGURE 1.1. Subtalar joint can be divided into anterior and posterior sections by the sinus tarsi, the tarsal canal, and its contents.

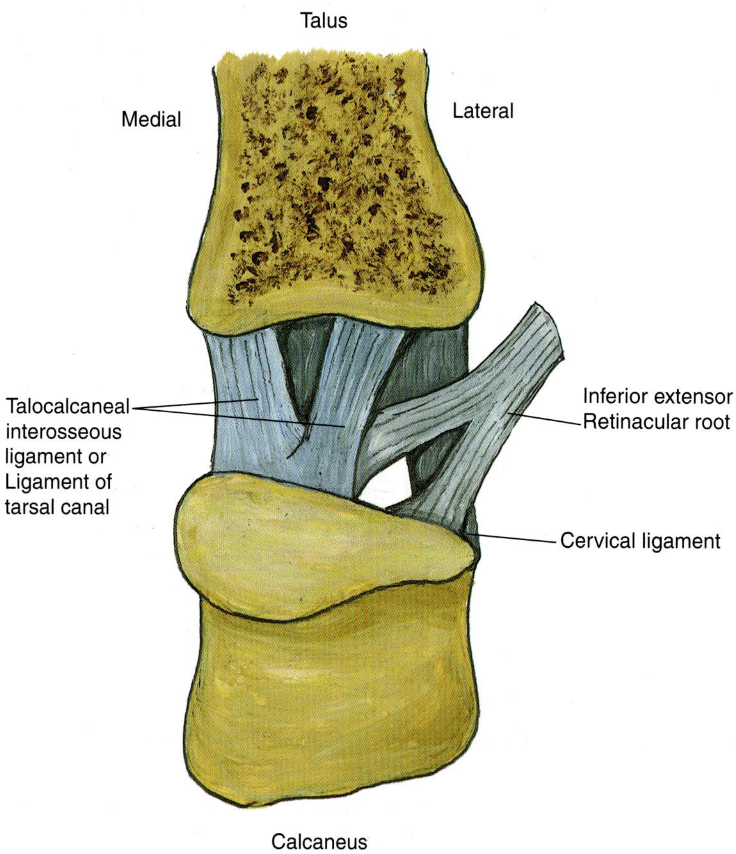

FIGURE 1.2. Contents of the tarsal canal include the cervical ligament, talocalcaneal interosseous ligament, medial root of the inferior extensor retinaculum, fat pad, and blood vessels.

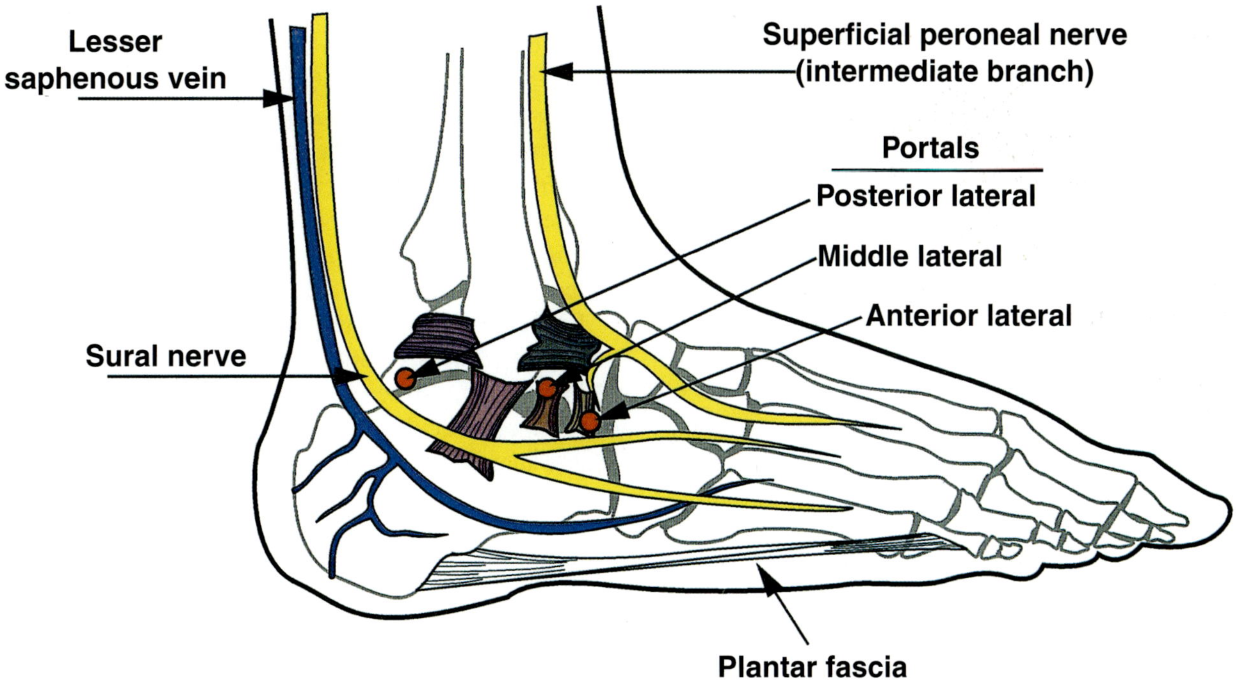

FIGURE 1.3. Location of the anterior, lateral, and middle portals for subtalar joint arthroscopy.

rior portal is associated with the highest risk, compared to other subtalar portals, of causing nerve or vessel damage. Structures endangered with posterior portal placement include the sural nerve, lesser saphenous vein, peroneal tendons, and Achilles tendon. Great care must be taken during posterior portal placement to avoid injury, especially to the sural nerve and lesser saphenous vein. After the skin incision, a hemostat should be used to spread the subcutaneous tissue gently down to the capsular level before inserting the arthroscope.

The sural nerve and lesser saphenous vein run parallel to each other along the posterolateral aspect of the ankle, the nerve lying posterior to the vein at the level of the ankle joint. In 7 of 10 cases reported by Frey et al.[3] the posterior portal was located posterior to the sural nerve, and in two cases it was found to be anterior to the nerve. The average distance from the sural nerve to the posterior portal was 4 mm (range 8 mm posterior, 6 mm anterior). In one case, the sural nerve was transected during portal placement; in another, a small laceration was made in the lesser saphenous vein. The peroneal tendon sheath was located an average of 11 mm (range 6–16 mm) anterior to the portal, and the Achilles tendon was an average of 15 mm posterior (range 10–20 mm) to the portal. Neither of these tendons was damaged in this series, but their proximity should be noted.

The point of entry for the anterior portal is described as being 2 cm anterior and 1 cm distal to the tip of the distal fibula, directing the instrument slightly upward and about 40 degrees posteriorly.[1,2] In the study by Frey et al. it was located an average of 28 mm (range 23–35 mm) anterior to the tip of the fibula. Structures at risk when placing this portal include the dorsal intermediate cutaneous branch of the superficial peroneal nerve, the dorsal lateral cutaneous branch of the sural nerve, the peroneus tertius tendon, and a small branch of the lesser saphenous vein. The dorsal intermediate cutaneous branch of the superficial peroneal nerve is located an average of 17 mm (range 0–28 mm) anterior to the portal. The dorsolateral cutaneous branch of the sural nerve, identified in 8 of 15 specimens reported by Frey et al., was located an average of 8 mm (range 2–12 mm) inferior to the anterior portal. The peroneus tertius tendon was located an average distance of 21 mm (range 8–33 mm) anterior to the portal. A small branch of the lesser saphenous vein consistently coursed along the anterolateral aspect of the foot in the vicinity of the anterior portal. It is located an average of 2 mm (range 0–5 mm) from the anterior portal and was lacerated in 20% of the cases reported by Frey et al. With use of the anterior portal, therefore, care must be taken to avoid injury to the dorsal intermediate cutaneous branch of the superficial peroneal nerve as it divides on the dorsum of the foot. A small branch of the lesser saphenous vein is also at risk, although damage to this structure is unlikely to cause significant problems.

The middle portal is described as being about 1 cm anterior to the tip of the fibula, directly over the sinus tarsi.[3] The middle portal was located an average of 10 mm (range 10–11 mm) anterior to the tip of the fibula. It is located directly over the sinus tarsi, and places no structures at risk during its placement. The middle portal is therefore considered relatively safe.

Mekhail et al.[6] described establishing a medial portal by placing a blunt-ended trocar into the sinus tarsi and then pushing it through the tarsal canal in a posteromedial and slightly cephalad direction (Fig. 1.4). The trocar should be angled about 45 degrees to the lateral border of the foot until exiting the skin. The ankle is in equinus and the foot inverted during placement of this portal. This position relaxes and slightly displaces the posteromedial neurovascular bundle posteriorly, thereby decreasing its risk of injury. Using blunt dissection, the portal entry lies along a line joining the tip of the medial malleolus to the medial calcaneal tubercle. The desired cannulation site is where the anterosuperior three-fourths joins the posteroinferior one-fourth of that line. Skeletal distraction can facilitate the use of this portal. It is thought that the posteromedial and anterolateral aspects of the posterior subtalar joint are better viewed from this portal than from the anterior or posterior portal. Specifically, the following intraarticular structures were thought to be better visualized: articular cartilage of the transverse portion and anterolateral slope of the posterior subtalar joint, calcaneofibular ligament, posterior pouch of the joint with its synovial lining, synovium covering the posterior aspect of the interosseous ligament, and joint capsule. One should be reminded, however, that these findings are the result of a cadaveric study, and no clinical trials have been reported using this portal. Moreover, in feet with significant edema or adipose tissue, the exit point for the trocar would be

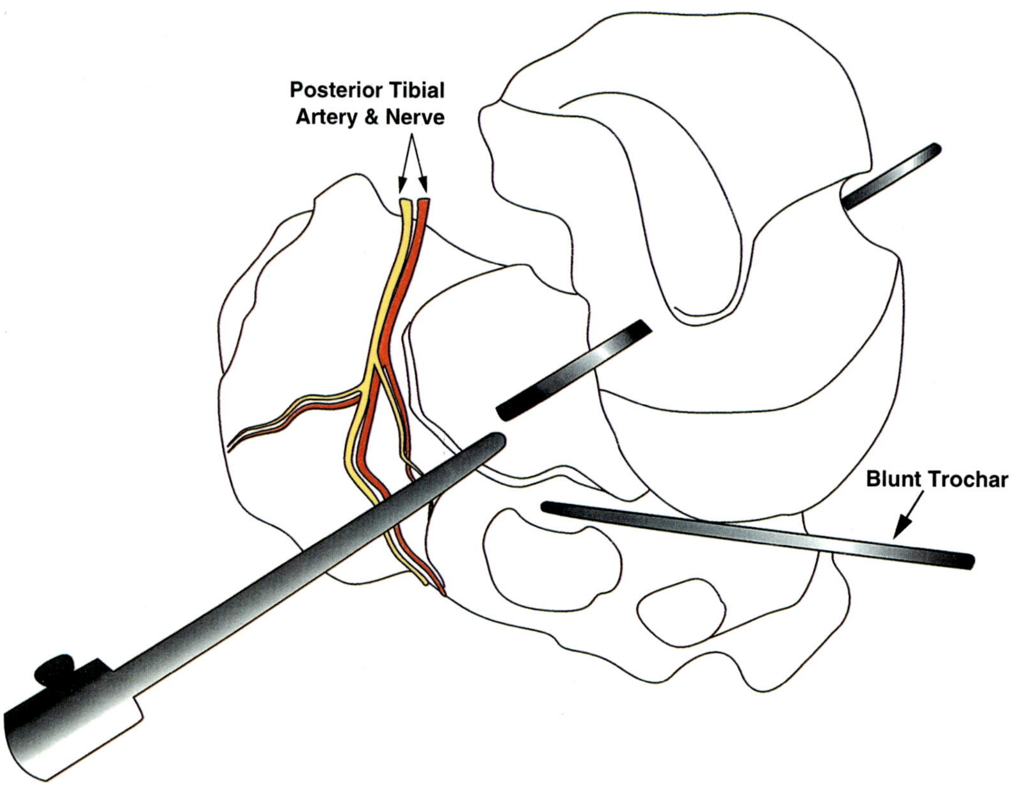

FIGURE 1.4. Medial portal is established by placing a blunt-ended trocar into the sinus tarsi, which is then pushed through the tarsal canal in a posteromedial and slightly cephalad direction. The trocar should be angled about 45 degrees to the lateral border of the foot until exiting the skin. Using blunt dissection, the portal entry lies along a line joining the tip of the medial malleolus to the medial calcaneal tubercle.

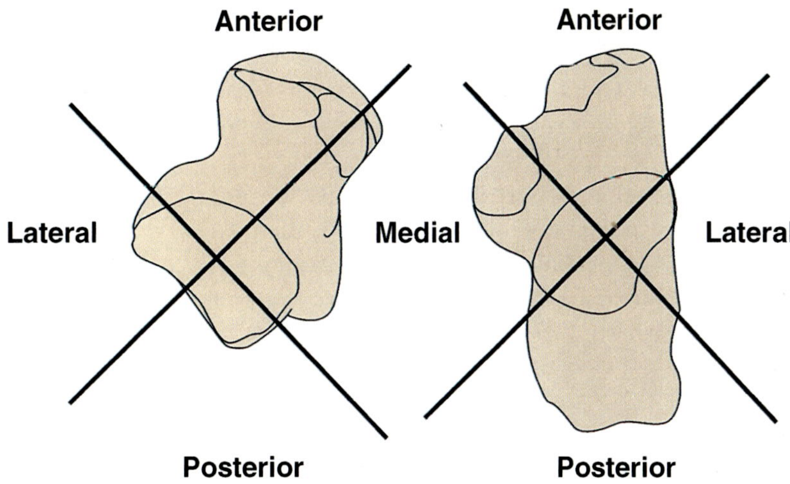

FIGURE 1.5. The posterior subtalar joint can be divided into four compartments: lateral, medial, anterior, and posterior.

more posterior than usual, which would potentially situate the portal closer to the posterior neurovascular bundle. This portal is rarely used.

Arthroscopic Anatomy

The posterior subtalar joint can be divided into four compartments: lateral, medial, anterior, and posterior (Fig. 1.5). The anterior and middle facets are located anterior and medial to the posterior facet, separated from it by the thick interosseous ligaments. It is difficult to visualize the middle and anterior facets unless there is a defect in the interosseous ligament structures. As the arthroscope enters the sinus tarsi, these ligaments block all access to the anterior joint and almost completely fill the tarsal canal. Only if the ligament is removed or torn can the anterior joint be accessed from laterally placed portals (Fig. 1.6).

The best portal combination for access to the cartilaginous posterior facet of the subtalar joint involves placing the arthroscope through the anterior portal and the instruments through the posterior portal. This allows direct visualization and instrumentation of nearly the entire cartilaginous surface of the posterior facet, posterior aspect of the in-

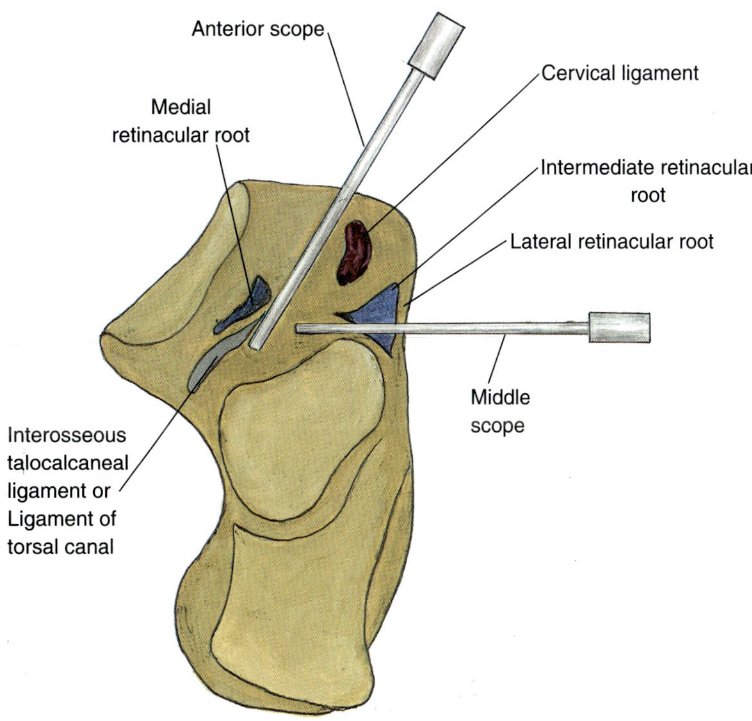

FIGURE 1.6. As the arthroscope enters the sinus tarsi, the interosseous ligaments almost completely fill the tarsal canal and block access to the anterior joint.

terosseous ligament, lateral capsule and its small recess (where it is possible to access the calcaneofibular and lateral talocalcaneal ligaments), and posterior pouch of the posterior joint with its synovial lining.

Instrumentation through the anterior portal provides access to the lateral compartment of the posterior facet. The medial, anterior, and posterior compartments cannot be reached through the anterior portal. In addition, there is significant risk of iatrogenic damage to the underlying subchondral bone; therefore it is not recommended that the anterior portal be used for instrumentation of the posterior facet.

The anterior and lateral compartments of the posterior facet and structures located in the extraarticular sinus tarsi are best accessed by placing the arthroscope through the anterior portal and the instruments through the middle portal. By avoiding posterior portal placement, potential damage to the sural nerve is averted. In addition, excellent visualization of the medial and posterior compartments of the posterior facet is possible, even though they cannot be instrumented via the middle portal. This portal combination is thus recommended for visualization and instrumentation of the sinus tarsi and the anterior and lateral compartments of the posterior subtalar joint, as well as when only visual inspection of the medial and posterior compartments is necessary.

OS TRIGONUM AND STIEDA'S PROCESS

Gross Anatomy

Terminology regarding the anatomy of the posterior aspect of the talus and subtalar joint can be confusing. The posterior surface of the talus, or "processus posterior," consists of the posteromedial and posterolateral processes, also known as tubercles (Fig. 1.7). Between these tubercles glides the flexor hallucis longus tendon in its small sulcus, which is directed obliquely downward and inward, angling anteriorly.[7] The larger posterolateral process, also called Stieda's process, can vary markedly in size. It is in direct continuity inferiorly with the posterolateral aspect of the articular surface of the talus, making it a partially intraarticular structure and thus possible to examine arthroscopically.[7] Its superior

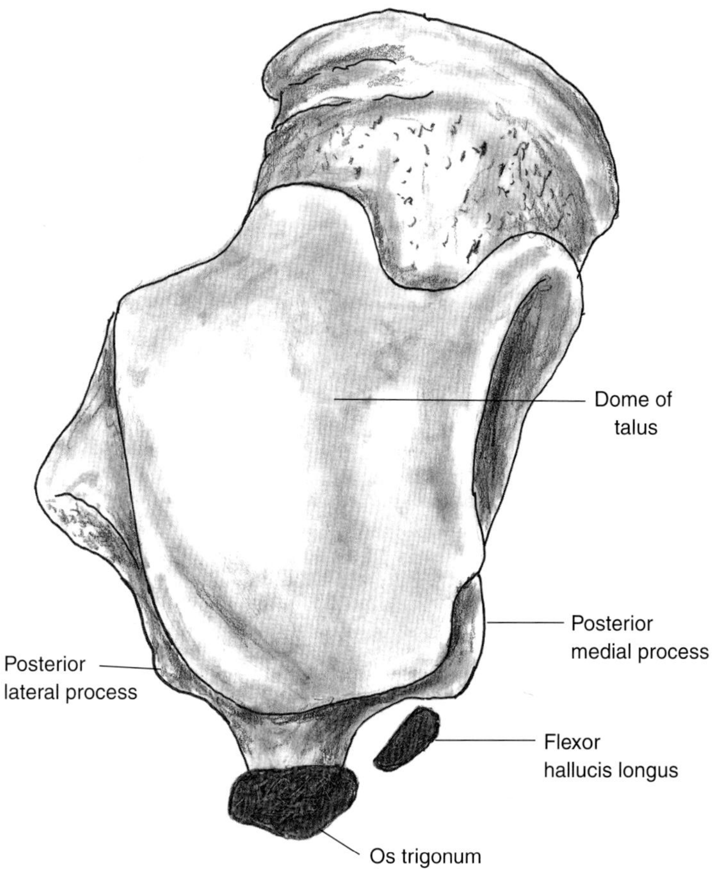

FIGURE 1.7. Posterior surface of the talus consists of both the posteromedial and posterolateral processes, also known as tubercles. Between the tubercles lies the flexor hallucis longus tendon in a small sulcus.

surface, however, is nonarticular, being part of the insertion of the posterior talofibular ligament and a portion of the fibuloastragalocalcaneal ligament of Rouviere and Canela Lazaro.[7] Occasionally, an accessory ossicle communicates with the posterolateral tubercle, and this is called the os trigonum. It too has multiple surfaces: anterior, inferior, and posterior. The anterior surface articulates with the posterolateral tubercle and the inferior surface with the os calcis. The posterior surface is nonarticular. When the os trigonum fuses, it is termed a trigonal process and becomes essentially a large lateral articulating tubercle.[7] It is often difficult to discern a fracture of Stieda's process from an os trigonum based on radiographs alone. Computed tomography (CT) scans and views of the opposite foot are sometimes helpful.[8]

The medial tubercle of the talus, an extension of the medial talar surface, provides an attachment site for a portion of the deep and superficial deltoid ligament, the medial talocalcaneal ligament, and part of the fibrous tunnel overlying the flexor hallucis.[7] When large enough, it is occasionally responsible for talocalcaneal coalitions. It should also be noted that posterior osteophytes can occur in the posterior region of the subtalar joint, which can be approached arthroscopically.

None of these terms should be confused with the lateral process of the talus, which is a distinctly different structure located on the mid-lateral aspect of the talus. It serves as the insertion of the lateral talocalcaneal ligament but is of arthroscopic importance because it is a palpable bony landmark and can be identified intraarticularly as the floor of the lateral gutter of the subtalar joint and capsule.

Arthroscopic Anatomy and Portals

Arthroscopic excision of the os trigonum is an advanced arthroscopic technique and has been reported to be a good alternative to open treatment for patients who require surgical intervention. Compared to open incisions, properly placed arthroscopic portals offer a decreased risk of skin necrosis, incisional neuromas, and cutaneous scarring.

Subtalar arthroscopy using standard portals is performed first. The borders of the os trigonum are carefully identified using specialized small-joint instrumentation. Care must be taken when working near the posterior and medial borders to avoid injury to the flexor hallucis longus and posterior tibial neurovascular bundle. When free of soft tissue attachments, the os is delivered with a grasper through an enlarged posterior portal. An accessory posterior subtalar portal is occasionally required under these circumstances (Fig. 1.8).

RETROCALCANEAL BURSA AND HAGLUND'S DEFORMITY

Gross Anatomy

The retrocalcaneal bursa is a consistently present, horseshoe-shaped structure located between the posterosuperior process of the calcaneus and the Achilles tendon[9] (Fig. 1.9). The distance from the calcaneal insertion of the Achilles tendon to the tip of the posterosuperior portion of the calcaneus is usually 2–3 cm. Although it is possible to obtain a bursogram of the retrocalcaneal bursa, the potential space usually contains only 1 ml or so of fluid, making it difficult to enter the bursa with an arthroscope. It can, however, be approached endoscopically.

Endoscopic Anatomy and Portals

Open procedures to remove the retrocalcaneal bursa and accompanying calcaneal exostosis have been described using single and double incisions. An endoscopic procedure has also been described. As with open procedures, to perform the endoscopic procedure well the anatomy of the retrocalcaneal space must be understood.

The superficial anatomy of the posterior aspect of the hindfoot is not complex. The medial and lateral borders of the Achilles tendon are easy to palpate in all patients, and the posterosuperior aspect of the calcaneus is easy to locate. The Achilles tendon inserts on the posterior margin of the calcaneus approximately 2 cm distal to its posterosuperior margin. The sural nerve runs, on average, 7 mm anterior to the anterior margin of the Achilles tendon.[10] Care must be taken when making the lateral portal, as the calcaneal branches of the lateral plantar nerve are also at risk in this region. Furthermore, the location of even a small portal in the area can cause a long period of postoperative tenderness aggravated by a firm heel counter when the patient returns to wearing shoes.

Endoscopy of the bursa is approached using a portal created just medial and lateral to the Achilles tendon at the level of the retrocalcaneal bursa

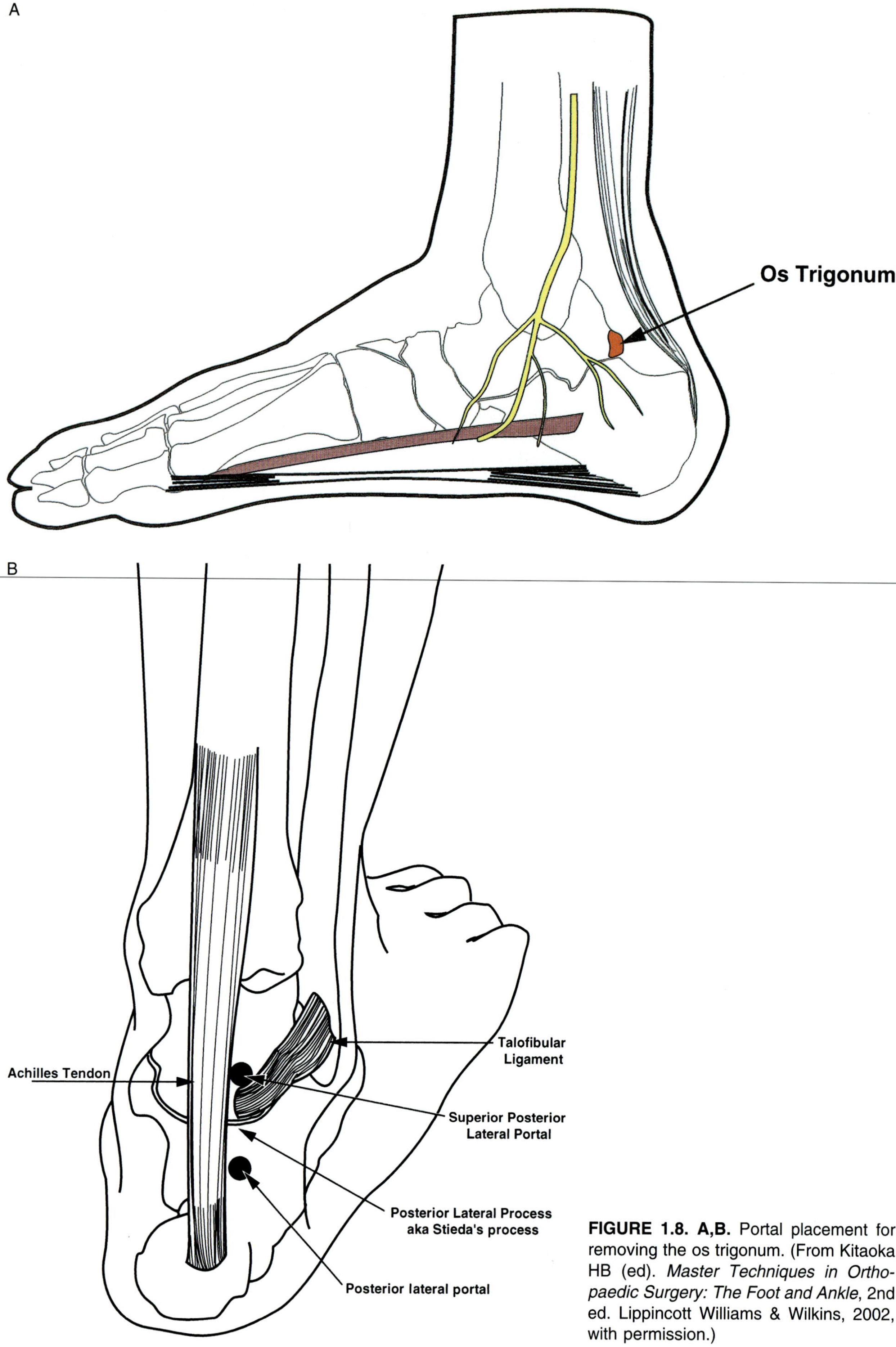

FIGURE 1.8. A,B. Portal placement for removing the os trigonum. (From Kitaoka HB (ed). *Master Techniques in Orthopaedic Surgery: The Foot and Ankle*, 2nd ed. Lippincott Williams & Wilkins, 2002, with permission.)

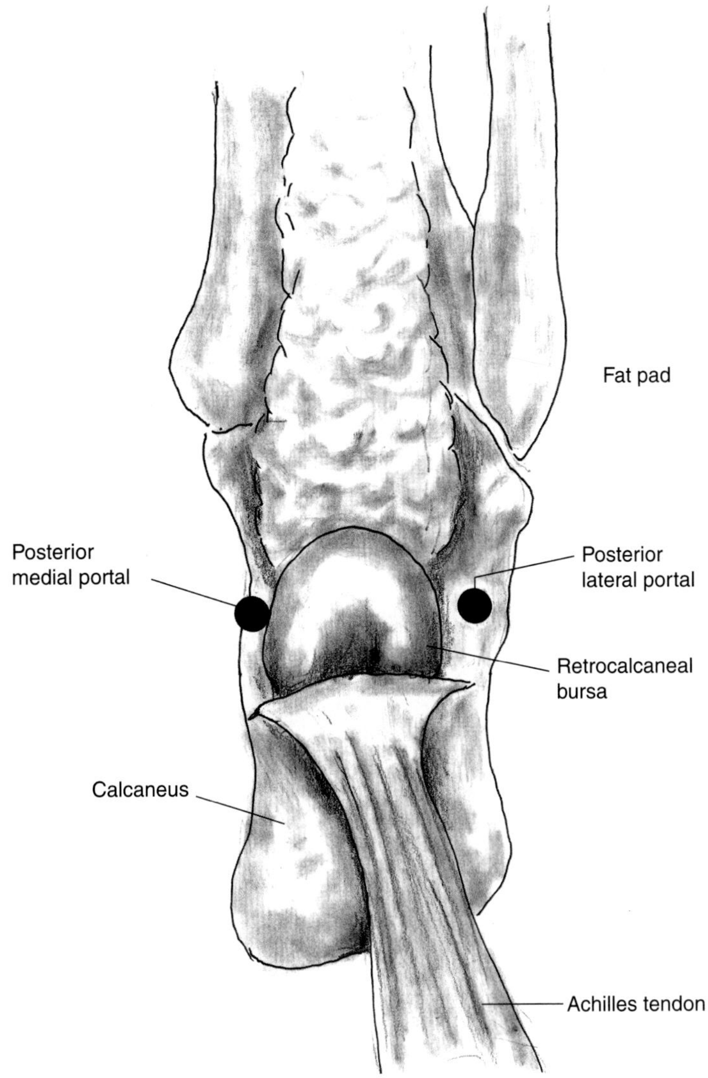

FIGURE 1.9. Retrocalcaneal bursa is a consistently present, horseshoe-shaped structure located between the posterosuperior process of the calcaneus and the Achilles tendon.

(Fig. 1.10). A 3-mm vertical incision is made in the skin, and the subcutaneous tissue is spread with a mosquito clamp. The bursa is then entered with a blunt trochar and cannula. Zimmer[11] believed that the bursa could be readily inspected arthroscopically along its entire course, from tendon insertion to the most superior and posterior aspects of the calcaneus.

Endoscopic calcaneoplasty has been described[12] as a reasonable alternative to open resection of Haglund's deformity and the retrocalcaneal bursa. Horizontal portals have been created just above the superior aspect of the calcaneus medial and lateral to the Achilles tendon. The arthroscope and any necessary instrumentation can be utilized interchangeably through these portals. The endoscopic procedure removes the posterior cortex of the calcaneus starting at the posterosuperior aspect of the calcaneus and moving inferiorly 2–4 cm beyond the superior attachment of the Achilles tendon. No complications have been reported with these incisions.

PLANTAR FASCIA

Gross Anatomy

The plantar fascia is the investing fascial layer of the plantar aspect of the foot[7,13] (Fig. 1.11). It consists of a network of connective and adipose tissues whose main function is to support and protect the underlying structures of the foot. The plantar fascia, a thick structure, originates from the medial calcaneal tuberosity, widens through the arch of the foot, and distally inserts into the plantar aspect of the bases of proximal phalanges. Proximally, it receives fibers from the Achilles and plantaris tendons. Histologically, it is composed of both colla-

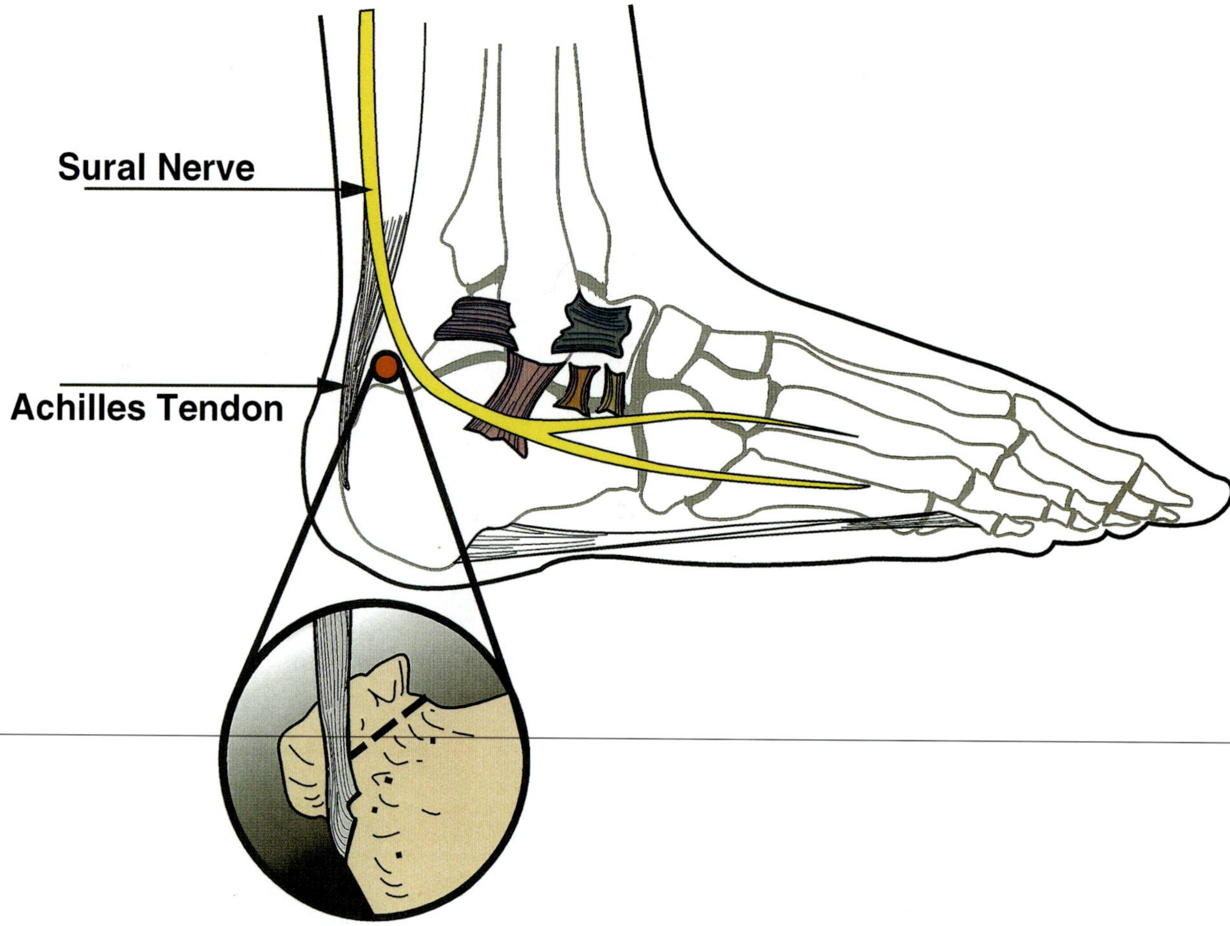

FIGURE 1.10. Endoscopy of the bursa is carried out using portals created just medial and lateral to the Achilles tendon at the level of the retrocalcaneal bursa.

gen and elastic fibers. The plantar fascia is subcutaneous and divides into three major components: central, lateral, and medial. The central fibers comprise the largest component. The plantar fascia is approximately 1.5–2.0 cm wide at its origin and expands distally to its insertional sites.[14] Its fibers are longitudinally oriented and adhere to the underlying flexor digitorum brevis muscle. On both sides it surrounds the flexor digitorum brevis muscle and thus forms the medial and lateral intermuscular septa.

It is at the level of the metatarsals that the fascia divides into five components that eventually insert distally at the bases of the toes and the overlying subcutaneous tissues and skin. Proximal to the metatarsophalangeal (MTP) joints, the longitudinal tracts are connected by transverse bands called the superficial transverse tract. The longitudinal tracts insert at the bases of the proximal phalanges via natatory and mooring ligaments. The longitudinal tracts, proximal to the metatarsal heads, also give off deep septa that pass on either side of the flexor tendons and insert onto the flexor tendon sheaths, the interosseous fascia, the fascia of the transverse head of the adductor hallucis, the deep transverse metatarsal ligament, and the plantar plate and collateral ligaments of the MTP joints.[14]

The lateral component is approximately 1.0–1.5 cm wide at its origin, before it extends toward the cuboid. Here, it divides into medial and lateral components, inserting into the base of the fifth metatarsal and the abductor digiti minimi fascia. The medial component, an extremely thin structure, forms most of the investing fascia of the abductor hallucis muscle. It is a more distinct structure distally.

The posterior tibial nerve provides multiple branches (medial calcaneal, medial plantar, and lateral plantar nerves) that cross the plantar medial as-

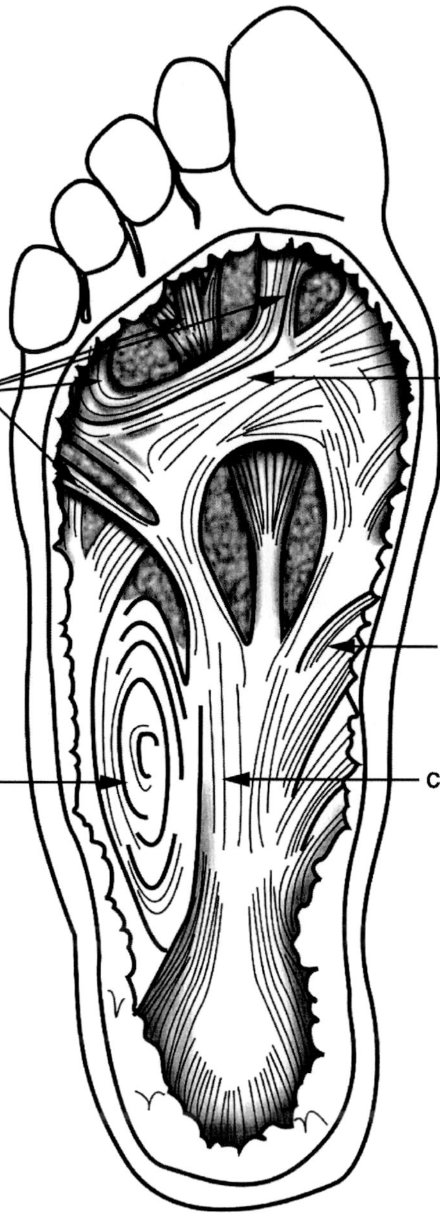

FIGURE 1.11. Plantar fascia is an investing fascial layer of the plantar aspect of the foot. It consists of a complex network of connective and adipose tissues that support and protect the underlying structures of the foot.

pect of the foot and heel. The first branch of the lateral plantar nerve (nerve to the abductor digiti quinti) passes just anterior to the medial calcaneal tuberosity (Fig. 1.12). The medial and lateral plantar nerves travel together under the abductor hallucis muscle. Distally, the medial plantar nerve travels under the abductor hallucis and then branches more superficially. The lateral plantar nerve emerges from under the abductor hallucis and follows an oblique course through the central compartment (Fig. 1.13). It lies between the flexor digitorum brevis and the quadratus muscle. Before beginning its course underneath the abductor hallucis, the lateral plantar nerve gives off a small branch, the nerve to the abductor digit minimi muscle. This nerve travels next to the medial calcaneal tubercle and passes laterally to innervate the abductor digiti minimi. There are also multiple calcaneal nerves, which may vary in number and course. Most of these nerves pass posterior to the lateral plantar nerve before terminating in the posteromedial aspect of the heel.

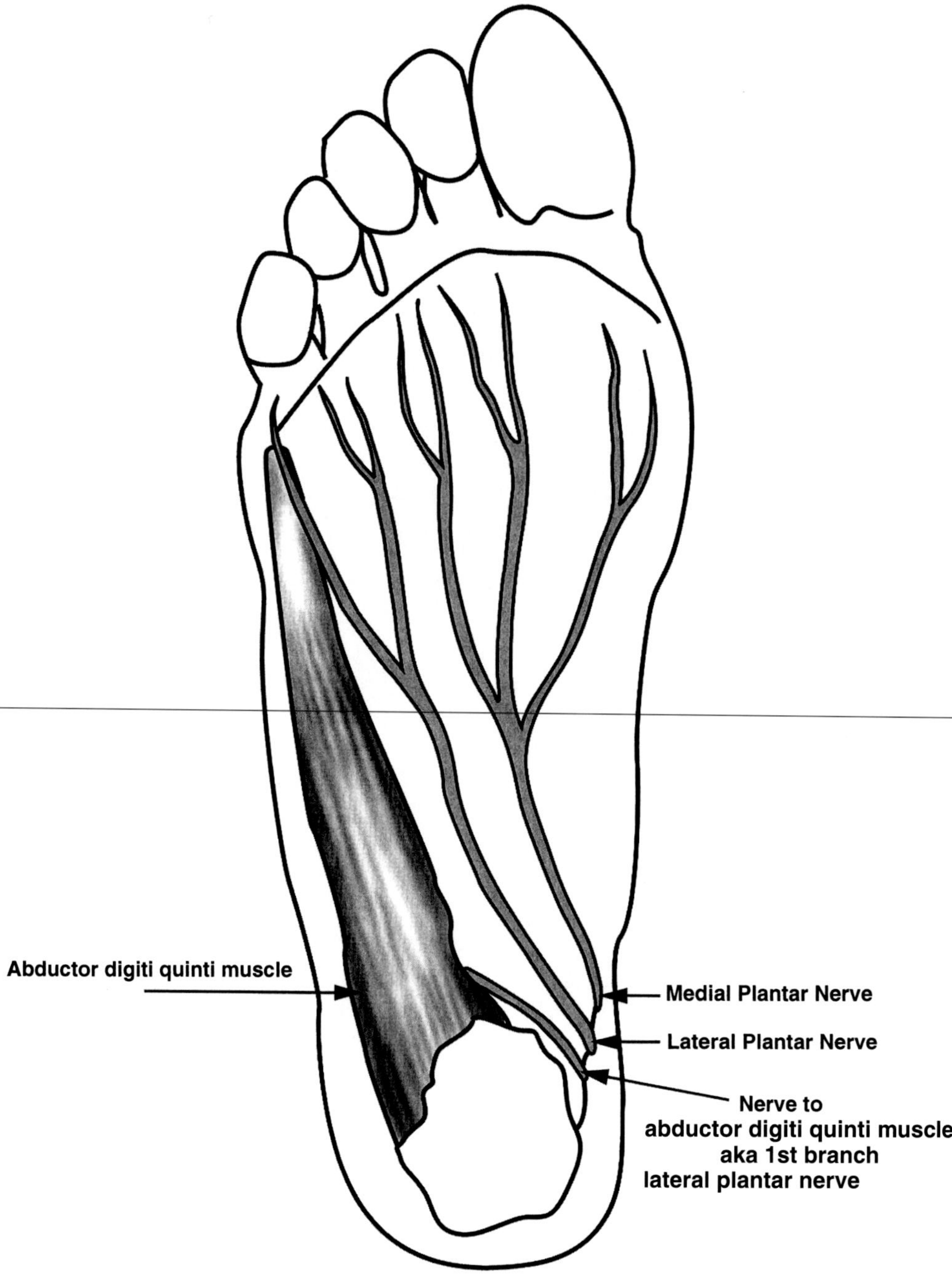

FIGURE 1.12. First branch of the lateral plantar nerve passes just anterior to the medial calcaneal tuberosity.

Arthroscopic Anatomy and Portals

Several structures are potentially at risk when using the endoscopic technique[15] for plantar fascial release, especially as most of these structures are not visualized during the procedure (Fig. 1.14). The structures at risk are the medial plantar nerve, lateral plantar nerve, nerve to the abductor digiti minimi, and intrinsic muscles. Hofmeister et al.[16] found that the calcaneal nerves were not at high risk for injury as they did not encounter any during dissection, although they did warn that the nerves have a variable course and should be carefully considered during endoscopy. The medial plantar nerve was found to be dorsal and medial to the area of dissection and was at low risk for injury. The lateral plantar nerve is not endangered so long as one is careful to keep both knife and en-

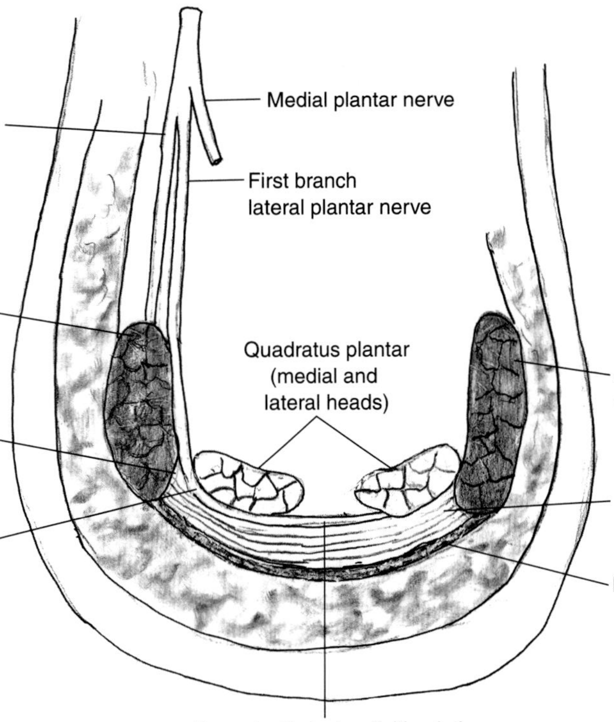

FIGURE 1.13. Course of the first branch of the lateral plantar nerve.

doscope in the superficial layers. The nerve to the abductor digiti minimi is also thought to be protected because of its proximity to the medial calcaneal tubercle. By placing the incision 1 cm distal to this tubercle, the nerve was not damaged in any of Hofmeister et al.'s specimens. The only structure injured while performing this technique was the flexor digitorum brevis, and damaged muscle fibers were clearly visualized through the endoscope. Great care must be exercised to avoid entering the central compartment where one may encounter intrinsic muscles and the lateral plantar nerve. Hofmeister et al.'s study also revealed that when using a one-portal technique for endoscopic plantar fascia release the average distances to the lateral plantar nerve and the nerve to the abductor digiti minimi are 10.5 and 12.3 mm, respectively. The flexor digitorum brevis muscle was partially transected in 46% of cases, and the average transection was 0.8 mm. Hofmeister et al. concluded that the endoscopic approach to release of the plantar fascia provides adequate release and does not appear to pose any danger to the underlying neurovascular structures.

Hawkins et al.[17] also studied the anatomy and structures at risk while performing an endoscopic plantar fascia release. They attempted 75% release using a two-portal technique. They found that partial release was possible, but controlling the exact percentage of the release was difficult. The release averaged 82% of the width of the fascia (range 53–100%). These authors noted that whereas the medial portion of the fascia was easy to identify through the endoscope the lateral border was not. They noted no damage to the first branch of the lateral plantar nerve in any specimen (the structure reported to be most at risk during the procedure). The release of the deep fascia of the abductor hallucis muscle was not possible in their study.

FIRST METATARSOPHALANGEAL JOINT

Gross Anatomy

Minimal stability is provided by the shallow ball-and-socket articulation between the proximal phalanx and the metatarsal head. The soft tissues,

A

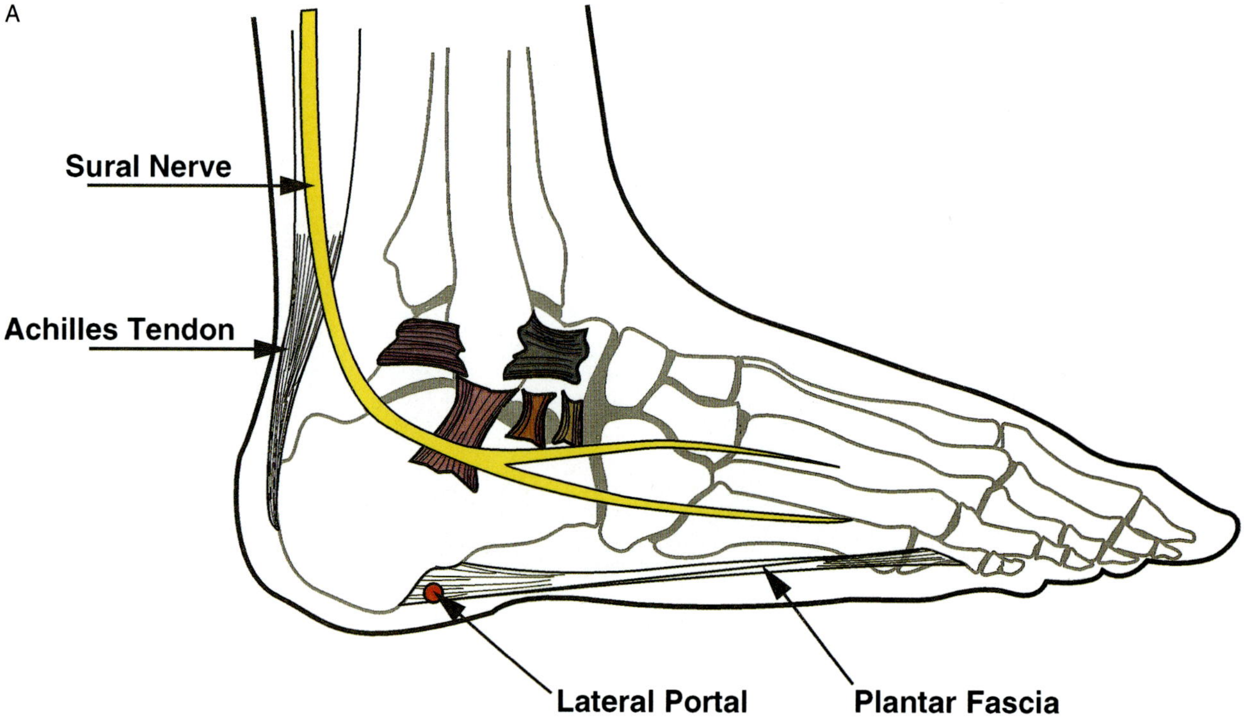

B

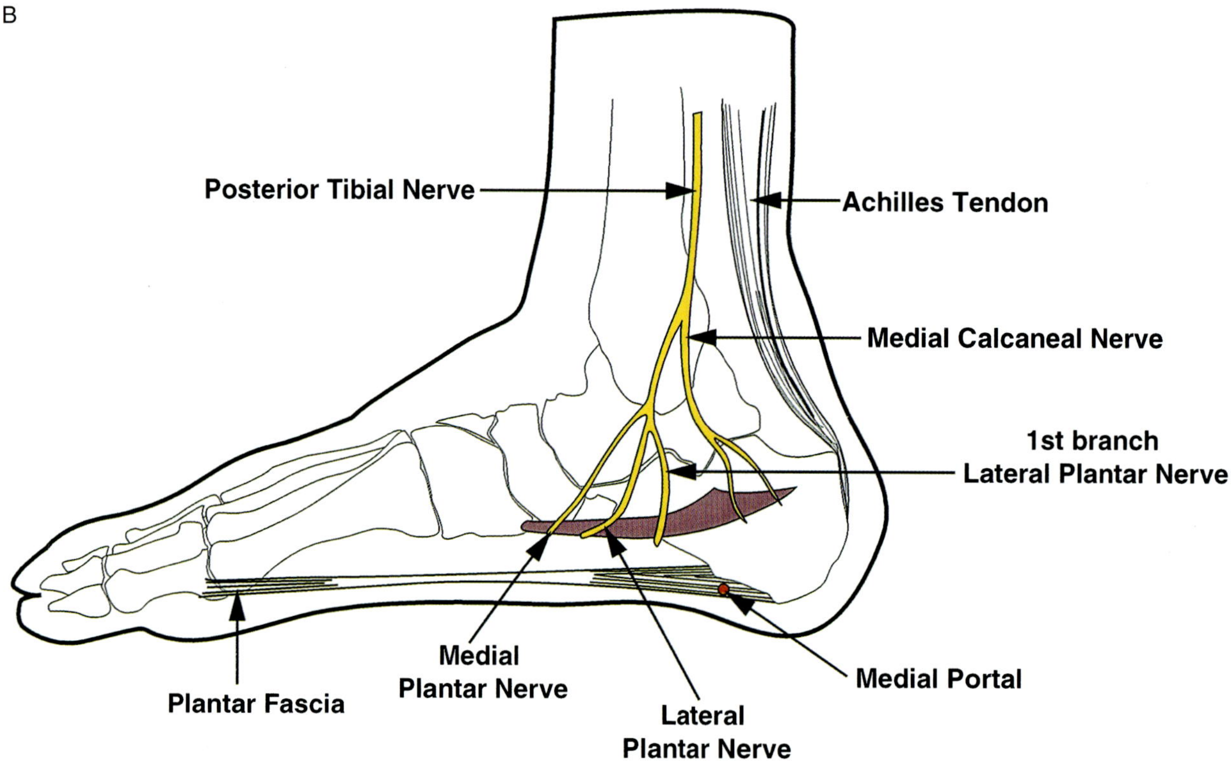

FIGURE 1.14 A,B. Several structures are at risk when performing endoscopic plantar fascia release, especially because most are not visualized during the procedure.

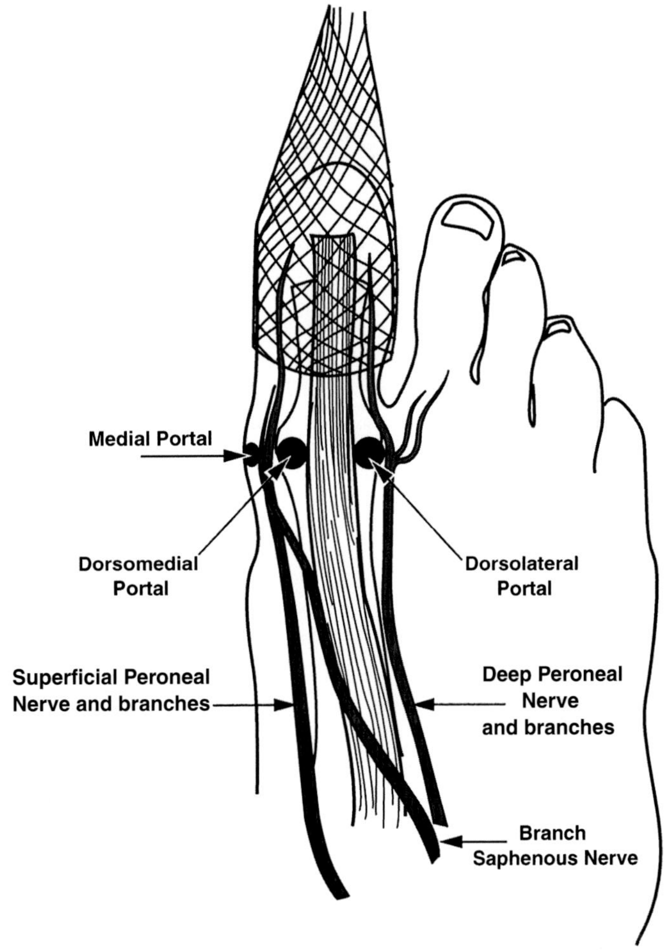

FIGURE 1.15. Structures at risk during portal placement for the first metatarsophalangeal joint.

including the capsule, ligaments, and musculotendinous structures, provide most of the support to the first MTP joint.

The extensor hallucis longus tendon divides the dorsum in half to the first MTP joint. Branches of the deep peroneal nerve innervate the lateral half, and branches of the superficial peroneal nerve innervate the medial half. The terminal branches of the saphenous nerve innervate the medial aspect of the great toe (Fig. 1.15).

The sesamoids are within the medial and lateral portions of the flexor hallucis brevis tendon on the plantar aspect of the first MTP joint. The sesamoids are enveloped by the split tendon of the flexor hallucis brevis, which sends fibers to the plantar plate and subsequently attaches to the proximal aspect of the proximal phalanx. The plantar plate is a strong fibrous structure that inserts on either side of the MTP joint. The flexor hallucis longus tendon is both superficial and between the two heads of the flexor hallucis brevis tendon.

Arthroscopic Anatomy and Portals

The dorsal medial, dorsal lateral, and straight medial portals are the most commonly used for the arthroscopic procedure. The dorsal medial and dorsal lateral portals are placed at the joint line and on either side of the extensor hallucis longus tendon (Fig. 1.16). The straight medial portal is placed through the medial capsule midway between the dorsal and plantar aspects of the joint, usually under direct visualization. Using a 4-mm longitudinal skin incision, the subcutaneous tissue is spread with a mosquito clamp to prevent neurovascular injury, and the joint is entered with an interchangeable cannula using a semiblunt trocar.

A 10-point arthroscopic examination of the MTP joint, performed through the dorsal lateral portal, includes the following: (1) lateral gutter; (2) lateral corner of the metatarsal head; (3) central portion of the metatarsal head; (4) medial corner of the metatarsal head; (5) medial gutter; (6) medial por-

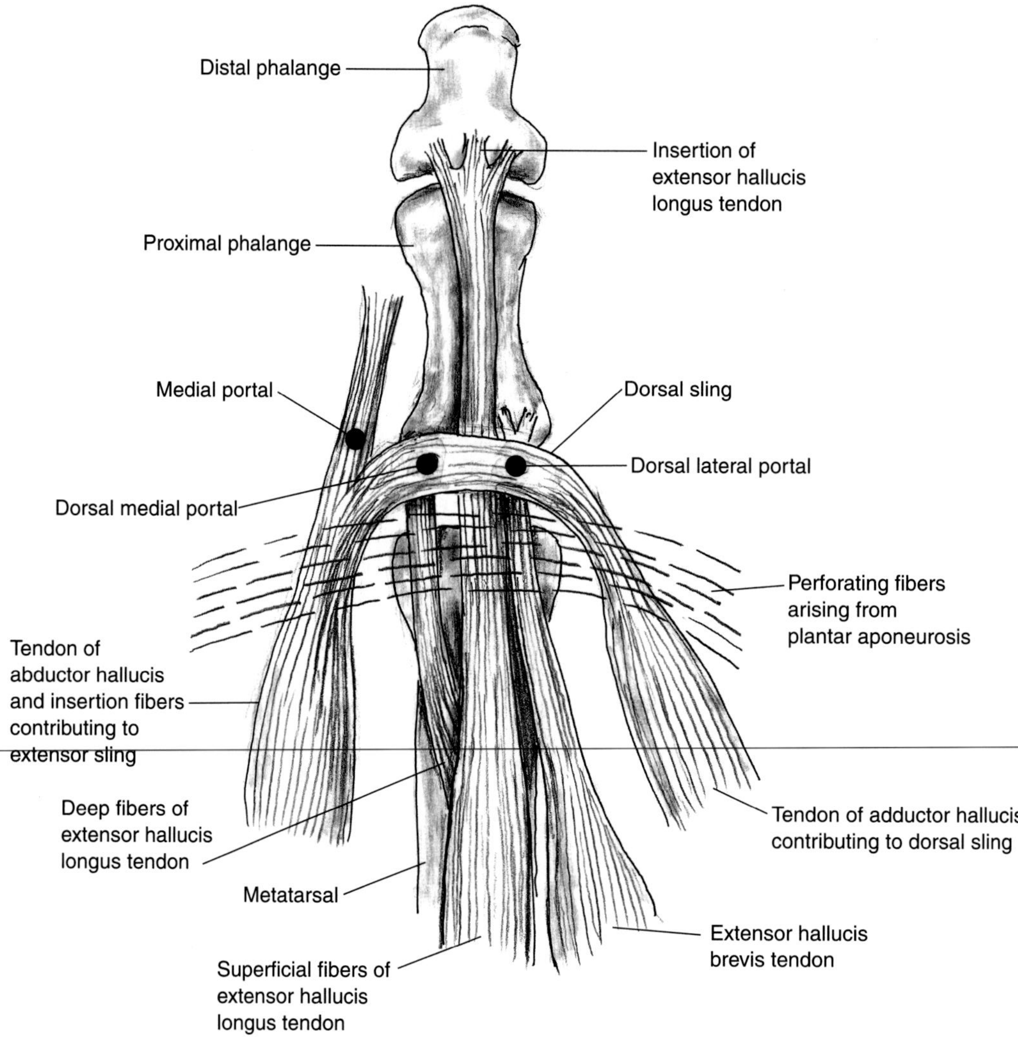

FIGURE 1.16. Portal placement for the first metatarsophalangeal joint.

tion of the proximal phalanx; (7) central portion of the proximal phalanx; (8) lateral portion of the proximal phalanx; (9) medial sesamoid; and (10) lateral sesamoid. The dorsal medial portal provides superior visualization of the dorsal aspect of the metatarsal head and proximal phalanx. The medial and lateral sesamoids are well visualized from the medial portal as well.

CALCANEOCUBOID JOINT

Gross Anatomy

The calcaneocuboid joint comprises part of Chopart's articulation in the midfoot. It is saddle-shaped, concave transversely and convex vertically, and plays a major role in midfoot motion as one of the transverse tarsal articulations. Medial and lateral calcaneocuboid ligaments help stabilize this joint, the former of which is part of the bifurcate ligament complex.[7] The inferior calcaneocuboid ligaments, known as the long and short plantar ligaments, are the stoutest of these and extend beyond the cuboid to attach to the bases of metatarsals 3–5, helping to maintain the longitudinal arch. There is also a small dorsal ligament of lesser significance. Inferiorly, the sural nerve and the peroneal tendons course through this region and must be protected. Superiorly, the extensor digitorum brevis and the peroneus tertius are in immediate proximity.

Arthroscopic and Portal Anatomy

Arthroscopic examination of the calcaneocuboid joint has recently been considered. Specifically, superior, middle, and inferior portals can be created

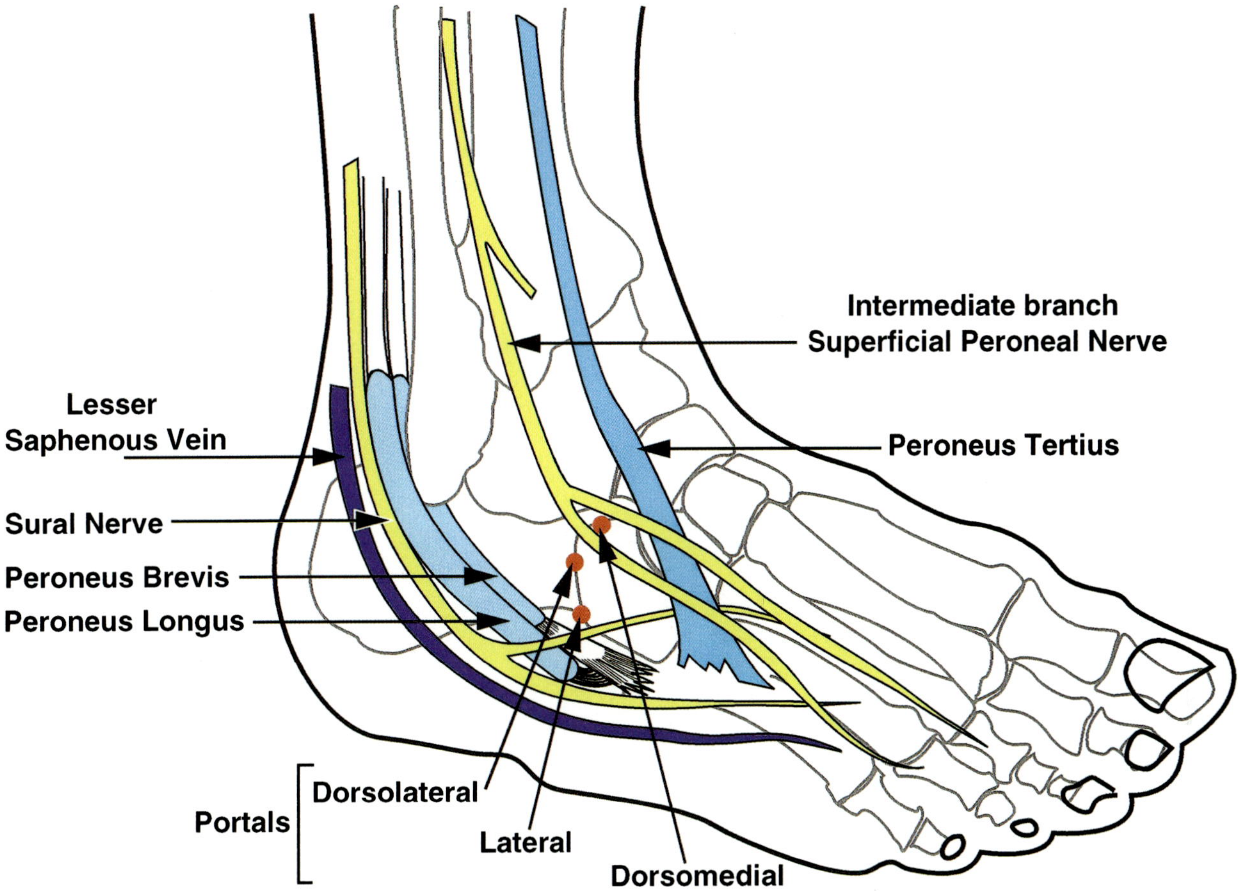

FIGURE 1.17. Portal placement and structures at risk in the calcaneocuboid joint.

for access to the joint (Fig. 1.17). Care must be taken with skin incisions to avoid penetration below the dermal layer to avoid damage to the underlying sural nerve and tendons. The peroneus tertius provides a good landmark for superior portal placement, as does the peroneus brevis for inferior placement.

BIBLIOGRAPHY

1. Parisien S. Arthroscopy of the subtalar joint. In: Guhl J (ed) *Foot and ankle arthroscopy*, 2nd ed. Thorofare, NJ: Slack, 1993;171–178.
2. Parisien S, Vangsness T. Arthroscopy of the subtalar joint: an experimental approach. *Arthroscopy* 1985;1:53–57.
3. Frey C, Gasser S, Feder K. Arthroscopy of the subtalar joint. *Foot Ankle Int* 1994;15:424–428.
4. Frey CC, Feder KS, DiGiovanni C. Arthroscopic evaluation of the subtalar joint: does sinus tarsi syndrome exist? *Foot Ankle Int* 1999;20:185–191.
5. Williams MM, Ferkel RD. Subtalar arthroscopy: indications, techniques, and results. *Arthroscopy* 1998;14:4.
6. Mekhail AO, Heck BE, Ebraheim NA, Jackson W. Arthroscopy of the subtalar joint: establishing a medial portal. *Foot Ankle Int* 1995;16:427–432.
7. Sarrafian S. Osteology. In: Sarrafian S (ed) *Anatomy of the foot and ankle*. Philadelphia: Lippincott, 1983;35–106.
8. Smith RW. Computerized sectional imaging: computed tomography and magnetic resonance imaging of the foot and ankle. In: Jahss M (ed) *Disorders of the foot and ankle*. Philadelphia: Saunders, 1991;155–204.
9. Frey C, Rosenberg Z, Shereff M, et al. The retrocalcaneal bursa: anatomy and bursography. *Foot Ankle* 1992;13:203–207.
10. Fiewell L, Frey C. Anatomic study of arthroscopic débridement of the ankle joint. *Foot Ankle Int* 1994;15:614–621.
11. Zimmer T. Arthroscopic surgery of the foot. In: Guhl J (ed) *Foot and ankle arthroscopy*, 2nd ed. Thorofare, NJ: Slack, 1993;179–183.
12. Van Dyk E. Endoscopic débridement of Haglund's deformity [abstract]. Presented at AOFAS Specialty Day, San Francisco, 1997.
13. Netter F. *The CIBA collection of medical illustrations, musculoskeletal system*. Summit, NJ: CIBA-Geigy, 1987.

14. Hedrick MR. The plantar aponeurosis. *Foot Ankle Int* 1996;17:646–649.
15. Barrett S, Day S. Endoscopic plantar fasciotomy for chronic plantar fasciitis/heel spur syndrome: surgical technique—early clinical results. *J Foot Surg* 1991;30:568–570.
16. Hofmeister EP, Elliott MJ, Juliano PJ, et al. Endoscopic plantar fascia release: an anatomical study. *Foot Ankle Int* 1995;16:719–723.
17. Hawkins BJ, Langerman DO, Gibbons T, et al. An anatomic analysis of endoscopic plantar fascia release. *Foot Ankle Int* 1995;16:552–558.

CHAPTER 2

Gross and Arthroscopic Anatomy of the Ankle

Richard J. Mason and Craig D. Morgan

Major technologic advances in fiberoptic light transmission, video cameras, and instrumentation have allowed great advances in small-joint arthroscopy.[1–5] Arthroscopy in particular is now a well established procedure for accurate diagnosis and operative management of certain ankle disorders.[1–12] The small size of the ankle and significant periarticular soft tissue structures make placement and advancement of the arthroscope and instrumentation more difficult than in larger joints. Successful arthroscopy of the ankle requires knowledge of the regional anatomy and a familiarity with the available arthroscopic portals. This chapter highlights the gross and arthroscopic anatomy of the ankle as it relates to current arthroscopic techniques. Particular emphasis is placed on the anatomic relations of the important osseous and soft tissue structures to assist the reader in developing a safe, reproducible approach to arthroscopic treatment of ankle pathology.

GROSS ANATOMY

Surface Anatomy and Soft Tissue Structures

Familiarity with surface anatomy and soft tissue structures of the ankle is imperative if complications are to be avoided during arthroscopy. Neurovascular structures and tendons are at risk if portals are improperly placed. This section reviews the topical anatomy as it pertains to arthroscopic approaches. We then review the neurovascular structures, tendons, ligaments, and plicae of the ankle.

Surface Anatomy of the Ankle

The anterior joint line is superficial and palpable, being separated from skin only by the subcutaneous layer, extensor tendons, anterior neurovascular structures, and the anterior capsule. The lateral aspect of the anterior joint line is found just lateral to the peroneus tertius tendon and just above the palpable lateral trochlear ridge of the talus. The medial side of the joint is identified by palpating the soft spot just medial to the anterior tibial tendon and inferior to the proximal corner of the medial malleolus (Figs. 2.1, 2.2). In contrast, the posterior tibiotalar joint is not easily palpated owing to 3–4 cm of thick fibroadipose tissue located between the Achilles tendon and the flexor tendons of the foot. There is, however, a constant 2-cm window located posterolaterally between the Achilles tendon, peroneal tendons, and flexor hallucis longus, where the posterior capsule is covered only by thin fibrous tissue and skin. The posterolateral approach is made in this area (Fig. 2.3).

Neurovascular Structures

Three major sensory nerves cross the ankle joint in the subcutaneous layer of the ankle: saphenous, superficial peroneal, and sural nerves. Most of these nerves are found with accompanying veins (Fig. 2.2B). These nerves are most vulnerable to injury

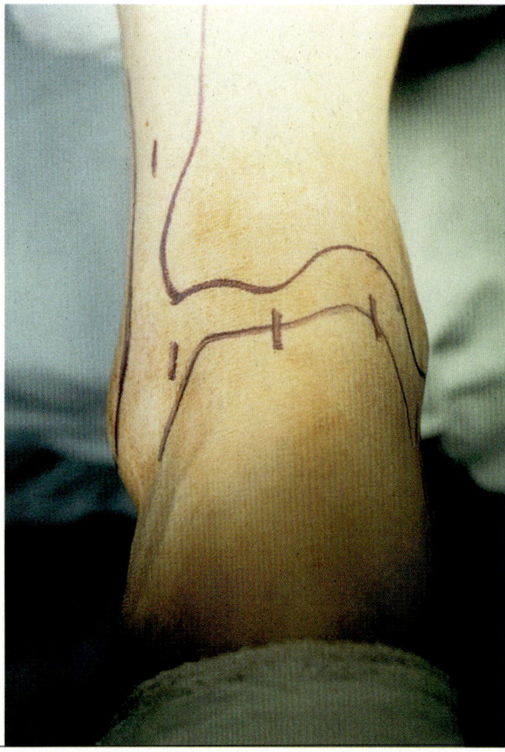

FIGURE 2.1. Anterior surface anatomy of the right ankle with the anterior portals marked.

during arthroscopy because they are small and have a somewhat variable location; each is located near a commonly established arthroscopic portal. Voto et al.[13] showed in cadaver studies that the location of the subcutaneous nerves about the ankle does not change significantly with ankle motion, distraction, or joint distension. However, their anatomic location is somewhat variable from specimen to specimen.

The saphenous nerve and great saphenous vein pass over the anterior edge of the medial malleolus (Fig. 2.4). Anteriorly, the nerve is located close to the site of the anteromedial portal, which falls 5 mm below the anteromedial joint line just medial to the palpable anterior tibialis tendon. The nerve and vein are at risk if the portal is made too far medially. The superficial peroneal nerve is a terminal branch of the common peroneal nerve. In the mid-anterolateral leg region, the terminal sensory portion of the superficial peroneal nerve becomes subcutaneous and bifurcates into medial and lateral branches. These branches further subdivide at the level of the ankle joint to supply sensation to the dorsum of the foot. With use of the anterolateral portal the lateral branch is at risk.

Posterolaterally, the sural nerve and short saphenous vein are located subcutaneously just posterior to the peroneal tendons behind the lateral malleolus (Fig. 2.5A). As the sural nerve curves distally under the lateral malleolus, it lies approximately 1.5–2.0 cm below the tip of the lateral malleolus and then proceeds distally along the lateral border of the foot, supplying sensation to this area. During ankle arthroscopy the sural nerve is vulnerable to injury at the posterolateral portal site[1,3,7,9] and the point of insertion of a laterally based calcaneal distraction pin.[3] To avoid the sural nerve when using the posterolateral approach, it is recommended that the skin portal be made adjacent to the lateral border of the Achilles tendon rather than straying laterally near the nerve (Fig. 2.6).

Two major neurovascular bundles cross the ankle joint. The dorsalis pedis artery (terminal branch of the anterior tibial artery) and the deep peroneal nerve make up the anterior neurovascular bundle. This bundle lies between the tibialis anterior and the extensor hallucis longus proximal to the joint. Roughly 2 inches above the ankle joint the bundle courses from the interosseous membrane to the anterior tibial margin and passes under the extensor retinaculum, lying just underneath the tendon of the extensor hallucis longus at the level of the anterior joint line. Distal to the joint the bundle lies between the extensor hallucis longus and the extensor digitorum longus[14,15] (Fig. 2.2B). This bundle is most likely to be damaged with use of the anterocentral portal, so the anterocentral portal is no longer recommended. The posterior neurovascular bundle is composed of the posterior tibial artery, venae comitantes, and posterior tibial nerve. This bundle passes behind the medial malleolus in the tarsal tunnel between the tendons of the flexor digitorum longus and flexor hallucis longus.[14,15]

Tendons

Beyond the subcutaneous layer lies the deep fascia, and deep to the fascia lie the tendons. Four sets of tendons cross the ankle joint: the anterior, posteromedial, posterolateral, and posterior tendons (Fig. 2.2). The anterior tendons (tibialis anterior, extensor digitorum longus, extensor hallucis longus, peroneus tertius) are the ankle dorsiflexors and toe extensors. The posteromedial tendons (tibialis posterior, flexor digitorum longus, flexor hallucis longus) pass behind the medial malleolus and plantar flex; they invert the ankle and

FIGURE 2.2. A: Superficial anatomy (anterior).

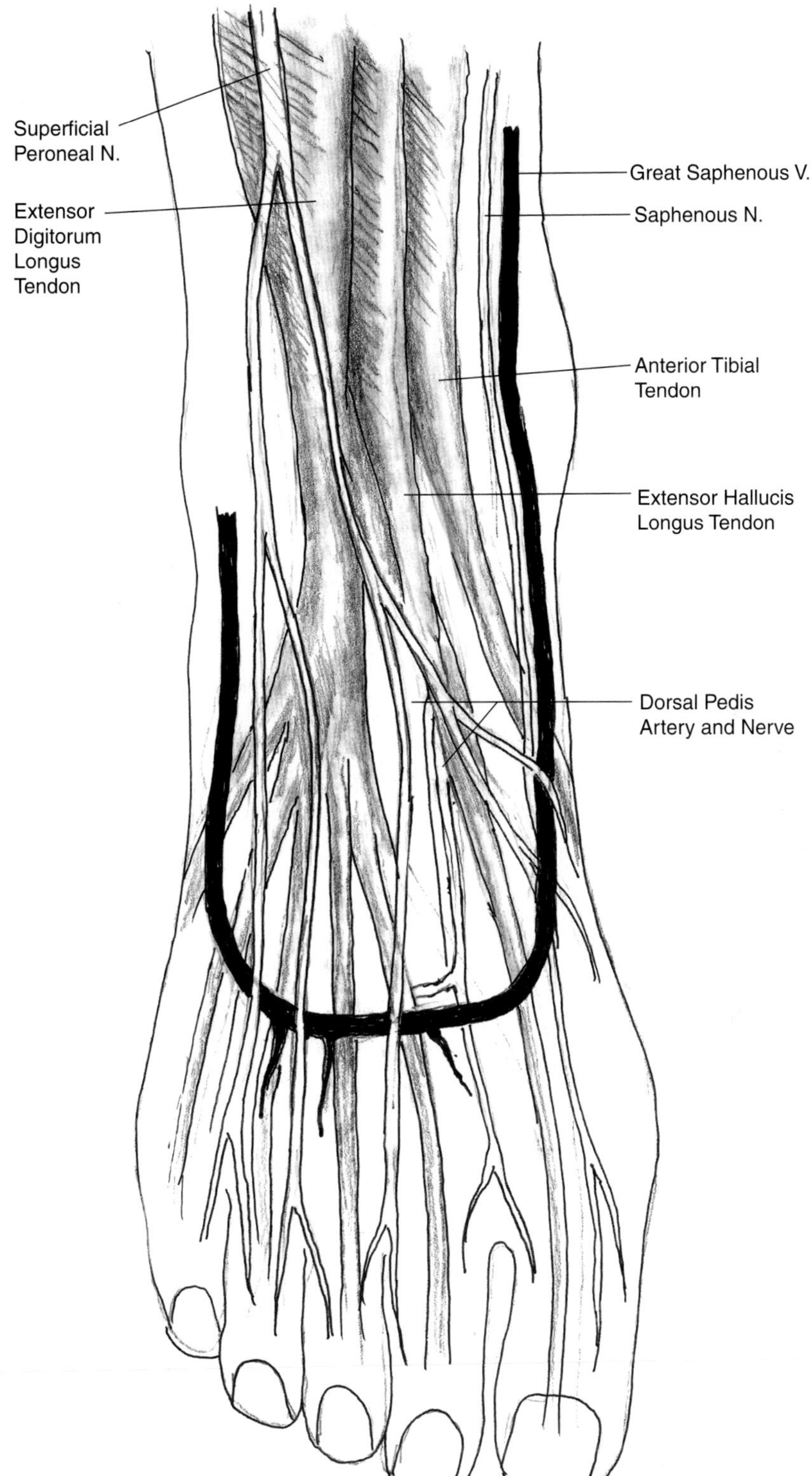

(Continued)

flex the toes. The posterolateral tendons (peroneus longus and brevis) pass behind the lateral malleolus and are evertors of the ankle. The posterior tendons (Achilles, plantaris) lie posteriorly in the midline and are flexors of the ankle joint.[14,15]

Ligaments

The ligaments of clinical and arthroscopic importance in the ankle originate from the medial and lateral malleoli. On the medial malleolus the anterior

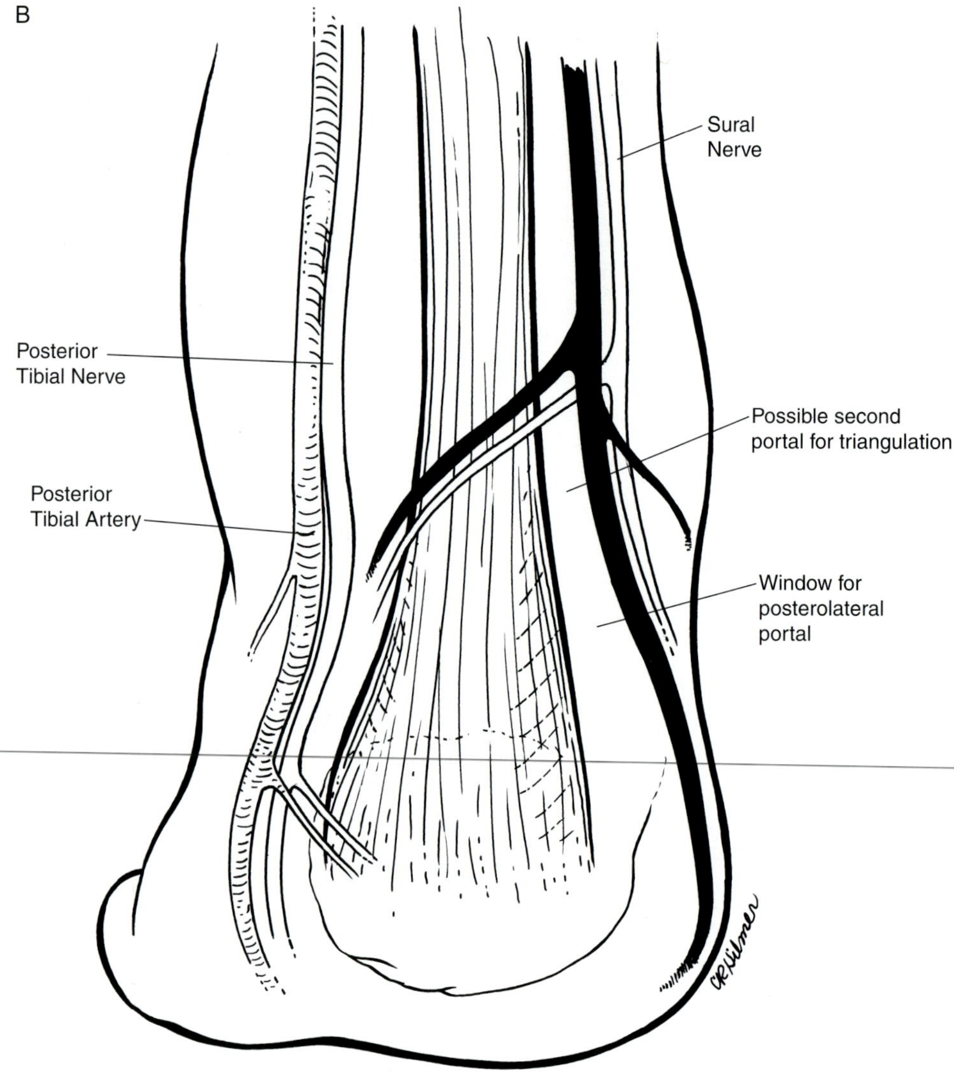

FIGURE 2.2 (*continued*). B: Posterior neurovascular structures and posterior portal sites of left ankle. Trans-Achilles tendon (TAT) and posteromedial (PM) portals are not recommended.

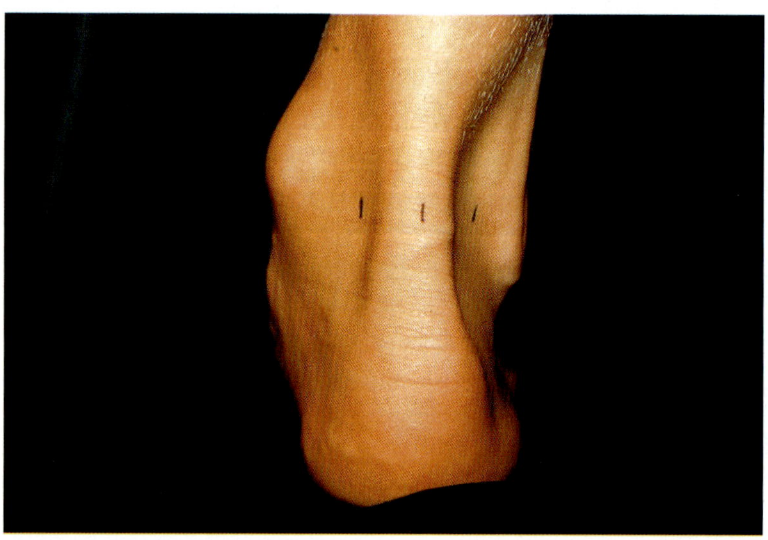

FIGURE 2.3. Posterior surface anatomy of the right ankle with posterior portals marked.

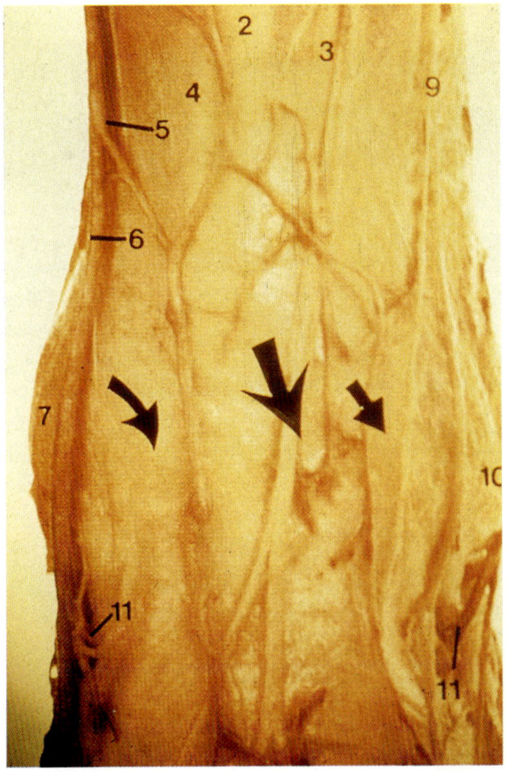

FIGURE 2.4. Cadaveric dissection of anterior left ankle. Note the lateral malleolus (10), lateral branch of the superficial peroneal nerve (9), saphenous vein and nerve (5, 6), and medial malleolus (7). Arrows mark anterior portal sites. The anterocentral portal is not recommended.

and posterior colliculi are two distinct distal medial prominences from which the deltoid ligament originates. The deltoid ligament is a thick, strong ligament that consists of superficial and deep fibers (Fig. 2.7). The superficial fibers originate primarily from the anterior colliculus and run extraarticularly as a continuous sagittal sheet. This sheet consists of four segments that insert on the talus, the calcaneus, the spring ligament, and the navicular, respectively. The deep portion of the deltoid ligament is intraarticular, is covered only by synovium, and is horizontally oriented, running from the intercollicular notch and posterior colliculus to the posteromedial surface of the talus.[3,14,15]

The lateral malleolus gives origin to five distinct, strong extraarticular ligamentous structures: (1) anterior talofibular ligament; (2) posterior talofibular ligament; (3) calcaneofibular ligament; (4) anteroinferior tibiofibular ligament; and (5) posteroinferior tibiofibular ligament with its most deeply located anterior extension, the transverse ligament or transverse tibiofibular ligament (Figs. 2.7, 2.8).[3,14] This transverse ligament is extraarticular and is covered with synovium, forming the posterior plica of the ankle (Fig. 2.9). This synovial covering may hypertrophy and cause pathologic hindfoot impingement pain when the transverse ligament is pinched between the posterior tibial lip and the posterior tibiofibular ligament during plantar flexion (Fig. 2.10). This entity usually responds well to partial resection.[3,16,17] This synovial lining over the transverse ligament is frayed or absent in up to 70% of older patients.[14]

Synovial Folds (Plicae)

Synovial folds, or plicae, are a normal part of the chondrosynovial interface in all movable joints. They allow the synovium to slide on the capsule or articular surface. In the ankle joint they are located at the anterior and posterior tibiotalar junctions and the talomalleolar spaces, and they project from the inferior, most intraarticular portion of the distal tibiofibular syndesmosis (Fig. 2.11). As mentioned, the posterior plica is simply the synovial covering of the transverse tibiofibular ligament (Fig. 2.12). Thickening and hypertrophy of the synovial folds due to trauma, adhesions, or chronic impingement may cause them to become a source of pathologic ankle pain and mechanical symptomatology. This is most commonly true for the synovial fold found in the anterosuperior aspect of the lateral talomalleolar joint, which causes the lateral synovial impingement lesion following traumatic inversion injury to the ankle.[2–4]

Osseous Structures

The ankle joint is formed by the distal articulations of the tibia, fibula, and talus. The medial malleolus, tibial plafond, and lateral malleolus form the mortise into which the talus articulates (Fig. 2.13). Its bony structure and strong periarticular ligaments stabilize this talocrural articulation.

Malleoli and Tibial Plafond

The medial and lateral malleoli are palpable subcutaneously and provide the primary fixed bony landmarks of the ankle. The tip of the lateral malleolus is located laterally, approximately 2 cm distally and 2 cm posteriorly compared to the medial position of the medial malleolus. The anterior joint line is located 2 cm proximal (cephalad) to the tip of the medial malleolus. The posterior articular margin of the

A

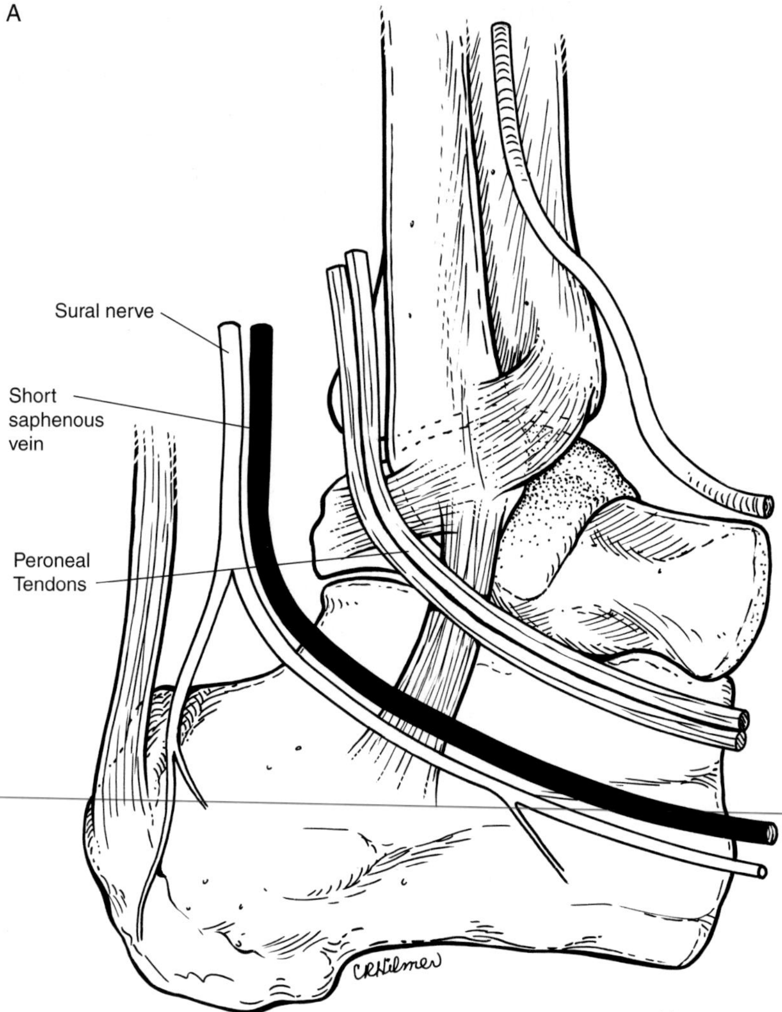

FIGURE 2.5. **A:** Lateral ankle and structures at risk. **B:** Medial ankle and structures at risk.

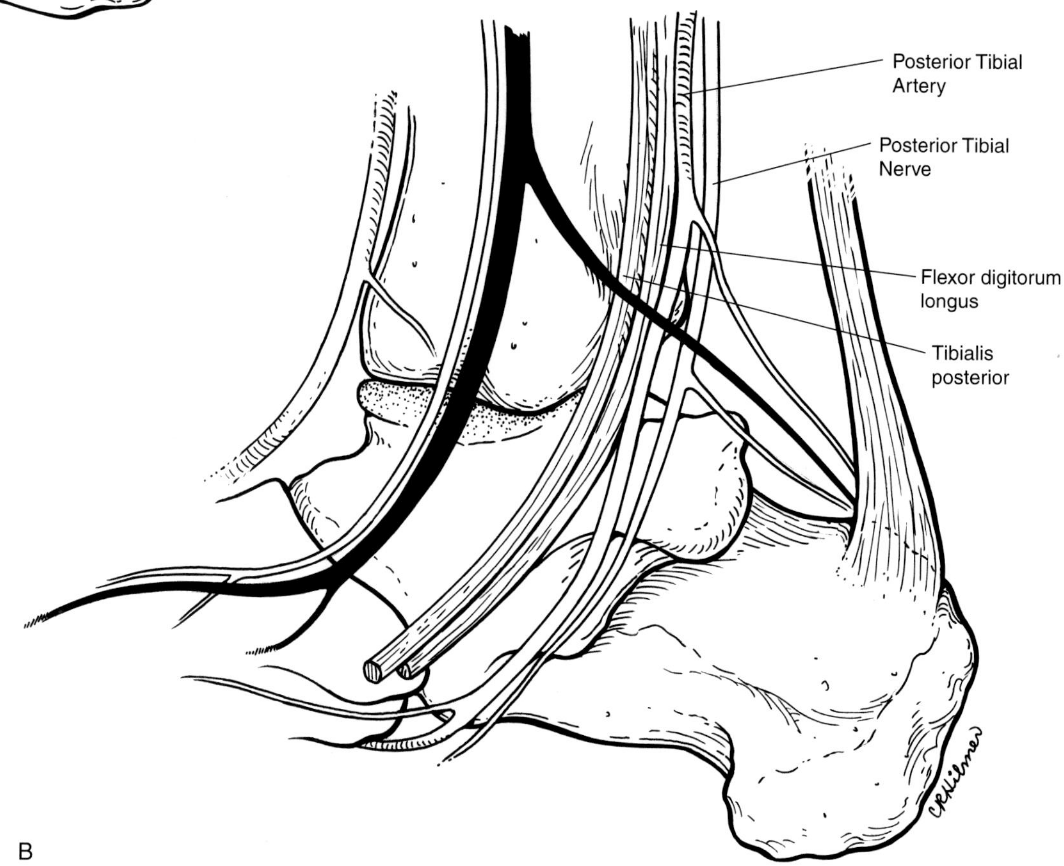

B

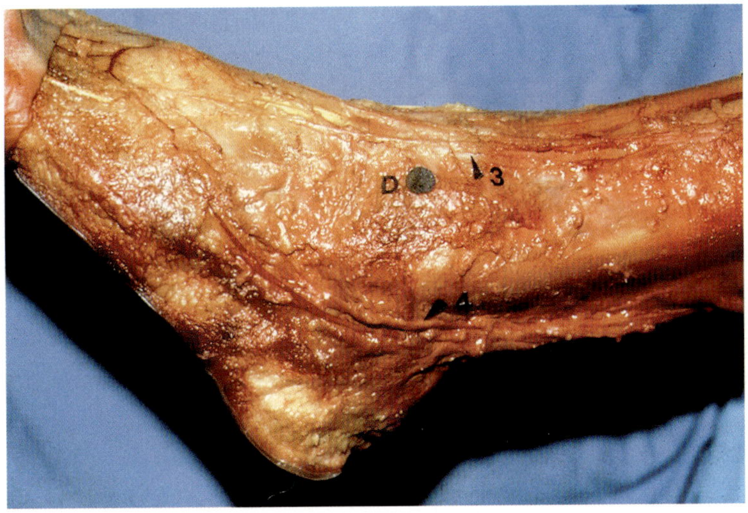

FIGURE 2.6. Cadaveric dissection of the lateral left ankle. Note the lateral branch of the superficial peroneal nerve (3), the sural nerve and short saphenous vein (4), and the anterolateral portal (D).

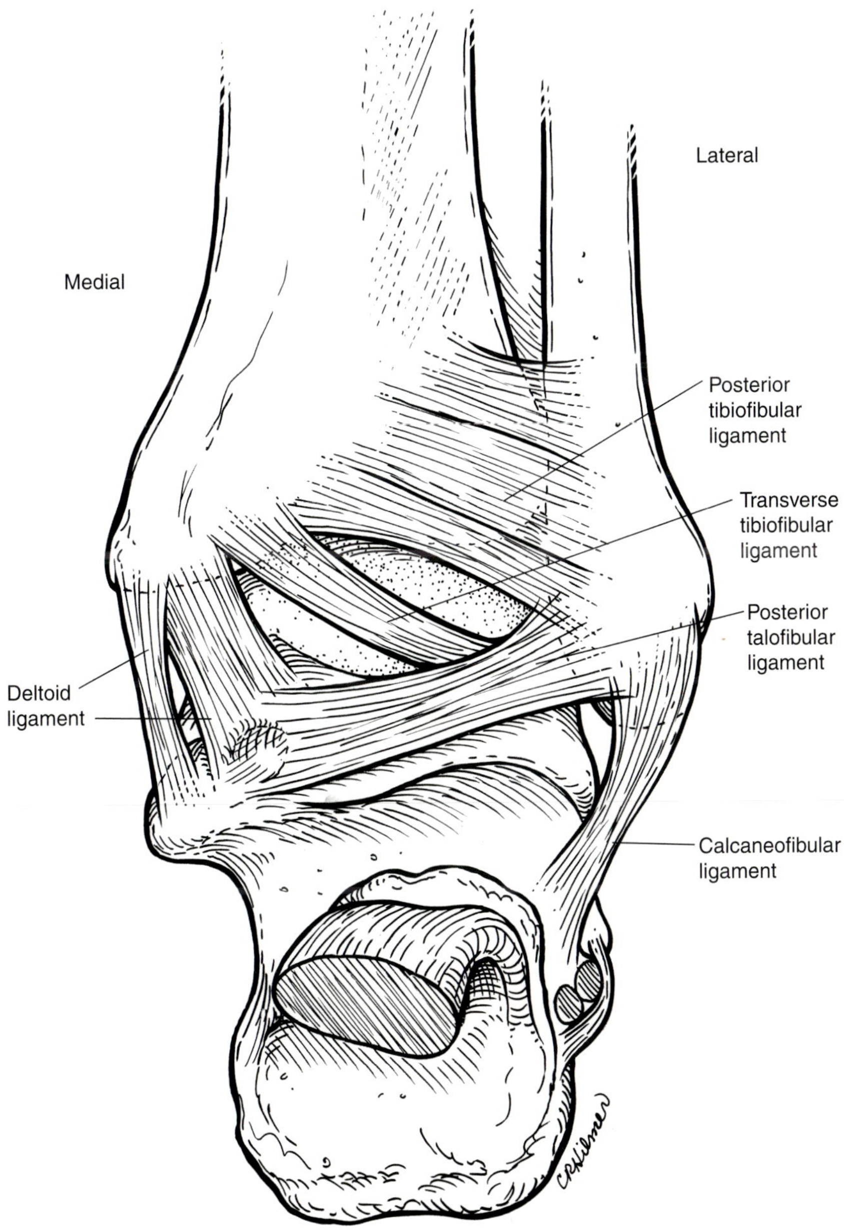

FIGURE 2.7. Ankle ligaments of the right ankle, posterior view.

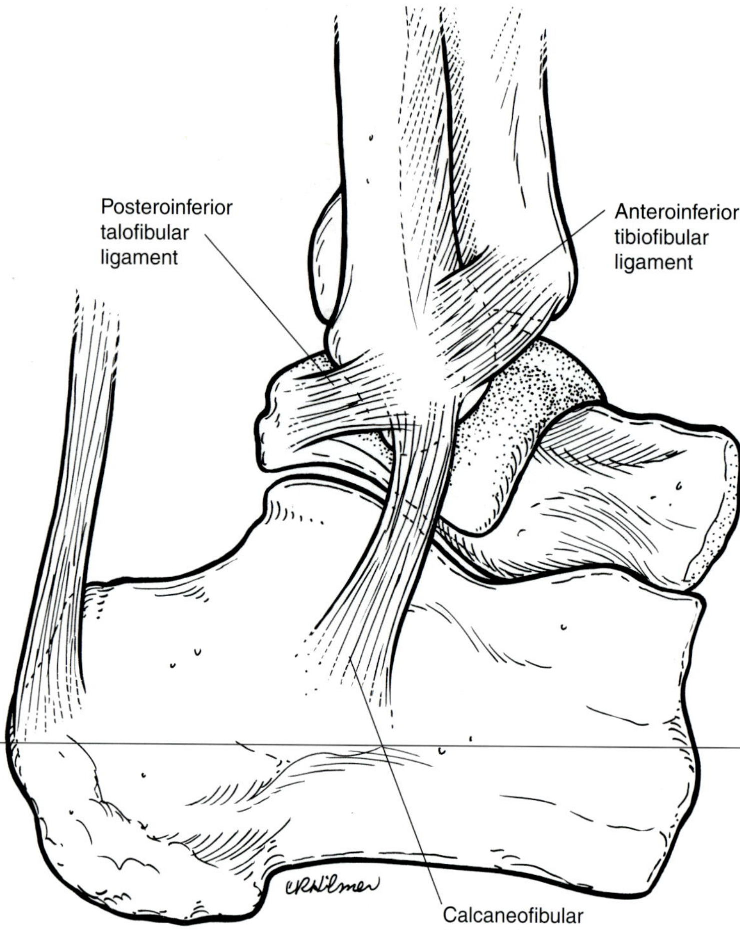

FIGURE 2.8. Lateral ligaments of the right ankle, lateral view.

tibia (posterior malleolus) projects 4–6 mm more distal than the anterior articular margin (Fig. 2.14). This relation is important in that posterior portals are made more distally than anterior portals. With inversion and eversion of the foot, in combination with plantar flexion, the medial and lateral ridges of the anterior talar dome are readily palpable just below the joint line adjacent to the anterior tibialis tendon medially and just lateral to the peroneus tertius tendon laterally. Palpation of these landmarks al-

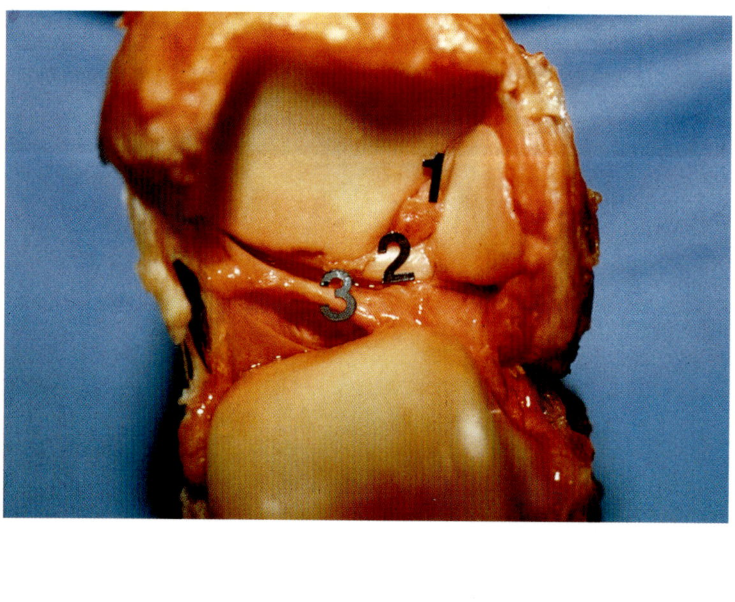

FIGURE 2.9. Intraarticular dissection of the left ankle. 1, syndesmosis; 2, posteroinferior tibiofibular ligament; 3, transverse tibiofibular ligament with overlying synovium.

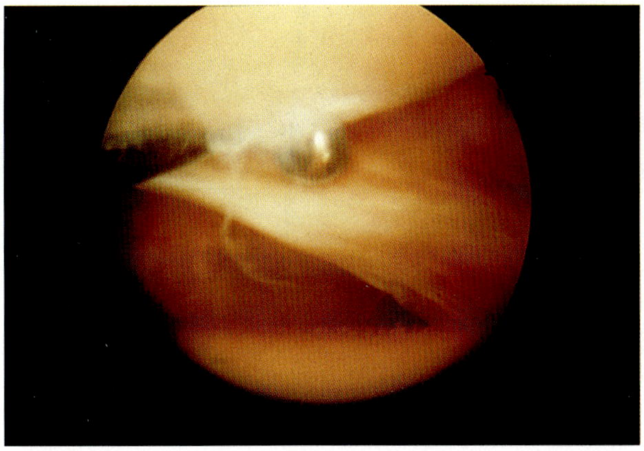

FIGURE 2.10. Arthroscopic view of the posterior plica and underlying transverse tibiofibular ligament of the left ankle. View is from the anterolateral portal with the probe from the anteromedial portal resting on top of the synovium covering the ligament.

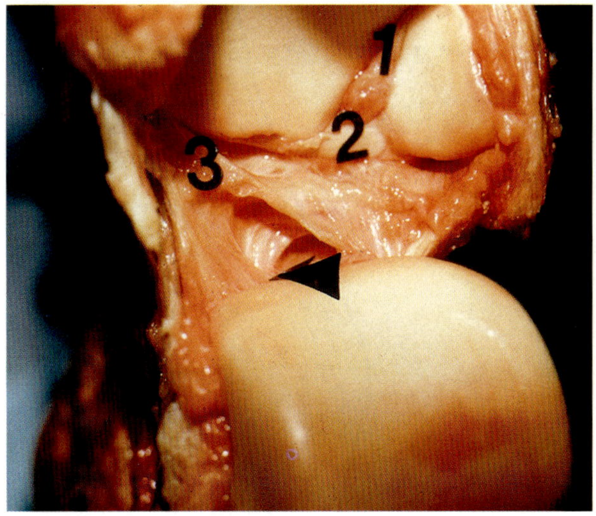

FIGURE 2.12. Arrow points to the medial talomalleolar plica below the origin of the transverse ligament (3).

lows reproducible identification of the anterior tibiotalar joint line, which is vital to proper anterior portal placement.

The anterior articular margin of the tibia appears as a relatively straight horizontal structure on mortise radiographs and has a constant 3- to 5-mm notch that recedes proximally near the junction of the medial malleolus. Harty defined this unnamed notch[14] and noted that it is best seen on anteroposterior (AP) radiographs. This notch is important, as it provides an extra space for passage of an instrument or arthroscope beyond the medial margin of the talar trochlear surface and into the middle and posterior aspects of the joint using the anteromedial approach (Figs. 2.13, 2.14).

Talus

The talar dome, also called the trochlear surface, is wider anteriorly than posteriorly; it is convex in the sagittal plane and slightly concave in the coronal plane (Fig. 2.15). The transverse concavity creates prominent medial and lateral margins to the dome that are an etiologic factor for transchondral and transcondylar fractures of the talar dome.[18,19] These prominent ridges can impede triangulation of in-

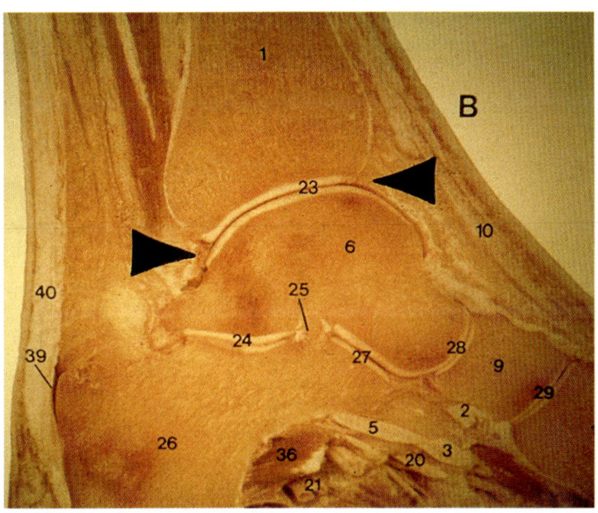

FIGURE 2.11. Sagittal section of ankle. Arrows point to the anterior and posterior synovial folds. Note the more distal position of the posterior joint line compared to the anterior joint line.

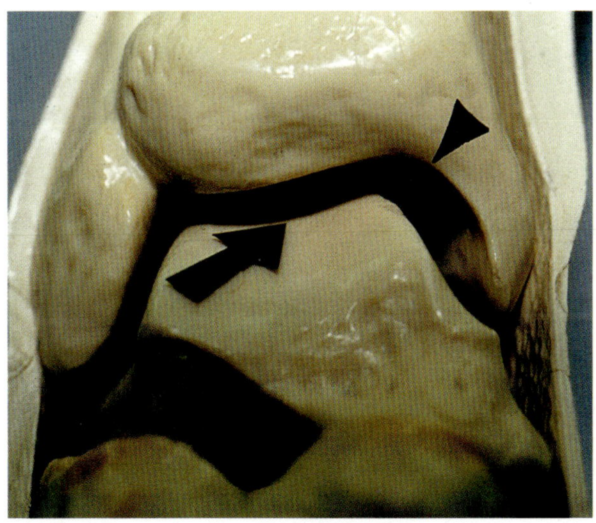

FIGURE 2.13. Anterior view of osseous structures of the right ankle. Arrowhead points to the anteromedial notch defined by Harty. Arrow points to the concavity of the trochlear surface of the talus.

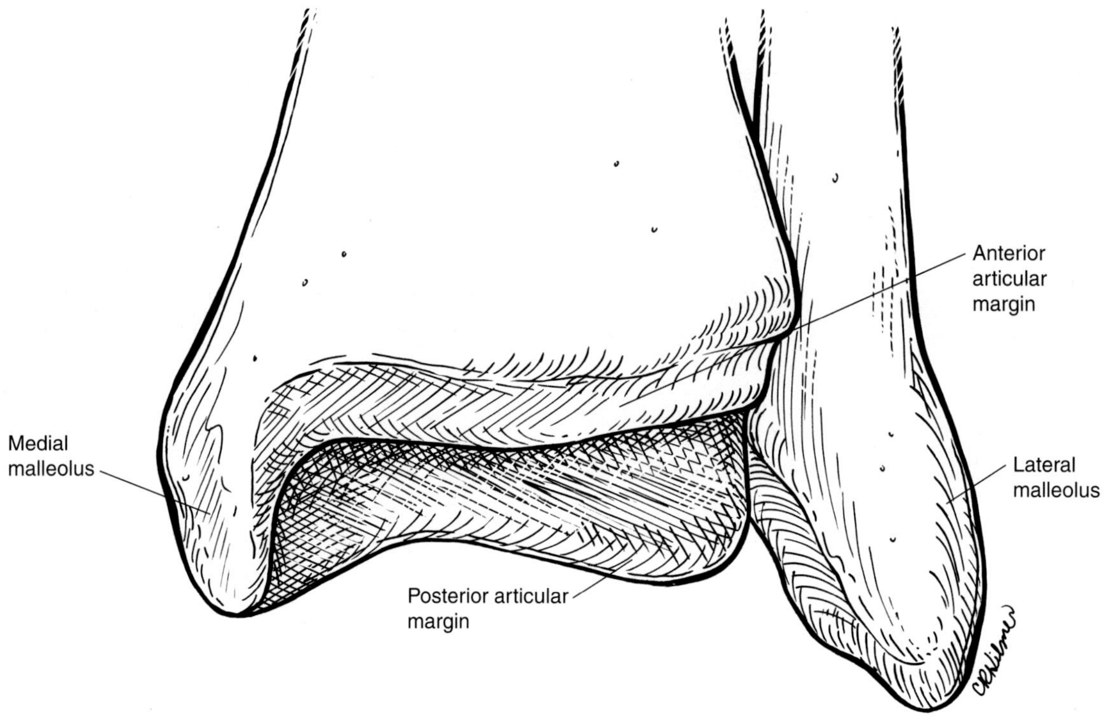

FIGURE 2.14. Anterior view of the malleoli and articular margins.

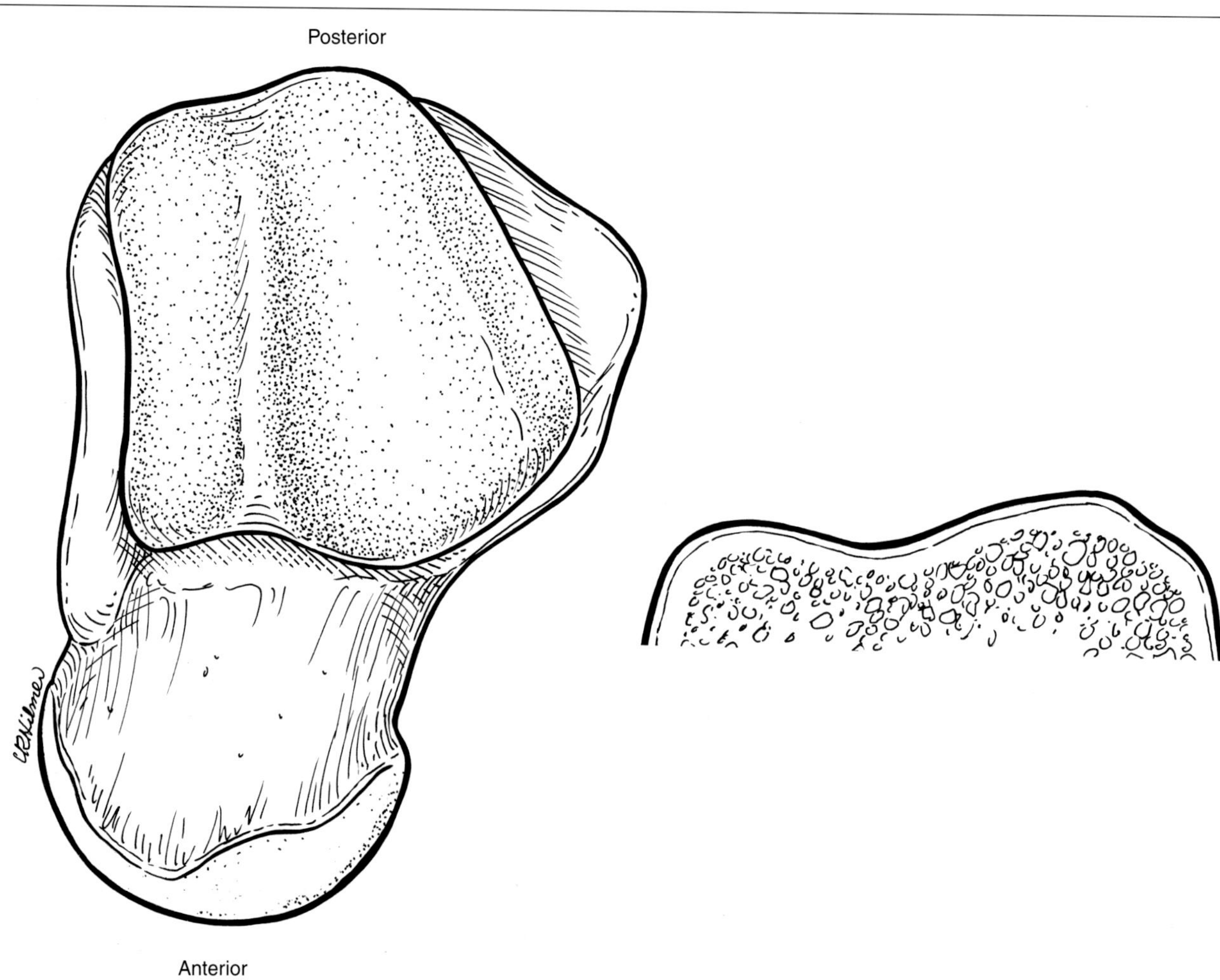

FIGURE 2.15. Superior view of the talus demonstrates a wider articular surface anteriorly. Coronal view shows trochlear ridges and a central concavity.

struments across the talus in the coronal plane when using the standard anteromedial and anterolateral portals.

ARTHROSCOPIC ANATOMY

Portal Anatomy

Arthroscopy has exposed the interior of the ankle from a perspective previously unobtainable with conventional open exposures. This exposure has revealed a surprising amount of previously unappreciated anatomy and pathology.[3,4,11,12] The described arthroscopic approaches to the ankle are divided into anterior, posterior, and transmalleolar.[2,10] The primary anterior portals are anterolateral and anteromedial. The anterolateral and anteromedial portal positions allow creation of adjacent accessory portals for instrumentation should this need arise. The posterior portals are rarely necessary with mechanical distraction. Their use may be necessary when pathology is located in the posterior compartment and triangulation is not possible from anterior portals. The most commonly used posterior portal is posterolateral, which allows instrumentation of the posterior compartment and is used by some surgeons to place a large-bore inflow cannula. The trans-Achilles tendon and posteromedial portals are of historic interest only and have been abandoned because of the risk of injury to neurovascular structures and tendons.[1–3,7–9,13,20] The posteromedial aspect of the ankle can be approached via the posterior tibial tendon sheath portal. The transmalleolar approaches are divided into the transmedial and translateral. These approaches are used primarily to treat osteochondritic lesions of the talar dome. An alternative to the transmalleolar portal is the transtalar approach, which is used when treating chondral and osteochondral pathology. This section reviews the extraarticular anatomy pertinent to portal placement and highlights the intraarticular anatomy visualized through the standard portals.

Careful technique is imperative when establishing arthroscopic portals around the ankle. The small joint space and close proximity of tendons, nerves, blood vessels, and important ligaments make the risk of iatrogenic injury much greater than in larger joints. Injury to these structures may be minimized by making vertical portal incisions through skin only. A small hemostat can then be used gently to spread the subcutaneous tissue vertically in line with the structures at risk. The subcutaneous and capsular layers are penetrated only by a cannula with a blunt trocar. Using this approach, any significant structure in close proximity to a given portal is pushed aside uninjured by the blunt trocar. Once in the joint, the cannula should not be removed until the end of the procedure, thereby avoiding multiple passes near the subcutaneous nerves and the risk of fluid extravasation. Skin closure of the portal should include skin and dermis only to avoid injuring the subcutaneous nerves during closure.[1,3,4]

Anterior Portals

Anterolateral Portal

As with arthroscopy of the knee, the anterolateral (AL) portal is the primary diagnostic one used for initially placing the arthroscope in the ankle (Fig. 2.16). The AL portal is made 5 mm below the joint line just lateral to the extensor tendons (Fig. 2.17). The lateral cutaneous branch of the superficial peroneal nerve lies near this portal region and can usually be visualized and palpated by inversion and plantar flexion of the ankle. From this approach one can visualize the anteromedial (Figs. 2.18, 2.19), anterocentral (Figs. 2.20, 2.21), and most of the anterolateral areas of the tibiotalar joint (Figs. 2.22, 2.23). With the assistance of a distraction device, the arthroscope is advanced posterocentrally and posterolaterally to visualize the central and posterior compartments (Fig. 2.24). The significant structures in these compartments are the intraarticular aspects and synovium of the distal tibiofibular syndesmosis, the posterior tibiofibular ligament, the transverse ligament, and the synovial plicae that overlie the transverse ligament (Figs. 2.25, 2.26).

Anteromedial Portal

Some arthroscopists establish the anteromedial (AM) portal as the primary diagnostic portal.[4,5] The AM portal is created 5 mm distal to the joint line, just medial to the anterior tibial tendon (Fig. 2.17). If the AL portal is established first, light from the arthroscope can be used to identify the course of the saphenous vein and nerve during establishment of the AM portal (Fig. 2.27). From this location, instrumentation may be advanced into the interior of the joint through the anterior tibial notch of Harty near the medial malleolus.[3,14] The AM portal is initially used for placing a diagnostic

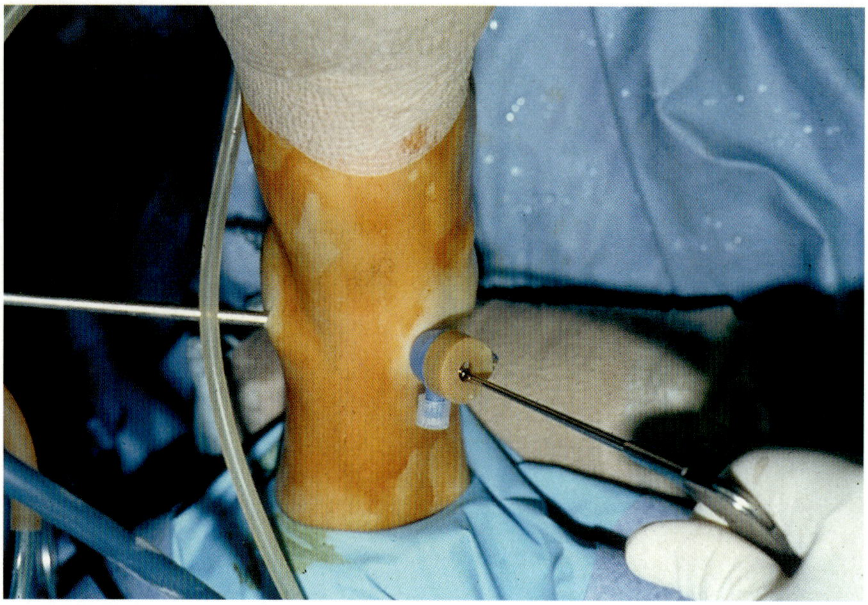

FIGURE 2.16. View of the right ankle during arthroscopy. Arthroscope is in the anterolateral (AL) portal; cannula is in the anteromedial (AM) portal.

probe or a motorized shaver, which is used to clear synovium that blocks visualization in the front of the joint. Following an accurate diagnosis, triangulation may be done by alternately switching the instruments and arthroscope between the AM and AL portals. In general, surgical instrumentation is inserted on the same side as the pathology, with the scope placed from the opposite anterior approach. Thus, visualization in the posterolateral compartment is best done with the arthroscope placed anteromedially.

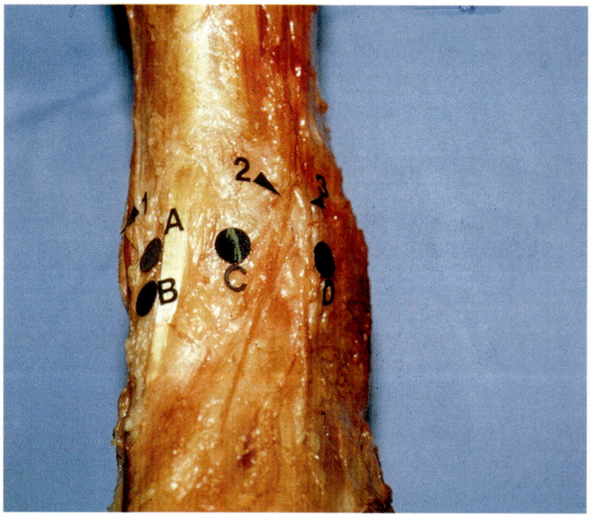

FIGURE 2.17. Superficial dissection of the anterior left ankle. **A:** AM portal. **B:** Accessory anteromedial (AAM) portal. **C:** Anterocentral (AC) portal. **D:** AL portal. 1, saphenous nerve and vein; 2, medial branch superficial peroneal nerve; 3, lateral branch of the superficial peroneal nerve.

Accessory Anteromedial and Anterolateral Portals

The accessory anteromedial (AAM) and anterolateral (AAL) portals are made approximately 1.5 cm below their respective standard portals (Fig. 2.17). They are used primarily for placing instruments in the talomalleolar spaces, with the scope placed in the ipsilateral standard anterior portal. When used in combination with their standard approaches, crowding is usually a problem. For this reason, accessory portals are avoided if possible.

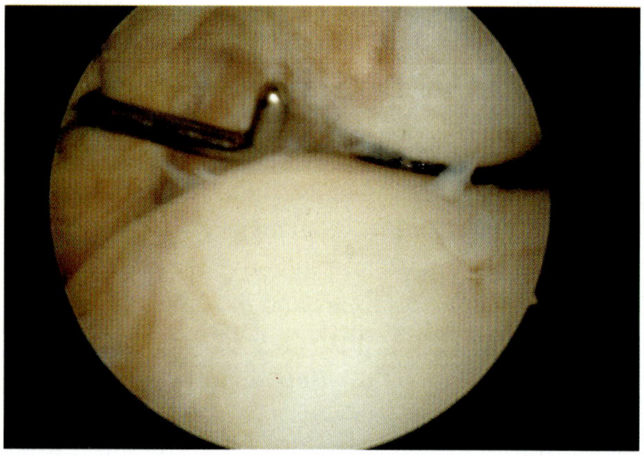

FIGURE 2.18. Anterior compartment, medial view. The probe is in the AM portal.

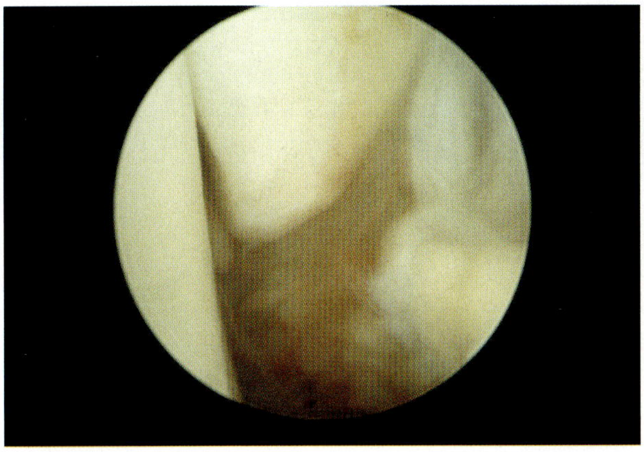

FIGURE 2.19. Tip of the medial malleolus and medial talar ridge viewed from the AL portal.

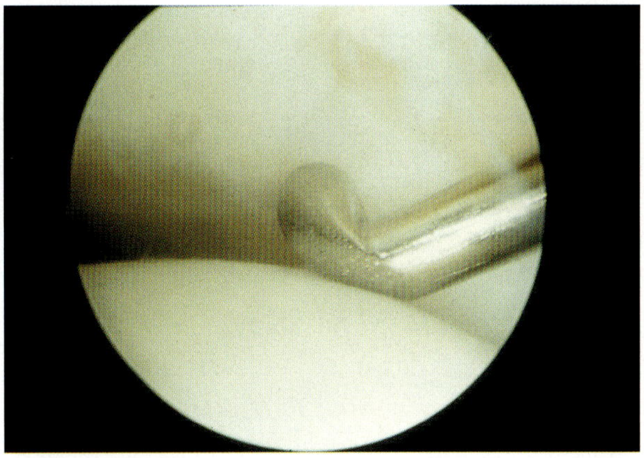

FIGURE 2.21. Middle compartment of the right ankle viewed from the AL portal.

Anterocentral Portal

The anterocentral (AC) portal is no longer recommended because of its close proximity to the dorsalis pedis artery and the terminal branch of the deep peroneal nerve (Fig. 2.2B). A pseudoaneurysm of the dorsalis pedis artery has been reported as a complication of this approach.[11,12] Other complications are inevitable should use of this portal be continued.

Posterior Portals

Posterolateral Portal

The posterolateral (PL) portal is made in the triangular space between the Achilles and peroneal ten-

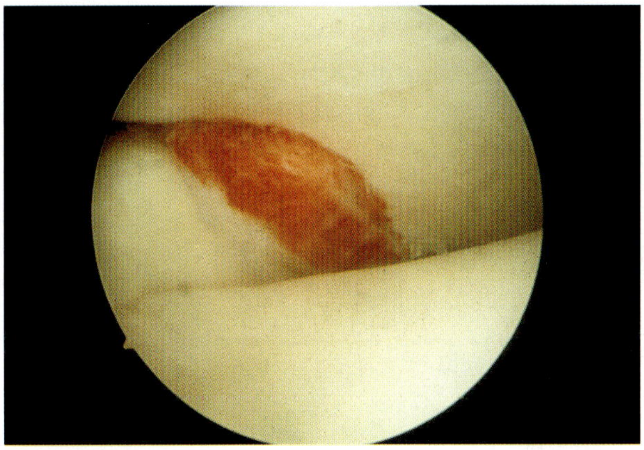

FIGURE 2.22. Midlateral view showing syndesmosis.

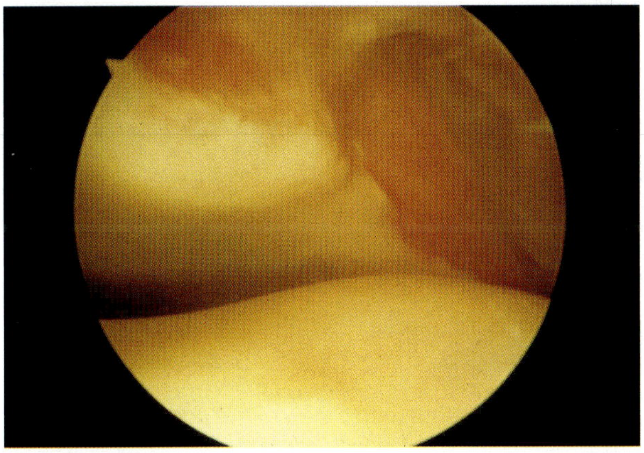

FIGURE 2.20. Anterocentral compartment viewed from the AL portal.

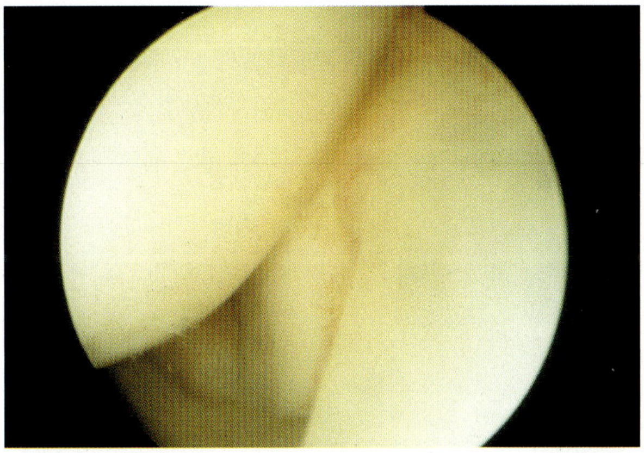

FIGURE 2.23. Lateral talomalleolar view showing the anteroinferior tibiofibular ligament running obliquely just lateral to the talar dome.

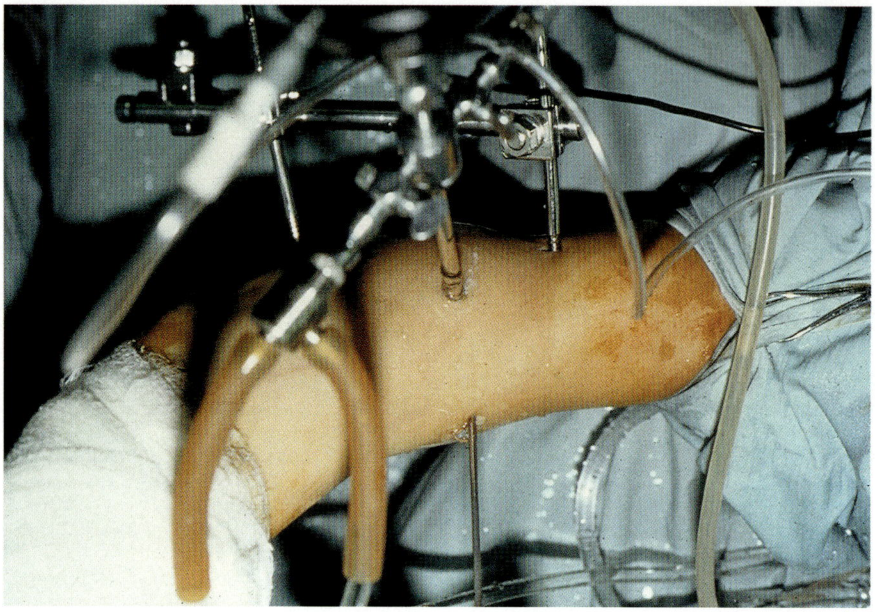

FIGURE 2.24. Right ankle with a lateral invasive distraction device. Arthroscope is in the AL portal; probe is in the AM portal.

dons. This portal is made roughly 1 cm more distal than the corresponding AL portal owing to the more distal location of the posterior joint line. The skin incision for the PL portal should be made adjacent to the lateral border of the Achilles tendon (Fig. 2.3). This reduces the risk of damage to the sural nerve and short saphenous vein, which lie farther laterally (Fig. 2.6). Care should also be taken to not stray too distally, as the subtalar joint may be entered inadvertently.

The PL portal is the only posterior portal recommended for routine use (Fig. 2.28). As discussed previously, it is used for instrumenting the posterior compartment when triangulation from anterior portals is unsuccessful (Fig. 2.29). It is also used for fluid inflow or for placing the arthroscope for viewing the posterior compartment[11,12] (Fig. 2.30).

Trans-Achilles Tendon Portal

The trans-Achilles tendon (TAT) approach, as of this writing, is not necessary. Improved methods of distraction and other approaches have made it obsolete.

Posteromedial Portal

The posteromedial (PM) portal is also not recommended by us. The posteromedial corner of the joint

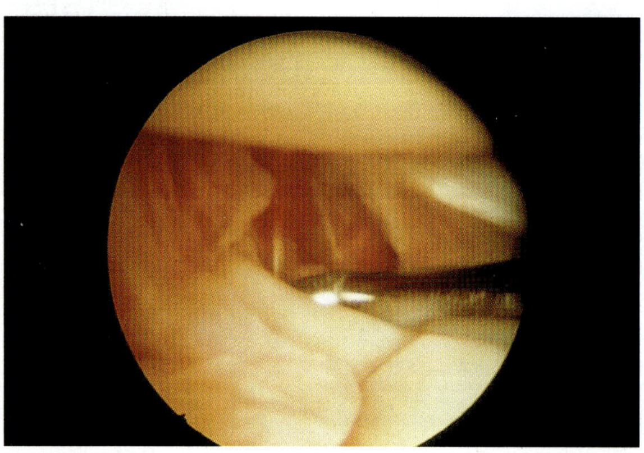

FIGURE 2.25. Arthroscopic view of the posterolateral compartment. Probe is under the posteroinferior tibiofibular ligament. Transverse ligament is under the probe at 4 o'clock.

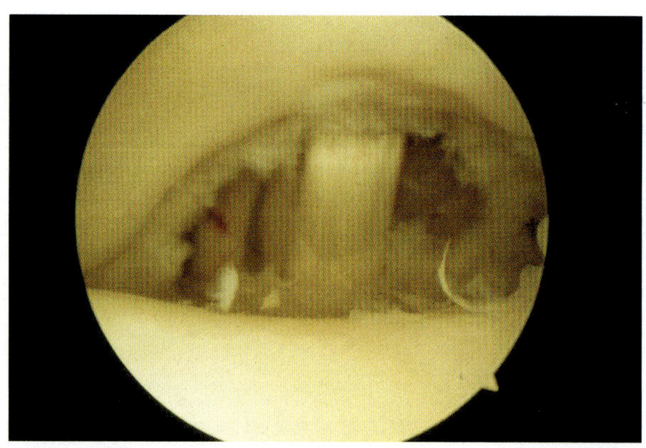

FIGURE 2.26. Arthroscopic view of the posterocentral and posteromedial left ankle with a torn posterior capsule. The flexor hallucis longus (FHL) is visualized centrally, with the posterior tibial artery and nerve just posteromedial to the tendon.

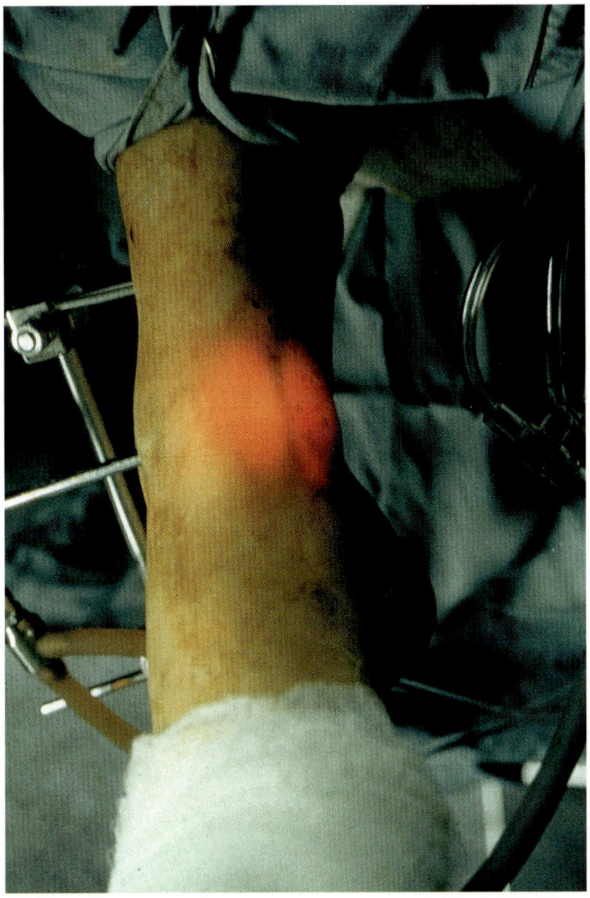

FIGURE 2.27. Right ankle with arthroscope in the AL portal transilluminating the position of the saphenous vein prior to establishing the AM portal.

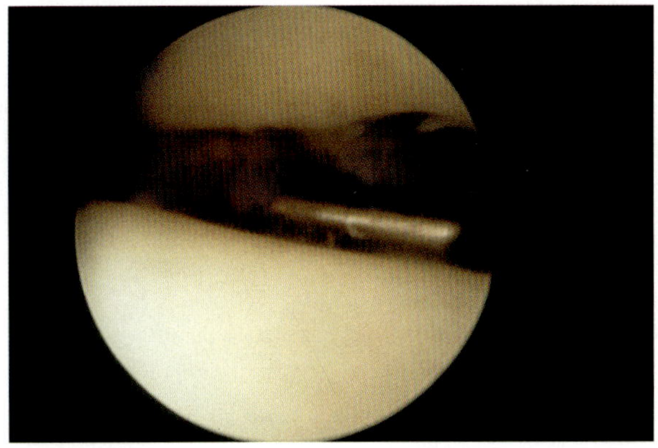

FIGURE 2.29. View of the shaver in the posterolateral compartment.

can be approached via the posterior tibial tendon sheath portal.

Posterior Tibial Tendon Sheath Portal

The posterior tibial tendon and its sheath course around and below the tip of the medial malleolus. Its sheath can be entered about 1.5 cm above the tip of the medial malleolus. Once inside the sheath from either direction, the obturator of a 2.7-mm cannula can be carefully and bluntly passed through the inner border of the sheath, penetrating the capsule and synovium to gain access to the ankle joint. Entry from the proximal position is preferred in most cases.

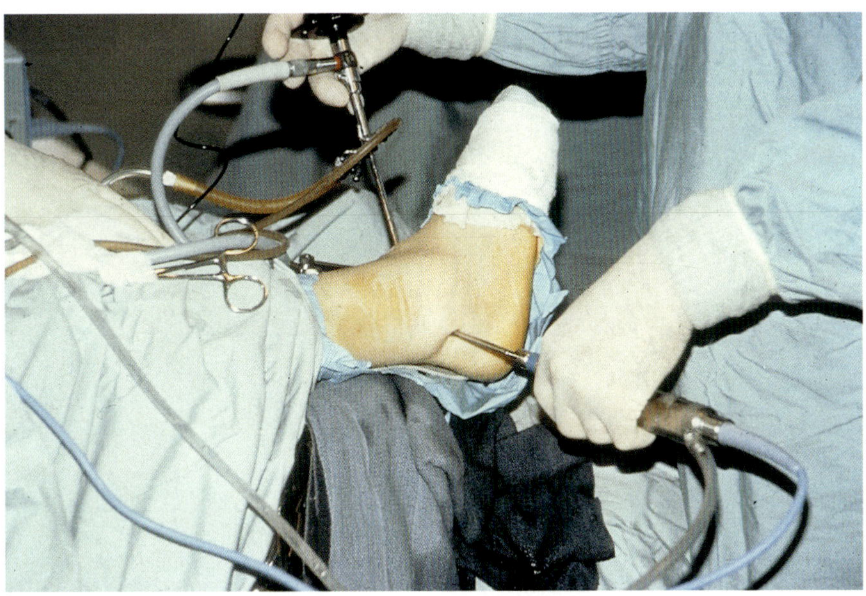

FIGURE 2.28. Positioning for use of the PL portal in the right ankle. Arthroscope is in the AM portal; shaver is in the PL portal.

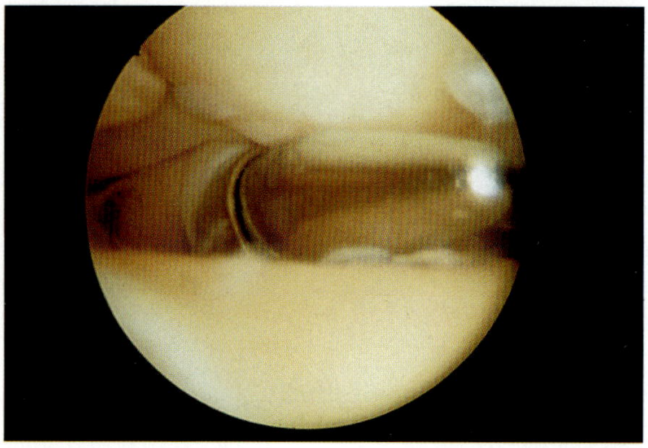

FIGURE 2.30. Arthroscopic inflow cannula in the PL portal.

Transmalleolar Approaches

The translateral and transmedial portals were developed to approach osteochondritic defects of the talar dome at an angle perpendicular to the base of the lesion. This approach decreases the risk of damaging adjacent healthy articular cartilage. The medial transmalleolar approach (MTM) is indicated more frequently than the lateral (LTM), as medial talar lesions are commonly located more posteriorly on the talar dome, and the medial malleolus is located more anteriorly than the lateral malleolus. An arthroscopic anterior cruciate ligament (ACL) drill guide facilitates accurate intraarticular pin place-

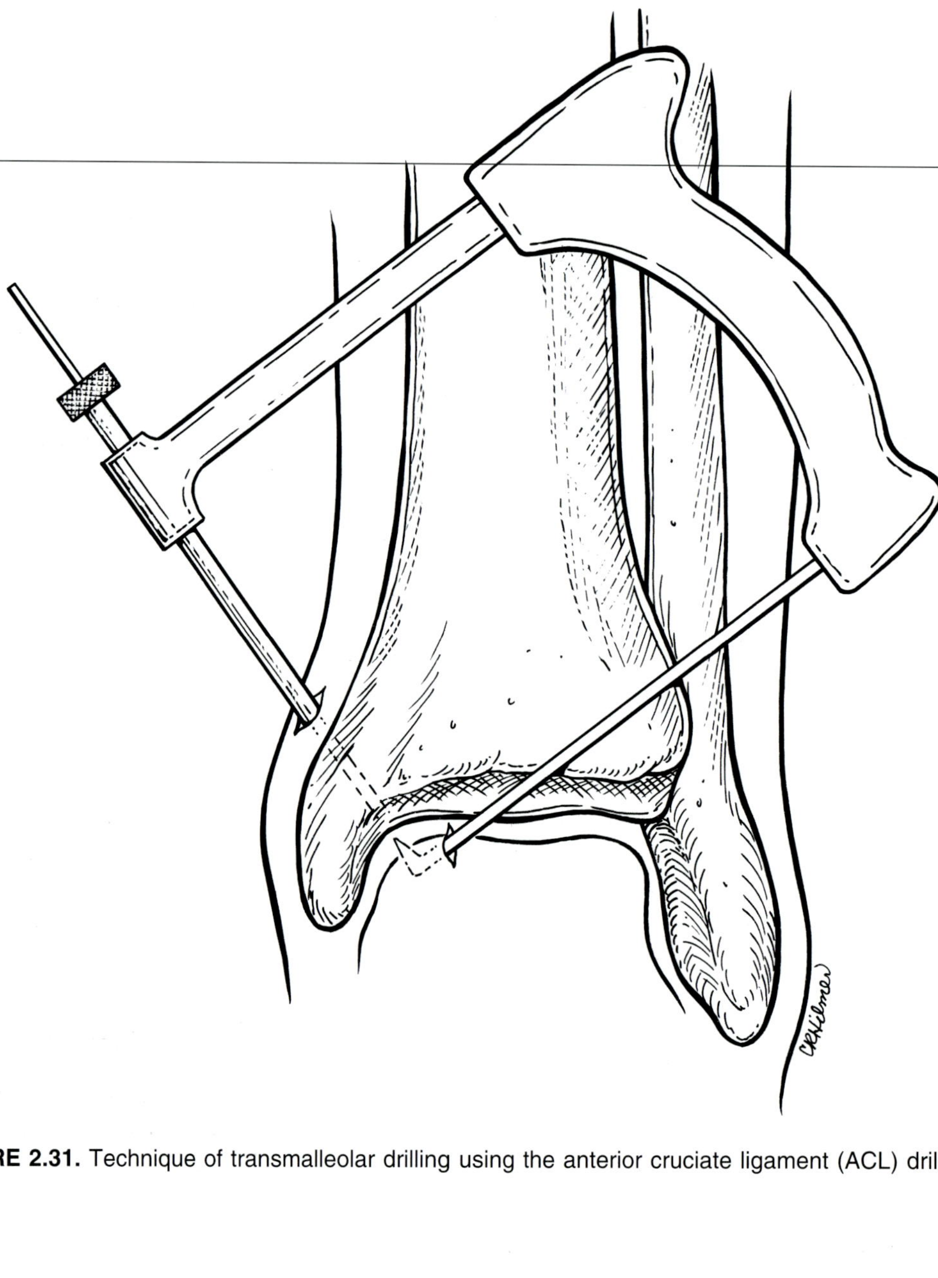

FIGURE 2.31. Technique of transmalleolar drilling using the anterior cruciate ligament (ACL) drill guide.

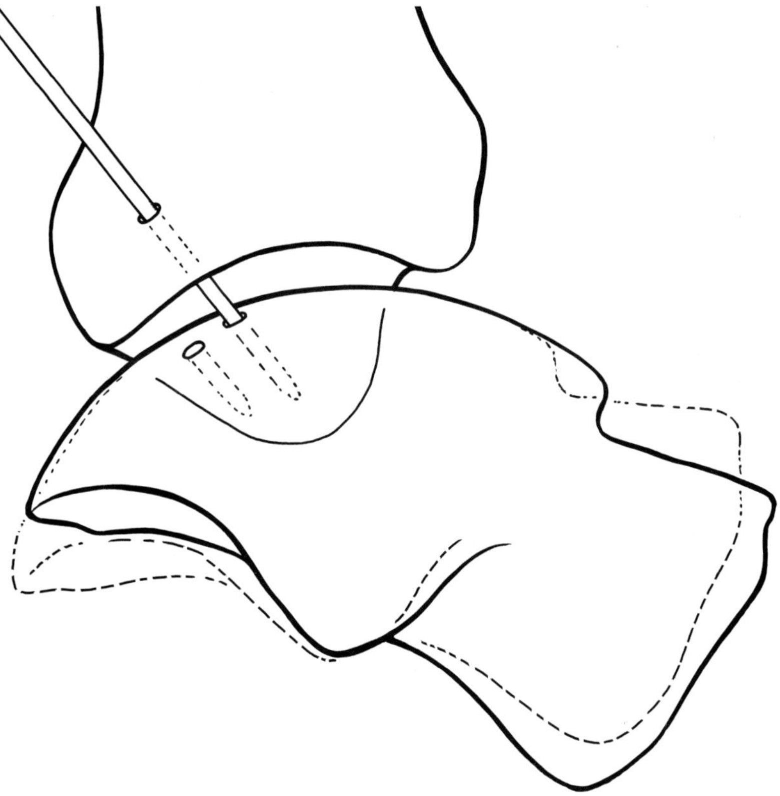

FIGURE 2.32. Lateral view of transmalleolar drilling demonstrating dorsiflexion and plantar flexion of the talus to position the lesion under the pin.

ment. The guide is placed through the anterior portal and placed on the tibial plafond over the talar lesion. A transmalleolar portal is then made 2–3 cm above the tip of the respective malleolus (Fig. 2.31). The pin is drilled through the malleolus until the tip is visualized intraarticularly. The talar lesion is positioned under the pin by dorsiflexion or plantar flexion of the foot, and multiple holes are drilled in the base of the crater[2–4,18,19] (Fig. 2.32).

ANKLE DISTRACTION

Many surgeons find ankle distraction a valuable technique that allows visualization and instrumentation of the posterior compartment of the ankle from the standard anterior portals. Invasive and noninvasive distraction devices are used for this purpose.[1,3,4,10] These devices and techniques are reviewed in Chapter 5. This section reviews the anatomy and structures at risk during placement of pins for medial and lateral invasive distraction.

Lateral distraction is well accepted and used more frequently than medial distraction.[3,4,10] This instrumentation requires a proximal tibial pin and a distal calcaneal pin. The tibial pin can be placed either just above or far above the joint line. The surgeon must be cognizant of the location of the anterior neurovascular bundle during tibial pin placement. The calcaneal pin is placed at least 3 cm distal to and on a 30- to 40-degree angle posteroinferiorly from the tip of the lateral malleolus. This decreases the risk to the sural nerve and small saphenous vein, which are located cephalad to the pin site (Fig. 2.33).

Medial distraction is occasionally used to approach posteromedial pathology from the AM portal. Medially based invasive distraction places the proximal tibial pin 1.5 cm above the joint and the distal pin in the talus. The distal pin is usually placed approximately 5 mm inferior and 5 mm anterior to the palpable tip of the medial malleolus.[3,11,12] The anterior neurovascular bundle is at risk if the proximal pin is placed too anteriorly. The posterior neurovascular bundle is jeopardized with excessive posterior placement of the distal pin. The more superficial saphenous nerve and vein are at risk with both proximal and distal pin placement. The nerve and vein run just posterior to the recommended proximal pin site and just anterior to the recommended insertion point for a medially based talar distraction pin (Fig. 2.34).

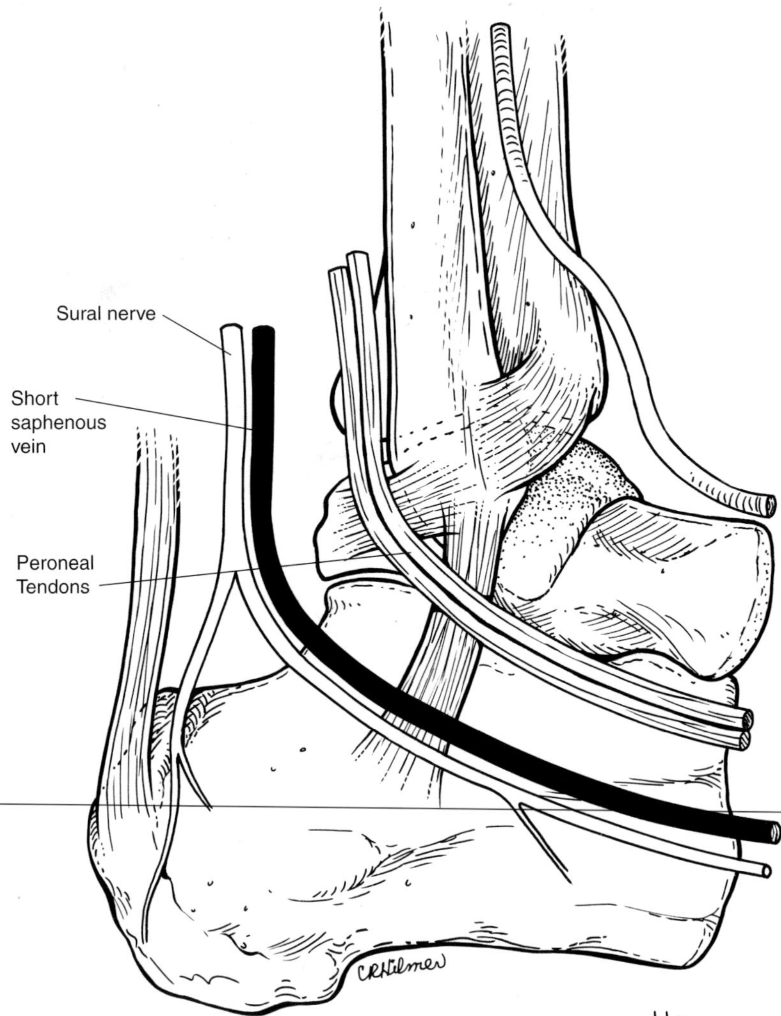

FIGURE 2.33. Structures at risk when laterally based invasive distraction is undertaken.

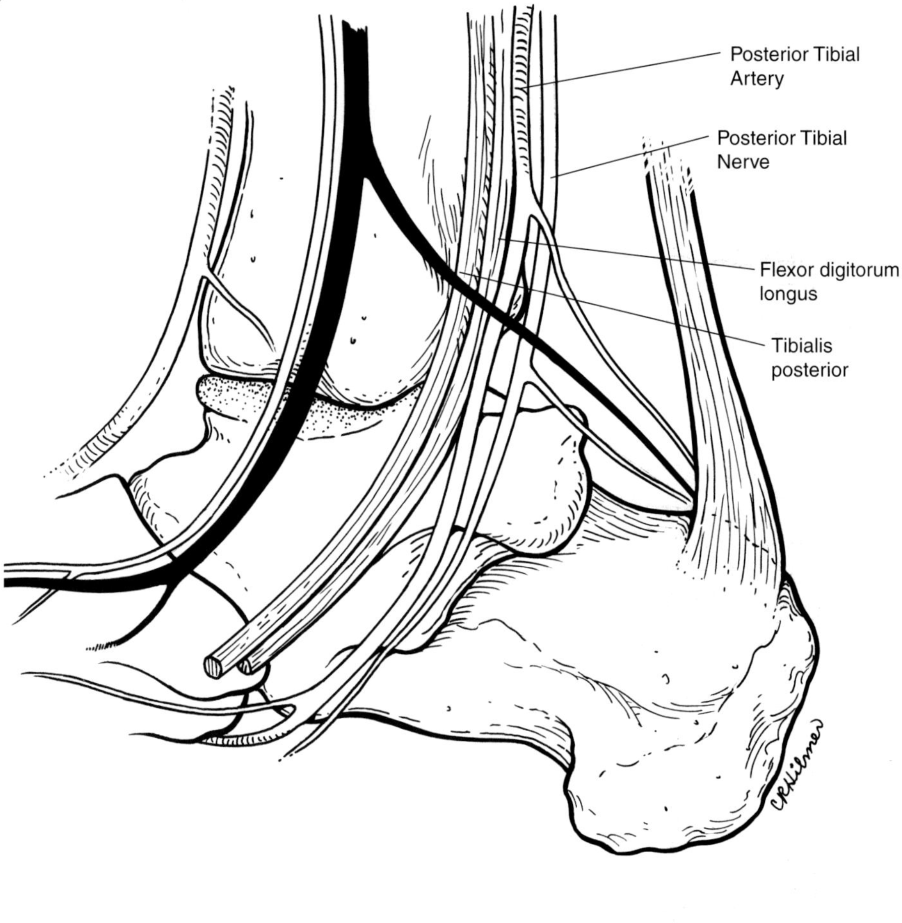

FIGURE 2.34. Structures at risk when medially based invasive distraction is undertaken.

BIBLIOGRAPHY

1. Stetson SB, Ferkel RD. Ankle arthroscopy. I. Technique and complications. *JAAOS* 1996;4:17–23.
2. Stetson SB, Ferkel RD. Ankle arthroscopy. II. Indications and results. *JAAOS* 1996;4:24–34.
3. Morgan CD. Gross and arthroscopic anatomy of the ankle. In: Meginty JB (ed) *Operative arthroscopy*. Philadelphia: Lippincott-Raven, 1996;1101–1117.
4. Ferkel RD. Arthroscopy of the ankle and foot. In: Mann RA (ed) *Surgery of the foot and ankle*. St. Louis: Mosby, 1993;1277–1310.
5. Parisien JS, Vangsness T. Operative arthroscopy of the ankle: three years experience. *Clin Orthop* 1985; 199:46–53.
6. Drez D, Guhl JF. Arthroscopy of the ankle. Presented at the Annual Meeting of the American Foot and Ankle Society, Las Vegas, 1981.
7. Drez D, Guhl JF, Gollehon DL. Ankle arthroscopy: technique and indications. *Foot Ankle* 1981;2:138–142.
8. Drez D, Guhl JF, Gollehon DL. Ankle arthroscopy: technique and indications. *Clin Sports Med* 1982;1: 35–45.
9. Gollehon DL, Drez D. Arthroscopy of the ankle. In: McGinty JB (ed) *Techniques in orthopaedics: arthroscopic surgery update*. Rockville, MD: Aspen, 1985;161–173.
10. Guhl JF. Arthroscopic advances: new techniques for arthroscopic surgery of the ankle. *Orthopedics* 1986; 9:261–269.
11. Morgan CD. Arthroscopic tibiotalar arthrodesis. In: Guhl JF (ed) *Ankle arthroscopy and surgical technique*. Thorofare, NJ: Slack, 1987;119–123.
12. Morgan CD. Arthroscopic tibiotalar arthrodesis. *Jefferson Orthop J* 1987;16:50–52.
13. Voto SJ, Ewing JW, Fleissner PR, et al. Ankle arthroscopy: neurovascular and arthroscopic anatomy of standard and trans-Achilles tendon portal placement. *Arthroscopy* 1989;5:41–46.
14. Harty M. Gross anatomy of the ankle joint. In: Guhl JF (ed). *Ankle arthroscopy: pathology and surgical technique*. Thorofare, NJ: Slack, 1987;7–12.
15. Hoppenfeld S, DeBoer P. The ankle and foot. In: Hoppenfeld S (ed) *Surgical exposures in orthopaedics*. Philadelphia: Lippincott, 1984;469–530.
16. Guhl JF. Soft tissue pathology. In: Guhl JF (ed) *Ankle arthroscopy: pathology and surgical technique*. Thorofare, NJ: Slack, 1987;79–94.
17. Hamilton WG. Differential diagnosis of ankle problems. In: Guhl JF (ed) *Ankle arthroscopy: pathology and surgical technique*. Thorofare, NJ: Slack, 1987; 69–78.
18. Baker CL, Andrews JR, Ryan JB. Arthroscopic treatment of trans-chondral talar dome fractures. *Arthroscopy* 1986;2:82–87.
19. Berndt AL, Harty M. Transcondylar fractures. *J Bone Joint Surg Am* 1959;41:988–1024.
20. Chen Y. Arthroscopy of the ankle joint. In: *Arthroscopy of small joints*. New York: Igaku-Shoin, 1985.

CHAPTER 3

Examination and Differential Diagnosis of the Foot and Ankle for Arthroscopic-Endoscopic Surgery

Lew C. Schon, Steven L. Haddad, and John T. Campbell

Physical examination is the most important technical skill in the arthroscopist's armamentarium. Physical examination and history taking represent the first and most critical steps in the process of formulating a diagnosis. The importance of interpreting the findings of other diagnostic tools such as radiography, computed tomography (CT), and magnetic resonance imaging (MRI) in the context of the clinical examination cannot be overemphasized. Similarly, the clinical significance of arthroscopic findings should be evaluated in light of the preoperative differential diagnosis established on the foundation of the carefully obtained history and physical examination. By reinforcing these basic components, this chapter strives to improve the ultimate diagnostic and therapeutic skills of arthroscopists who treat foot and ankle disorders.

PRINCIPLES OF EXAMINATION

The physical examination consists of seven steps conducted sequentially: observation, palpation, range of motion testing, strength evaluation, neurovascular assessment, disorder-specific maneuvers, and dynamic assessment.

Observation

The first step when evaluating the foot and ankle is a global visual inspection of the patient's body habitus, gait pattern, and lower extremity alignment. As the patient enters the examination room, gait pattern is observed to detect any gross abnormality, such as an antalgic limp, varus or valgus thrust, slapping (steppage) gait, or circumduction. The patient's habitus can also provide clues to pathophysiologic conditions, with obesity often associated with symptomatic mechanical problems of the lower extremities. A slender build may indicate a generalized level of fitness, particularly in athletes, but may also suggest subtle metabolic or endocrinologic abnormalities (e.g., female distance runners with anorexia, amenorrhea, or osteopenia).

Adequate assessment of the feet and ankles requires removing trousers (or rolling up the pant legs) to examine the lower thigh and removing shoes and socks from both feet to allow side-by-side comparison. Next, the overall alignment of the body is assessed. Proximally, one looks for scoliosis, pelvic obliquity, and excessive anteversion or retroversion of the hips. Other observations include looking for deformity of the knee (e.g., flexion contracture, genu varum, genu valgum, procurvatum, recurvatum) and varus or valgus malalignment of the ankle. Limb length discrepancy is noted, and determinations are made at which level the discrepancy occurs. Systematic assessment of the alignment of the foot proceeds from proximal to distal, assessing heel valgus or varus, tarsal abduction or adduction, and relative pronation or supination of the forefoot. Assessment of toe alignment includes identifying hallux valgus, hallux varus, and claw, hammer, mallet, or splaying deformities. Relative toe lengths are noted, especially short first metatarsals and long second metatarsals. The global shape of the foot, such as a pes planus or a pes cavus deformity, is also considered. Subtle differences in the shape of the foot may provide insight into diagnosis. For example, pes plano valgus due to insufficiency of the posterior tibialis tendon typically encompasses heel valgus with forefoot pronation and abduction. Conversely, pes planus with foot abduction without heel valgus may be due to instability or arthrosis of the tarsometatarsal joint complex after a traumatic injury. Comparison of the symptomatic and asymptomatic sides is useful because symmetric deformity may represent physiologic or "normal" alignment, whereas asymmetry typically suggests a pathologic process.

The final phase of inspection focuses on local phenomena of the foot and ankle. Edema is often the most apparent clinical sign consistent with an acute injury or a chronic local disease process, although it can be present with systemic disorders as well. The location must be carefully noted: If the edema is focal in nature, it may indicate injury to underlying structures. For example, doughy edema over the shaft of a metatarsal may indicate a stress fracture of that bone. Similarly, ecchymosis may localize the site of an acute injury. In some cases, however, the injury is remote from the bruising; for example, ecchymosis near the plantar skin of the heel may be due to an ankle fracture. Skin lesions such as ulcers, calluses, or fracture blisters and the presence of previous surgical incisions are noted because they may be part of underlying pathology and may have an impact on subsequent surgical approaches. Erythema can indicate infection and other inflammatory conditions such as arthritis or gout. Finally, skin color changes accompanied by shininess, hair loss, swelling, and soft tissue atrophy suggest nerve dysfunction or reflex sympathetic dystrophy, although these conditions often present more subtly without these physical findings.

Palpation

The first step when palpating the extremity is to assess skin temperature. Warmth may be found directly over a fracture site or in association with synovitis or tenosynovitis. A more localized zone of increased warmth may also be found in association with an acute nerve injury. Diffuse warmth is characteristic of infection, such as cellulitis, but may also be found with reflex sympathetic dystrophy. With more chronic nerve injuries, the zone of damage may be relatively colder than surrounding skin owing to autonomic dysfunction.

Pain on palpation of a structure or region is one of the most critical findings during the orthopedic examination. While palpating a painful area, the clinician considers the local anatomy and various structures that may be producing the discomfort. For example, pain with palpation over the anterolateral ankle may indicate injury to the anterior talofibular ligament, the lateral process of the talus, a chip fracture of the anterior aspect of the fibula, or an injury to a branch of the superficial peroneal nerve. The patient's response during palpation and the character of the pain can help determine the structure involved. A patient with a nerve injury may describe pain as burning, shooting, tingling, or radiating along the course of that nerve. Conversely, the lack of such a complaint would make a diagnosis of nerve injury less likely. Painful crepitus detected during motion of a joint could indicate a fracture, arthritis, loose body, chondral tear, or overlying tenosynovitis. It is also important to realize that palpating certain structures may be painful in the absence of pathology, so side-to-side comparison can be helpful. An overriding principle during the orthopedic examination is that palpating the offending structure should reproduce some of the patient's symptoms, particularly the character, quality, and intensity of the pain. Because multiple etiologies can coexist, careful palpation to assess all structures in the area is necessary.

Range of Motion

The joints of the foot and ankle should be individually examined for passive and acting range of motion. Diminished passive range of motion can be due to soft tissue contractures of the joint, mechanical blocks, or severe arthritis. Decreased active range of motion in the presence of a normal passive range could be due to weakness, tendinopathy, or guarding from pain.

To assess passive motion of a joint accurately, the examiner must position his or her hands to mobilize the joint of interest while immobilizing adjacent joints. To measure dorsiflexion and plantar flexion of the ankle joint, the heel is held in a neutral position to lock the subtalar joint (Fig. 3.1). Subtalar motion is tested with inversion/eversion of the hindfoot while stabilizing the ankle in neutral position (Fig. 3.2). Transverse tarsal motion is noted with supination and pronation while stabilizing the heel and mid-tarsus (Fig. 3.3), whereas motion of the mid-foot complex can be elicited with supination, pronation, and dorsiflexion-plantar flexion stresses, with one hand stabilizing the hindfoot and transverse tarsal joints and the other hand securing

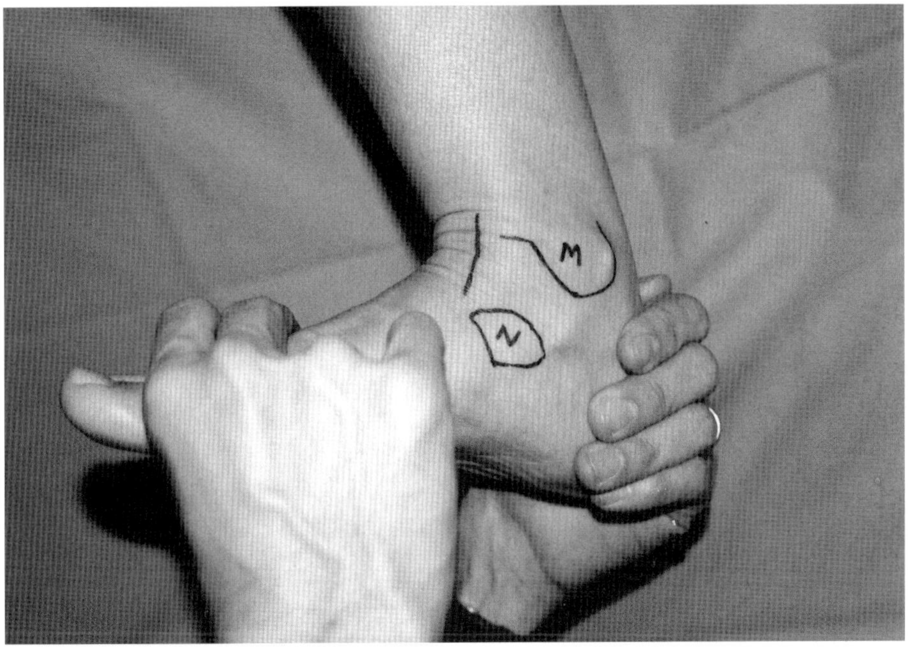

A

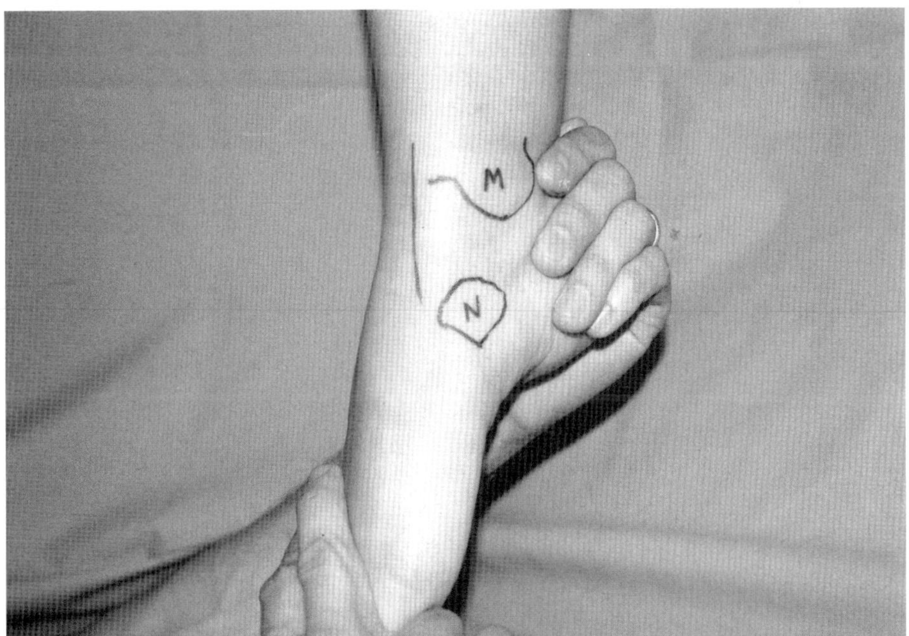

B

FIGURE 3.1. Dorsiflexion **(A)** and plantar flexion **(B)** of the ankle. M, medial malleolus; N, navicular. Vertical line indicates the medial border of the tibialis anterior tendon.

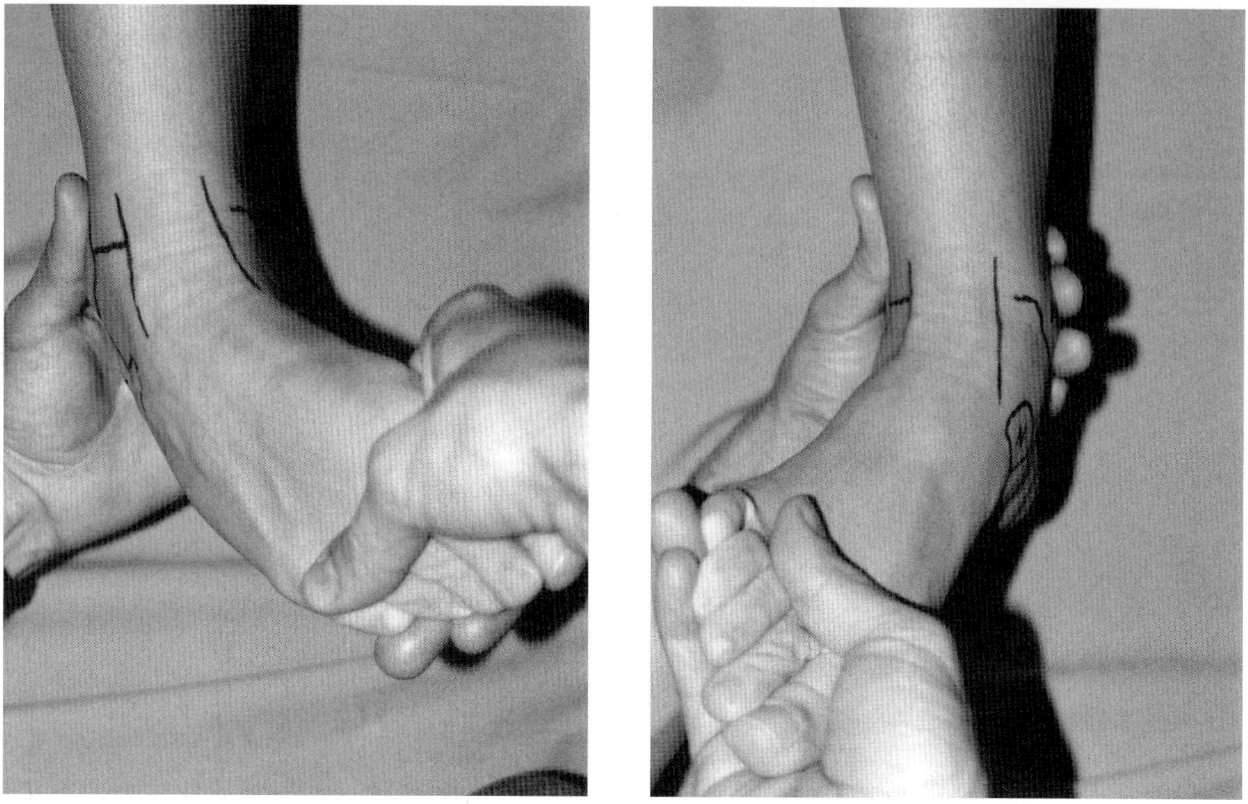

A B

FIGURE 3.2. Inversion **(A)** and eversion **(B)** of the subtalar joint. Vertical lines indicate the medial and lateral borders of the extensor tendons. Horizontal lines indicate the talotibial articulation.

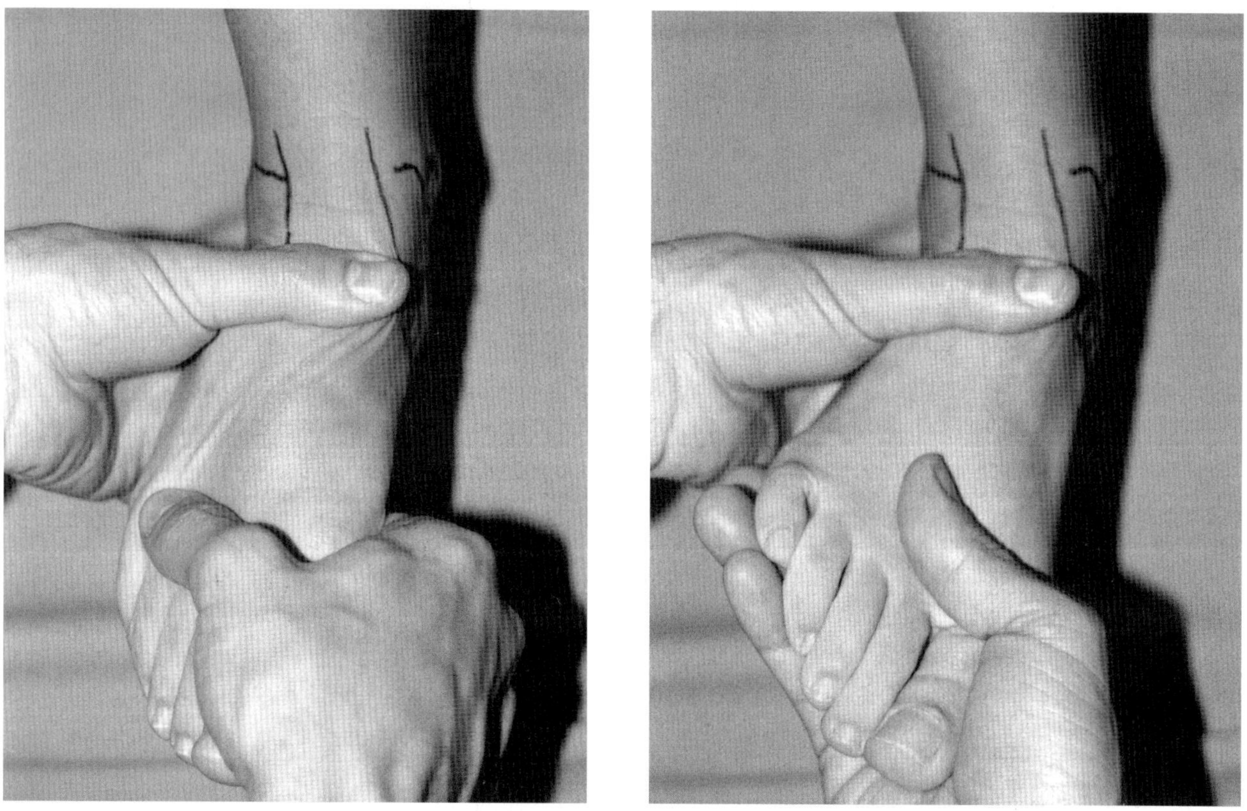

A B

FIGURE 3.3. Pronation **(A)** and supination **(B)** of the transverse tarsal joints while stabilizing the hindfoot. Vertical lines indicate the medial and lateral borders of the extensor tendons. Horizontal lines indicate the talotibial articulation.

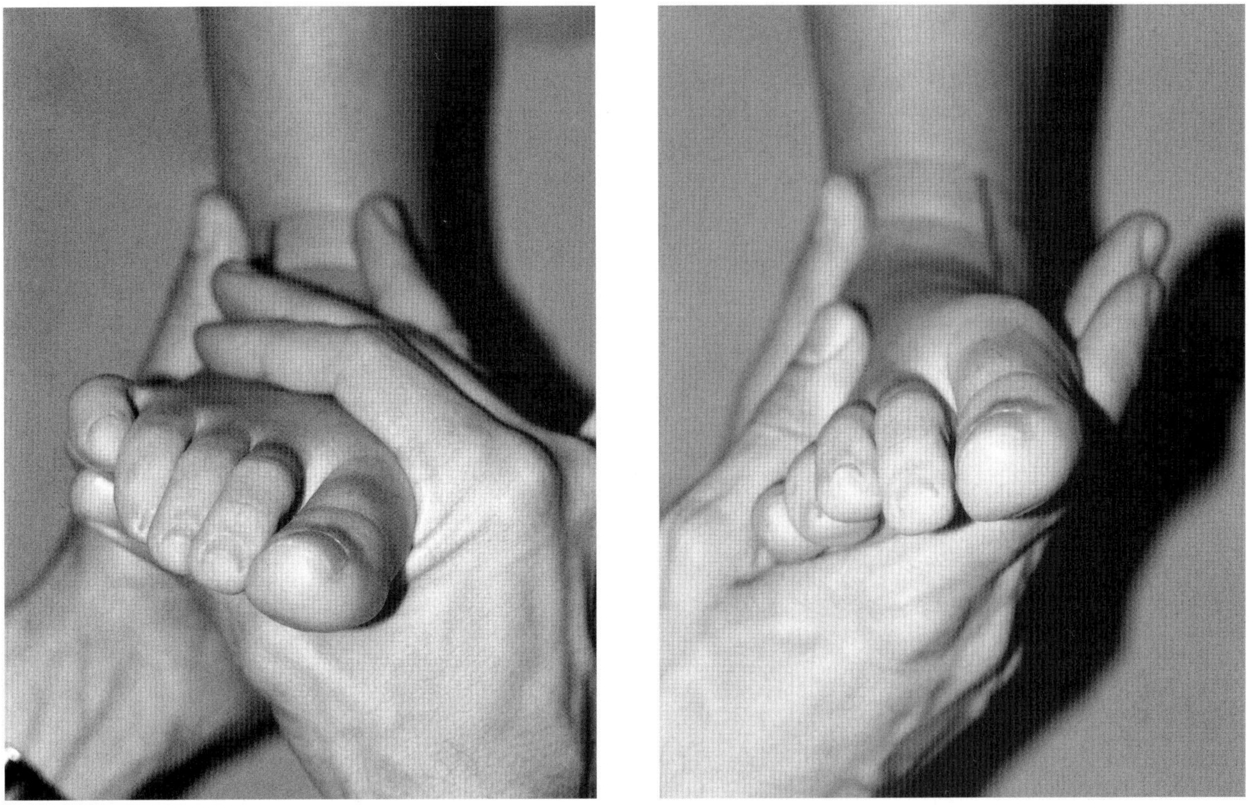

A B

FIGURE 3.4. Pronation **(A)** and supination **(B)** of the mid-foot.

the forefoot (Fig. 3.4). Motion of the metatarsophalangeal (MTP) and interphalangeal (IP) joints of the toes should also be recorded, including dorsiflexion and plantar flexion (Fig. 3.5). Finally, generalized systemic laxity can be assessed by the ability to approximate the thumb to the volar forearm, hyperextension of the metacarpophalangeal joints, hyperextension of the elbow, and increased lateral translation of the patella.

Strength Testing

The clinician should assess the strength not only of each group of muscles and tendons but also of specific tendons depending on the patient's complaints. Weakness or pain noted during examination of a particular tendon is an important diagnostic finding. Dorsiflexion against resistance can test the tibialis anterior, extensor hallucis longus (EHL), and extensor digitorum longus (EDL). Inversion in the plantar-flexed position tests the posterior tibialis tendon primarily (Fig. 3.6) and the flexor hallucis longus (FHL) and flexor digitorum longus (FDL) secondarily. Inversion of the foot with the ankle in neutral position tests the tibialis anterior and tibialis posterior tendons. Plantar flexion of the ankle primarily tests the gastrocnemius–soleus complex as well as the tibialis posterior, FHL, and FDL tendons. Eversion assesses the peroneal tendons, with peroneus brevis acting as the primary everter of the ankle and peroneus longus contributing secondarily, in addition to its main role as plantar flexor of the first ray.

The long and short tendons to the toes are also examined. The strength of the EHL is tested by applying resistance against dorsiflexion at the level of the distal phalanx of the hallux. The extensor hallucis brevis (EHB) is tested at the MTP joint and does not provide a dorsiflexion power at the IP joint of the hallux. Similarly, the FHL permits flexion of the IP and MTP joints, whereas the flexor hallucis brevis (FHB) provides flexion of the MTP joint alone. Anatomically, it is important to note that the FHL has tendinous branches to the second toe FDL tendon. Consequently, testing the FHL may involve the patient curling the second toe as well as the hallux against resistance. An assessment of functional strength is also useful. The ability to rise up on the toes tests both the posterior tibialis tendon and the

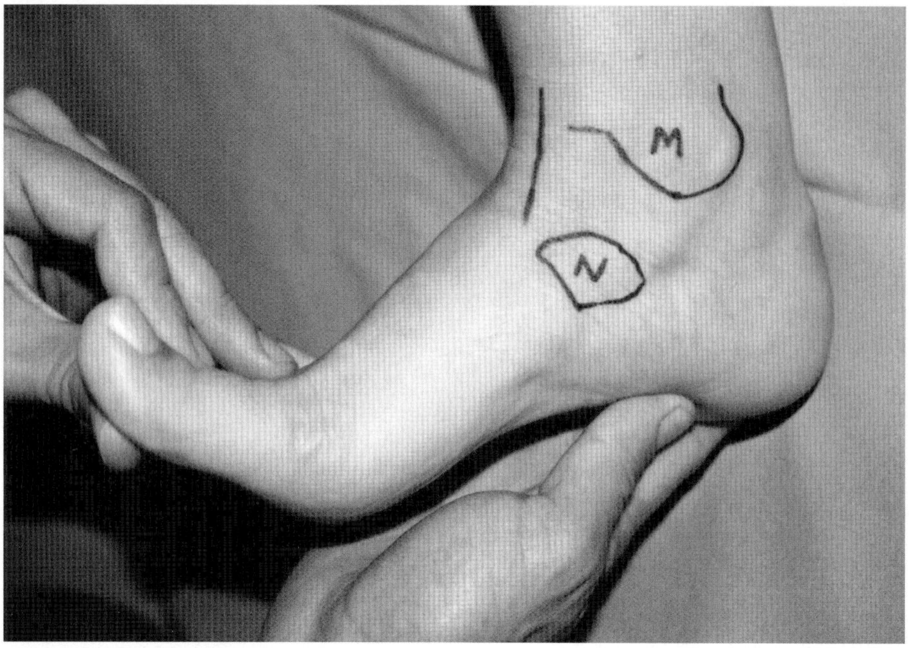

A

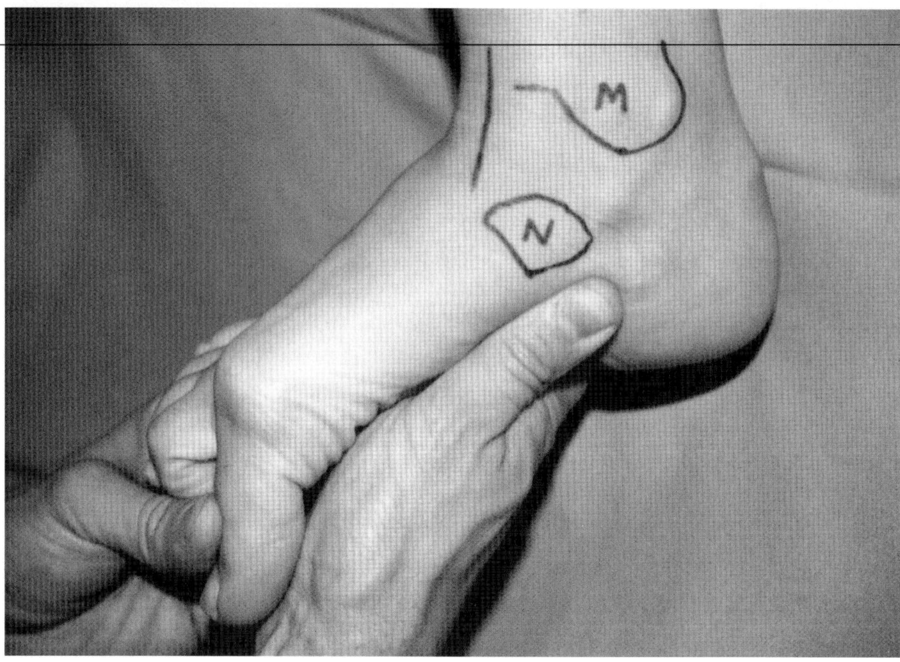

B

FIGURE 3.5. Dorsiflexion **(A)** and plantar flexion **(B)** of the hallux metatarsophalangeal (MTP) joint. M, medial malleolus; N, navicular. Vertical line indicates the medial border of the tibialis anterior tendon.

gastrocnemius–soleus complex. The posterior tibialis initiates early heel rise by inverting the heel and locking the subtalar complex. The gastrocnemius–soleus complex then powers further heel rise. An inability to perform multiple single limb heel rises or the lack of heel inversion may indicate posterior tibialis weakness. The ability to walk on the heels with the toes elevated from the ground tests the anterior compartment musculature, including the anterior tibialis, EHL, and EDL.

Neurovascular Examination

Palpation of the dorsalis pedis artery is performed between the first and second metatarsals on the dorsum of the foot; it can also be identified more proximally at the level of the ankle between the EHL and EDL tendons. The posterior tibial artery is palpated behind the medial malleolus just posterior to the tibialis posterior and FDL tendons. In some cases a distal branch of the peroneal artery can be

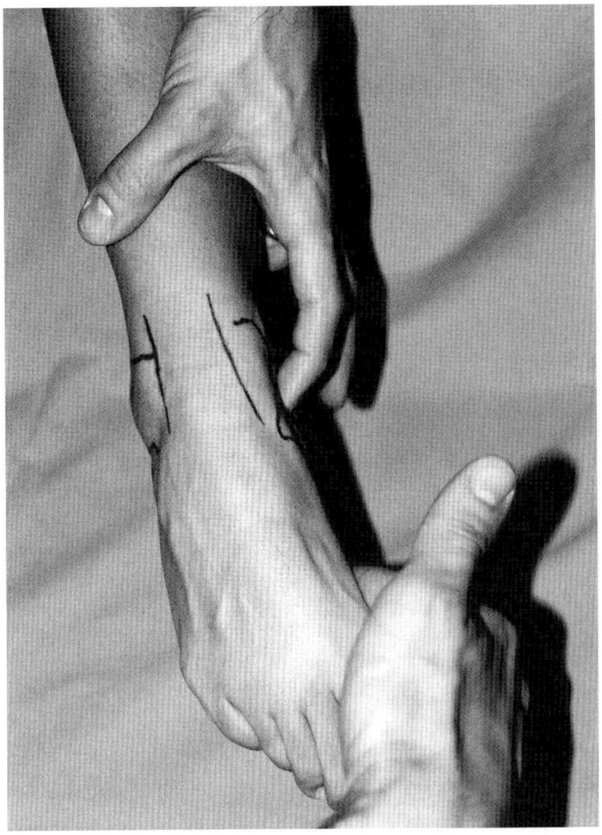

FIGURE 3.6. Testing the posterior tibialis tendon with direct palpation and resisted plantar flexion-inversion. Vertical lines indicate the medial and lateral borders of the extensor tendons. Horizontal lines indicate the talotibial articulation.

palpated over the anterolateral aspect of the fibula. Distally, capillary refill can be assessed at the tip of the digits or at the nail beds.

Neurologic evaluation includes routine palpation over all the nerves of the foot, including the superficial peroneal, deep peroneal, saphenous, sural, and tibial nerves. The dermatome of each nerve is tested for light touch sensation and, if indicated, pinprick sensation. Semmes-Weinstein monofilaments can be used to help identify an underlying neuropathy, and proprioception and vibratory sensation can be assessed for subtle neurologic deficits. Percussion along a peripheral nerve causing radiating pain, burning, tingling, or shock-like sensation (positive Tinel's sign) usually indicates neurologic pathology, such as compression or a neuroma.

Disorder-Specific Maneuvers

Several specialized tests are considered standard when evaluating the foot and ankle. In general, these maneuvers are performed with the patient relaxed, as guarding may preclude a positive finding. The anterior talofibular ligament is tested by the anterior drawer maneuver. This is performed by the examiner cupping the patient's heel in one hand and placing the other hand on the anterior aspect of the distal leg. The heel is firmly drawn toward the examiner, and counterpressure is applied to stabilize the distal leg (Fig. 3.7). The ankle must be stressed in the neutral position with the foot at right angles to the leg, as this position is typically the most stable for the anterior talofibular ligament. The calcaneal fibular ligament can be assessed by applying inversion stress to the ankle (Fig. 3.8). Similarly, insufficiency of the deltoid ligament can be tested with valgus or rotatory stress on the ankle. It is sometimes difficult to determine instability of the subtalar joint on a clinical basis, although in rare cases of severe instability there is gross gapping of the subtalar joint when varus stress is applied to the hindfoot.[1] When performing all of these ligamentous maneuvers, it is helpful to place one's fingers along the joint line being studied to detect any clunking or subluxation that occurs. Additionally, it is critical to compare the degree of stability on the involved side with that of the contralateral extremity.

Thompson's test specifically evaluates the integrity of the gastrocnemius–soleus complex and the Achilles tendon. The patient lies prone on the examination table or kneels on a stool with the feet relaxed and hanging free. A gentle squeeze to the patient's calf should cause a small degree of passive plantar flexion of the foot (Fig. 3.9). Disruption of the integrity of the gastrocnemius–soleus muscle group or an Achilles tendon rupture typically results in a lack of plantar flexion from this calf squeeze, although false-negative tests may occur owing to the secondary plantar flexors of the ankle or the plantaris tendon. The squeeze test is performed to identify injuries to the syndesmotic ligaments. During this maneuver the examiner gently squeezes the tibia and fibula together in the proximal portion of the calf. As this is performed, pain elicited along the course of the calf or at the level of the syndesmosis is highly suspicious for syndesmotic injury.

Dynamic Assessment

A dynamic functional assessment of the patient to reproduce the symptoms in question is critical, particularly in the athlete. Having the patient perform

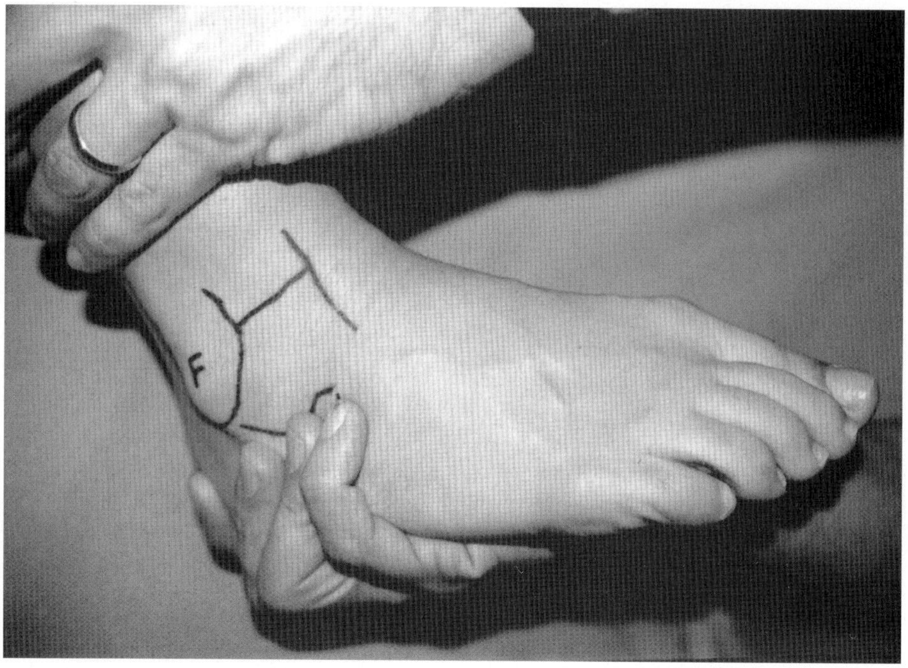

FIGURE 3.7. Anterior drawer test of the ankle. F, lateral malleolus of the fibula. Vertical line indicates the lateral border of the tibialis anterior tendon. Horizontal line indicates the talotibial articulation.

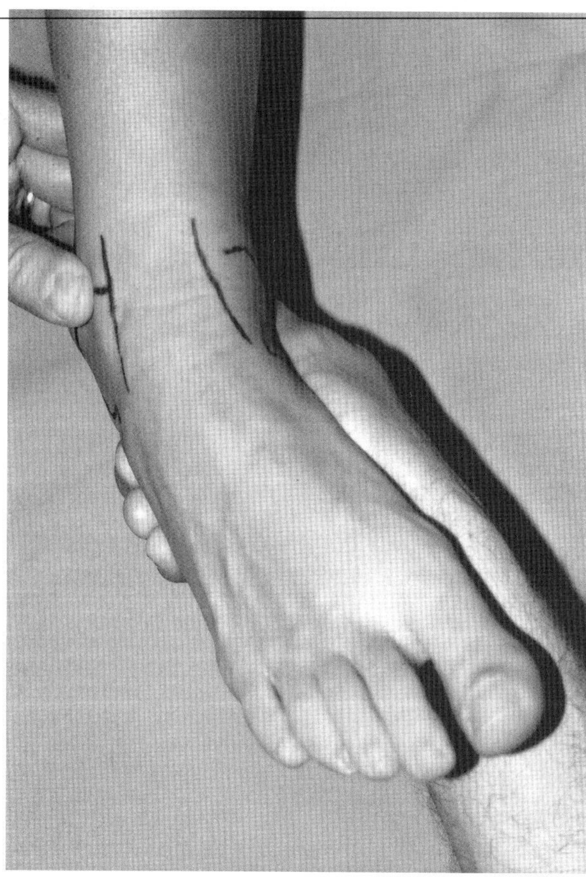

FIGURE 3.8. Inversion stress test of the ankle. Concurrent palpation of the lateral aspect of the talus during inversion stress testing may identify subtle varus laxity. Vertical lines indicate the medial and lateral borders of the extensor tendons. Horizontal lines indicate the talotibial articulation.

the activity, movement, or sport-specific maneuver that causes symptoms is essential. Thus the tennis player who complains of a painful toe during the serve should simulate his serving technique during palpation of the hallux. Other athletes are similarly examined during performance of the specific maneuver that causes their problem. Ballet dancers in particular require functional assessment during the five classic ballet positions and while performing steps, including relevé, demi-plié, grand plié, and developpé à la seconde (Fig. 3.10). Testing is also performed during jumps and pirouettes.[2,3] The swimmer complaining of posterior ankle pain on push-off may be suffering from posterior impingement. These examples highlight the need to examine the athlete during a performance of the symptomatic maneuver, which may unmask a faulty technique or subtle abnormality not otherwise elicited on static examination.

REGIONAL EXAMINATION

When examining a patient for a foot and ankle problem, it is useful to organize the thought process by specific region and point of maximum tenderness. Thus a patient with anterolateral ankle pain could have chronic lateral ligament instability, anterolateral synovial impingement, superficial peroneal neuritis, or chondral injury. Next, the examiner must focus mentally on the various anatomic structures

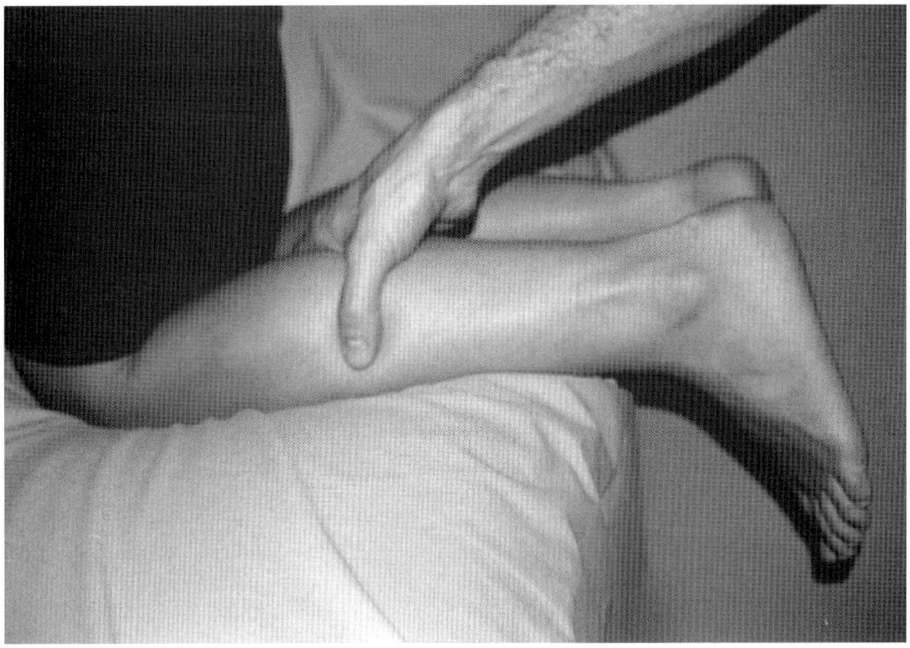

A

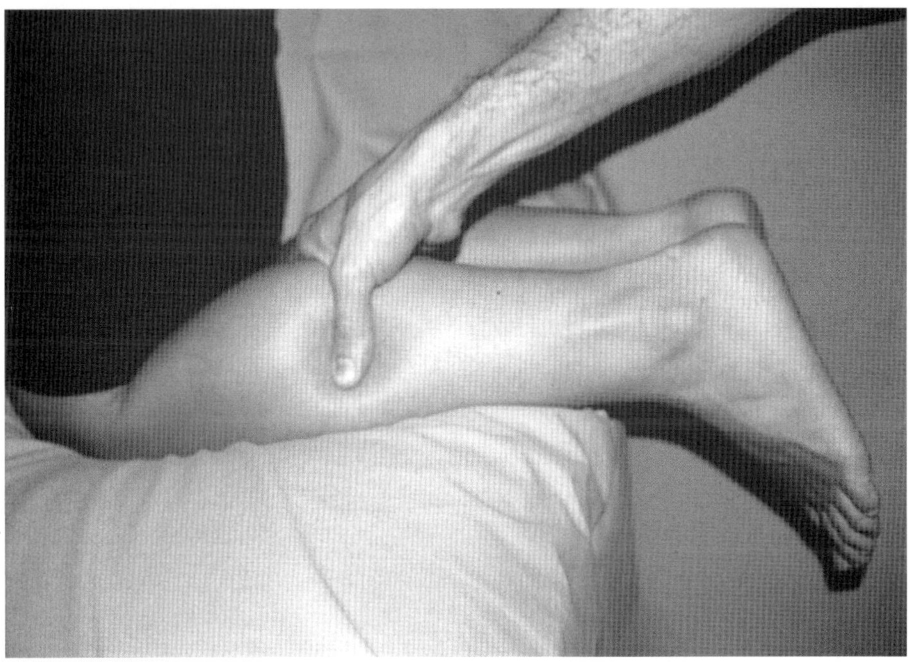

B

FIGURE 3.9. Thompson's test of Achilles tendon integrity. **A:** Relaxed position. **B:** Squeezing the calf musculature causes plantar flexion of the ankle.

that may elicit pain when compressed. It is helpful to recall the local anatomy, both topographic and cross-sectional, to identify injured structures that may be potential causes of symptoms (Fig. 3.11). Noting the character of the pain helps differentiate between damaged structures.

When examining a painful region, the physician must exclude not only local causes but other distant or systemic conditions as well.[4] For example, referred pain from a herniated lumbar disc may mimic superficial peroneal neuritis and symptoms associated with ankle instabilities, such as pain, weakness, and giving way. In addition, systemic conditions, including connective tissue diseases, systemic arthritis, Marfan's endocrine disorder, or a nutritional disorder, must be considered. Although some of these conditions (e.g., rheumatoid arthritis) are uncommon in the young, athletic population, others (e.g., seronegative arthropathies) are often diagnosed in this age group.

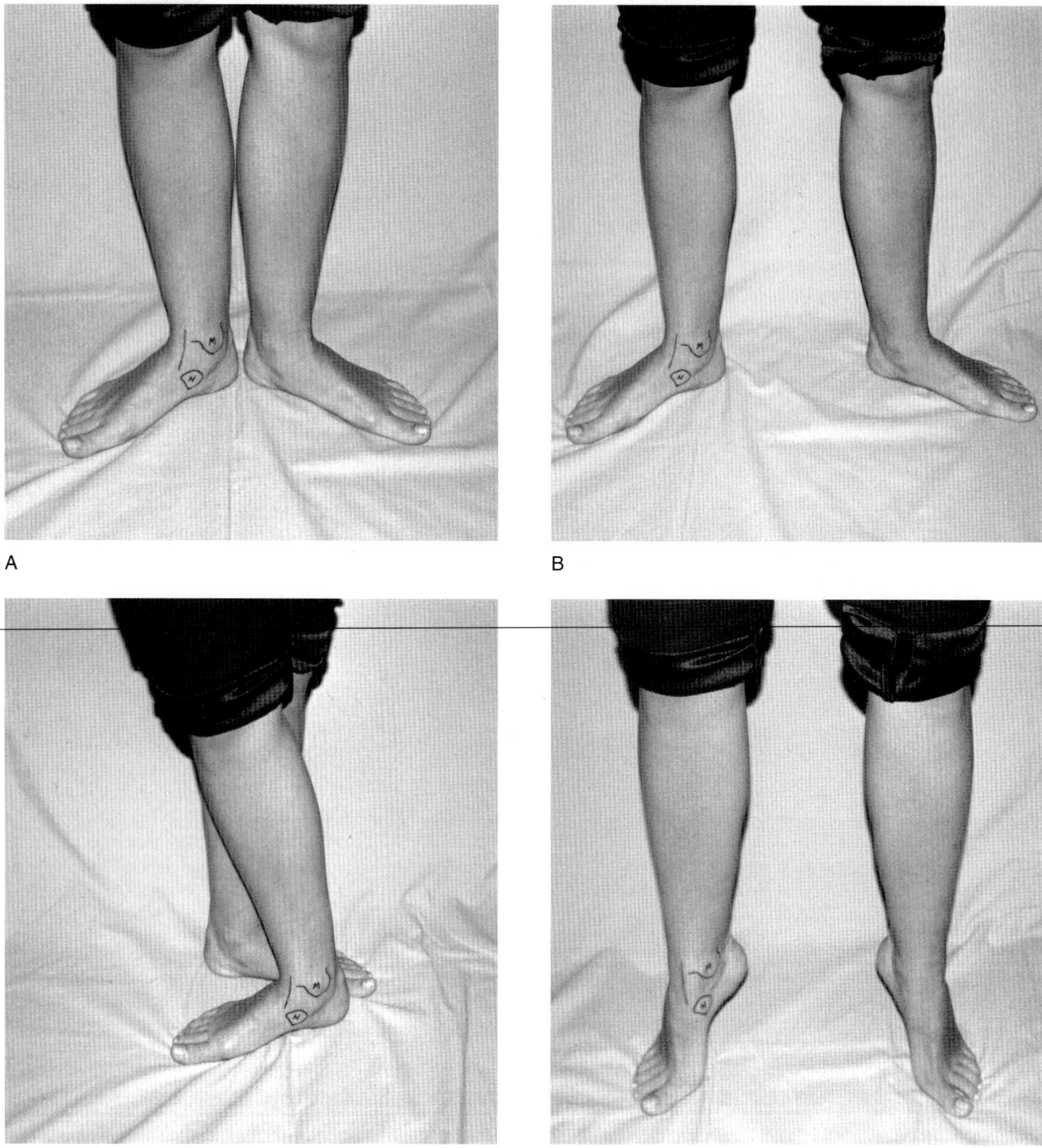

FIGURE 3.10. Ballet dance positions and steps. **A:** First position. **B:** Second position. **C:** Fifth position. **D:** Relevé. M, medial malleolus; N, navicular. Vertical line indicates the medial border of the tibialis anterior tendon.

Finally, it is critical to recall that secondary or compensatory pathology can arise in the setting of an initial process. A patient with peroneal tendinitis may be suffering primarily from chronic lateral ankle instability but may not have specific peroneal tendinitis manifestations. Patients can also develop symptoms secondarily owing to compensatory mechanisms as they "push through" the inciting pain. For example, an athlete with pain in the first MTP joint may begin to unload that area by walking or running on the side of the foot. This then leads to secondary symptoms of peroneal tendinitis, ankle instability, or

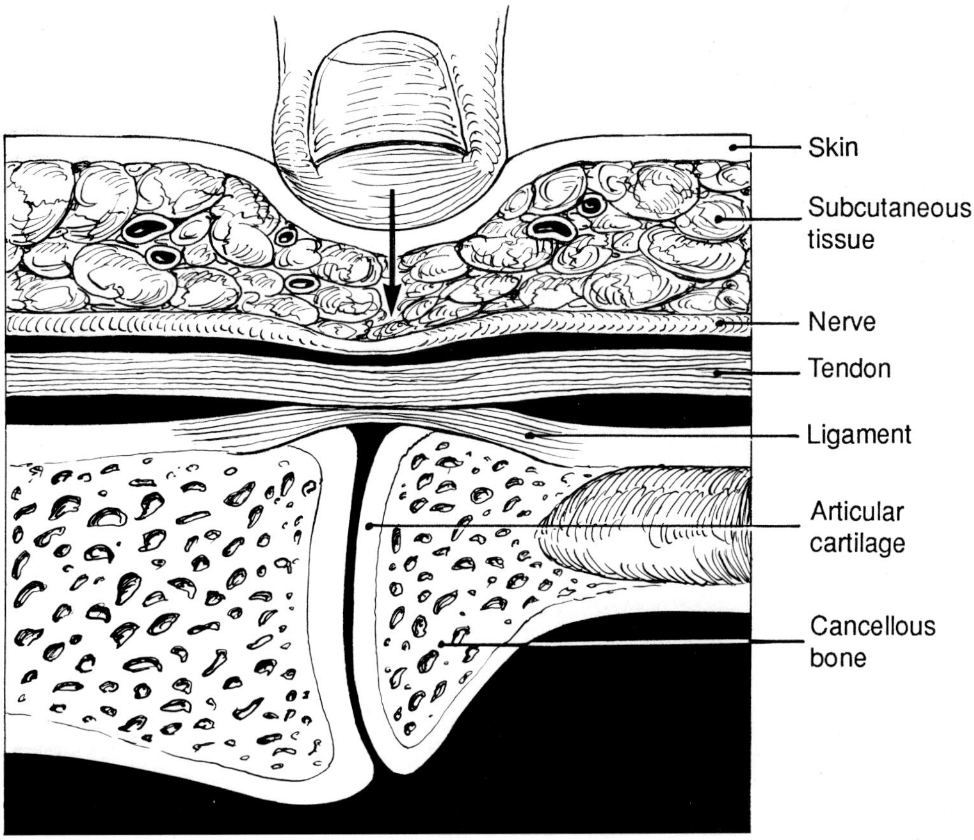

FIGURE 3.11. Cross-sectional view of various tissues and structures compressed during regional palpation.

lateral stress fracture even though the primary problem relates to the first MTP joint. Focusing attention only on the secondary symptoms may result in recurrence, as the primary process remains untreated.

Ankle

Diagnosing pathologic processes in the ankle can be frustrating for the examiner. The breadth of articular and nonarticular processes that create pain and dysfunction in this confined space may create confusion during attempts to define a specific entity. However, using a systematic approach, the physical diagnosis augmented by a careful history may point the examiner toward entities amenable to arthroscopic treatment. We find it useful to divide the ankle into quadrants: anteromedial, anterolateral, posteromedial, and posterolateral. In each region, specific pathologic entities may occur: some that are unique to that particular quadrant and others that may be found anywhere about the ankle joint. What follows is a symptom-oriented exploration by quadrant, as defined by historical and physical features.

Anteromedial Quadrant

Specific palpation within the anteromedial quadrant is the key to localizing particular entities. Common in this location is osteochondral pathology. This label encompasses the entity known as osteochondritis dissecans (OCD) as well as transchondral fractures of the talus. Many of these lesions are initially noted when the patient with an ankle sprain or ankle fracture undergoes radiographic evaluation. Although most of these injuries are thought to occur secondary to trauma, a substantial portion may present in the absence of any distinct traumatic event. Because most of the lesions are localized in the posterior or central portion of the medial talus, they may be diagnosed by firmly plantar-flexing the ankle and directly palpating the medial talus. More posterior lesions can be palpated behind the medial malleolus while dorsiflexing the ankle. Forced inversion stress may also create deep medial ankle pain as the lesion affects the tibial plafond. With advanced disease (less common on the medial side), a mobile fragment may be palpable, and crepitus or limited motion may be noted with passive dorsiflexion and plantar flexion.

A loose body is the final common pathway of osteochondral lesions. Other sources of loose bodies include synovial chondromatosis, fracture of osteoarthritic spurs (both traumatic and degenerative), and fragmented bone from previous fractures. Typically, a loose body in the ankle causes intermittent symptoms, including swelling, crepitus or clicking, locking, decreased motion, pain, or any combination of these symptoms. Loose bodies are often harbored in the medial, anterior, or lateral gutters of the ankle joint. The loose body itself may be difficult to palpate, although occasionally it is mobile enough to roll between the examiner's fingers, causing pain in the patient. Concurrent passive motion of the ankle may assist in making the fragment more palpable. Painful crepitus and limited motion may also be noted.

It is important to remember that symptoms such as pain, crepitus, and decreased motion can be due to other, less common etiologies, including a ruptured anterior tibialis tendon, a thrombosed saphenous vein, or intraarticular soft-tissue lesion (e.g., pigmented villonodular synovitis, ganglion cysts, chondromatosis, hemangioma, or even synovial cell sarcoma).

Degenerative joint disease often creates anteromedial ankle pain. Typically, the ankle demonstrates warmth and bogginess. Degenerative or posttraumatic osteophytes are palpable subcutaneously along the anterior tibial lip, medial malleolus, or talar neck and are often tender to palpation. The ankle range of motion is limited compared to the opposite extremity, as the "kissing" osteophytes impinge. More importantly, a patient with degenerative joint disease experiences pain with forced dorsiflexion of the ankle. Intraarticular injection of local anesthetic, resulting in relief of symptoms, is effective for confirming the joint as the source of pain.

Deltoid insufficiency is a rare cause of medial ankle findings. A rupture of the deep deltoid ligament (generally due to violent trauma or falls from a height with the heel in valgus) is necessary to produce such instability. Acutely, one must rule out lateral malleolus fracture, syndesmotic injury, or proximal fibular (Maisonnneuve) fracture. In the chronic setting, clinical instability may be difficult to elicit. Patients have point tenderness over the deltoid (which must be distinguished from the posterior tibial tendon by the tests mentioned below) and pain with valgus stress of the ankle and subtalar joints or abduction of the transverse tarsal joint. Stress radiographs are frequently normal, and an MRI scan may be necessary to determine the extent of ligamentous damage.

Posterior tibial tendinitis can be present with anteromedial ankle pain, although the more typical form is retromalleolar pain. The tendon courses inferior to the joint line and may have associated swelling or bogginess due to tenosynovitis. A palpable gap in the tendon may be present. A painful single-limb heel rise or an inability to perform a single-limb heel rise points more specifically toward this condition, as does pain with resisted plantar flexion and inversion.

Neuritis of the saphenous or deep peroneal nerves may present as pain in the anteromedial quadrant. Patients may be extremely sensitive to light touch, rubbing from shoewear, or pressure from bed linen. Paresthesias are a common complaint, but frank numbness is rare. Extreme plantar flexion creates nerve traction and often exacerbates the symptoms. This tenderness differs from the above-mentioned conditions by occurring more superficially in the ankle. Tinel's sign is useful, as such a test is rarely positive when intraarticular conditions are causing the pain.

Finally, a navicular stress fracture may present as pain in the anteromedial quadrant of the ankle. Although symptoms of this condition are often diffuse, pain over the medial mid-foot during gait and difficulty with single-limb heel rise can mimic posterior tibialis tendinitis or insufficiency. Careful palpation reveals maximal tenderness over the navicular rather than along the tendon itself. Maximum passive pronation and active supination of the forefoot against resistance may also cause pain. A radiograph or radionuclide bone scan is helpful for this assessment.

Anterolateral Quadrant

There is obvious crossover in pathologic entities between the anteromedial and anterolateral quadrants. OCD lesions or transchondral fractures may occur on the lateral border of the talus. When the lesion is on the lateral talus, it is generally anterior on the dome of the talus. Because of their anterior location, these lesions are more accessible to direct palpation than are medial lesions. Extreme valgus of the ankle joint can create intraarticular impingement, eliciting pain. The presence of effusion and clicking are intermittent, similar to that with medial lesions. Degenerative joint disease laterally has a presentation similar to that on the medial side. Again, the "kissing" osteophytes impinge with extreme dorsiflexion of the foot, resulting in pain and crepitus.

Severe inversion ankle sprains may cause persistent symptoms in the anterolateral quadrant. Acutely in the lateral quadrant, one can find ecchymosis and palpable tenderness over the injured ligaments. The anatomic course of each ligament [including the anterior talofibular (ATF), calcaneofibular (CF), and posterior talofibular (PTF) ligaments] is palpated for localized tenderness. In acute cases where the ankle was rested, elevated, and iced, there is little edema, and the tender areas are located directly over the ligaments. During a typical examination, however, the entire region may be tender due to swelling. In this case, the examiner's finger must compress the edematous tissue to disperse the fluid, allowing more specific deep palpation of the ligaments. In addition, acute presentations demonstrate limited range of motion and a painful anterior drawer sign (see below) rather than evidence of gross laxity due to guarding.

In the child or adolescent patient, inversion injuries often present with fracture of the distal fibula (e.g., Salter Harris I or II) or avulsion fracture of the anterolateral tubercle of the distal tibia (juvenile Tillaux fracture). This is because the ligamentous structures of the ankle are stronger than the adjacent physes. Consequently, the growth plates typically fail before ligamentous or capsular structures do so. In such cases, the point of maximum tenderness is over the corresponding bony structure rather than the ligaments.

With chronic presentations after inversion injury, patients complain of functional instability, or "giving way," of the ankle with less dramatic swelling or pain. On examination, these patients may have mild tenderness over the ligaments. Functional laxity, however, is more pronounced than with acute presentations and is elicited with an anterior drawer sign. To assess ATF ligament laxity, the anterior drawer test is performed by flexing the knee 90 degrees, grasping the heel with one hand, providing resistance against the tibia with the other hand, and pulling the heel forward. A soft endpoint, no endpoint, or dimpling over the anterolateral gutter strongly suggests instability (Fig. 3.12). To assess CF ligament laxity, the talar tilt test is performed by grasping the heel with one hand, placing the second hand against the tibia for countertraction, and forcing inversion with the ankle in neutral. Again, lateral dimpling or a soft endpoint suggests instability. Radiographic evaluation via stress views may confirm clinically diagnosed instability.

As common as injuries to the lateral ankle ligaments are, several other etiologies must be kept in mind when examining the patient with anterolateral ankle pain. Among them is the development of chronic scar tissue in the anterolateral gutter after inversion-type injuries. This thickened "meniscoid" tissue typically creates anterolateral pain, which is maximally tender to palpation over the gutter. Related to this condition is anterolateral impingement by a thickened distal fascicle of the anteroinferior tibiofibular ligament. As described by Bassett et al.,[15] hypertrophy of this inferior fascicle can impinge against the anterolateral aspect of the talar dome, particularly in extremes of dorsiflexion. On examination, the patient may show tenderness over this ligament and over the anterolateral dome of the talus corresponding to the lesion. The symptoms can also be reproduced by maximum dorsiflexion of the ankle.

Unrecognized bony trauma can similarly result in anterolateral symptoms after an inversion-type injury. Occult fracture of the lateral process of the talus may produce a frustrating, long-term source of pain that can be difficult to diagnose. The lateral portion of the talocalcaneal ligament attaches to the lateral process of the talus, and repetitive traction on the bone from this ligament may be responsible for persistent pain at the site of the fibrous nonunion. Again, inversion and dorsiflexion of the ankle may allow the fibula to impinge into the lateral talar process, creating pain. Additionally, a mortis radiograph of the ankle, obtained at the time of the initial inversion injury or subsequently, may demonstrate a chip fracture of the lateral process. CT scanning can also be used to identify a fracture of this often poorly visualized bony process.

Another bony injury that may result in anterolateral symptoms is fracture of the anterior process of the calcaneus. Like the lateral process of the talus, the anterior process of the calcaneus is typically injured by an inversion mechanism. Soft tissue attachments to this bony process of the calcaneus include the bifurcate and talocalcaneal ligaments and the inferior extensor retinaculum. Similar chronic symptoms may be produced by ligament traction on an unrecognized fracture fragment. This pain is localized more anterior and distal to the lateral malleolus than is typically seen with injury to the anterotalofibular ligament (ATFL). Symptoms are also

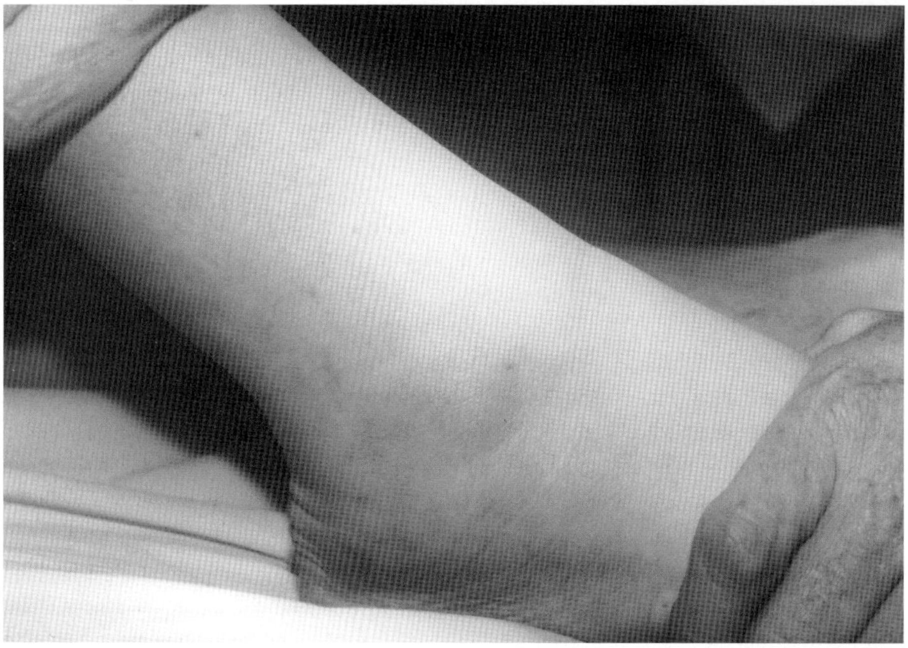

A

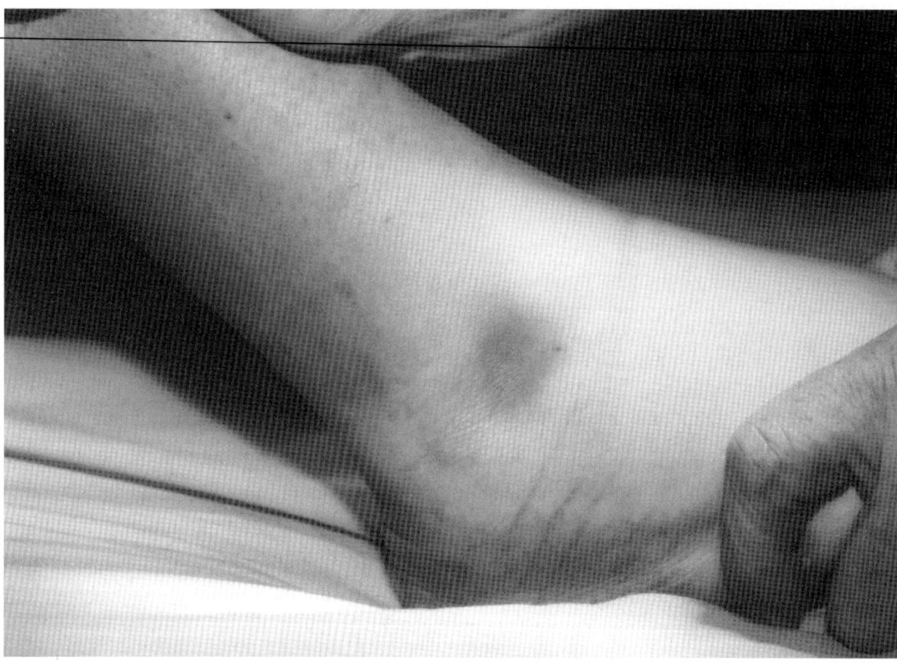

B

FIGURE 3.12. Clinical photographs of positive anterior drawer test findings demonstrating a positive "suction sign." **A,** unstressed; **B,** stressed. (From Clanton TO, Schon LC. Athletic injuries to the soft tissues of the foot and ankle. In: Mann RA, Coughlin MJ (eds) *Surgery of the Foot and Ankle*, 6th ed. St. Louis: Mosby-Year Book, 1993;1125, with permission from Elsevier.)

reproduced with inversion stress of the foot. Plain radiographs, including lateral and oblique views, can demonstrate the avulsion fragment. CT scanning is useful for confirming the diagnosis and assessing the magnitude of the fracture fragment and the degree of intraarticular involvement of the calcaneocuboid joint. Finally, referred pain from a fracture at the base of the fifth metatarsal occasionally presents as anterolateral ankle symptoms. This injury is more distant from the ankle than the above-mentioned bony injuries and should be more readily identified on examination with direct palpation over the base of the metatarsal reproducing the maximum point of tenderness.

Anterolateral ankle pain may also be due to impingement of the region of the sinus tarsi. Typically, injuries to the medial structures of the ankle, such as the posterior tibial tendon or deltoid ligament, may allow sufficient dynamic valgus instability of the hindfoot to create impingement between the distal fibula and the calcaneus in the region of the sinus tarsi. On examination, point tenderness is located in the region of the sinus tarsi. Forced eversion of the hindfoot increases point tenderness in that area, differentiating it from injury to the lateral ankle ligaments, which usually indicate pain on a varus stress or anterior drawer-type maneuver. Resisted extension of the phalanges may also accentuate pain in the sinus tarsi, as the origin of the extensor digitorum brevis muscle arises in the area of inflammation. A diagnostic injection with local anesthetic can be helpful for confirming the sinus as the source of the pain.

Lastly, nerve injury may also present as anterolateral pain.[6,7] There may be traction injuries to the superficial peroneal nerve (SPN) during inversion ankle sprains. The injury may occur anywhere along the course of the nerve about the lateral portion of the ankle but often is located where the nerve exits the deep fascia, approximately 10–12 cm proximal to the tip of the lateral malleolus. Direct compression of the nerve and a positive percussion sign (Tinel's sign) are diagnostic. The SPN divides into the intermediate and medial dorsal cutaneous branches, supplying most of the dorsum of the foot. Consequently, the symptoms may be present not only in the anterolateral quadrant but also on the dorsum of the foot or even the toes. Additional provocative tests, such as resisted dorsiflexion and eversion or passive plantar flexion and inversion of the foot, may elicit the symptoms.

Posterolateral Quadrant

The posterolateral quadrant is similarly affected by a specific set of injuries localized by diagnostic tests. Intraarticular pathology, such as osteochondral fractures of the talus or tibia and degenerative arthritis, can produce posterolateral symptoms. OCD lesions in the posterolateral zone are relatively uncommon. Degenerative changes in that zone would produce findings as described above, including swelling, bogginess, possible crepitus, and localized pain in response to palpation. Additionally, pain may be elicited with active and passive motion of the ankle joint.

A symptomatic os trigonum can present with posterolateral symptoms. Persistent motion at the fibrous union between the ossicle and the posterior talus or overt fracture through such a synostosis can result in focal pain. Symptoms may be located primarily posterolaterally or posteromedially. Deep palpation in the retrotalar region should elicit discomfort accentuated by extreme plantar flexion of the ankle. It is important to examine the stability of the lateral ankle ligaments because primary ankle instability may lead to a secondary symptomatic os trigonum as the talus subluxes anteriorly and impingement of the ossicle against the posterior lip of the tibia occurs. Lateral radiographs, including maximum plantar flexion views, may demonstrate an os trigonum; this is a relatively common finding, and most are asymptomatic. Consequently, a triple-phase bone scan with increased uptake in that area is a supportive finding.

Pain in the retrocalcaneal region may also be due to bursitis in conjunction with insertional Achilles tendinitis or Haglund's deformity of the posterior tuberosity of the calcaneus. These etiologies may represent a continuum of a pathophysiologic process resulting in inflammation and pain (see Heel section). Under these conditions, the pain is typically more posterior and superficial than that due to an os trigonum.

A calcaneal stress fracture may present with pain in the posterolateral quadrant. Like other stress fractures, a calcaneal stress fracture may be caused by an increase in the magnitude or duration of activity or a recent alteration in an athlete's training regimen. Such an overuse injury presents with an acutely tender lateral wall of the calcaneus. It must be distinguished from involvement of the sural nerve or peroneal tendons, as described below. Clinical suspicion is critical because the patient's history may be vague. A calcaneal squeeze test, or direct horizontal compression of the medial and lateral walls of the calcaneus, can elicit pain (Fig. 3.13). The pain can be severe with weight-bearing, and patients often state that they walk on their toes to experience relief. Lateral radiographs can assist in diagnosing this condition by demonstrating disruption of the normal trabecular pattern seen within the body of the calcaneus. However, because radiographs are often normal, a bone scan or MRI scan may be necessary to diagnose an occult stress fracture.

Pathology of the peroneal tendons is a common source of posterolateral ankle symptoms. The peroneal tendons course behind the fibula within a groove, traveling anterior to the peroneal tubercle toward their insertions on the base of the first and fifth metatarsals. The superior peroneal retinaculum functions in conjunction with the fibular groove to maintain the position of the tendons behind the fibula. Peroneal tendinitis can be seen as an overuse

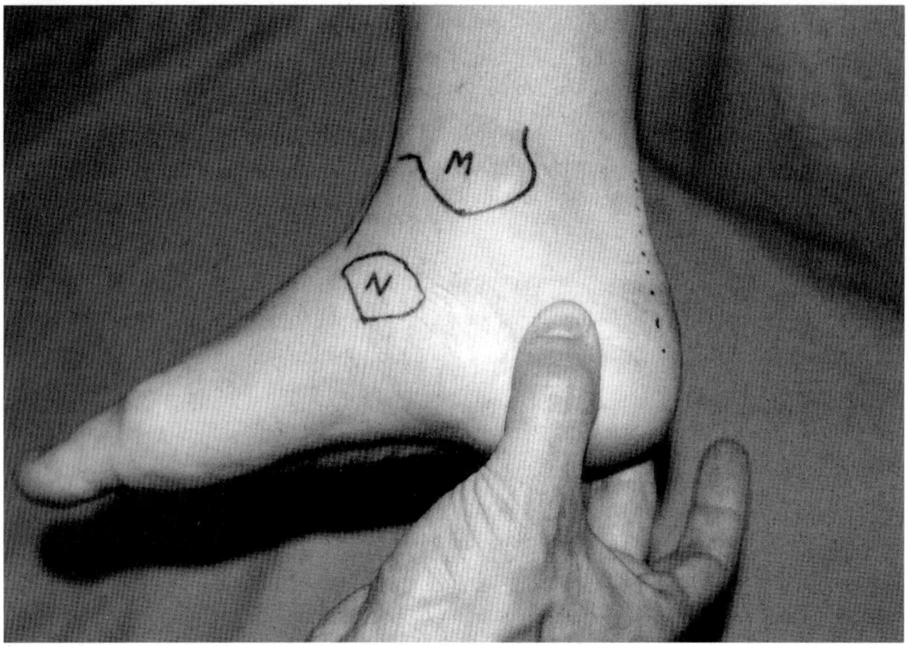

FIGURE 3.13. Calcaneal squeeze test with medial and lateral compression of the calcaneus to diagnose a calcaneus stress fracture. M, medial malleolus; N, navicular. Vertical line indicates the medial border of the tibialis anterior tendon. Dotted line indicates the Achilles tendon border.

injury after excessive strain or increased activity level, particularly in athletes. This tenderness is easily discernible when a lateral ligament sprain of the ankle is present because of its location posteriorly about the fibula. Pain is typically elicited with resisted eversion of the forefoot or passive inversion of the foot. Injuries resulting in excessive contraction of the tendons while in dorsiflexion can result in rupture of the superior peroneal retinaculum, which can then produce recurrent subluxation or even frank dislocation of the tendons from the fibular groove. Patients may complain of a popping or snapping sensation as well as pain usually located directly over the lateral malleolus. Subluxation or dislocation of the tendons can be detected by positioning the ankle in dorsiflexion and having the patient evert the foot against resistance. With the other hand, the examiner palpates the area as the tendon subluxes over the border of the fibula. Apprehension and pain with this maneuver are typical. Circular motion of the ankle and hindfoot may cause subluxation, even in the absence of resistance.

Finally, the sural nerve courses halfway between the distal fibula and the Achilles tendon in the posterolateral quadrant. Severe inversion injuries may cause traction neuritis of the nerve, resulting in burning/shooting pain or parethesias. Other causes of sural nerve involvement include calcaneal fractures with lateral wall entrapment and impingement of the nerve. Surgical incisions in the posterolateral hindfoot can also result in laceration of the sural nerve or one of its branches, causing a stump neuroma. Direct compression along the course of the nerve as well as percussion of the nerve results in sensitivity or pain. Diagnostic injection with local anesthetic can once again confirm the diagnosis.

Posteromedial Quadrant

As with other regions of the ankle, the posteromedial quadrant can have involvement of the intraarticular processes, such as osteochondral lesions or degenerative arthritis. OCD lesions of the medial talus typically present in the posterior portion of the dome, as described above. Symptoms may include pain with weight-bearing or active motion of the joint and a sensation of clicking or locking. On examination, the ankle may be swollen medially with mild synovitis and warmth. The posteromedial portion of the talar dome may be tender to direct palpation, although maximum dorsiflexion of the ankle may be required to uncover this portion of the talus from behind the medial malleolus. Similar findings may be present with arthritic involvement of the medial aspect of the ankle, although usually in a more diffuse pattern.

As described in the previous section, retrocalcaneal bursitis and insertional Achilles tendinitis may present with symptoms primarily posteromedially. There may be swelling and warmth in the area as well as pain during direct palpation of the retrocalcaneal bursa or the attachment site of the tendon. Similarly, a calcaneal stress fracture may present primarily with medial-side pain, which is best demonstrated with direct mediolateral compression of the bone.

Pathology of the posterior tibial tendon is a common cause of medial-side ankle symptoms, ranging from mild strain of the tendon to tendinitis to gross insufficiency and even frank rupture of the tendon. These conditions can be due to chronic overuse or acute trauma. On examination, the medial portion of the ankle is typically swollen, inflamed, and boggy. There is usually pain with palpation along the course of the posterotibialis tendon, most commonly directly posterior and inferior to the malleolus where strain to the tendon is concentrated. When viewed from behind, the heel may be in excessive valgus with respect to the tibia, resulting in the often described "too many toes sign."[8] On muscle testing, the patient may have normal strength or severely decreased power if significant tendinosis or rupture is present. Often the patient has difficulty performing a double-heel rise and may be completely unable to perform a single-limb heel rise on the affected side. Resistance to inversion and plantar flexion elicits pain and noticeable weakness. This diagnosis is clear clinically, and MRI scanning is not necessary in most cases.

Conditions of the flexor hallucis longus tendon can also result in posteromedial symptoms. Tendinitis of the FHL tendon often occurs in dancers and may be associated with an os trigonum lesion as the FHL tendon enters the fiber osseous tunnel behind the posterior aspect of the ankle. Because the symptoms of both conditions are located deep within the retrotalar compartment, differentiation by palpation can be difficult. Specific tests for the FHL include resistance to plantar flexion of the distal phalanx of the hallux, which should result in pain. The hallux may also demonstrate triggering similar to that seen with stenosing tenosynovitis of the digits of the hand, a condition known as hallux saltans. Thomasen's sign similarly implicates the FHL tendon along the course behind the talus (Fig. 3.14). This test involves pain with passive dorsiflexion of the hallux that is accentuated by dorsiflexing the ankle. Placing the ankle in a dorsiflexed position causes increased excursion of the tendon with resulting impingement of the FHL muscle belly as it enters the fibroosseous sheath. Passive extreme plantar flexion of the ankle, especially if combined with inversion and eversion, induces pain in a patient with a symptomatic os trigonum but not in one with an FHL lesion. Lateral radiographs may reveal no obvious bony pathology or may demonstrate a large posterolateral trigonal process or an os trigonum. MRI scanning may reveal swelling and intratendinous changes consistent with tendinosis, indicating the FHL.

Finally, tarsal tunnel syndrome is classically present in the posteromedial quadrant of the ankle. Patients complain of diffuse pain on the plantar aspect of the foot that is often described as burning or tingling in nature. Although the pain may worsen with weight-bearing, it can present while the patient is at rest or asleep. There may be associated proximal radiation along the calf as well. Direct pressure over the tibial nerve in the retromalleolar area elicits extreme sensitivity and pain. Percussion over the nerve often produces a positive Tinel's sign with stabbing, radiating pain into the plantar foot. Patients may not demonstrate frank numbness on examination. The symptoms may be exacerbated by passive eversion of the hindfoot as the nerve is placed under tension. Electrodiagnostic studies can be helpful in establishing a diagnosis. Diagnostic injection with local anesthetic can also confirm the diagnosis but is not completely specific owing to anesthesia of other structures that may be causing these symptoms. As a result, tarsal tunnel syndrome must still be considered a diagnosis based primarily on clinical grounds.

Subtalar Pathology

Subtalar problems are uncommon in the athletic population. There are four common conditions that present in this area: (1) chip fractures or avulsion fractures of the anterolateral shoulder of the talus or anterior process of the calcaneus; (2) tarsal coalitions; (3) subtalar instability; and (4) subtalar synovitis, with or without impingement. Palpating various regions along the subtalar joint complex helps establish a diagnosis.

Tenderness over the Anterolateral Shoulder of the Talus

Tenderness over the anterolateral shoulder of the talus, just anterior to the fibula is found in patients with tibial fractures of the lateral process of the talus. Lateral talocalcaneal ligament injury or tears of the lower fibers of the anterior talofibular ligament may also manifest with tenderness. With the examiner's finger over the spot, subtalar excursions may produce clicking or accentuate a small, loose, or irregular fragment of bone in this location. Ten-

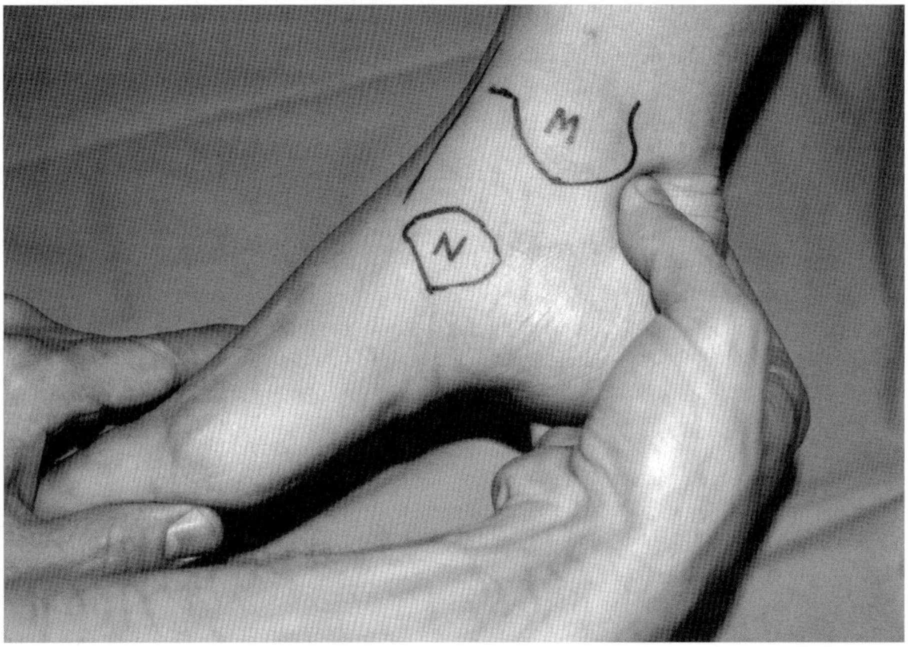

A

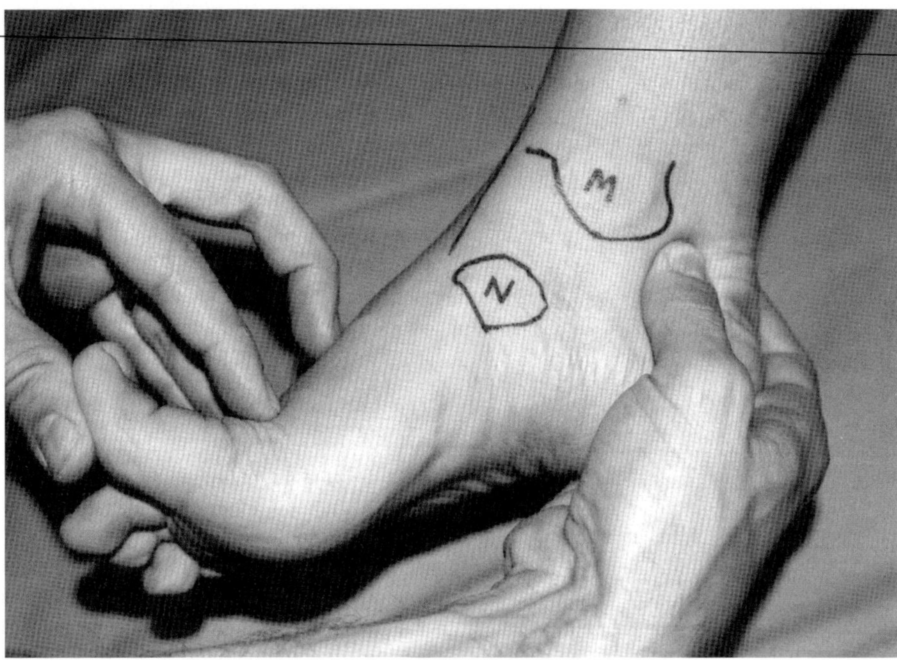

B

FIGURE 3.14. Thomasen's sign. **A:** Resting position. **B:** Passive dorsiflexion of the hallux to elicit triggering of the flexor hallucis longus (FHL) tendon at the posteromedial ankle. M, medial malleolus; N, navicular. Vertical line indicates the medial border of the tibialis anterior tendon.

derness deeper in the sinus tarsi or more laterally along the talocalcaneal junction is consistent with a sprain of the talar ligaments or posttraumatic synovitis of the subtalar joint. If there is sinus tarsi impingement, the patient has more pain with palpation of the sinus tarsi when the foot is everted. This positioning brings the anterolateral portion of the body of the talus into direct contact with the calcaneus in the region of Gissane's angle. Tenderness in the spot aggravated by inversion of the foot is characteristic subtalar instability. Patients with instability may have increased subtalar excursion compared to the opposite side or may have palpable gapping of the subtalar joint with eversion/inversion manipulation.

Tenderness over the Anterior Process of the Calcaneus

Tenderness over the anterior process of the calcaneus may signify a chip fracture of the anterior process of the calcaneus, a tear of the bifurcate ligament, or a calcaneonavicular coalition. An athlete with a coalition would be expected to have (1) decreased inversion/eversion, (2) a palpable bony prominence in this location, (3) possible crepitus with range of motion or (4) warmth in association with a stress fracture of the coalition or mechanical friction at the junction of the calcaneus and navicular.

Tenderness medially over the subtalar joint just distal to the medial malleolus over the sustentaculum tali is found in patients with subtalar synovitis or a medial facet tarsal coalition. Tenderness to palpation in this region may also be found in patients with tendinitis of the posterior tibialis, FDL, or FHL. Distinguishing between these and subtalar pathology requires specific testing of the affected tendons.

Heel

Examination of the heel should begin at the Achilles tendon proximally and proceed to the dorsal aspect of the calcaneus and then extend inferiorly and finally plantarly. For ease of examination, these positions have been organized into several regions: the Achilles tendon 1–5 cm above the dorsal posterior border of the calcaneus, the posterior border of the calcaneus, and the plantar aspect of the posterior calcaneus.

Achilles Tendon

A thickened appearance of the Achilles tendon associated with warmth, bogginess, and tenderness often represents an intrasubstance Achilles tendon tear, chronic tendinosis, or stenosing tenosynovitis. An acute Achilles tendon tear presents after a traumatic event during which the patient felt that he or she was shot or kicked in the back of the ankle. Ecchymosis often accompanies acute tears. If the tendon is totally disrupted, squeezing the calf does not cause plantar flexion of the foot (Thompson test). If the disruption is partial, the foot plantar-flexes when the calf is squeezed. With a partial rupture, there is pain and weakness with plantar flexion against resistance, and there may be some increased passive dorsiflexion due to stretching of the tendon. Careful palpation along the course of the tendon may identify a defect or a gap where the rupture occurred.

With Achilles tendinosis (intrasubstance degeneration of the tendon), usually there is a gradual onset of swelling and pain that is exacerbated by activity. There often is nodular thickening of the tendon, which is tender to palpation and squeezing (Fig. 3.15). The tendon power is good, although it may be slightly decreased owing to pain. The continuity of the tendon should be assessed to rule out a tear.

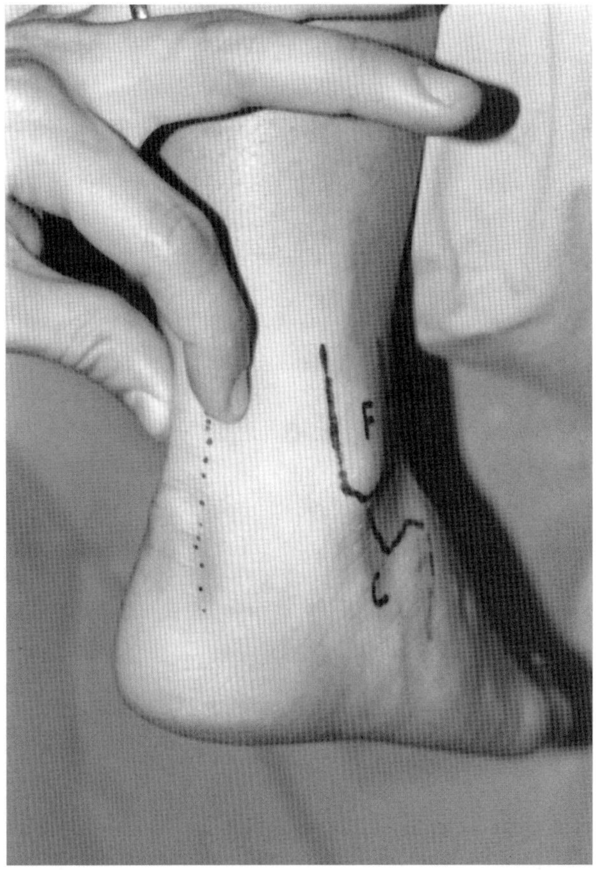

FIGURE 3.15. Palpation of the Achilles tendon proximal to the calcaneus to identify noninsertional tendon pathology. Dotted line indicates the Achilles tendon border.

With stenosing tenosynovitis, there may or may not be a visible or tender nodule. There is often a 1- to 2-cm zone of fullness along the tendon 2–5 cm above its insertion. The size of the nodule and the degree of associated tenderness depends on the degree of coexistent active tendinosis. With stenosing tenosynovitis, the hallmark is painful crepitance on range of motion testing of the Achilles tendon when the fingers squeeze the tendon.

Posterior Border of the Calcaneus

The tenderness in the retrocalcaneal region may represent insertional Achilles tendinitis, retrocalcaneal bursitis, Haglund's deformity, or superficial Achilles bursitis. It is important to be aware that these conditions may coexist, which has implications regarding prognosis and treatment. Tenderness and warmth directly posterior to the dorsal half of the calcaneus is characteristic of insertional Achilles tendinosis (Fig. 3.16). In advanced cases there may also be thickening of the tendon in this location that begins at the insertion of the Achilles and at times extends more proximally. Pain is increased with plantar flexion against resistance or with passive

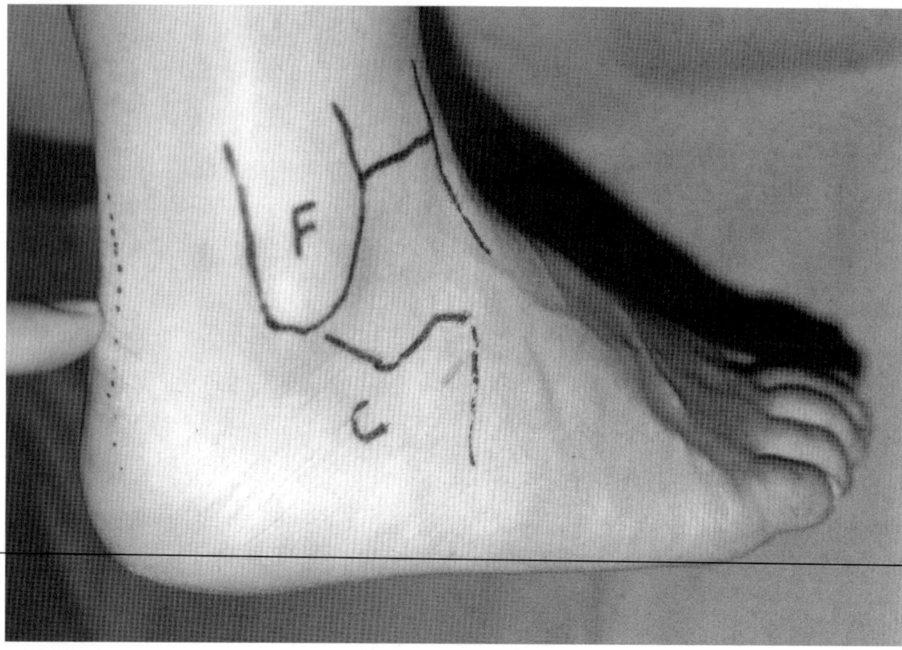

A

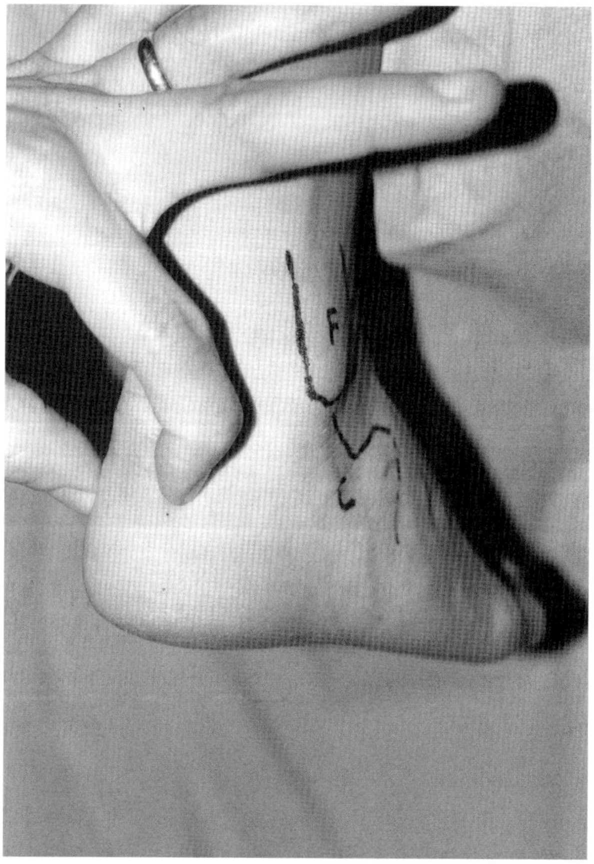

B

FIGURE 3.16. Palpation of the Achilles tendon where it passes by the posterosuperior process of the calcaneus **(A)** and mediolaterally at its insertion **(B)**. F, lateral malleolus of the fibula; C, calcaneus. Vertical line indicates the lateral border of the tibialis anterior tendon. Horizontal line indicates the talotibial articulation. Dotted line indicates the Achilles tendon border.

dorsiflexion stretch of the tendon. Lateral radiographs may demonstrate osseous deposits within the insertion of the Achilles (spurring).

Retrocalcaneal bursitis typically manifests with tenderness and swelling along the sides of the Achilles between the Achilles tendon and the posterior border of the calcaneus (Fig. 3.17). Patients have pain during both passive dorsiflexion and active plantar flexion against resistance. There may be warmth and erythema in the region of the bursa.

Patients with Haglund's deformity have prominence of the posterosuperior edge of the calcaneus. This may be palpable both medial and lateral to the tendon or just on one side of the tendon. In symptomatic cases, pain is reproduced with palpation over the bony edge or where the tendon or bursa encounters the prominence. Patients usually feel better without a shoe or with a backless shoe. The pain in this condition is aggravated by walking or running with a heel counter compressing the spot. Radiographs demonstrating the posterosuperior prominence of the calcaneus support this diagnosis. Not uncommonly, a patient with long-standing symptomatic Haglund's deformity have retrocalcaneal bursitis and Achilles tendinosis in association with a bony prominence. In these situations the bony prominence acts as a constant irritant for these more superficial tissues.

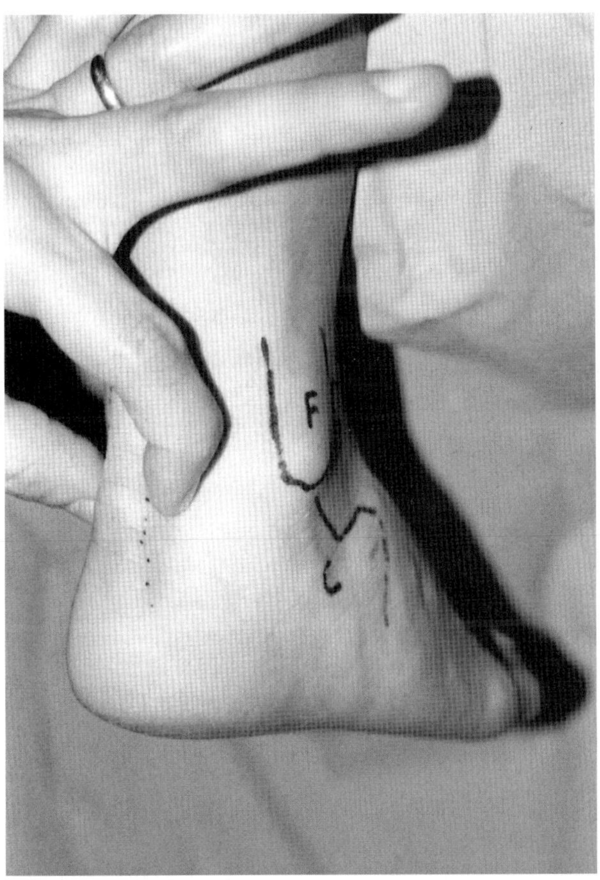

FIGURE 3.17. Palpation of the retrocalcaneal bursa. Dotted line indicates the Achilles tendon border.

Two final conditions warrant mentioning. Some patients have posterior heel pain associated with a large, protuberant posterior and inferior process of the calcaneus. In these patients the prominence is distal to the Achilles insertion. This lower bulging of the posterior calcaneus (the "pregnant heel") often makes shoewear difficult, as with a Haglund's prominence. Resection of the posterosuperior prominence does not reduce the bony prominence because it involves the entire posterior portion. The clinician inspects this entire posterior region for scars because they may be a source of pain. Given the lack of fat tissue padding and the presence of thickened scars in this area, the occasional sural neuroma can be symptomatic.

Plantar Heel Pain

Plantar heel pain may represent several entities: plantar fasciitis, calcaneal stress fracture, fat pad insufficiency or atrophy, or first branch lateral plantar neuritis. There are, however, differentiating characteristics. Pain with palpation and compression of the medial and lateral walls of the posterior tubercle of the calcaneus is indicative of calcaneal stress fracture. Point tenderness at the junction of the plantar-medial aspect of the calcaneus and the proximal medial origin of the plantar fascia is indicative of plantar fasciitis (Fig. 3.18). Tenderness elicited along with neuritic symptoms (i.e., burning, shooting, tingling, radiating pain) while palpating along the proximal medial aspect of the abductor hallucis muscle is indicative of irritation or entrapment of the first branch of the lateral plantar nerve. More proximal tenderness along the course of the tibial nerve also would lead the examiner to consider nerve entrapment as a cause of, or contributing factor to, the heel pain. Tenderness located proximal to the plantar fascia insertion, along the course of the plantar bony tubercle, may represent plantar fasciitis; but more often it represents a fat pad insufficiency. In such cases the fat pad is typically soft, and the bone is readily palpable plantarly through the atrophic fat pad.

With plantar fasciitis, it is important to note that testing the windlass mechanism by hyperex-

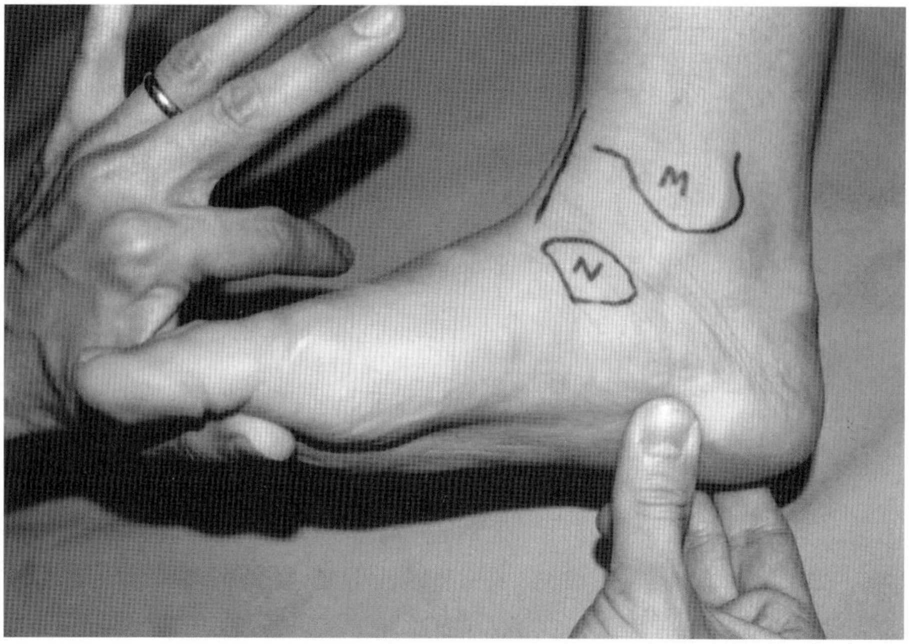

FIGURE 3.18. Palpation of the plantar fascia origin on the calcaneus. M, medial malleolus; N, navicular. Vertical line indicates the medial border of the tibialis anterior tendon.

tending the toes and dorsiflexing the ankle may not induce or increase the pain. This is an infrequent finding. Similarly, palpation along the entire plantar fascia with diffuse tenderness represents a more diffuse fasciitis than the typical plantar fasciitis, which is probably more like a plantar fasciosis or insertional degenerative fascial deterioration.

MTP Joint

Dorsal MTP

Tenderness over a dorsal prominence of the metatarsal head in conjunction with localized skin changes consistent with acute or chronic irritation (i.e., redness, blistering, or thickening of the skin) is typical of hallux limitus or rigidus. Decreased range of motion of the great toe on one side versus the other and pain with extremes of dorsiflexion or plantar flexion are characteristic of this condition. Radiographs demonstrate dorsal joint space narrowing and osetophytic changes of the metatarsal head or base of the proximal phalanx. Loose bodies in the MTP joints are most likely to be palpated dorsally, where there is some redundant capsule and where the skin is relatively thin. Occasionally, a loose body is appreciated plantarly by palpating this area while supinating and pronating the toe, adding varying degrees of flexion and extension during the maneuver.

Medial MTP

Tenderness over a medial prominence of the metatarsal head and hallux valgus are typical findings associated with a bunion deformity. The prominence may show signs of acute or chronic skin irritation due to mechanical pressure from the shoe. Dorsomedially, the distal branch of the medial dorsal cutaneous nerve can be irritated. Similarly, plantar-medially, the medial hallucal nerve can be irritated, compressed, or stretched where the nerve rides over the abductor tendon just proximal to the medial sesamoid. An acutely erythematous, warm, tender MTP joint with medial (or occasionally dorsal) prominence may signify podagra or gouty arthritis/synovitis of the first MTP joint. In these cases the toe is exquisitely tender, and any attempted range of motion produces extreme pain.

Plantar MTP

Plantarly, tenderness over the sesamoid exacerbated by extreme dorsiflexion of the MTP is typical of sesamoid or flexor brevis mechanism overuse or tear. Buildup of skin callus underneath one or both sesamoids may be indicative of overloading or excessive weight-bearing on the sesamoids. Flexion weakness of the proximal phalanx is typical of an injury to the flexor brevis mechanism, whereas flexion weakness of the distal phalanx is indicative of an FHL injury. Additional causes of sesamoid tenderness include injury, nonunion, sprain, osteochondrosis, or osteoarthritis. After acute athletic injury, stability of the great toe should be assessed with varus and valgus stress and a modified anterior drawer maneuver. This maneuver is performed by stabilizing the first metatarsal head with one hand, grasping the base of the proximal phalanx with the other, and then stressing the toe from a plantar to dorsal direction. With a plantar capsular injury, excessive translation is noted relative to the contralateral side.

BIBLIOGRAPHY

1. Clanton TO, Schon LC, Baxter DE. An overview of subtalar instability and its treatment. *Perspect Orthop Surg* 1990;1:103–113.
2. Schon LC, Biddinger KR, Greenwood P. Dance screen programs and development of dance clinics. *Clin Sports Med* 1994;13:865–882.
3. Schon LC, Weinfeld SB. Lower extremity musculoskeletal problems in dancers. *Curr Opin Rheumatol* 1996;8:130–142.
4. Clanton TO, Schon LC. Athletic injuries to the soft tissues of the foot and ankle. In: Mann RA, Coughlin MJ (eds) *Surgery of the foot and ankle*, 6th ed. St. Louis: Mosby-Year Book, 1993;1095–1224.
5. Bassett FH, Gates HS, Billys JB, et al. Talar impingement by the anteroinferior tibiofibular ligament: a cause of chronic pain in the ankle after inversion sprain. *J Bone Joint Surg Am* 1990;72:55–59.
6. Schon LC. Nerve entrapment, neuropathy, and nerve dysfunction in athletes. *Orthop Clin North Am* 1994; 25:47–59.
7. Schon LC, Baxter DE. Neuropathies of the foot and ankle in athletes. *Clin Sports Med* 1990;9:489–509.
8. Funk DA, Cass JR, Johnson KA. Acquired adult flat foot secondary to posterior tibial-tendon pathology. *J Bone Joint Surg Am* 1986;68:95–102.

CHAPTER 4

Imaging Techniques

Richard D. Ferkel and Gregory R. Applegate

After a careful history and physical examination, radiologic evaluation is critical to the proper treatment of ankle disorders. Advances in imaging techniques have given us the opportunity to understand better soft tissue and bony pathology and, in some cases, to diagnose conditions previously unknown. This chapter describes current methods for imaging the ankle and suggests which method is most appropriate in specific situations.

CONVENTIONAL RADIOGRAPHY

Plain radiographs are still the easiest, least expensive way to evaluate the problems of the ankle initially. At least two projections at right angles to each other are needed, and frequently a third or fourth view is indicated, depending on the abnormality suspected. Proper exposure and technique vary by region, and it is important that the radiology technician understands the area of interest and what the physician suspects may be the problem.

Routine Views of the Ankle

Anteroposterior View

The articular surface of the malleoli, mortise, syndesmosis, and body of the talus are outlined by the anteroposterior (AP) view. The fibula lies in the tibial groove, and the anterior and posterior tibial tubercles obscure the syndesmosis. The medial clear space is the distance (in millimeters) between a line drawn tangential to the medial articular margin of the talus and that drawn tangential to the articular margin of the medial malleolus. This distance defines the integrity of the ankle mortise and is normally 2–3 mm. An increased distance (>3–4 mm) is associated with ankle fractures or syndesmotic injuries in which the talus shifts laterally. It also indicates that there has been a rupture of the deltoid ligament (Fig. 4.1).

Weight-bearing AP radiographs of the ankle can reveal information not readily apparent from non-weight-bearing films. As in the knee, a weight-bearing radiograph of the ankle can demonstrate significant joint space narrowing, varus or valgus angulation, or subluxation (Fig. 4.2).

Lateral View

The articular space between the talus and the tibia is seen with the lateral view, as is the articulation of the talus with the navicular and calcaneus. The calcaneocuboid joint, mid-foot joints, and the base of the fifth metatarsal can also be identified. The subtalar joint, tarsal canal, and sinus tarsi can be seen at the junction of the declining angle of the posterior facet of the calcaneus (45 degrees) and the inclining angle of the anterior facet. A portion of the sustentaculum tali can also be seen. A "true" lateral radiograph is necessary to evaluate the extent of anterior and posterior distal tibial and talar osteophytes, the Stieda process, and loose bodies (Fig. 4.3). A weight-bearing lateral radiograph of the ankle is also important to demonstrate joint space narrowing, anteroposterior subluxation, and incongruity of the distal tibia with the talus and the talus to the calcaneus.

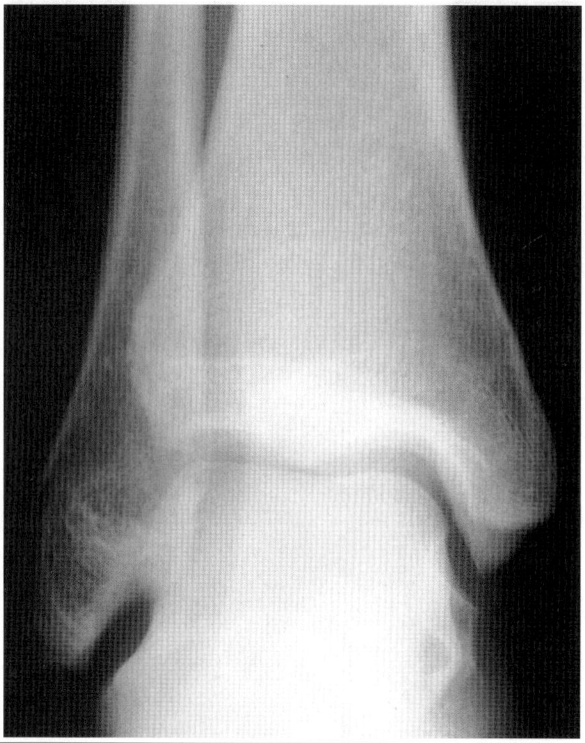

FIGURE 4.1. Anteroposterior (AP) view of the ankle. Note the medial clear space and the overlap of the fibula with the distal tibia and talus.

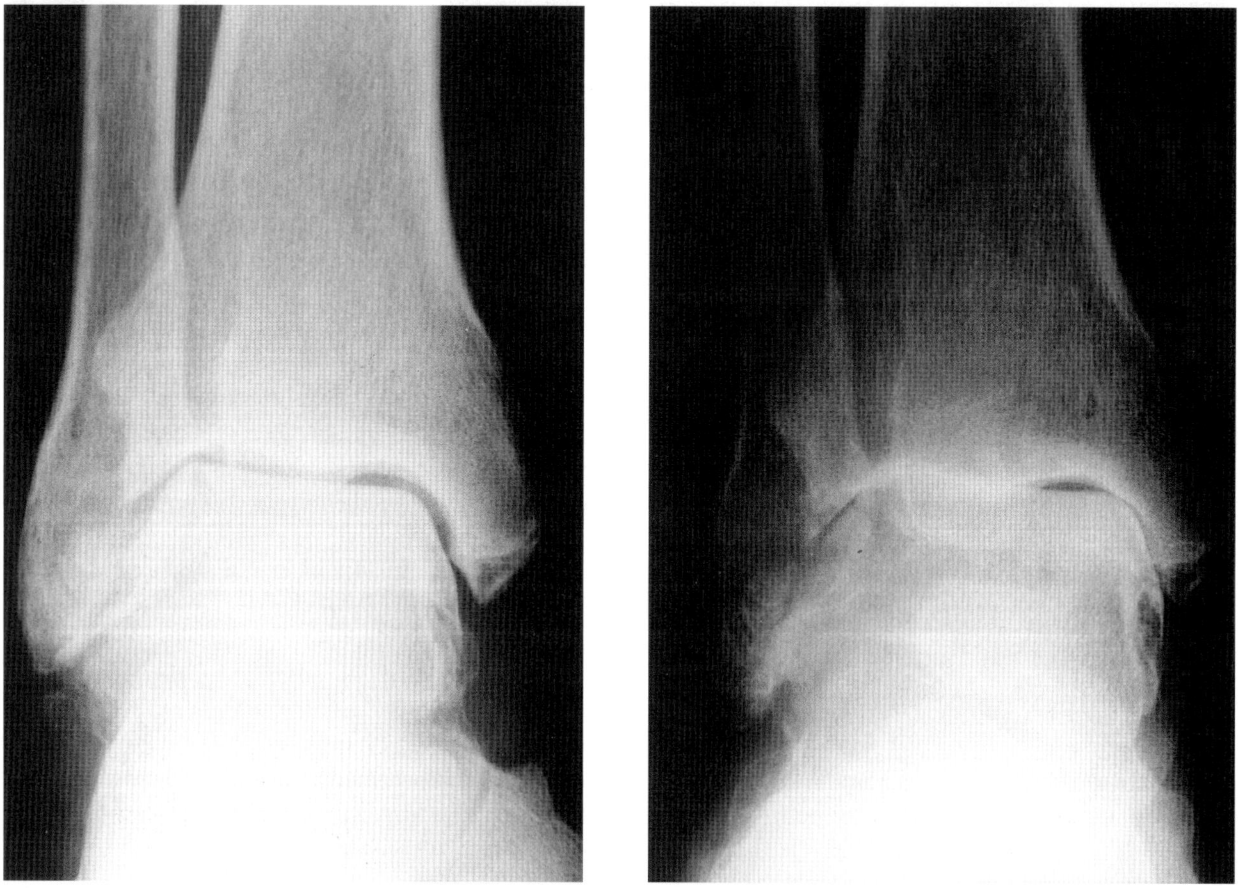

A B

FIGURE 4.2. Importance of the weight-bearing radiograph. **A:** Non-weight-bearing AP view of the ankle. **B:** Weight-bearing AP view of the ankle. Note the loss of joint space and valgus angulation on the weight-bearing radiograph.

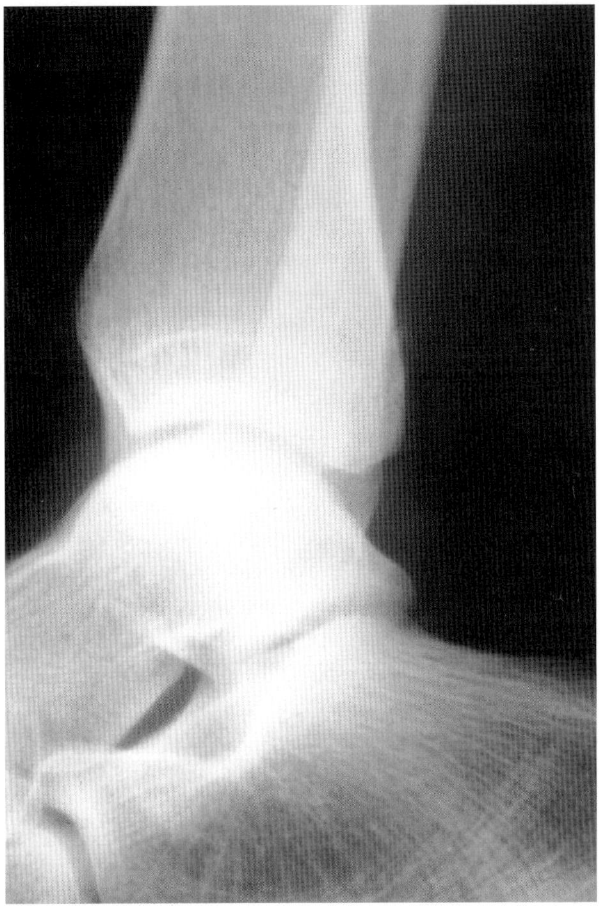

FIGURE 4.3. Lateral view of the ankle. The distal anterior and posterior portions of the tibia are clearly seen, as is the space between the distal tibia and talus and subtalar joint. A portion of the sustentaculum tali is seen through the sinus tarsi and tarsal canal. The declining angle of the posterior facet of the calcaneus and incline angle of the anterior facet meet at the tarsal canal (i.e., sinus tarsi).

Mortise (Oblique View)

The mortise, or oblique, view is obtained by having the patient recumbent, with the leg and foot rotated internally 20–30 degrees. When properly done, this view allows visualization "around" the talus. The medial and lateral clear spaces and distal tibiofibular syndesmosis are well seen and measured. This view is particularly helpful when evaluating ligamentous injuries at the syndesmotic area and detecting subtle shifts in the talus. Normally, the distal tibiofibular syndesmosis has a width of 2 mm; and an increase in the width indicates ligamentous injury. The mid-tarsus is obscured, but the zone of rarefaction in the talus clearly shows the posterior facet of the subtalar joint (Figs. 4.4, 4.5).

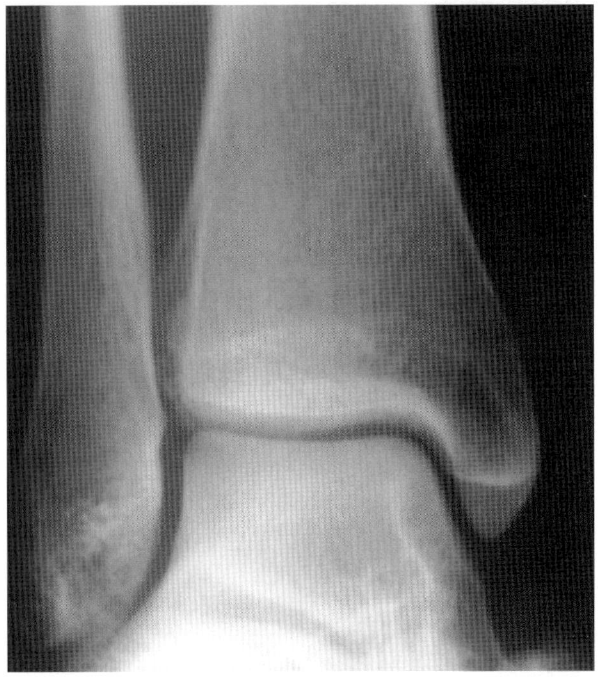

FIGURE 4.4. Mortise view of the ankle. The medial clear space measures 2 mm, as does the tibiofibular syndesmosis, which is within the normal range. The zone of rarefaction in the talus shows the posterior facet of the subtalar joint.

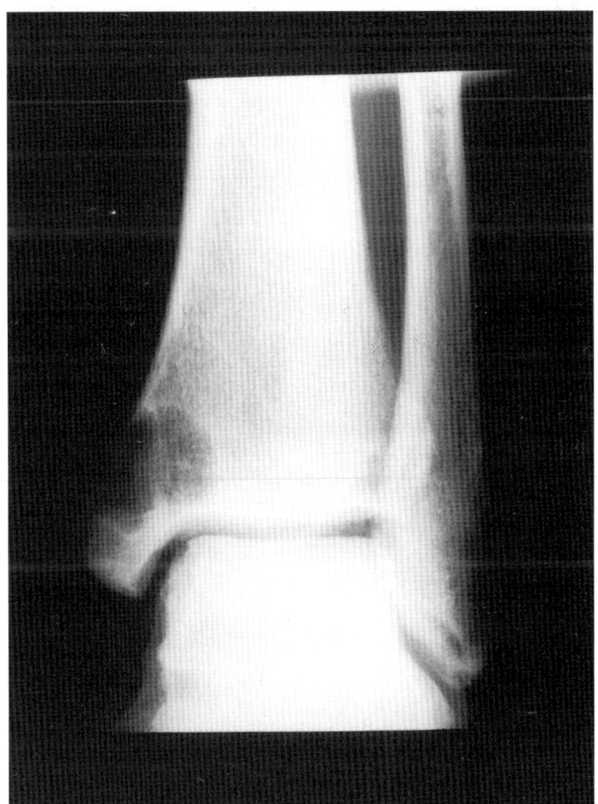

FIGURE 4.5. Mortise view of the ankle demonstrating an interosseous ganglion of the medial malleolus.

Both AP and mortise radiographs are important for assessing the integrity of the syndesmosis and judging the adequacy and stability of the reduction of a fracture or ligamentous injury to the distal lower extremity syndesmosis (DLES). Two radiographic dimensions are particularly important for evaluating the syndesmosis. The first is the tibiofibular clear space, which is the distance between the medial border of the fibula and the lateral border of the posterior tibia, measured 1 cm above the distal tibial articular surface. The second measurement is the tibiofibular overlap (i.e., the maximum amount of overlap of the distal fibula and the anterior tibial tubercle).[1] Studies have revealed some variance in the exact measurements that indicate an injury to the syndesmosis. In patients without an ankle injury, the tibiofibular clear space is never more than 5–6 mm on the AP and mortise views. More variance exists regarding the appropriate amount of tibiofibular overlap that indicates syndesmotic injury.[1]

Subtalar Joint. It is important to evaluate carefully the integrity of the subtalar joint, especially in cases of trauma or postsprain ankle pain. A portion of the subtalar joint can be seen using a 45-degree wedge under the outer border of the foot with the central x-ray beam directed at the sinus tarsi. This projection outlines the anterior portion of the subtalar joint, the calcaneus, the cuboid, and the talonavicular joint.[2]

The Broden view is helpful for visualizing the posterior facet of the subtalar joint and the talofibular and tibiofibular joints. This view is obtained with the patient supine and the foot rotated medially 45 degrees. The foot is extended and a central x-ray is pointed at the lateral malleolus and angled cephalad at 10 degrees. This maneuver shows the most posterior portion of the posterior facet. If the angle is increased to 20–30 degrees, the middle facet is better visualized. The anterior portion of the posterior facet is best seen at 40 degrees (Fig. 4.6).

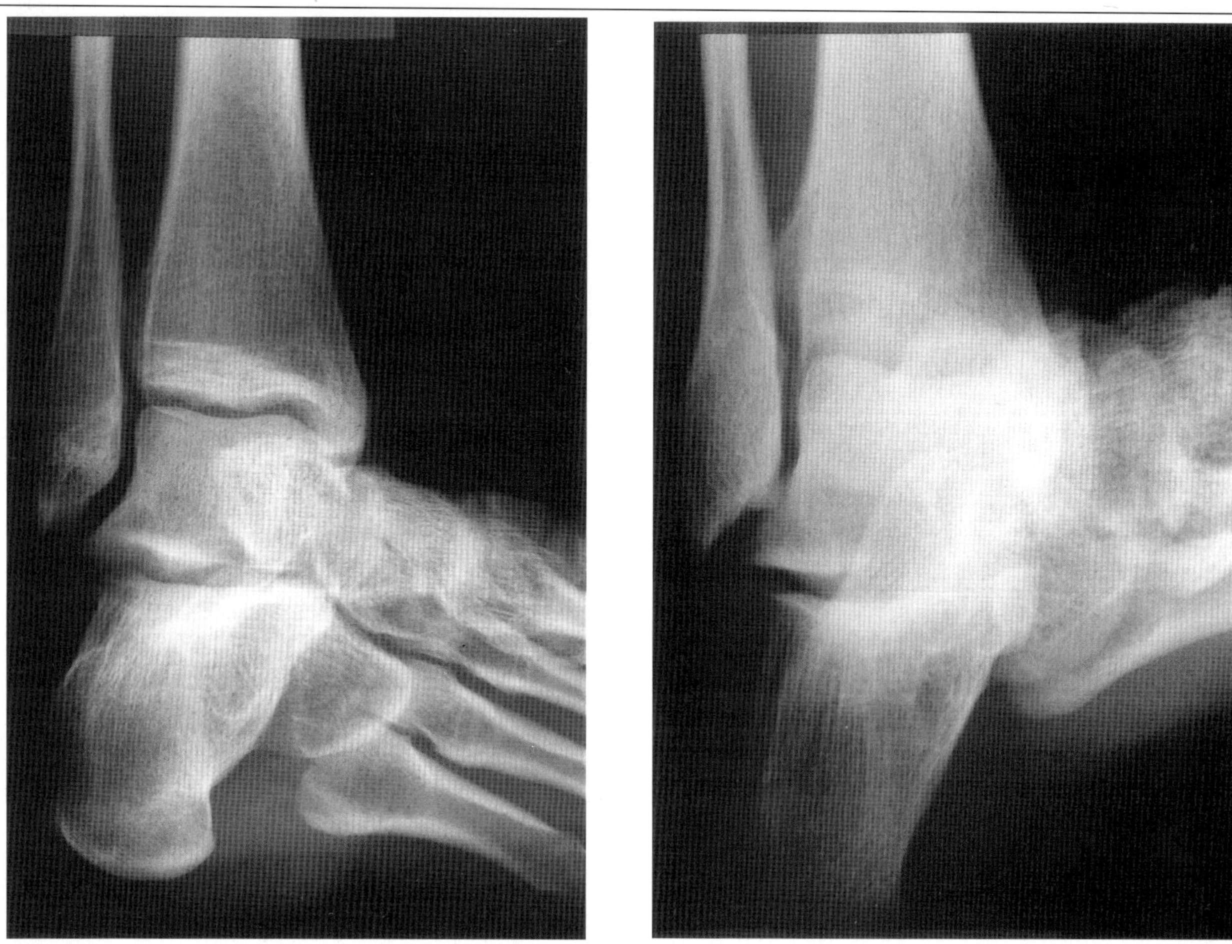

A B

FIGURE 4.6. Broden views of the subtalar joint. **A:** The most posterior portion of the posterior facet is seen at 10 degrees angulation. **B:** The anterior portion of the posterior facet is seen at 40 degrees.

The Cobey view is good for evaluating the position of the calcaneus relative to the tibial axis and the ankle joint. It is particularly helpful when looking at varus and valgus alignment.

The Isherwood view shows the calcaneus in an oblique projection. This view allows visualization of the posterior portion of the subtalar joint, the sustentaculum tali, the sinus tarsi, and a portion of the anterior subtalar joint.

Heel. The posterior tangential (Harris-Beath) view is excellent for evaluating fractures of the calcaneus, injuries to the subtalar joint, and talocalcaneal coalitions.[3] This view is obtained with the patient erect and the sole of the foot flat on the film cassette. The central beam is usually angled 45 degrees toward the midline of the heel. The middle facet of the subtalar joint is seen oriented horizontally in this projection; the sustentaculum tali projects medially. The posterior facet projects laterally and is parallel to the middle facet. The body of the calcaneus is well seen (Fig. 4.7).

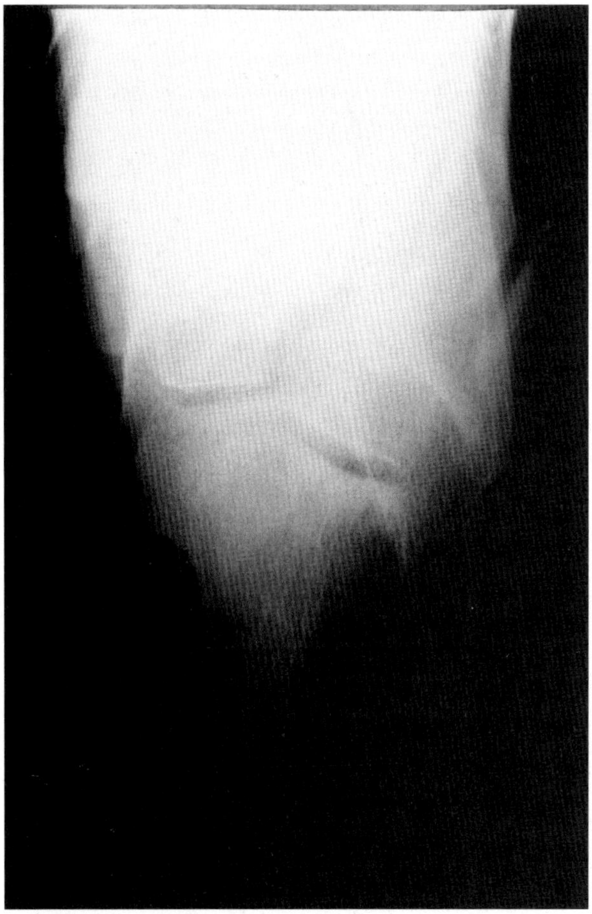

FIGURE 4.7. Posterior tangential (Harris-Beath) view of the foot. The middle facet of the subtalar joint is seen oriented horizontally, and the sustentaculum tali projects medially. The posterior facet projects laterally and is parallel to the middle facet; the body of the talus is well seen.

Stress Views

Stress radiographs are used to evaluate ligamentous integrity about the ankle and subtalar region. The major ligaments about the ankle are described elsewhere in this book (see Chapter 2). Ligamentous injuries are quite common about the ankle, but 20–40% of patients following ankle sprains have chronic pain. One cause of this pain and "giving way" is laxity of the ligaments surrounding the tibiotalar joint. When stress radiographs are obtained, it is important that both the injured and normal extremity be evaluated and the difference between them calculated. In the acute situation, some advocate injection of anesthetic in the area of the injured ligament. However, it has been our experience that most advanced grade I and II ankle sprains are still too painful to subject them to stress accurately in the acute situation. However, when a grade III or complete tear of the ankle ligaments occurs, particularly on the lateral side, minimal gentle stress is needed to demonstrate significant talar tilt. This can usually be done without anesthesia, as people with complete grade III tears frequently have little pain during stress radiography.

Stress radiography can be done manually by the physician, an experienced assistant, or a mechanical device, although many of the devices are cumbersome and inaccurate. In addition, it may be difficult to generate a reproducible force by either manual or mechanical methods.

The method we prefer for stress testing is the Telos stress device.[4] It has several advantages. It (1) causes no radiation exposure to the examining physician, (2) provides reproducible patient motion, (3) allows gradual, accurate application of stress to avoid muscle splinting, and (4) allows reproducible fixation and 18-degree internal rotation to approximate the mortise view during stress.

The apparatus is composed of a U-shaped frame connected to two parallel bars that slide to adjust for differences in leg length. A pressure bar and calcaneal attachment are placed on the top of the frame, and the pressure bar is equipped with a screw-threaded shaft (Fig. 4.8). As the handle of the shaft is turned, the amount of pressure is observed on the light emitting diode (LED) readout. The force is shown in kiloponds (kp: a force equal to 1 kg of

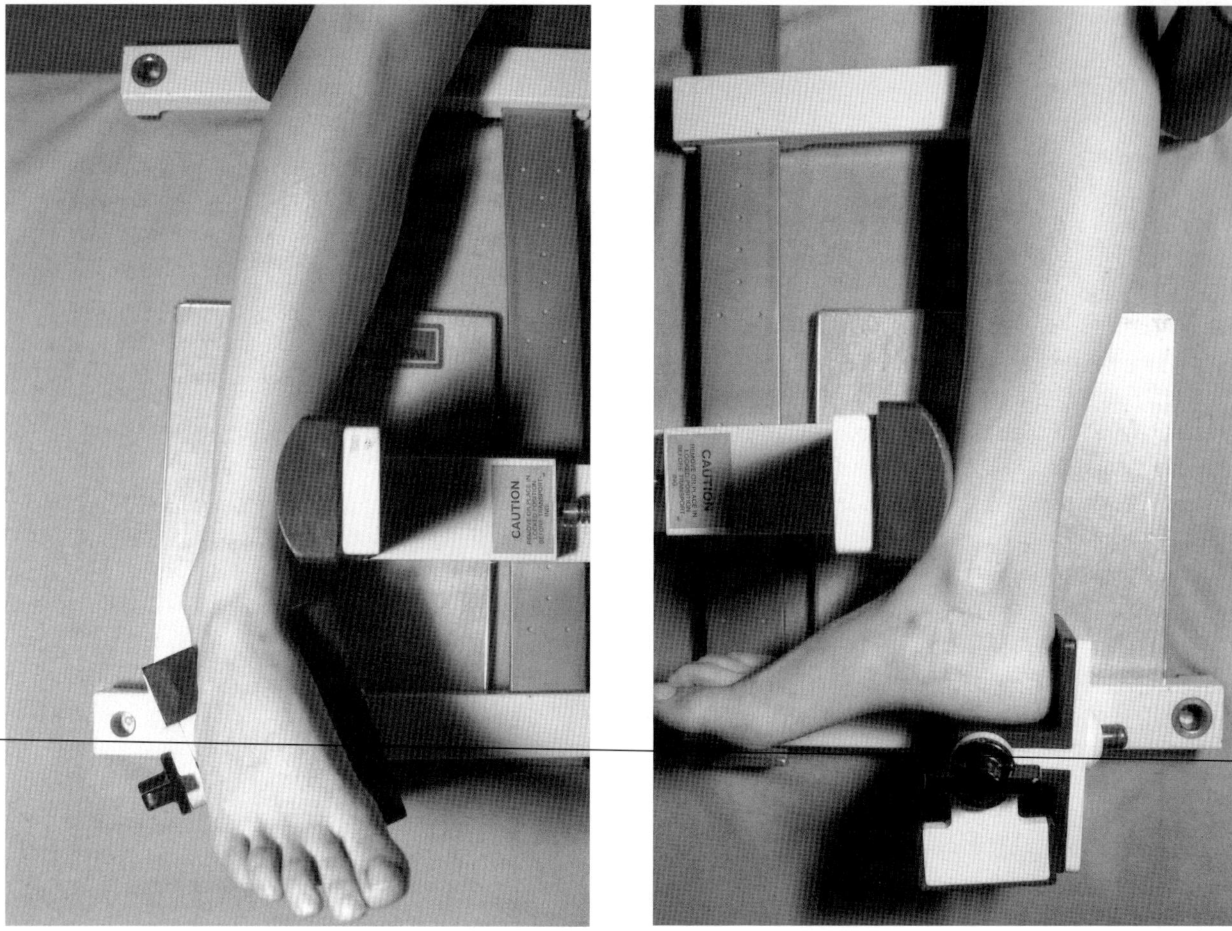

A B

FIGURE 4.8. A: Patient in Telos device positioned for the inversion stress test. The calcaneal attachment is positioned at 18 degrees to approximate a mortise view. **B:** Patient positioned in Telos device for anterior drawer stress test. Force is applied in a posterior direction on the distal tibia while the heel and foot are secured.

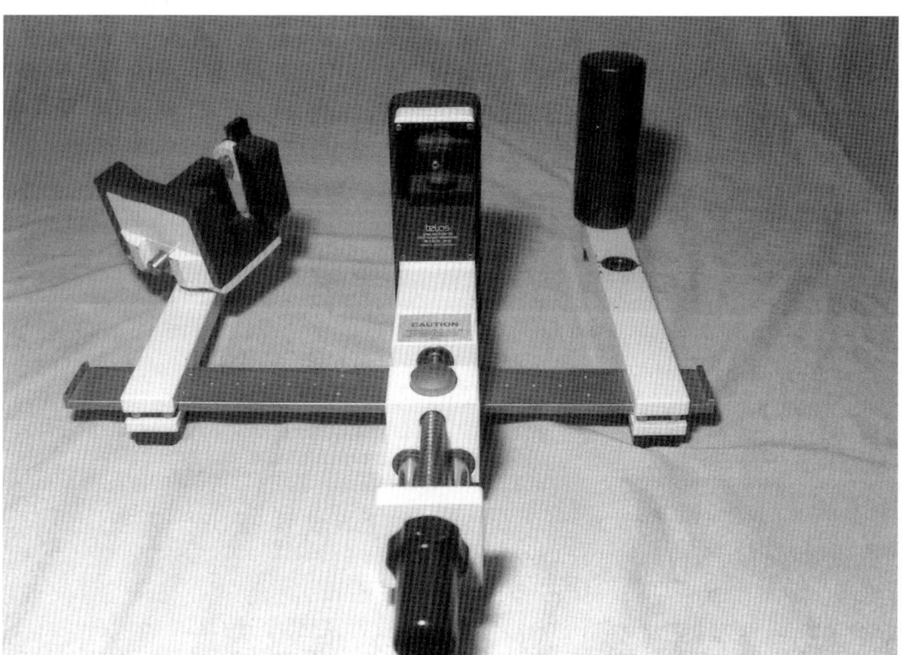

FIGURE 4.9. Telos pressure bar with LED digital readout. The force is applied by rotating the handle of the shaft up to 20 kiloponds.

mass under the influence of gravity). Usually the force is steadily increased over a 30- to 45-second period to avoid muscle splinting until a pressure of 20 kp is obtained (Fig. 4.9). This pressure is considered to be near the maximum amount tolerated by most patients. Inversion, eversion, and anterior drawer testing can be done with this apparatus. Poor technique by the examining technician is the usual cause for nonreproducible results. Careful attention to all technical aspects of using this device is necessary.

Inversion Stress Test. The inversion stress test is done utilizing the Telos device or manually with the patient supine and the foot mounted in internal rotation. It has been shown that plantar flexion inversion stress is a better indicator of the integrity of the anterior talofibular ligament, and dorsiflexion inversion stress is thought best to test the calcaneofibular ligament. Various values have been calculated for normal and abnormal talar tilt, but no standards are universally accepted. As stated above, it is important that stress radiographs be compared with views of the uninjured ankle. Some believe that a maximum variation of 10 degrees between the right and left ankles occurs in normal people.[5]

Using the Telos stress device, Sauser and coworkers found a talar tilt of 10 degrees or more to be associated with a lateral ligament injury in 99% of cases.[6] Normal values for talar tilt have been reported to range from 5 to 23 degrees.[7] Chrisman and Snook noted that a difference of more than 10 degrees between ankles was significant when measuring the anterior talofibular and calcaneofibular ligaments[8] (Fig. 4.10).

Anterior Drawer Stress Test. The anterior drawer stress test specifically tests the integrity of the anterior talofibular ligament (ATFL). In general, this test is the most reliable indicator of injury to the ATFL. The test is done using manual pressure or a mechanical testing device, such as the Telos machine. Force is applied to the distal tibia in a posterior direction, and a lateral radiograph of the ankle is obtained. With injury to the ATFL, the talus is anteriorly displaced in relation to the tibia. As with the inversion stress test, absolute values for normal and abnormal are not well established. Gould et al.

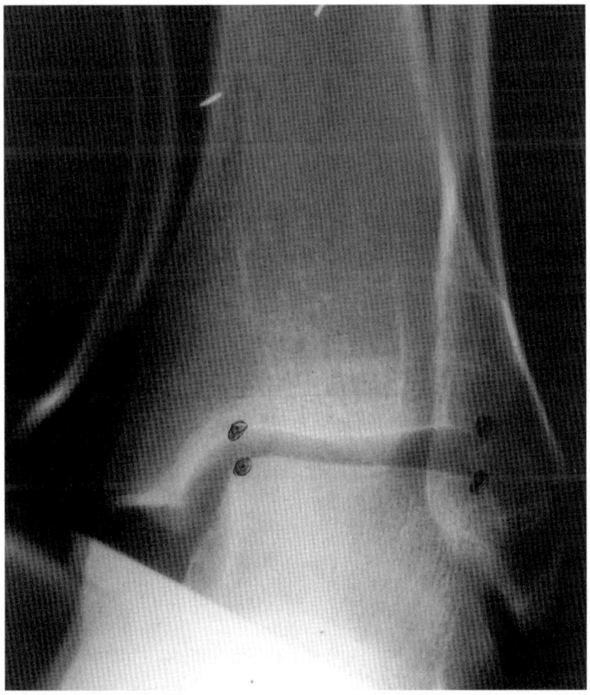

A

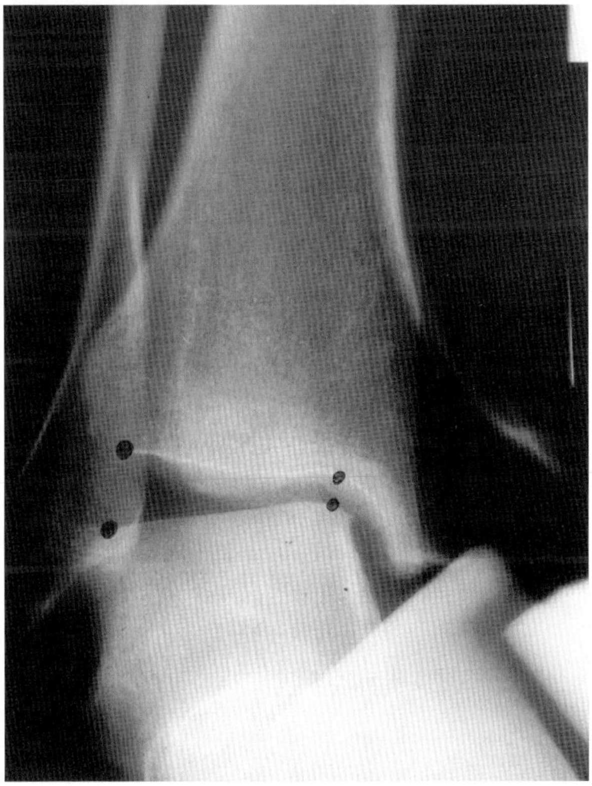

B

FIGURE 4.10. Inversion stress radiographs of the ankle. **A:** Uninjured ankle opens 4 mm during the stress test. **B:** Injured ankle opens 11 mm with inversion stress testing, indicating a positive test for ankle stability.

thought that, with the anterior drawer test an increase of 4 mm was indicative of instability,[9] whereas Laurin and colleagues thought that more than 9 mm was abnormal.[5] Overall, values up to 5 mm separation between the talus and distal tibia are considered normal; values between 5 to 10 mm are abnormal in most cases; and values higher than 10 mm are grossly abnormal (Fig. 4.11).

Eversion Stress Test. The eversion stress test evaluates the integrity of the deltoid ligament. This test is used infrequently, as plain films usually reveal widening of the medial clear space, an indicator of deltoid ligament injury. The test can be done manually or using a mechanical device. Complete tears are associated with a talar tilt of 35–45 degrees.

Subtalar Stress Test. Subtalar instability can also be tested with the Telos device. Although it can be difficult to diagnose, stress radiographs can detect laxity in the joint when done properly. A special foot piece and a change in position is necessary for the subtalar stress test. The results should always be compared with those of the opposite side.[10]

ARTHROGRAPHY

Ankle arthrography is mainly indicated when it is necessary to evaluate the integrity of the ankle ligaments. It is also useful for evaluating degenerative joint disease, loose bodies, and adhesive capsulitis. Double-contrast arthrography usually gives better resolution of noncalcified intraarticular loose bodies. When combined with tomography, arthrotomograms may be helpful when evaluating osteochondral pathology and synovial surface abnormalities. Diffuse synovial disorders such as inflammatory disease, pigmented villonodular synovitis, synovial ganglia, and adhesive capsulitis are readily evalu-

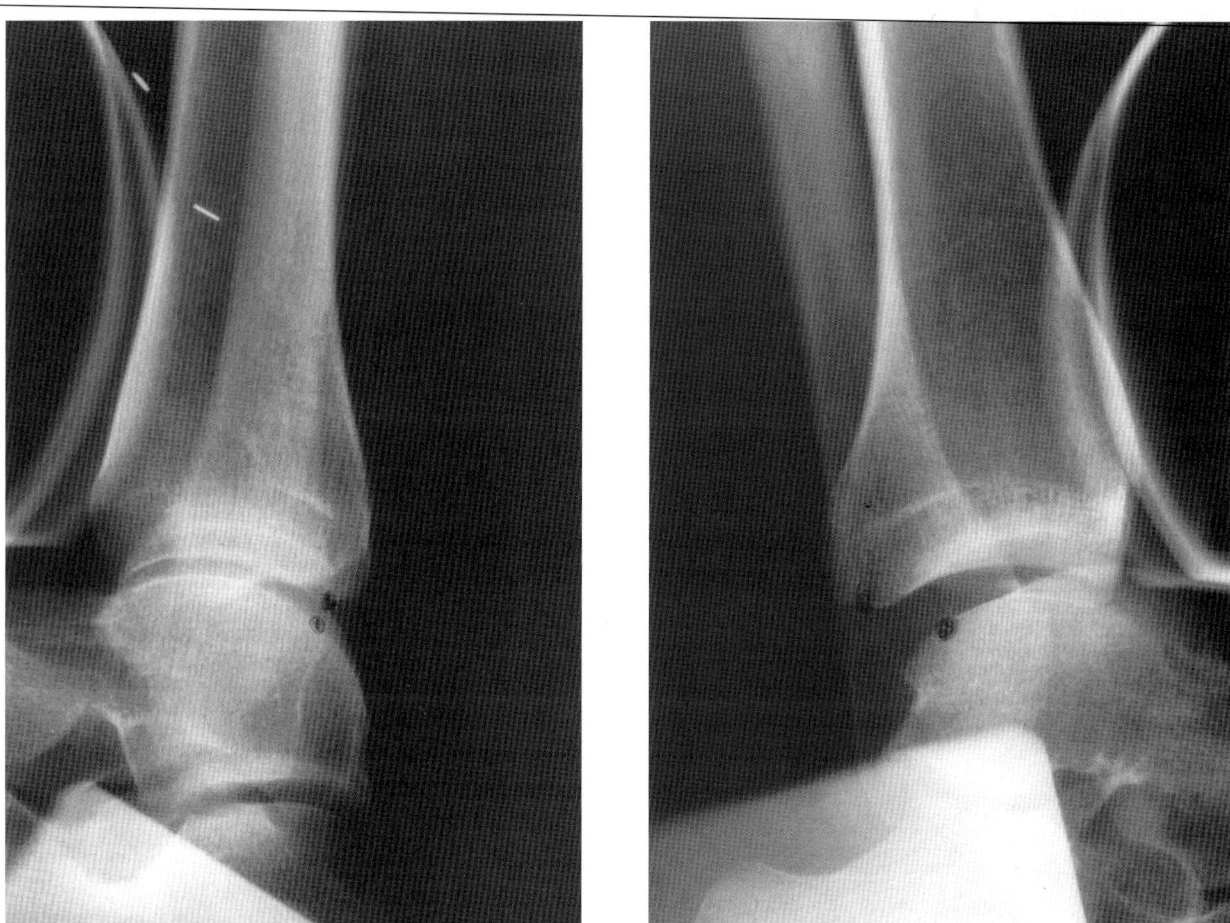

A B

FIGURE 4.11. Anterior drawer stress test. **A:** Uninjured ankle shows minimal widening of the posterior tibiotalar joint space with stress. **B:** Injured ankle demonstrates 10 mm of anterior displacement.

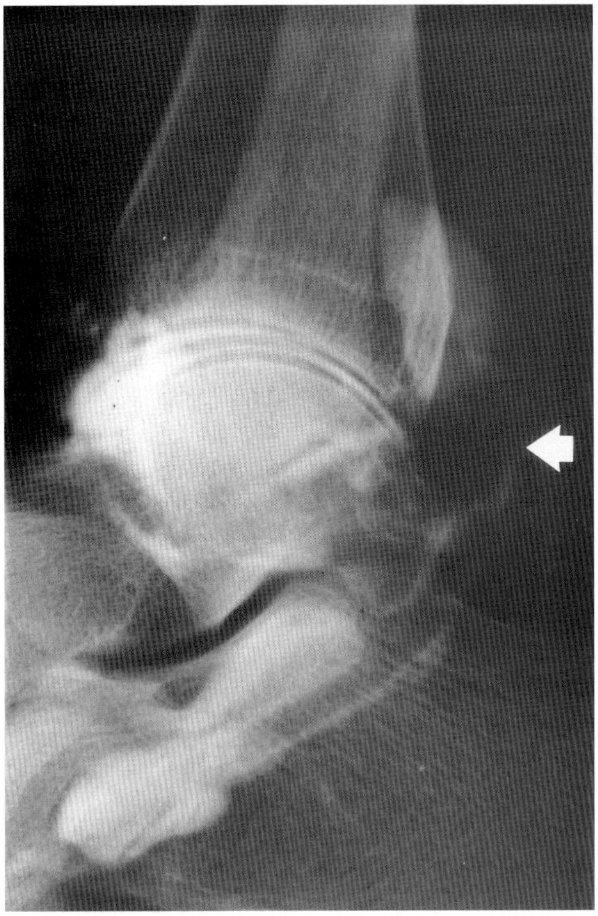

FIGURE 4.12. Arthrogram of the ankle. On this sagittal view a filling defect (arrow) in the posterior capsule represents a hyperplastic synovial nodule of pigmented villonodular synovitis (PVNS).

ated using arthrography (Fig. 4.12). Ankle tomography currently has limited usefulness in our practice, having been replaced by computed tomography (CT) and magnetic resonance imaging (MRI), unless contraindicated.

TENOGRAPHY

Tenography can be useful for evaluating tendons and their sheaths, and it is occasionally helpful when assessing ankle joint ligament tears. It is particularly helpful for evaluating peroneal tendon disease including tenosynovitis and tendon rupture.

Tenography has some disadvantages. It is an invasive procedure that may be difficult to perform when a large amount of swelling obscures normal ankle landmarks. Furthermore, fibrosis and scarring may block the tendon sheath and prevent the introduction of contrast fluid. Currently, tenography has limited indications, and it has been supplanted by CT and MRI, unless contraindicated.

XERORADIOGRAPHY

Xeroradiography is most commonly utilized for mammography. Occasionally, it is helpful when evaluating bone and soft tissue pathology of the extremities. The disadvantages of the procedure are that (1) it requires high radiation exposure and (2) there are broad areas of contrast suppression in which large regions of relatively uniform density may be indistinguishable from one another. Today, xeroradiography has been supplanted by CT and MRI.

NUCLEAR MEDICINE

Radionuclide imaging is an excellent modality for evaluating diseases of the foot and ankle.[11] The technique's high sensitivity (which allows it to identify bone disease in patients whose radiographs are normal) and low radiation dose requirement results in a good screening test. Although nuclear medicine studies have less spatial resolution than MRI or CT, they are still clinically helpful for evaluating benign or malignant tumors, septic arthritis, osteomyelitis, osteonecrosis, stress fractures, metabolic bone disease, plantar fasciitis, and tarsal coalition.

The most commonly used radiopharmaceutical for bone imaging is the technetium-99m phosphate compound methyl diphosphonate (MDP). After intravenous injection, the phosphate compound appears to adsorb to the hydroxyapatite crystal within the bone matrix. Imaging can be performed as a routine bone scan or a three-phase examination. For the latter, the first phase (perfusion) of imaging is performed during isotope injection. The second (venous pool) phase is obtained 60–90 seconds after the injection. The third phase is usually performed 3–4 hours after the injection. Some have added a fourth phase at 24 hours to increase the specificity.

Routine bone scan imaging is adequate for structural abnormalities (i.e., trauma, arthritis, and metastatic disease) (Fig. 4.13). Enthesopathy (bony proliferation at ligamentous insertions) is a type of stress syndrome. Bone scans are particularly sensitive for detecting stress fractures, and a grading system is sometimes used[12] (Fig. 4.14). Bone scintigraphy is a sensitive tool for evaluating early stages

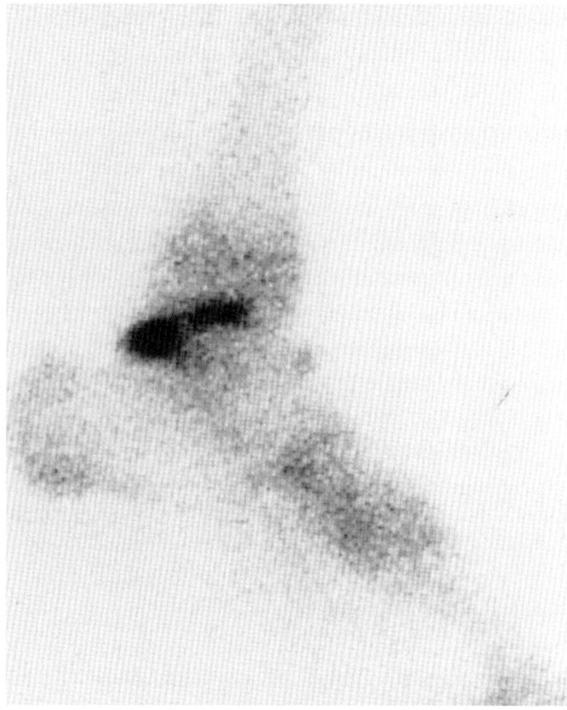

FIGURE 4.13. Bone scan demonstrating increased activity in the medial dome of the talus and the os trigonum, consistent with an osteochondral lesion of the medial dome of the talus and nonunion of the os trigonum.

of bone production of any etiology.[13] Bone scans are also helpful for evaluating subtle or occult trauma, delayed union, reflex sympathetic dystrophy, and metastatic disease.[14] The three-phase bone scan is used in patients with avascular necrosis to evaluate both hyperemia within primary bone tumors and reflex sympathetic dystrophy, and it is critical for assessing inflammatory conditions of soft tissue and bone.[15] For most of these indications, MRI is preferred at present because the specificity of bone scintigraphy is limited.

Additional scintigraphic procedures used to identify soft tissue abscesses and osteomyelitis are gallium-67 citrate and indium-111 white blood cell (WBC) scans. When correlated with the three-phase images, these tests help differentiate osteomyelitis from cellulitis. Indium-111 WBC imaging appears to be the superior technique, although with some chronic bone infections gallium imaging is positive when the indium scan is negative.[16] However, when the cost of multiple scintigraphic studies and the added time necessary are considered, MRI may be the procedure of choice for evaluating osteomyelitis, particularly in patients with underlying neuropathic disease.

TOMOGRAPHY

Conventional tomography can be useful for defining the exact anatomic location of a lesion detected on regular radiographs. Whereas plain film radiography superimposes one structure on another, tomography provides a sharp definition of the particular area of interest without superimposition of adjacent overlying structures. Tomograms can be

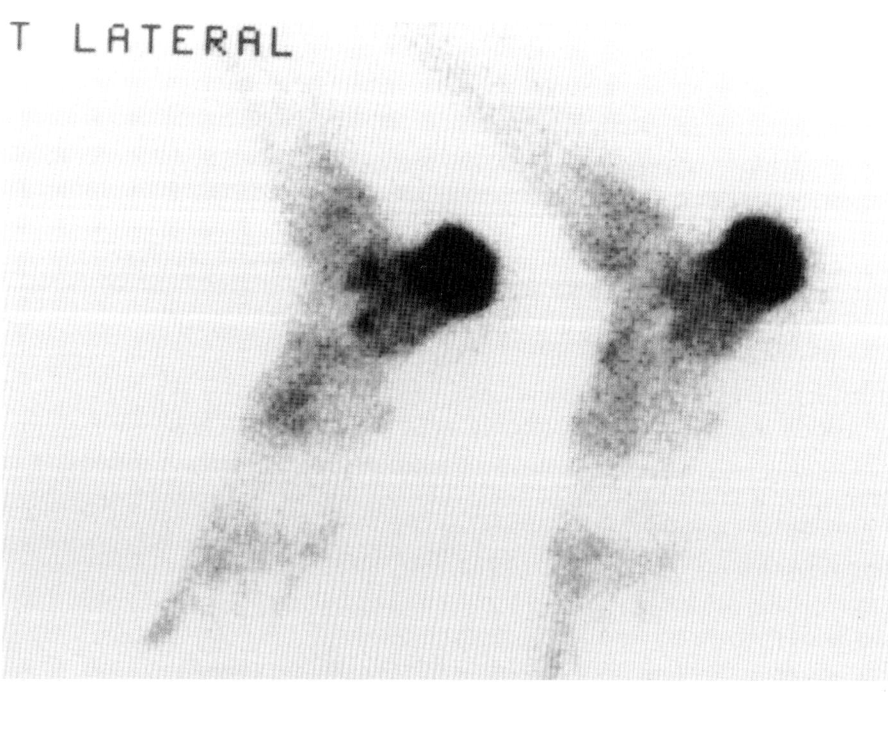

FIGURE 4.14. Bilateral calcaneal stress fractures in a 30-year-old marathon runner.

unidirectional (linear tomography) or pluridirectional. The slice thickness can vary from 2 to 5 mm and can be obtained in both the AP and lateral projections. Tomographic sections should be contiguous and the kilovoltage low enough (80 kVp or less) to allow adequate contrast.

The main indications for tomography are to evaluate nonunions, arthrodesis, osteochondral fractures of the talus, and Lisfranc's fracture-dislocations. It also can be used to evaluate navicular stress fractures, calcaneal fractures, and subtalar arthritis.

The disadvantages of tomography include high radiation exposure and absorption. The planes must be exactly perpendicular; otherwise the pictures are not accurate. In addition, tomographic studies can take a long time for completion, particularly when images are obtained in multiple planes.

Arthrotomography can also be done by injecting contrast material into the ankle. This procedure is particularly useful for determining if an osteochondral lesion of the ankle is loose. Today conventional tomography has been replaced by CT, and at the present time tomography is rarely used in our practice.

COMPUTER TOMOGRAPHY

Sectional Planes

To understand computerized sectional imaging, it is critical that one have an accurate understanding of the sectional planes for scans. Most images are produced in one or more of the following orthogonal planes: coronal, transverse (axial), sagittal. The coronal view is perpendicular to the planar surface of the foot, whereas the transverse or axial plane is parallel to the plantar surface of the foot and ankle. The sagittal view resembles the lateral view of the ankle. These sectional planes are shown in Figure 4.15.

Advantages

Computed tomography produces images based on tissue densities and individual differences in radiation absorption. It is superior to MRI for evaluating joint surfaces and the cortical outlines of individual bones. A hindfoot scan can be done unilaterally or bilaterally (for comparison with the opposite side). This scan gives a clear picture of the distal tibia, ankle, and subtalar articulations as well as the medial and lateral gutters in two planes. It also distinguishes the talus and calcaneus, which are superimposed on conventional radiographs. Some soft tissue outlines can be appreciated and differentiated on the scan, although MRI is better for most soft tissue abnormalities.

The indications for CT include evaluation of osteochondritis dissecans, osteochondral fractures, loose bodies, subtalar and ankle arthritis, tarsal coalition, and all fractures involving the hindfoot.

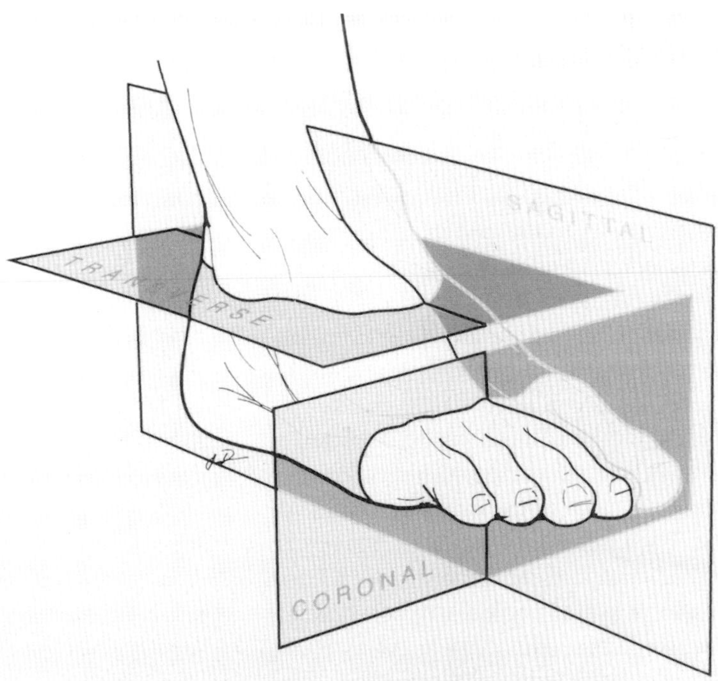

FIGURE 4.15. Sectional plane drawing indicating the lines of axis for the coronal, transverse (axial), and sagittal views.

Peroneal tendons can also be seen on transverse imaging images, which are particularly well suited to evaluate shallow fibular grooves in patients with peroneal subluxation.

Disadvantages

The disadvantages of the CT scan include its high radiation dosage, its inability to image directly in various planes, and its low spatial resolution compared with conventional radiography and tomography.

Technique

Positioning the patient for CT scanning is extremely important.[17] Symmetry between the two extremities must be maintained, and the plantar aspects of the feet should be pressed against the flat surface with a mild amount of pressure simulating weight-bearing. The patient is supine, with hips and knees flexed sufficiently to allow full insertion of the hindfoot in the scanner aperture. A foot holder is particularly helpful for maintaining the appropriate position of the hindfeet to obtain symmetric images on bilateral scans.

The transverse (axial) plane images are done with the foot at a 90-degree angle to the end of the table extension. The gantry is tilted either 0 or 20 degrees (Fig. 4.16A,B). For coronal plane images, the patient is supine, with the feet placed in extension with a 20-degree incline plane (Fig. 4.16C). If this is not comfortable, a 40-degree incline plane can be used. The gantry is tilted 20 degrees to compensate for the incline plane of 20 degrees and is maintained in perpendicular alignment with the plantar aspect of the foot.

The sequence of the sections is from the posterior surface of the talus to the body of the navicular. The slice interval is usually 3–5 mm, but the scanner capability can be as little as 1 mm. The slice thickness varies also but is generally 4 mm. For ankle and hindfoot pathology, generally the coronal and transverse planes are utilized. The computer reconstructions in multiple planes may be obtained at the termination of the examination, although they lack the spatial resolution of the direct transverse or coronal scans. With newer software the image can also be recreated with a three-dimensional picture that occasionally is useful particularly for evaluating patients with fracture pathology.

Clinical Applications

The CT scans can be extremely useful when evaluating and treating numerous disorders of the ankle. Normal anatomy must be appreciated to understand pathologic conditions. A detailed discussion of normal anatomy is beyond the scope of this chapter, and the reader is referred elsewhere for further in-depth presentations.[18,19]

Computed tomography scans are particularly useful for evaluating osteochondral lesions of the talus. By examining both the coronal and transverse planes, the size and location of the lesion can be assessed in AP and mediolateral directions (Fig. 4.17). A staging system for osteochondral lesions has been developed based on our experience (more than 150 cases) with pre- and postoperative CT scans and arthroscopic verification[20] (Table 4.1). Other applications of CT scanning include evaluation of tarsal coalition and fractures (Figs. 4.18, 4.19).

Contraindications

Metallic implants provide a reflection pattern that obscures images. However, sometimes, despite the blurring of these images from such things as screws, staples, and plates, the specific point of interest is still visible if the metallic implant is not too close to the target anatomy. In addition, the newer hardware is able to eliminate some of these problems. Thus in the future it will be easier to scan these areas.

MAGNETIC RESONANCE IMAGING

Magnetic resonance imaging is indicated for evaluating ligamentous and tendon injury, osteochondral injuries, stress fractures, coalition, bone and soft tissue tumors, ischemic necrosis, infection, and postoperative complications.[21–25] Routine radiography remains the initial screening procedure of choice when imaging the foot and ankle. MRI, however, is proving to be the procedure of choice for evaluating soft tissue injuries of the capsule, ligaments, tendons, cartilage, and muscle as well as radiographically occult conditions. The advantages of MRI include lack of ionizing radiation, the ability to scan clearly in a multiplanar fashion, and superb soft tissue contrast with the ability to distinguish fat, ligamentous tendons, bone marrow, and fluid. There is

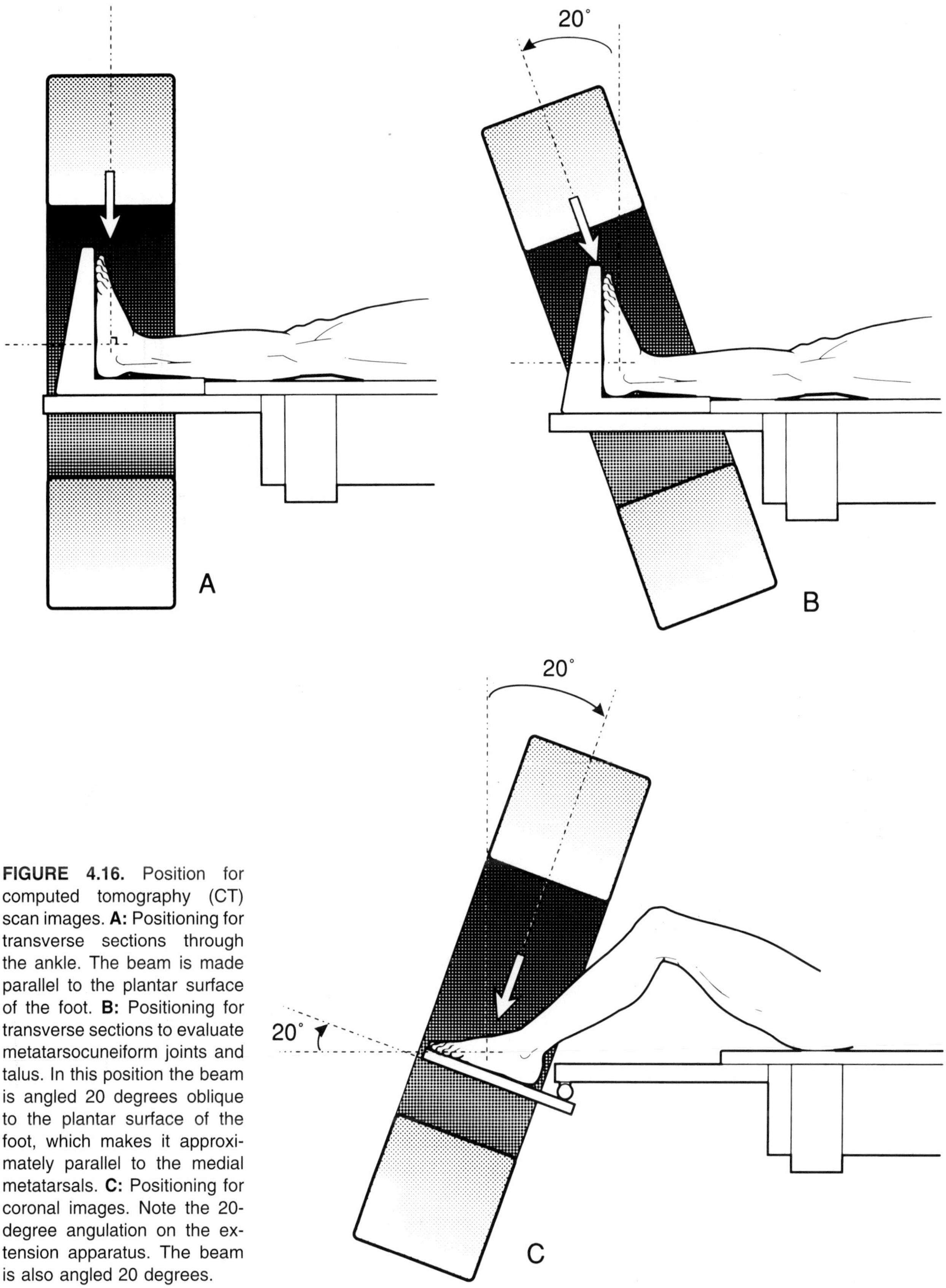

FIGURE 4.16. Position for computed tomography (CT) scan images. **A:** Positioning for transverse sections through the ankle. The beam is made parallel to the plantar surface of the foot. **B:** Positioning for transverse sections to evaluate metatarsocuneiform joints and talus. In this position the beam is angled 20 degrees oblique to the plantar surface of the foot, which makes it approximately parallel to the medial metatarsals. **C:** Positioning for coronal images. Note the 20-degree angulation on the extension apparatus. The beam is also angled 20 degrees.

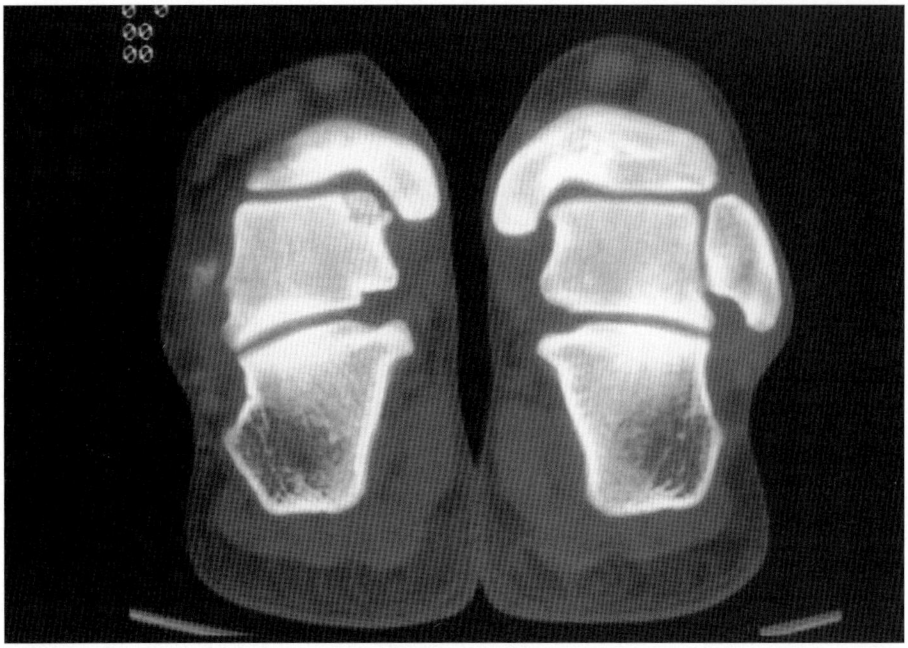

A

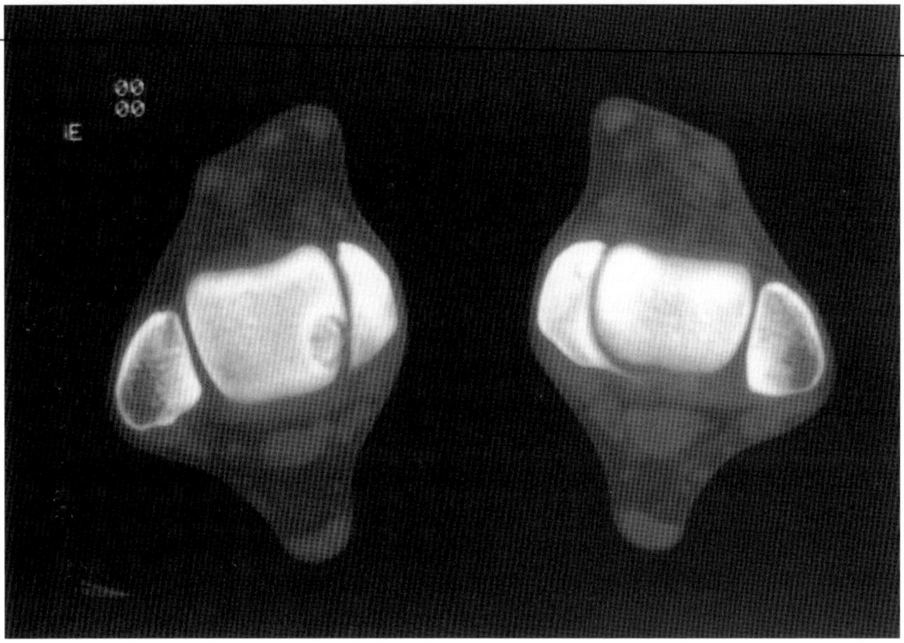

B

FIGURE 4.17. Osteochondral lesion of the medial dome of the talus. **A:** Bilateral coronal images demonstrating a stage 3 lesion with lucency surrounding the lesion on the right. **B:** Bilateral axial images showing the posteromedial extent of the lesion on the right with the sclerotic line surrounding it.

excellent resolution of the ankle, subtalar joint, foot, and surrounding soft tissue.

The magnetic resonance phenomenon involves an atomic nucleus. Those imaged are usually hydrogen nuclei, which consist of a single proton and are most abundant in water. A strong magnetic field is used to align these protons uniformly. Frequency pulses are then applied that change the orientation of the aligned protons. After the pulse, the protons relax back to their initial state. This relaxation process may be described by two time characteristics: T1 and T2. We can emphasize either of these two characteristics by altering two variables: echo time (TE) and recovery time (TR). Images with short TE and TR are relatively T1-weighted; those with long TE and TR are T2-weighted. The third type of image is a "balanced," or intermediate-weighted, image, with a long TR

TABLE 4.1. *Classification of osteochondral lesions of the talus*

Stage	*Description*
I	Cystic lesion within dome of talus, intact roof on all views
IIA	Cystic lesion with communication to talar dome surface
IIB	Open articular surface lesion with overlying nondisplaced fragment
III	Undisplaced lesion with lucency
IV	Displaced fragment

From Ferkel RD, Sgaglione NA. Arthroscopic treatment of osteochondral lesions of the talus: long term results [scientific exhibit]. Presented in part at the 60th annual meeting of the American Academy of Orthopaedic Surgeons, San Francisco, 1993.

and a short TE. This is also referred to as a proton density image.

The characteristics just described apply to the most commonly used sequence, the spin echo technique. There are many other sequences, including gradient echo and short tau inversion recovery (STIR) imaging.

The patient is usually positioned supine, preferably on a 1.5-tesla MR imager, the highest field strength available for clinical imaging today. This high field strength allows the highest signal-to-noise ratio, helping to optimize overall image quality and permitting high-resolution imaging. Imaging of only one foot or ankle is preferred, utilizing a dedicated extremity coil. We utilize a custom-built hindfoot

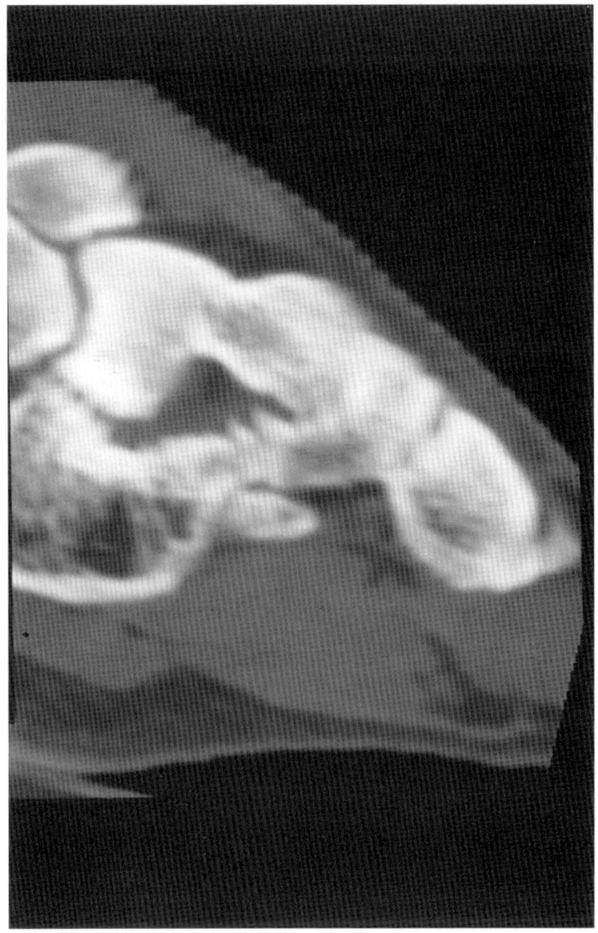

FIGURE 4.18. Talonavicular coalition is best demonstrated on sagittal CT scan reconstruction in a patient with recurrent ankle sprains.

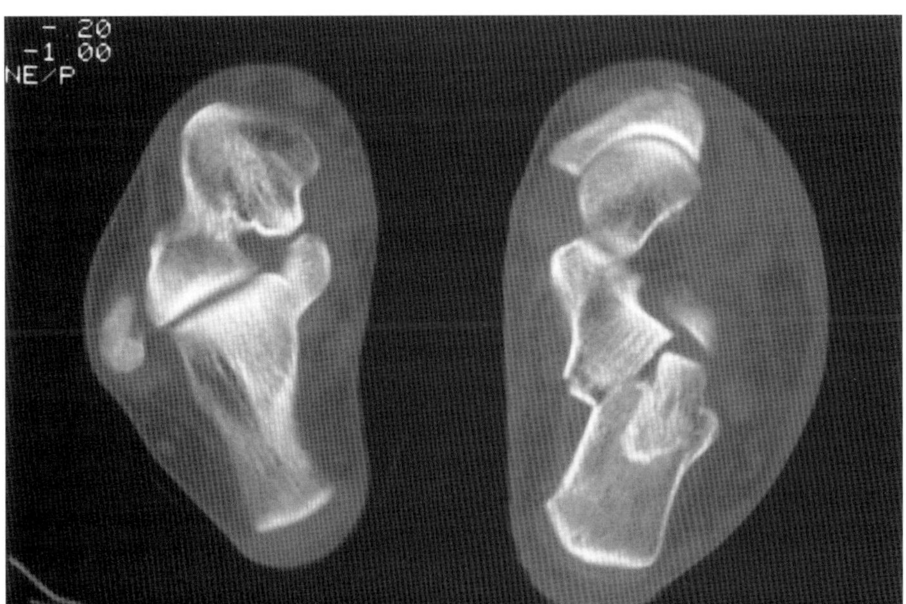

FIGURE 4.19. Comminuted calcaneal fracture of the left foot is best demonstrated on this axial CT scan.

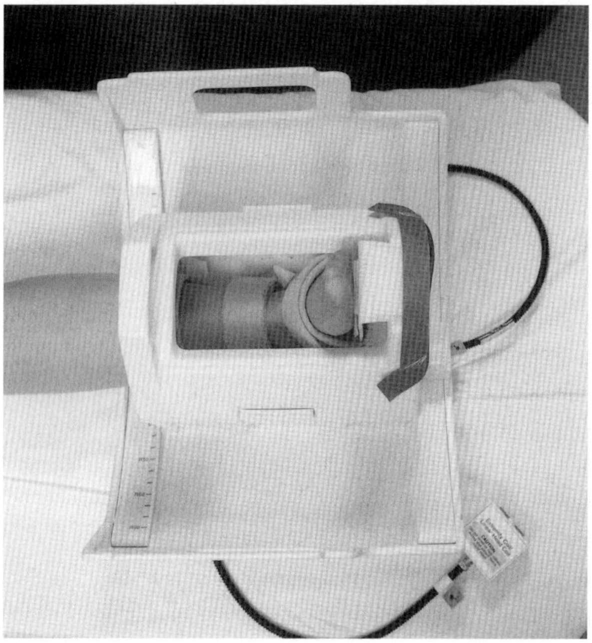

FIGURE 4.20. Custom built hindfoot positioning device for magnetic resonance imaging (MRI) scans. The device is worn while scanning is done inside the extremity coil.

positioning device and a separate custom-built foot-holding device for imaging the midfoot and forefoot (Fig. 4.20). To maximize resolution, we image a small anatomic area utilizing thin (3–4 mm) sections with an interslice gap of 0–1 mm.

The MRI scans provide dramatic tissue contrast. Pulse sequences can be selected to maximize this soft tissue contrast. Fluid gives a low signal intensity on T1-weighted (T1W) images and high signal intensity on T2-weighted (T2W) images. Fat saturation techniques such as the STIR sequences allow exquisite detection of bone marrow edema and are essential for the earliest detection of osseous pathology. Table 4.2 highlights the key sequences for MR imaging of the foot and ankle.

Osteochondral Lesions of the Talus

The MRI technique is useful for diagnosing numerous pathologic conditions of the foot and ankle.[26,27] Whether CT or MRI is the study of choice for evaluating osteochondrosis dissecans (OLT) (osteochondral lesions of the talus) is still controversial. MR is more accurate than CT for detecting cartilaginous abnormalities and their communication with the subchondral bone. A thin layer of fluid may extend into the bed of the OLT, with full-thickness chondral defects that communicate with the joint. This results in potential instability of the osteochondral fragment. MRI may overestimate the size of the osteochondral lesion if the associated subchondral cystic changes are not described separately. We advocate MRI for OLT if the routine radiographs are negative; we suggest CT if an OLT is demonstrated on the radiographs. CT more accurately defines the cortical marginations and calcified loose bodies but may not detect cartilaginous loose bodies, early OLT, or isolated cartilaginous lesions (R.D. Ferkel et al., unpublished observations).

Ligament Injuries

The lateral ankle sprain is the most common ankle injury. Most acute ankle sprains require only conventional radiography. MRI may be helpful for detecting associated osteochondral lesions or establishing the degree of ligamentous injury.[28] With a chronic ankle sprain that fails to respond to therapy, MR may be helpful for evaluating associated injuries, including osteochondral lesions of the talus and anterolateral impingement.

The intact lateral ligaments are best demonstrated on axial and coronal sequences as low signal intensity. Mild sprains demonstrate increased signal in-

TABLE 4.2. *Preferred MRI sequences for the foot and ankle*

Area of pathology	*Key plane(s)*	*Sequence(s)*
Achilles tendon	Sagittal, axial	T2 with F/S and/or STIR
Medial or lateral flexor tendons	Axial, coronal	PD and T2
Anterolateral impingement	Sagittal	T1 and STIR
	Axial	T2
Ankle ligaments	Axial	PD and T2
	Oblique coronal	PD with F/S
Soft tissue	Axial	PD and T2
Bone	Sagittal	T1, STIR

F/S, fat saturation; MRI, magnetic resonance imaging; PD, proton density or balanced images; STIR, short tau inversion recovery, a fat saturation technique.

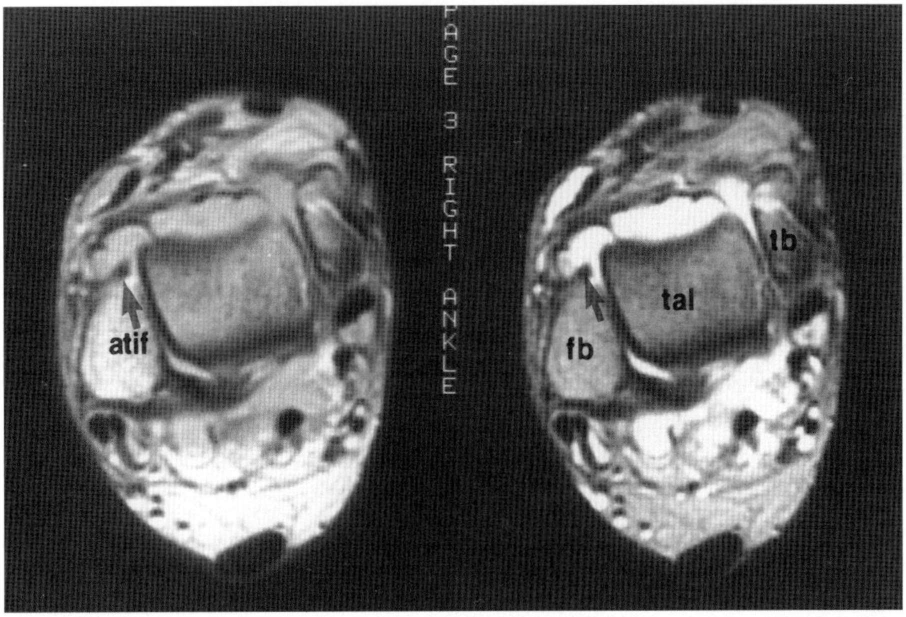

FIGURE 4.21. Acute tear of the anterior tibiofibular ligament. These T2-weighted double echo axial images demonstrate rupture of the right anterior tibiofibular ligament and an extensive amount of fluid. atif, anterior tibiofibular ligament; fb, fibula; tal, talus; tb, tibia.

tensity with irregular thinning or thickening. Complete discontinuity is seen with complete grade III ligament injuries (Fig. 4.21).

The deltoid ligament demonstrates a series of low signal intensity bands extending from the medial malleolus to the talus, sustentaculum talus, and spring ligament and navicular. The posterior tibiotalar component normally demonstrates a striated appearance.

To evaluate injuries to the syndesmotic complex, all imaging sequences must be extended at least 4 cm above the talar dome. The components of the syndesmotic complex are normally of uniformly low signal intensity and follow an oblique course. Complete disruption may be evident and is best depicted on axial sequences. Tables 4.3 and 4.4 list the sequences and anatomic orientations recommended for MR evaluation of the ankle, hindfoot, mid-foot, and forefoot.

Coalition

Osseous, fibroosseous, and osteocartilaginous coalitions are a frequent cause of ankle and foot pain. Traditionally, plain radiography and CT scans have been the studies of choice to evaluate coalition. Properly performed, MRI demonstrates osseous coalitions (Fig. 4.22). In addition, MRI has the advantage of depicting the bone marrow edema that may be present at sites of fibroosseous and osteocartilaginous coalitions. The latter two conditions may be difficult to detect with CT.

Soft Tissue Impingement

The MRI technique is useful for diagnosing soft tissue impingement of the ankle and tears of the ankle ligaments (Fig. 4.23).[29] Abnormal soft tissue can be seen in the anterolateral gutter in patients with soft tissue impingement. In our experience, this is best demonstrated on sagittal images through the fibula.

Tendon Injuries

Tendon pathology is best demonstrated with MRI (Fig. 4.24).[30,31] Tendon injuries may be described as grade I, with increased size and signal intensity

TABLE 4.3. *Ankle and hindfoot MRI protocol*

Key Plane(s)	*Sequence(s)*
Axial	PD and T2
Coronal	T2
Sagittal	T1
Sagittal	STIR
Oblique coronal[a]	PD with F/S

[a]35–45° along the talar dome.

TABLE 4.4. *Forefoot and mid-foot MRI protocol*

Key plane(s)	*Sequence(s)*
Sagittal	T1
Sagittal	STIR
Coronal	T1
Coronal	STIR
Oblique axial	PD with F/S

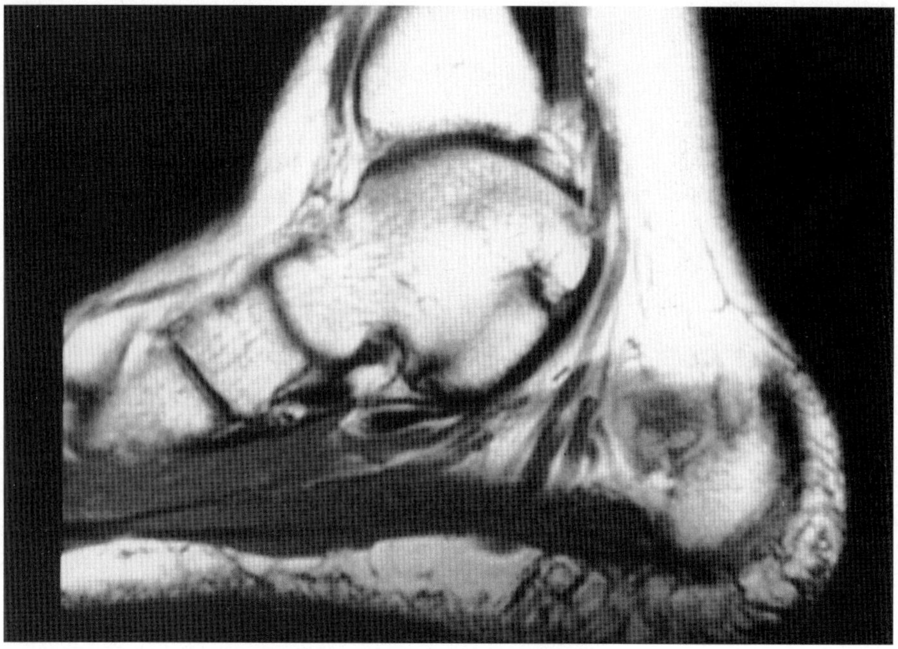

A

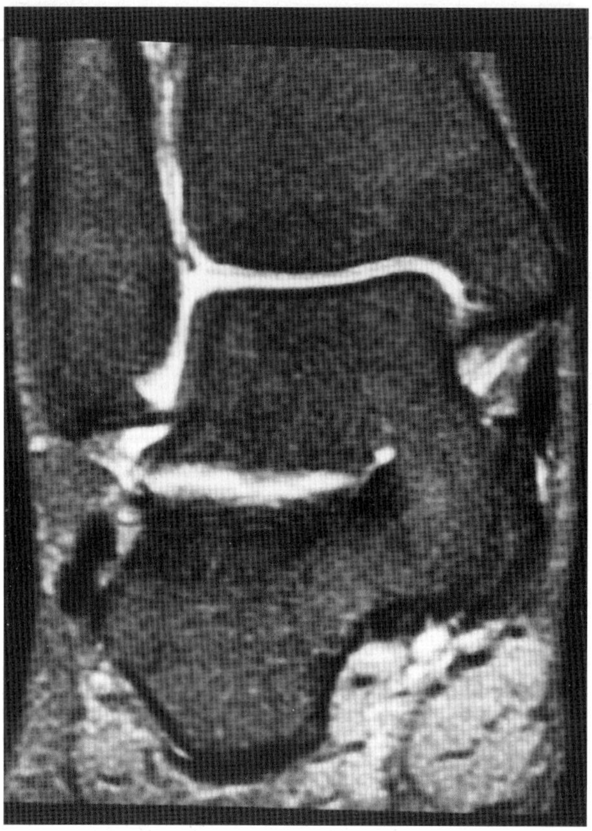

B

FIGURE 4.22. Talocalcaneal coalition. **A:** Sagittal T1-weighted sequence demonstrates talocalcaneal osseous coalition. **B:** Oblique coronal proton density-weighted image demonstrates talocalcaneal osseous coalition.

of the tendon representing partial tearing. With grade II tendon injuries, the tendon has a thin, attenuated appearance and may or may not have altered signal intensity. Grade III tendon injuries represent complete tendinous disruption. The peroneus split syndrome has been described, characterized by a longitudinal split tear of the peroneus brevis. The peroneus longus is usually intact and is located between the two split portions of the peroneus tendon, which may form an inverted V (Fig. 4.25).[32]

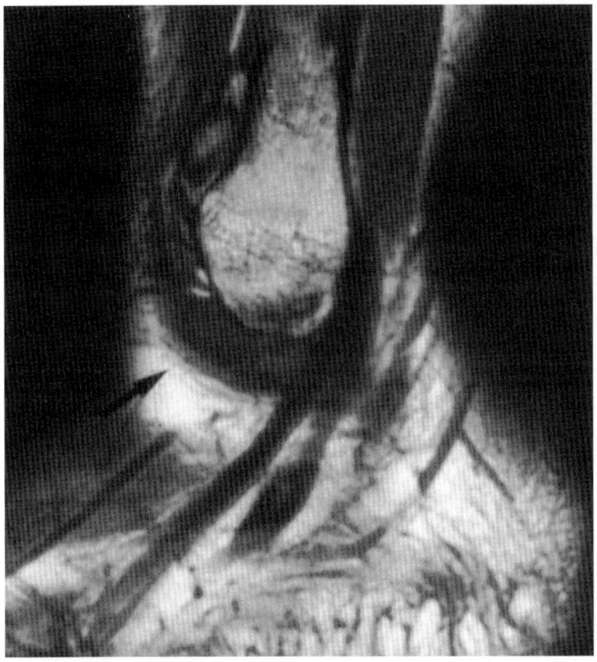

FIGURE 4.23. Soft tissue impingement. A sagittal T1-weighted image demonstrates a low signal density mass in the anterolateral gutter (arrow) consistent with soft tissue impingement.

Infection

The MRI procedure is the study of choice following routine radiography for detecting infection.[33,34] Although evaluating osteomyelitis in the diabetic foot is a challenge on all radiographic studies, MRI is the most accurate imaging technique. Areas of cortical destruction or fluid collections in the medullary cavity of bone are the key imaging features of osteomyelitis. MRI is also helpful for delineating soft tissue abscesses. Fat saturation techniques, including STIR imaging, are extremely sensitive for detecting early bone marrow edema. The presence of marrow edema may be encountered only with neuropathic changes and marrow edema related to regional hyperemia; alone it is not sufficient for a diagnosis of osteomyelitis.

Tumors

The MRI technique is also the imaging study of choice following plain radiography for evaluating osseous and soft tissue tumors (Figs. 4.26, 4.27).[35]

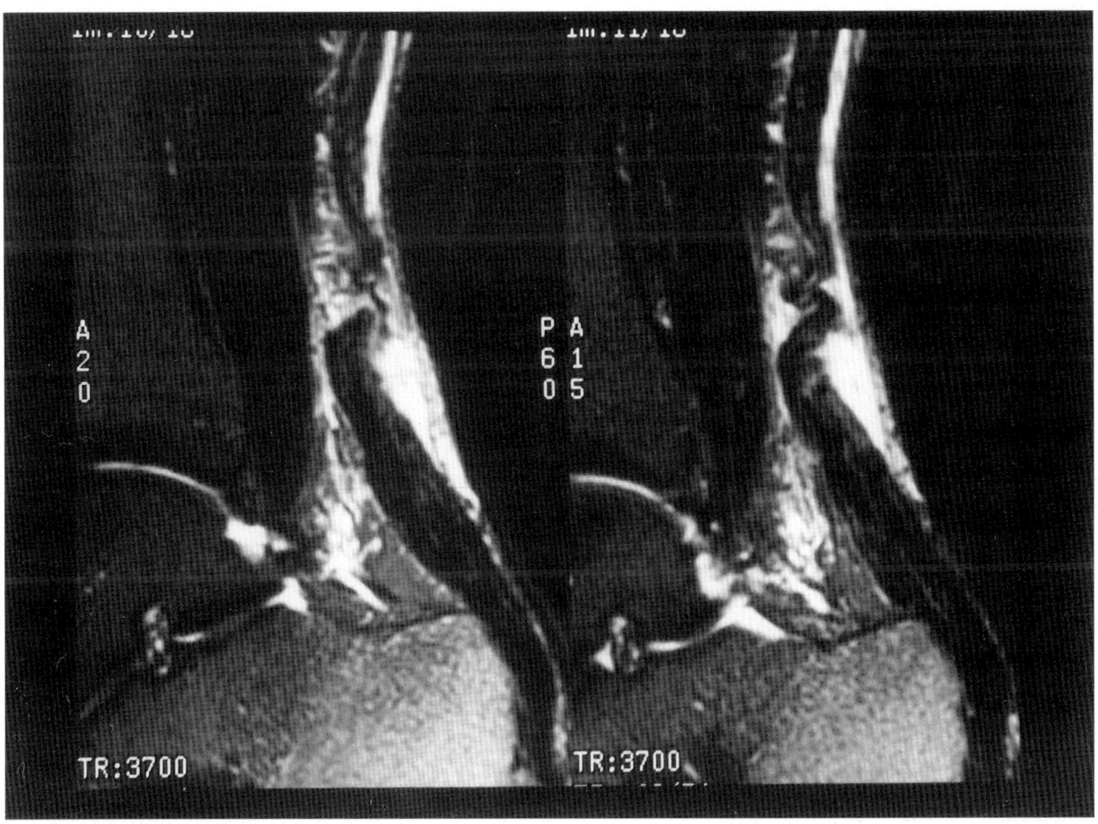

FIGURE 4.24. Achilles rupture. Sagittal T2-weighted images demonstrate rupture of the Achilles tendon at the musculotendinous junction.

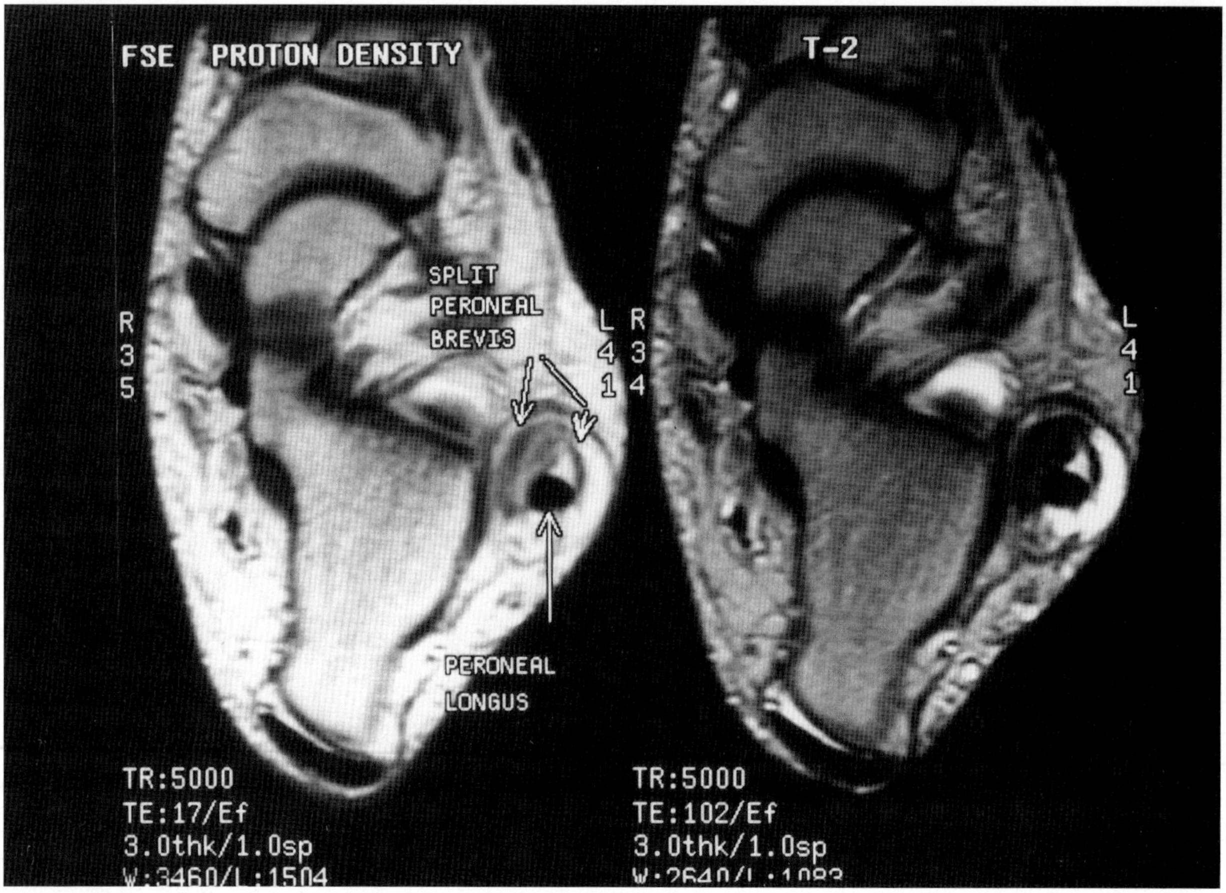

FIGURE 4.25. Axial proton density (left) and T2 images demonstrate a split tear of the peroneus brevis. Accompanying fluid is best seen in the T2 image on the right. The peroneal longus is intact.

Some soft tissue masses (e.g., lipomas and ganglions), have typical homogeneous imaging features; and osseous masses (e.g., enchondromas) have typical MR features. The primary role of MRI evaluation in the presence of malignant osseous neoplasms is diagnostic staging. Evaluating the extent of soft tissue involvement and neurovascular bundle involvement is critical in the diagnostic workup of malignant neoplasms. Whole-body bone scans to detect additional lesions are also indicated. Radiographic evaluation of the chest may be necessary as well.

Kinematic MRI

Kinematic MRI studies may be useful for evaluating osseous and soft tissue impingement and peroneal subluxation. Further research is necessary to confirm the utility of this developing MRI application.

Three-dimensional MRI Applications

Three-dimensional (3D) MR imaging currently allows contiguous 0.7 mm slices. These high resolution sequences improve MRI's role in evaluating chondral lesions. Currently, 3D gradient echo acquisitions with fat saturation are being utilized for cartilaginous detection. The 3D data sets may also be useful when evaluating ankle ligaments with oblique reconstruction techniques. It is likely that in the future several 3D data sets will be acquired, and all imaging data will be reconstructed from those data sets after the patient scan has been completed.

MR Arthrography

Direct MR arthrography using dilute gadolinium solutions (1:100) have demonstrated improved accuracy for detecting ligamentous injuries in patients with chronic ankle instability.[36] Institutional Review Board approval is recommended, as the intraarticular administration of gadolinium has not received Food and Drug Administration (FDA) approval. Our experience with MR arthrography suggests improved visualization of chondral lesions (Fig. 4.28), loose bodies, and the deep component of the deltoid ligament. Further investigation is needed to determine the

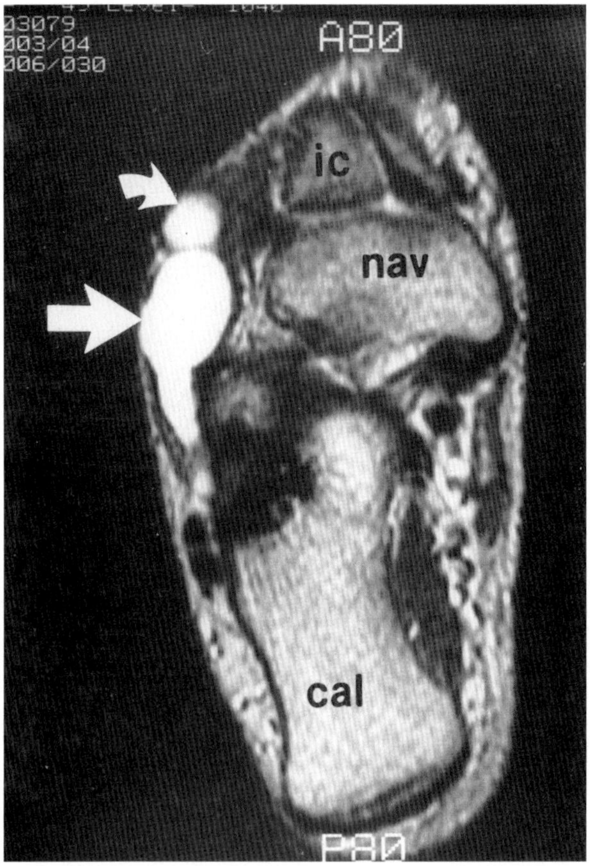

FIGURE 4.26. Axial T2-weighted image demonstrates a ganglion cyst on the dorsolateral surface of the foot associated with the extensor digitorum brevis muscle. ic, intermediate cuneiform; nav, navicular; cal, calcaneus.

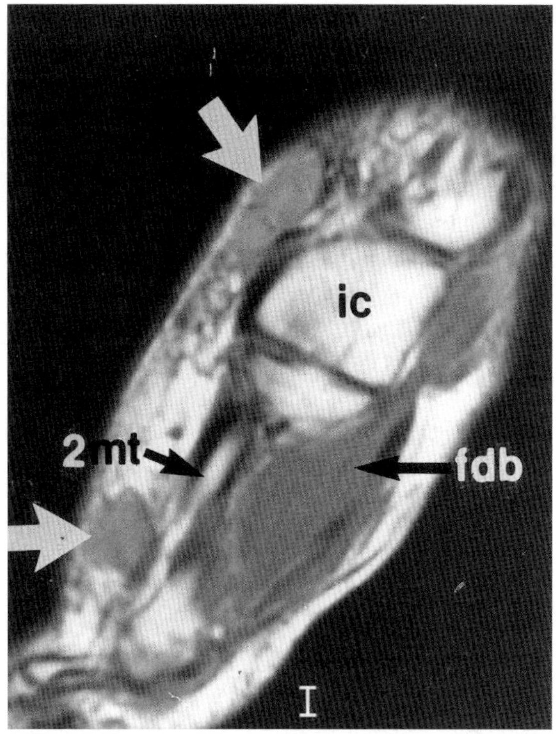

FIGURE 4.27. Two lesions, one dorsal to the second metatarsal and the other dorsal to the intermediate cuneiform, are seen on this sagittal T1-weighted image. The patient was diagnosed as having angiosarcoma following surgical biopsy of both tumors. ic, intermediate cuneiform; 2mt, second metatarsal; fdb, flexor digitum brevis.

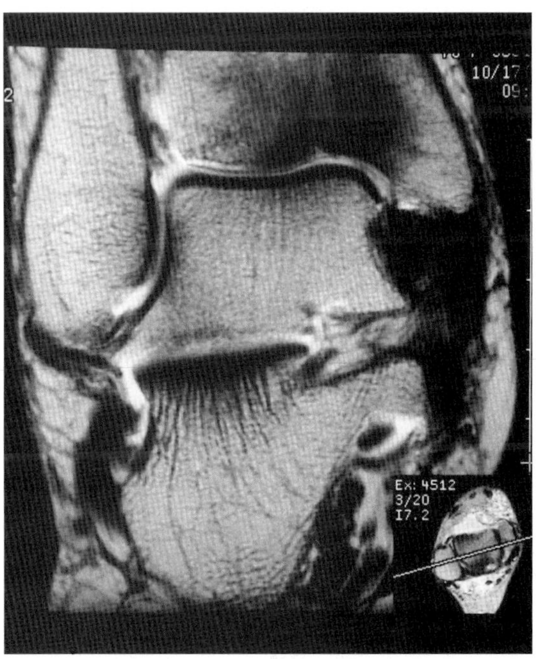

A

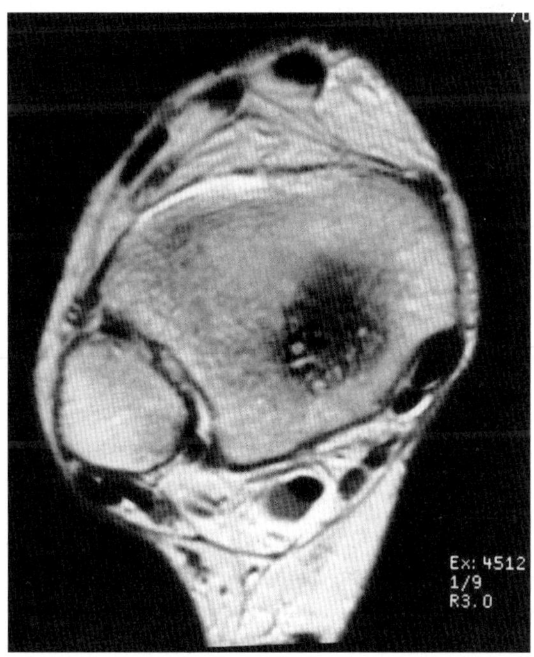

B

FIGURE 4.28. Magnetic resonance (MR) arthrography. **A:** High-resolution T1-weighted oblique coronal MR arthrogram demonstrates an osteochondral lesion of the plafond. Cartilaginous faces are well demonstrated. **B:** Axial T2-weighted image through the plafond demonstrates the osteochondral lesion with multiple small cystic components.

ultimate role of MR arthrography in evaluation of the foot and ankle. We do not advocate the use of indirect MR arthrography. Indirect arthrography utilizes intravenous gadolinium with a time delay following exercise, allowing the contrast to accumulate in the joint fluid. The major drawback to this technique is the simultaneous enhancement of areas of increased vascularity and synovium. No joint distension is achieved with indirect techniques.

BIBLIOGRAPHY

1. Wuest TK. Injuries to the distal lower extremity syndesmosis. *J Am Acad Orthop Surg* 1997;5:172–181.
2. Feist JH, Mankin HJ. The tarsus. I. Basic relationships and motions in the adult and definition of optimal recumbent oblique projection. *Radiology* 1962; 79:250.
3. Kleiger B, Makin HJ. A roentgenographic study of the development of the calcaneus by means of the posterior tangential view. *J Bone Joint Surg Am* 1961; 43:961.
4. Christensen JC, Dockery GL, Schuberth JM. Evaluation of ankle ligamentous insufficiency using the Telos ankle stress apparatus. *J Am Podiatr Assoc* 1986; 76:527.
5. Laurin CA, Ouellet R, St Jacques R. Talar and subtalar tilt: an experimental investigation. *Can J Surg* 1968;11:270.
6. Sauser DD, Nelson RC, Laurine MH, et al. Acute injuries of the lateral ligaments of the ankle: comparison of stress radiography and arthrography. *Radiology* 1983;148:653.
7. Rubin G, Witten M. The talar tilt ankle and the fibular collateral ligaments: a method for the determination of talar tilt. *J Bone Joint Surg Am* 1960;42A:311.
8. Chrisman OD, Snook CA. A reconstruction of lateral ligament tears of the ankle: an experimental study and clinical evaluation of seven patients treated by a new modification of the Elmslie procedure. *J Bone Joint Surg Am* 1969;51:904.
9. Gould N, Seligson D, Glassman J. Early and late repair of lateral ligaments of the ankle. *Foot Ankle* 1980;1:84.
10. Clanton TO, Schon LC. Athletic injuries to the soft tissues of the foot and ankle. In: Mann RA, Coughlin MJ (eds) *Surgery of the foot and ankle*. St. Louis: Mosby, 1992;1153–1167.
11. Maurice HD, Newman JH, Watt I. Bone scanning of the foot for unexplained pain. *J Bone Joint Surg Br* 1987;69:448–452.
12. Matin P. Basic principles of nuclear medicine techniques for detection and evaluation of trauma and sports medicine injuries. *Semin Nucl Med* 1988; 18:90.
13. Rupani HP, Holder LE, Espinola DA, Engin SI. Three-phase radionuclide bone imaging in sports medicine. *Radiology* 1985;156:187.
14. McDougall IR, Keeling CA. Complications of fractures and their healing. *Healing* 1980;18:113.
15. Park CH, Kapadia D, O'Hara SE. Three phase bone scan findings in stress fracture. *Clin Nucl Med* 1981;6:587.
16. Gupta NC, Prezio JA. Radionuclide imaging in osteomyelitis. *Semin Nucl Med* 1988;18:287.
17. Smith RW, Staple TW. Computerized tomography (CT) scanning technique for the hindfoot. *Clin Orthop* 1983;177:34.
18. Solomon MA, Gilula LA, Oloff LM, et al. CT scanning of the foot and ankle. I. Normal anatomy. *AJR Am J Roentgenol* 1986;146:1192.
19. Soloman MA, Gilula LA, Oloff LM, et al. CT scanning of the foot and ankle. II. Clinical applications and review of the literature. *AJR Am J Roentgenol* 1986;146:1204.
20. Cheng MS, Ferkel RD, Applegate GR. Osteochondral lesions of the talus: a radiologic and surgical comparison. Presented at the annual meeting of the American Academy of Orthopaedic Surgeons, New Orleans, February 1995.
21. Stoller DW, Ferkel RD. The ankle and foot. In: Stoller DW (ed). *Magnetic resonance imaging in orthopaedics and sports medicine*. Philadelphia: Lippincott-Raven, 1997;443.
22. Deutsch AL, Mink JH, Kerr R (eds). *MRI of the foot and ankle*. New York: Raven, 1992.
23. Ho CP. Magnetic resonance imaging of the ankle and foot. *Semin Roentgenol* 1995;30:294–303.
24. Link SC, Erickson SJ, Timins ME. MR imaging of the ankle and foot: normal structures and anatomic variants that may simulate disease. *AJR Am J Roentgenol* 1993;161:607–612.
25. Roberts DK, Pomeranz SJ. Current status of magnetic resonance in radiologic diagnosis of foot and ankle injuries. *Orthop Clin North Am* 1994;25:61–68.
26. Ferkel RD, Flannigan BD, Elkins BS. Magnetic resonance imaging of the foot and ankle: correlation of normal anatomy with pathologic conditions. *Foot Ankle* 1991;11:289.
27. Mink JH, Deutsch AL (eds). *MRI of the musculoskeletal system*. New York: Raven, 1990.
28. Rijke AM, Goitz HT, McCue FC III, Dee PM. Magnetic resonance imaging of injury to the lateral ankle ligaments. *Am J Sports Med* 1993;21:528–534.
29. Rubin DA, Tishkoff NW, Britton CA, et al. Anterolateral soft-tissue impingement in the ankle: diagnosis using MR imaging. *AJR Am J Roentgenol* 1997; 169:829–835.
30. Rosenberg AZ, Beltran J, Cheung YY, et al. MR features of longitudinal tears of the peroneus brevis tendon. *AJR Am J Roentgenol* 1997;168:141–147.
31. Tjin A, Ton ER, Schweitzer ME, Karasick D. MR

imaging of peroneal tendon disorders. *AJR Am J Roentgenol* 1997;168:135–140.

32. Schweitzer ME, Eid ME, Deely D, et al. Using MR imaging to differentiate peroneal splits from other peroneal disorders. *AJR Am J Roentgenol* 1997;168: 129–133.
33. Modic MT, Pflanz W, Feiglin DNI, et al. Magnetic resonance imaging of musculoskeletal infections. *Radiol Clin North Am* 1986;24:247.
34. Beltran J, McGhee RB, Shaffer PB, et al. Experimental infection of the musculoskeletal system: evaluation with MR imaging and Tc-99m MPP and Ga-67 scintigraphy. *Radiology* 1988;167:167.
35. Seale KS, Lange TA, Monson D, Hackbarth DA. Soft tissue tumors of the foot and ankle. *Foot Ankle* 1988;9:19–27.
36. Chandnani VP, Harper MT, Ficke JR, et al. Chronic ankle instability: evaluation with MR arthrography, MR imaging, and stress radiography. *Radiology* 1994;192:189–194.

CHAPTER 5

Setup, Distraction, and Instrumentation

Melbourne D. Boynton, J. Serge Parisien, James F. Guhl, and Carole S. Vetter

OPERATING ROOM SETUP

Ankle arthroscopy, as for most arthroscopy, requires a large operating room essentially dedicated to arthroscopy. The room requires special attention to electrical control with appropriate grounding. All electric cables must have adequate shielding to prevent macro- or microshocks. The operating room must be large enough to accommodate all arthroscopy equipment and operating room personnel. Ankle arthroscopy requires a significant amount of equipment, including the operating table and distraction device, arthroscopy cart, first and second instrument tables, suction and pump systems, and instrument storage cart. Occasionally, fluoroscopy is needed; therefore the room must be large enough to accommodate this additional equipment and personnel. Operating room personnel must be able to move around the room freely and maintain appropriate sterile and unsterile areas. The anesthesiologist must have the necessary equipment for general, regional, or local anesthesia. The arthroscopy cart should be mobile such that it can be moved about the room and contain the video camera, video monitor, motorized shaver, light source, and video recorder or printer. The instrument cart should be equipped with a full supply of motorized tools, extra sterile light cords, an extra camera and arthroscope, and backup instruments in case of malfunction or contamination.

It is ideal if the circulating nurse, scrub nurse, and assistant are specialized in arthroscopic surgery. They must be familiar with all arthroscopic equipment and be able to troubleshoot any problems. It is extremely important that the scrub nurse be familiar with the goals of the procedure so he or she is able to anticipate the needs of the surgeon. Performing ankle arthroscopy often requires several coordinated steps with both hands; therefore the surgeon cannot be distracted by having to show the scrub nurse what instruments are needed next. A new scrub nurse should be supervised by a nurse or operating room (OR) technician who is experienced in ankle arthroscopy until the new scrub nurse has sufficient experience.

All personnel, including the surgeon, must have a thorough knowledge of how the camera, monitor, recorder/printer, and distension fluid system functions. They must also be able to clean, inspect, and appropriately care for all instruments.

The Mayo stand contains sharp instruments and the most commonly used diagnostic instruments, such as trocars, cannulas, and probes. The back table contains the therapeutic instruments, such as graspers, baskets, and curettes.

PATIENT POSITIONING

Ankle arthroscopy can be performed with general, regional, or local anesthesia. If general anesthesia is used, the patient should be paralyzed to allow easier distraction and visualization. Local anesthesia (ankle block) (see Chapter 21) can provide excellent anesthesia and is often combined with intravenous sedation for ankle arthroscopy. If a tourniquet is required for hemostasis/visualization, conversion to a general anesthetic may be necessary.

The position of the patient varies depending on the surgeon's preference and the anticipated mode of distraction. Ankle arthroscopy can be performed in three positions: supine using a thigh and ankle holder; supine using a leg holder with the end of the operating table dropped 90 degrees; and lateral decubitus using a bean bag. Figure 5.1 shows four positions of the foot and leg for ankle arthroscopy using noninvasive distraction.

To use the thigh and leg holder, the patient is positioned supine with the hip and knee flexed 45–50 degrees. A tourniquet is placed around the proximal thigh, and the thigh is placed on a nonsterile holder that supports the thigh superior to the popliteal fossa. Foam pads are placed under the thigh to prevent injury to the hamstrings or sciatic nerve. The extremity is secured in the thigh holder with an Ace wrap and is then prepared with a sterilization solution and draped. If needed, a sterile ankle holder or noninvasive distraction strapping device is applied and attached to a sterile clamp as in Figure 5.2. The clamp is attached to the table over the drapes. The foot of the operating room (OR) table can be lowered 10–20 degrees if required to make room to work through the posterolateral portal.

An alternative method has the patient in a supine position with the leg in a knee holder and the end of the OR table dropped 90 degrees. The leg and ankle hang over the end of the table, allowing some distraction by gravity. Additional noninvasive distraction can be applied by an assistant using a Kerlix wrap clove-hitch knot around the ankle or prefabricated straps held under the foot.[1]

Parisien described a 45-degree lateral position.[2] The patient is placed in a lateral decubitus position with the body supported by a bean bag and tilted slightly posteriorly, as shown in Figure 5.3. The ankle is elevated on a well-padded box. The ipsilateral hip is externally rotated for anterior portals access and internally rotated for posterolateral portals access. Plantar flexion of the foot and ankle allow better anterior visualization and instrumentation. This position is particularly useful for subtalar arthroscopy through lateral portals.

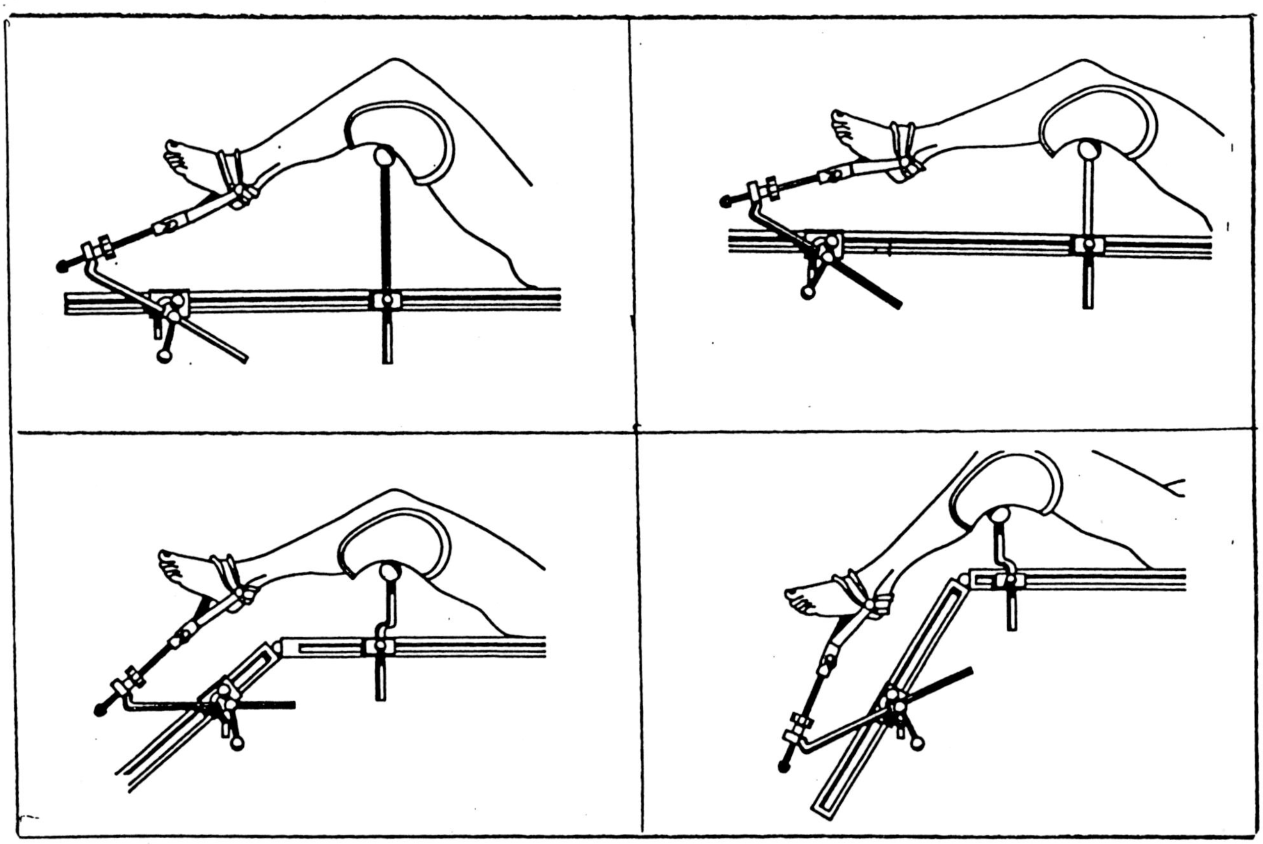

FIGURE 5.1. Four positions of the leg and foot for ankle arthroscopy using the Guhl noninvasive ankle distractor. (Smith & Nephew Inc./Arthroscopy—Andover, MA.)

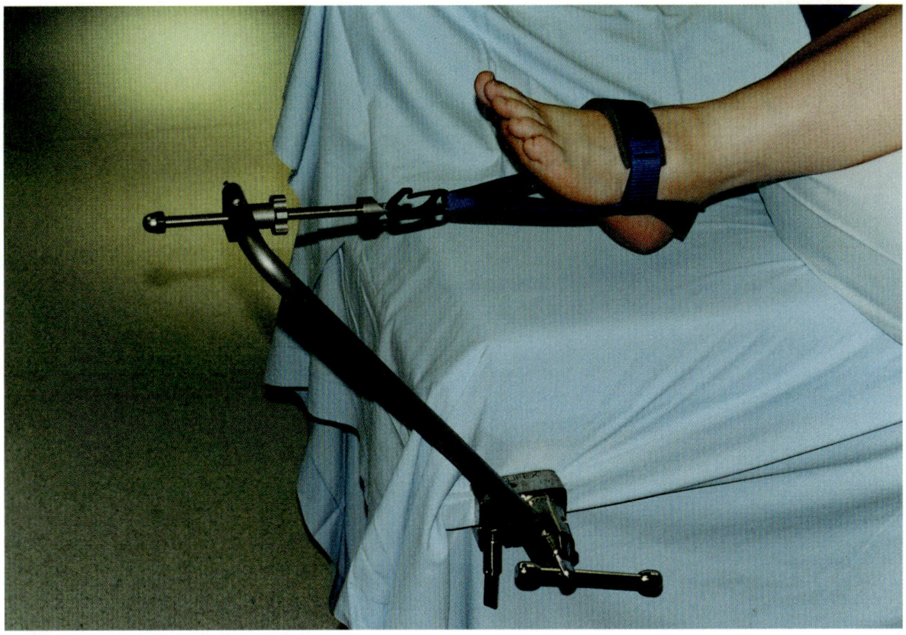

FIGURE 5.2. Noninvasive distraction with the ankle in the Guhl noninvasive distractor. (Smith & Nephew Inc./ Arthroscopy—Andover, MA.)

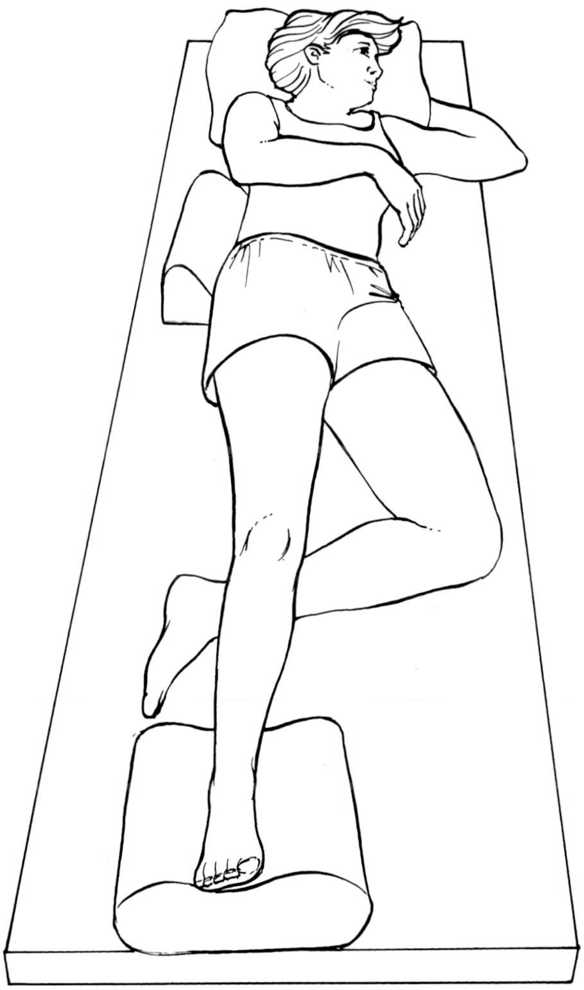

FIGURE 5.3. Ankle and subtalar arthroscopy can be performed with the patient positioned supine and a bolster at the end of the operating table. Manual distraction is maintained by an assistant.

DISTRACTION

Visualization and manipulation of the ankle can be significantly improved by the use of distraction, which increases the space between the tibia and the talus. It allows better visualization of all compartments while decreasing the risk of scuffing the articular cartilage and breaking the instruments or arthroscope. Without distraction, it is difficult to place a rigid arthroscope over a curved structure such as the talar dome, as seen in Figure 5.4.

Distraction methods applied to the ankle may be invasive or noninvasive. In our experience it is rare that invasive distraction is required. With the current methods of securing the patient to the OR table, the commercially available noninvasive distractors, use of small joint instruments, the 2.7 mm arthroscope, and use of the posterolateral portal, we have not needed invasive distraction for ankle or subtalar arthroscopy for at least 5 years.

Noninvasive Distraction

Noninvasive techniques such as manual distraction and gravity are considered "uncontrolled" methods because the amount of force applied cannot be measured, monitored, or maintained. Certainly, gravity-only distraction is safe, whereas manual distraction is associated with the possibility of damaged ligaments, although to our knowledge this complication has not been reported. Noninvasive techniques

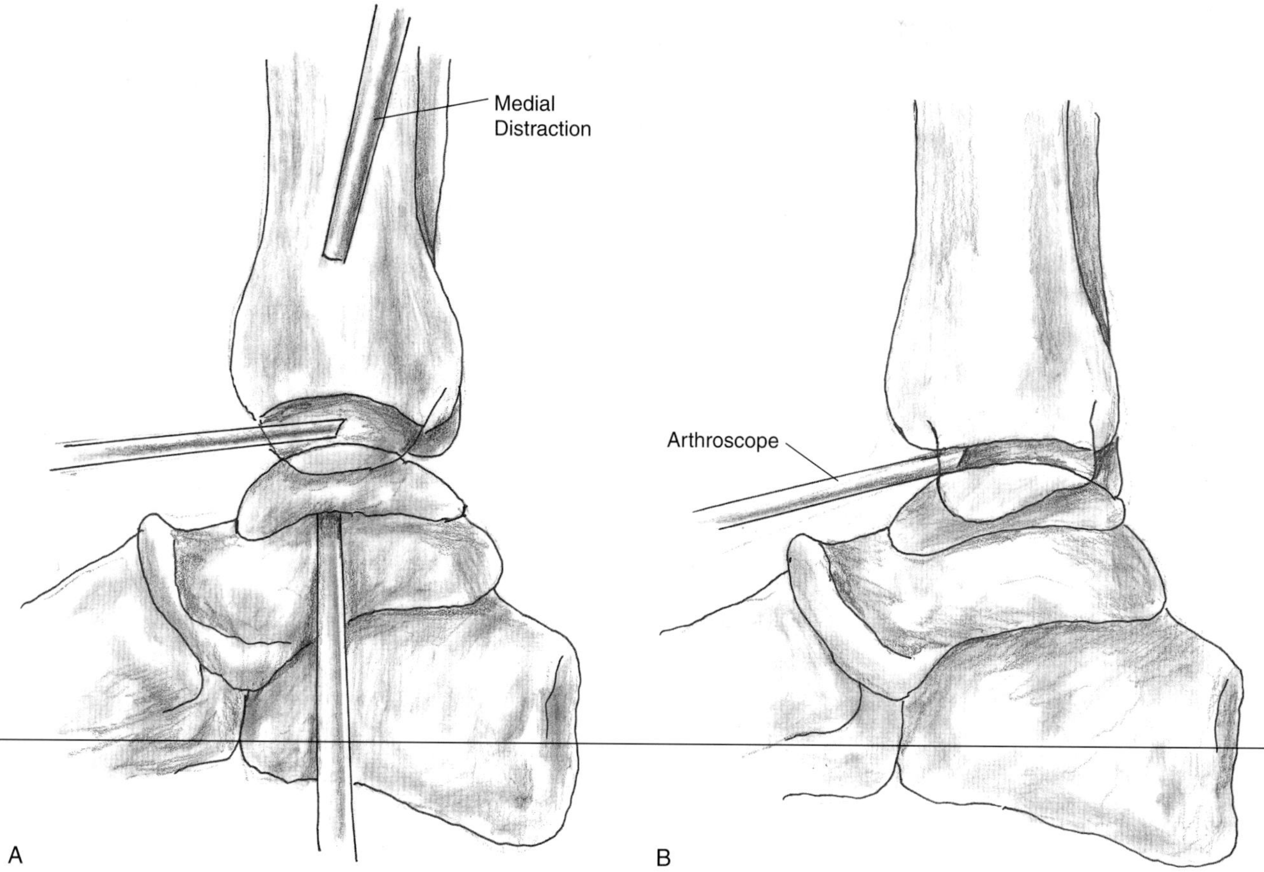

FIGURE 5.4. A: Distraction helps prevent iatrogenic injury to the articular cartilage during arthroscopy. **B:** Without distraction it is difficult to visualize the posterior structures of the ankle.

such as the Kerlix clove-hitch knot with pressure applied by stepping on the end is considered a "semi-controlled" method of distraction. A "controlled" method of noninvasive distraction developed by Guhl involves prefabricated straps that hook across the foot and behind the heel and attach to an outrigger, which applies a distraction force. The Guhl noninvasive distractor is seen in Figures 5.2, 5.5, and 5.6. The distraction maintained should be no more than 30 lb (135 N) of force and should be applied for no more than 30–45 minutes without periodic relaxation. Dowdy et al. demonstrated reversible nerve conduction changes with 30 lb (135 N) of force applied for 1 hour.[3] Exceeding these limits can result in paresthesias or neurapraxia in the peripheral nerves of the foot. In practice, we do not use a device to measure the distraction force but frequently release and readjust the noninvasive distraction strap during the procedure. Often no distraction is needed for anterior ankle joint arthroscopic surgery.

Contraindications to noninvasive distraction include impaired circulatory status, diabetes, ankle edema, and fragile skin. Disadvantages include inadequate distraction and therefore increased potential for missing the pathology, scuffing articular cartilage, and breaking instruments. The disadvantages are minimized by attention to detail, as mentioned earlier.

Invasive Distraction

Invasive distraction, although rarely required, is indicated if noninvasive distraction does not provide adequate visualization or enough room to perform the arthroscopic procedure. Skeletal or invasive distraction is performed by placing pins (medial or lateral) in the tibia and talus or calcaneus. A threaded distraction device is placed on the pins and is used to open the joint a controlled amount.

Contraindications for invasive distraction include reflex sympathetic dystrophy, open physis, osteopenia, and infection. Disadvantages include a risk to neurovascular structures, infection, pin breakage, and stretching of ligaments beyond their elastic limit or ligamentous disruption. Another significant dis-

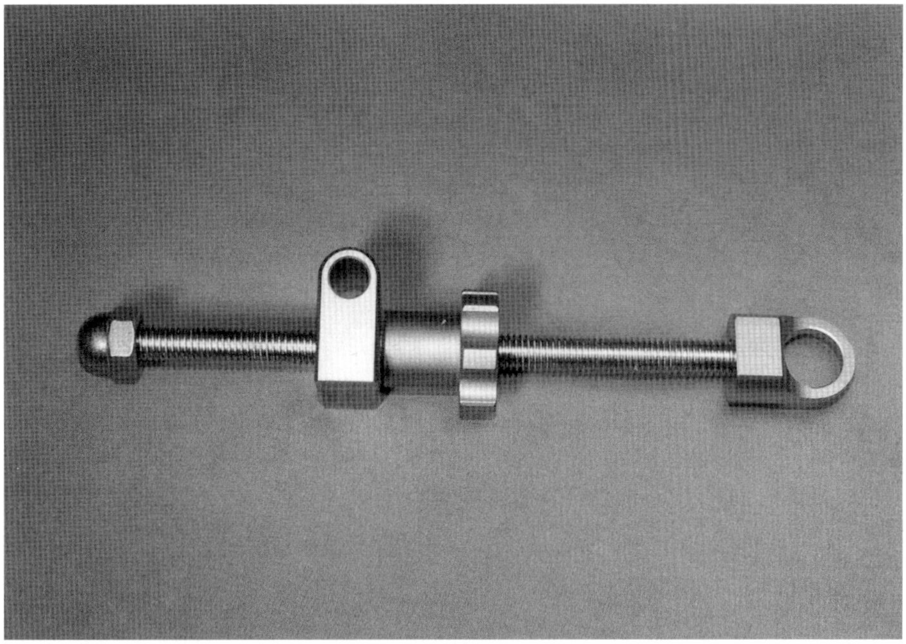

FIGURE 5.5. This device is part of the Guhl noninvasive distractor. It allows fine adjustment of distraction interoperatively.

advantage of invasive distraction is the inability to manipulate the ankle position easily while maintaining distraction during the procedure. Invasive distraction can be performed using unilateral medial or lateral pins or double distraction using through-and-through pins and two distractors.

Lateral Distraction

Two threaded trochar-tipped Steinmann pins measuring 4–5 inches long and 3/16 inch in diameter are used for lateral distraction. The tibial pin is placed 2.5–3.0 inches (6.5–7.0 cm) proximal to the ankle joint line and a thumb's-breadth below the anterior tibial crest. A soft-tissue trocar is used to tunnel through the subcutaneous tissue anterior to the tibialis anterior tendon. A Steinmann pin is placed through the trocar and is drilled across the lateral cortex but not through the medial cortex. The calcaneal pin is placed approximately 1 inch (2.5 cm) anterior and 1 inch (2.5 cm) superior to the posteroinferior calcaneal margin and directed at a 20-

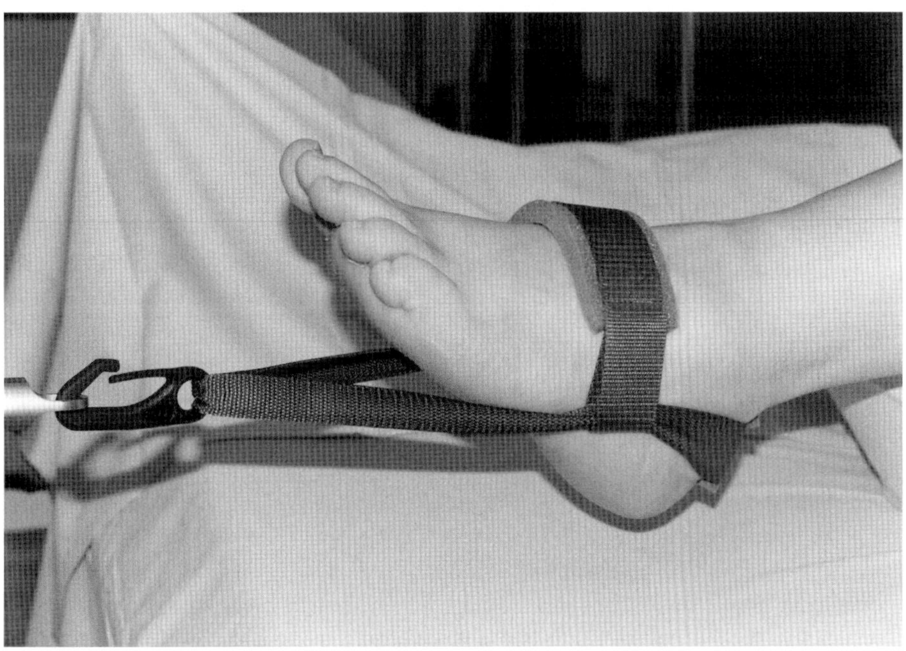

FIGURE 5.6. This prefabricated sterile strap allows ankle arthroscopy using both anterior and posterior portals. (Smith & Nephew Inc./ Arthroscopy—Andover, MA.)

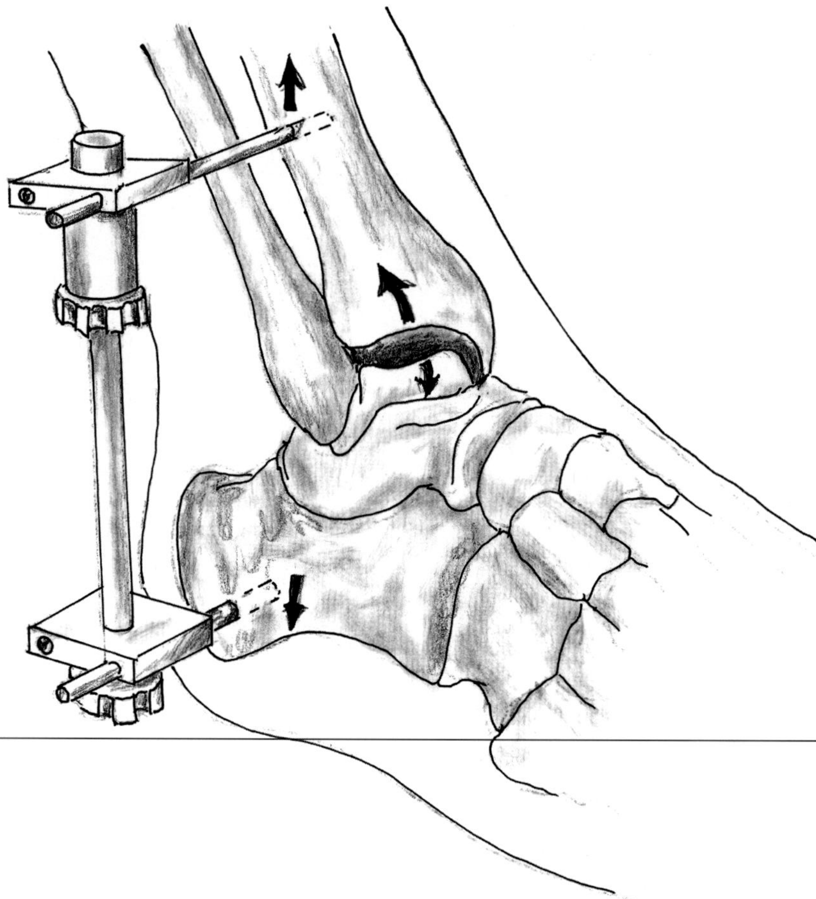

FIGURE 5.7. Invasive distraction is performed by placing threaded pins laterally and applying an external fixator device, as illustrated. Most ankle arthroscopy procedures can be performed with noninvasive distraction.

to 30-degree caudal inclination. This pin should be drilled through the lateral cortex up to but not through the medial cortex. The joint is slowly distracted 4–5 mm. Additional traction is applied as the capsular tissues relax. The pins then assume a near-parallel position. Distraction should not exceed 7–8 mm or 50 lb of force for more than 1.5 hours. Care should be taken to minimize bending of the pins.[4] Figure 5.7 illustrates pin placement for invasive distraction on the lateral side. The superficial peroneal nerve and anterior tibial tendon are at risk of injury with proximal pin placement. The sural nerve, lesser saphenous vein, and peroneal tendon are at risk of injury with distal pin placement.

Medial Distraction

The technique for medial distraction is performed by placing the proximal pin in the medial bare area of the tibia approximately 1.5 inches proximal to the ankle joint line. The distal pin is placed into the talar body just anterior and inferior to the palpable tip of the medial malleolus. This pin should be drilled through the medial cortex up to but not through the lateral cortex. Both pins should be directed 10 degrees anterior and superior while parallel to the joint to avoid the subtalar joint and neurovascular bundle.[5]

INSTRUMENTATION

Arthroscopes

Originally, the 4.0 mm standard rod-lens system arthroscope was exclusively used in the ankle. In some cases, however, this arthroscope is too large in diameter and has too long a lever arm and too large a sheath to allow complete visualization of the ankle joint. This larger arthroscope is thought to allow higher irrigation fluid flow rates through the sheath and therefore continues to be preferred by some surgeons. We now use exclusively 2.7 mm diameter arthroscopes for ankle and foot arthroscopy. This more delicate 2.7 mm arthroscope is required for tight ankles, improving visualization of the gutters, posterior ankle, and subtalar joint. Angulations of 25 or 30 degrees and 70 degrees are useful for visualization in the ankle. The future development and improvement in image quality of smaller-diameter arthroscopes will result in the application of arthroscopic procedures to smaller joints in the foot. Development of a flexible arthroscope may assist the ankle surgeon in the future.

Also important for ankle arthroscopy is an interchangeable cannula system that allows the arthroscope to be switched from portal to portal without reinstrumentation of the portals, thereby decreasing potential injury to the tissue or local nerve branches. A disposable cannula system can be used for arthroscopy of the ankle. The presence of a double seal prevents leakage of fluid medium, and the side port allows inflow or outflow, eliminating the need for accessory portals. These features help protect soft tissues when inserting and removing instruments.

Video Cameras/Monitors/Light Source

Video cameras are of two types: tube and solid state. The older video tube camera is not suitable for ankle arthroscopy because of its large size and weight. Having significant weight on the end of a small-diameter arthroscope can result in breakage due to the lever effect and makes delicate surgery difficult. Currently available solid-state charge-coupled device (CCD) chip cameras are lightweight (2 oz) and provide a high-resolution image when used with a powerful light source. Single-chip and three-chip cameras are available. The three-chip camera offers slightly better image quality. Both types are relatively reliable; but, as with all surgical instruments/equipment, a spare camera should always be available.

A video monitor compatible with the video format of the video camera used for arthroscopy is required. Three video formats are used worldwide but are not compatible. The National Television Systems Committee (NTSC) is the standard for North America, most of South and Central America, and several countries in the Far East. Phase alternating line (PAL) is the standard in most of Europe, Asia, and Africa. Sequential Couleur à Mémoire (SECAM) is used in France and a few other European countries. Some video camera/monitor systems have the capacity to record, monitor, or play in all three formats. These systems are useful for sharing or presenting information with colleagues in other countries.

The resolution of the monitor is another consideration. The better the resolution, the better is the image quality for arthroscopic viewing. Monitors are available with as many as 750 lines of horizontal resolution. However the ultimate image resolution is only as good as the resolution of the imaging device with the least resolution. For example, if a video camera with 300 lines of horizontal resolution is coupled with a monitor with 750 lines of horizontal resolution, the image resolution is only 300 lines. A videotape recorder or video printer can be used for documentation purposes. Currently, the American Board of Orthopaedic Surgery (ABOS) requires pictorial documentation of arthroscopic findings for cases reviewed at the oral examination. Commercially available video printers provide a convenient means for documenting the postoperative explanation of surgical findings to the patient and a means to meet the ABOS requirement.

The light source is extremely important for arthroscopy. The operating room personnel must know how to change the light bulb in the source during the procedure and to operate the source adequately. The light source cable to the arthroscope is a fiberoptic cable that is flexible and easy to sterilize. However, the light-conducting fibers in the cable break and fail to conduct light adequately with time; hence the fiberoptic cables should be checked frequently and replaced if the light transmission capacity is diminished.

Inflow System

Irrigation fluid is required for visualization during foot and ankle arthroscopy. We have no experience with gas (CO_2) for distension but suspect that it would not be suitable because of poor visualization secondary to bleeding or synovial fluid, the inability to irrigate away debris, and the inability to distend the joint secondary to leakage.

Various irrigation solutions can be used for ankle arthroscopy. We use and suggest lactated Ringer's solution because it is physiologically and osmotically compatible with articular cartilage and is rapidly reabsorbed if it extravasates from the joint. Lactated Ringer's solution is also compatible with radiofrequency devices if the surgeon wishes to use them for foot or ankle arthroscopy.

Gravity inflow or an arthroscopic pump can be used for joint irrigation. Gravity works well when the fluid is elevated as high as possible above the patient and is run through a separate inflow cannula or when the arthroscopic sheath cannula has a large enough diameter to provide reasonable flow. High flow tubing and 3-liter fluid bags provide an appropriate pressure head when elevated. Ferkel reported that an inflow cannula with 3.0 mm inner diameter provides a flow rate of 750 ml/min with an inflow fluid bag height of 3 feet.[6] If the 2.7 mm scope is placed in this 3.0 mm cannula, the flow decreases to 75 ml/min. The flow of a 3.7 mm cannula with a 2.7 mm scope in it is 500 ml/min at the same bag height. The 4.5 mm "high flow" cannula with a 4.0 mm scope in it produces a flow rate of 110 ml/min.

Arthroscopic pump systems can provide excellent visualization but require pressure-regulating devices to prevent overdistension or extravasation into soft tissues. Extreme extravasation could result in a compartment syndrome in the foot or leg. We have excellent visualization with gravity inflow and therefore presently cannot justify the risk or expense of the pump systems.

Hand Instruments

Probes

The probe functions as a palpating finger during ankle arthroscopy. Flat-ended and curved-handle probes are designed to evaluate chondral lesions and to adjust to the multiple curvatures and multicompartment aspects of the ankle. Probes for ankle arthroscopy should be 1.0–1.8 mm in diameter and be able to be used through interchangeable cannulas (Fig. 5.8). Probes can have markings to help determine the size of intraarticular lesions, but the markings should be inked on to the metal and not scored into it. Scoring creates stress concentration that can result in breakage.

Knives

Special blades have been designed for the small confines of the ankle joint. The blades are sharp, are resistant to breakage, have magnetic properties, and are disposable. They are short and can be delivered through a cannula system. The blades are either straight or hooked and are sharp on one or both sides. These knives are used for sectioning fibrous bands, plicae, capsular tissue, and ligaments and for excising osteochondral fragments and articular cartilage.

Basket Forceps

Small-joint, short, basket forceps with a variety of tip designs are useful as cutting instruments for débridement. They may be straight, angled right or left, and angled up or down. Figure 5.9 is a basket forceps with suction.

Currettes

Various small-joint, sharp curettes are particularly useful for removing osteochondral lesions, trimming articular cartilage edges, or removing articular cartilage for arthrodesis. They can be straight or curved

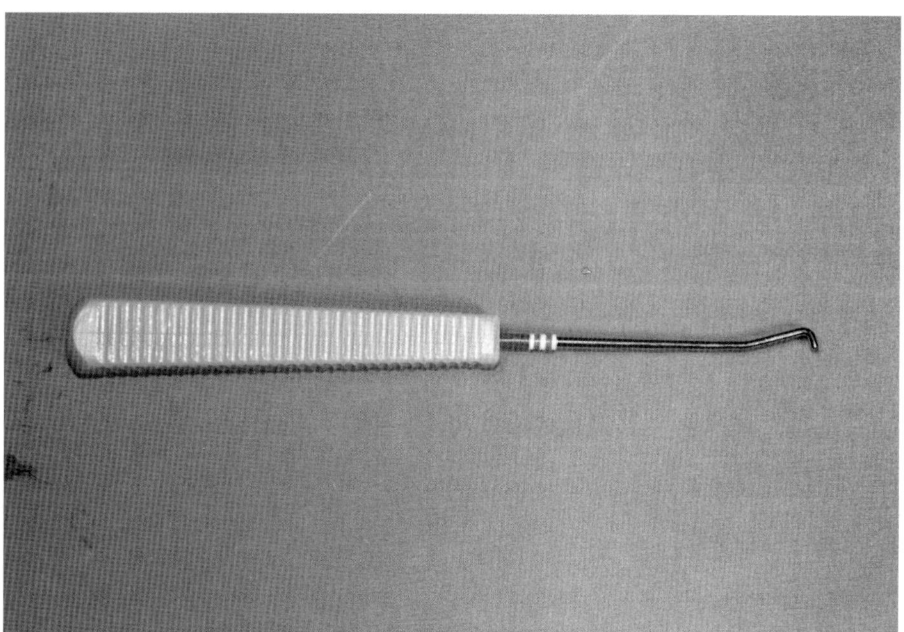

FIGURE 5.8. Ideal probe for ankle arthroscopy is as stout as a probe for a knee joint but shorter.

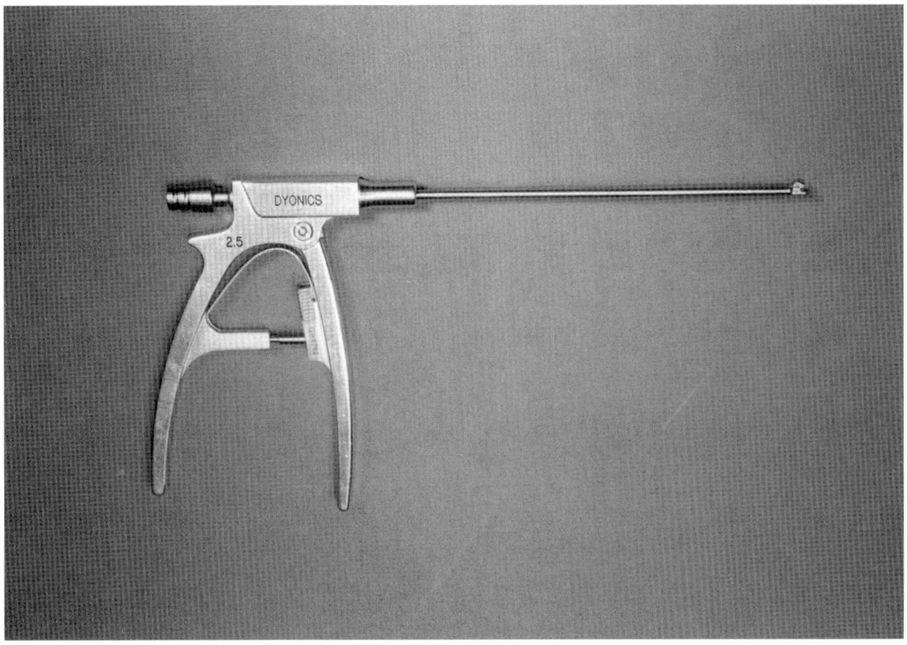

FIGURE 5.9. This instrument is a basket forceps or punch that is cannulated for suction. The suction punch helps prevent the tissue being resected from getting loose in the joint.

and of an open-ring or closed-cup design. They should resist bending and breakage. Small ring curettes are used in only approximately 10 cases and then are discarded before intraarticular fatigue failure occurs. Curved Freer elevators are useful for disrupting adhesions and loosening osteochondral fragments. Three hand instruments are shown in Figure 5.10.

Rasps

Small rasps, both curved and straight, are particularly valuable for modeling areas of the joint surface after excising osteophytes or for abrading tissue and smooth uneven surfaces of exposed cortical bone.

Graspers

The optimal grasper has a flat head, is 2.7–3.0 mm in diameter, and is able to reach all areas of the ankle easily. Graspers are used primarily to remove loose bodies and soft tissue fragments. Pituitary forceps are also useful not only for grasping loose debris but for trimming osteophytes and débriding scar

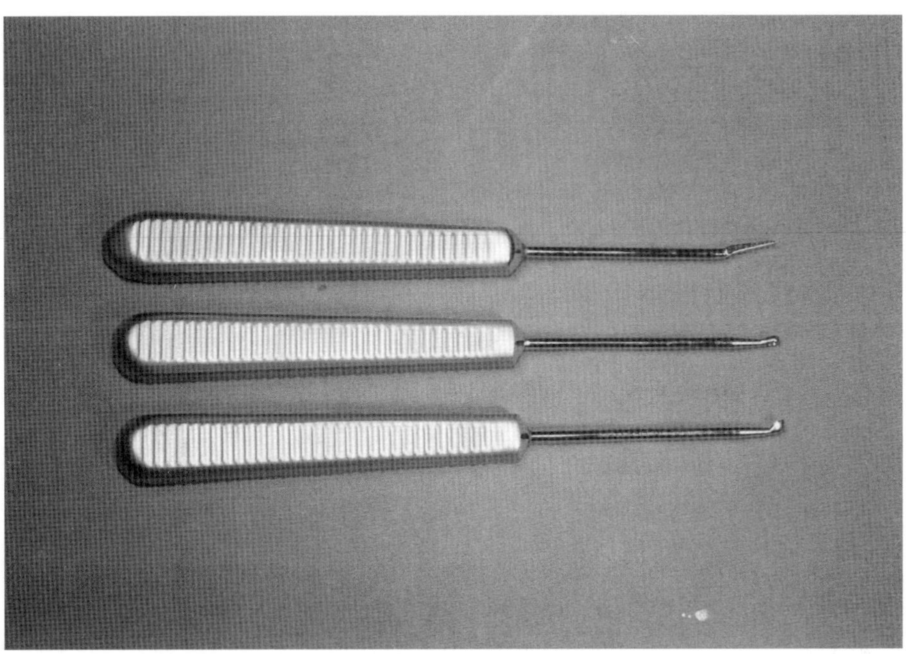

FIGURE 5.10. Hand instruments for tissue resection and elevation between tissue planes.

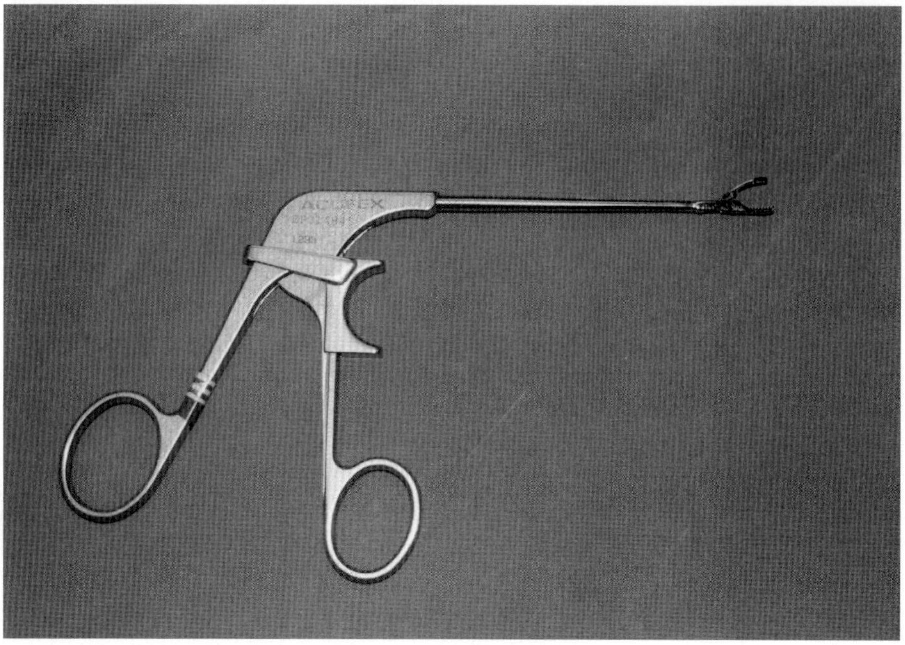

A

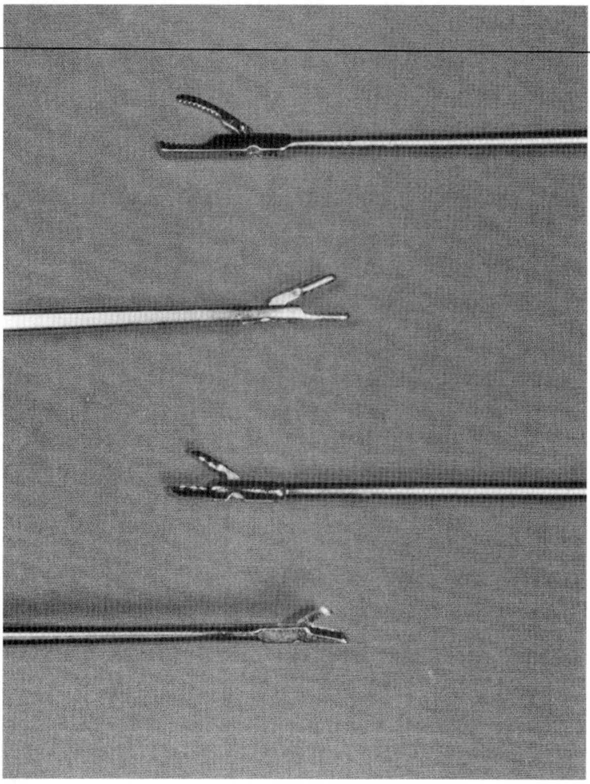

B

FIGURE 5.11. **A:** Arthroscopic tissue grasper. **B:** Four styles of grasping tip for loose body removal and tissue excision.

tissue especially from the medial and lateral gutters. Figure 5.11 shows various graspers.

Osteotomes

Small, sharp osteotomes are useful for removing osteophytes and elevating capsular or periosteal tissue.

Aiming Devices

Aiming devices, such as those used for anterior cruciate ligament reconstruction, are useful for accurate placement of guide pins, drills, and screws. Although the devices designed for the knee work adequately in most instances, a small joint device is available commercially and can be helpful in tight spaces.

Motorized Instruments

Small joint intraarticular shaving systems with 2.0–3.5 mm diameter instruments are used for ankle arthroscopy. As with the larger motorized instruments, suction is applied to the instrument to facilitate drawing the tissue to be cut into the cutting blade or removing the tissue that is being abraded away. The device is helpful, as it can débride the joint of soft tissue more efficiently than simple hand instruments. It is helpful to have a selection of cutting blades readily available in the operating suite. The blades can be divided into three types: full radius resectors, cartilage cutters, and abraders. Motorized instruments are useful for performing synovectomy, débriding adhesions, resecting osteophytes, and abrading exposed cortical surfaces. A power drill and selection of Kirshner wires should be available, as they are useful for drilling the bases of defects or osteocartilaginous craters that are impossible to reach with the motorized shaver.

Retrieving Instruments

Metallic tubes with suction and magnetic properties on one end are crucial during emergency situations for immobilizing and retrieving broken instruments. The combination magnetic tip with suction can greatly simplify removal of a broken instrument tip and can decrease patient morbidity by preventing exploratory arthrotomy.

Repair Instrumentation

Several systems are available for repairing ligamentous injuries. Stapling systems and suture anchor systems can be used to tighten the anterior talofibular ligament. Biodegradable pins can be used to reattach osteochondral lesions of the tibia or talus. The advantage of this device for osteochondrial fixation is its ability to repair small lesions and minimal iatrogenic damage to the articular cartilage. Moreover, there is no need for hardware removal. The disadvantage is its relatively poor fixation strength compared to a screw.

BIBLIOGRAPHY

1. Yates CK, Grana WA. A single-distraction technique for ankle arthroscopy. *Arthroscopy* 1985;4:103–105.
2. Parisien JS. Arthroscopic treatment of osteochondral lesions of the talus. *Am J Sports Med* 1986;14:211–217.
3. Dowdy PA, Amendola A, Brown J, Watson B. Non-invasive ankle distraction: relationship between force, magnitude of distraction and nerve conduction abnormalities. *Arthroscopy* 1996;12:64–69.
4. Guhl JF. New concepts: distraction in ankle arthroscopy. *Arthroscopy* 1988;4:160.
5. Skie MC, Ebraheim NA, Hannum SQ, Podeszwa DA. Anatomic considerations for the placement of distraction pins in the talus. *Foot Ankle* 1994;15:221.
6. Ferkel RD. Instrumentation. In: Ferkel RD (ed) *Arthroscopic surgery: the foot and ankle*. Philadelphia: Lippincott-Raven, 1996;47–48.

CHAPTER 6

Soft Tissue Pathology

Melbourne D. Boynton and James F. Guhl

Soft tissue lesions are usually synovial or fibrocartilaginous in origin and chronic in nature. Soft tissue pathology accounts for approximately 40% of the lesions in the ankle joint amenable to arthroscopic treatment. Most soft tissue lesions amenable to arthroscopic treatment are secondary to trauma and are localized. However, arthroscopic surgery can also be useful for rheumatoid synovitis, chronic synovial chondromatosis, and pigmented villonodular synovitis. Soft tissue lesions can occur coincidentally with or secondary to chondral pathology and may be associated with joint instability.

Arthroscopy is a major advance in the treatment of soft tissue lesions of the ankle. Previously, many disabling soft tissue impingement lesions were considered untreatable sequelae of a severe ankle sprain. Arthroscopy not only allows identification of soft-tissue impingement lesions but is a minimally invasive technique for excision.

POSTTRAUMATIC LESIONS

Sprains or fractures of the ankle joint can result in localized synovitis and fibrous scar formation. Ankle sprains are an extremely common injury, occurring during sports and activities of daily living. Ankle sprains account for 45% of basketball injuries, 25% of volleyball injuries, and 31% of soccer injuries.[1] In a survey of 32 health care providers associated with professional athletic teams, lateral ankle sprains were the most common injury of the foot and ankle among the athletes.[2] Chronic symptoms are seen in 40–50% of patients with moderate to severe ankle sprains.[3,4] Although some patients develop painful instability after an inversion injury to the ankle, others have pain alone, with no feeling of instability. A localized soft tissue reaction can occur after an ankle sprain.[3,4] With a localized synovial or hyalinized fibrocartilaginous scar reaction, motion of the ankle can cause impingement by the talus or distal tibia. These space-occupying soft tissue lesions cause pain and occasionally swelling with impingement. Chronic impingement can result in further hypertrophic synovium or fibrocartilage formation.

Injury of the anterior talofibular ligament and inferior band of the anterior tibiofibular ligament can result in fibrocartilaginous scar formation at the anterolateral corner of the ankle joint. The hemarthrosis that occurs with these injuries can result in a fibroblastic response with fibrous tissue hypertrophy. The hemarthrosis can also result in a synovitis that can become chronic.[5]

Chronic synovitis and fibrocartilaginous hypertrophy results in a mass of inflamed tissue that is most often seen in the anterolateral gutter of the ankle joint. The same painful mass is occasionally seen anteromedially, posteriorly, or at the interarticular portion of the syndesmosis. Most often with posterior impingement symptoms, there is loose chondral debris in the posterior recess responsible for the chronic irritation that leads to the synovitis.

Anterolateral Impingement

Soft tissue impingement of the ankle is most often seen anterolaterally. At this location, any reactive synovitis or fibrocartilaginous scar can be impinged upon by the talus between the anterior tibia, the corner bounded by the anterior tibia and fibula, or both. This phenomenon was described in 1950 by Wolin et al., who treated nine patients with chronic pain and swelling at the anterolateral corner of the ankle after an ankle sprain.[6] They described a mass of hypertrophied fibrocartilaginous scar tissue that was being impinged upon with motion of the ankle. They termed this scar tissue a "meniscoid lesion" because it was similar in appearance to a knee meniscus. Open excision of this tissue resulted in relief of pain in all of their cases (Figs. 6.1, 6.2).

The development of localized hypertrophied synovium or hyalinized-appearing scar tissue after an ankle sprain can be due to two causes. Reactive synovium can form and become chronically painful secondary to the hemarthrosis of a single injury or repeated injuries. Second, the instability that results from disruption of the anterior tibiofibular ligament can result in altered ankle joint kinematics. Such instability allows the scar tissue at the anterolateral corner of the ankle to be pinched between the talus and tibial plafond or in the lateral gutter between the talus and the fibula. Instability of the ankle is not required for anterolateral soft tissue impingement to occur, but it can be a cause of impingement symptoms.

Impingement of the talus on the anteroinferior tibiofibular ligament's most distal fascicle was described by Bassett et al. after a rear foot inversion injury.[7] During arthroscopy this ligament is sometimes seen below the articular edge of the distal tibia. It can be a primary cause of impingement symptoms if it is thickened or scarred from injury. The fascicle can also predispose an ankle to impingement. After a mild inversion injury, an ankle with a large distal fascicle of the anteroinferior tibiofibular ligament can develop significant symptoms due to mild hypertrophy of the synovium simply because of the space-occupying effect of the fascicle.

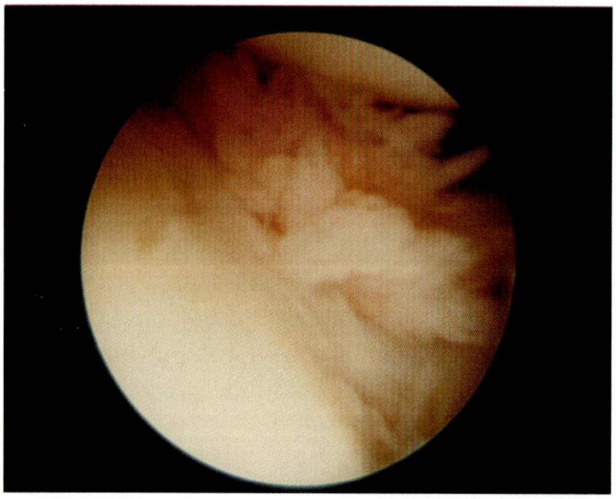

FIGURE 6.1. Local subacute synovitis typical of what occurs a few months following a sprain of the right ankle. At a later date it may become chronic and develop into a synovial impingement lesion.

The typical chief complaint of anterolateral impingement lesions is pain with activities of daily living after an inversion ankle injury (or more) that has not resolved over several months. Often the inciting sprain is described as mild. The pain is made worse by climbing stairs or prolonged standing or walking, and sometimes the patient complains of an inability to run. The patient may have a feeling of instability, but this complaint is not a diagnostic prerequisite. A complaint of instability or "giving way" can be confusing, as the symptom may be due to true mechanical instability secondary to ligamentous insufficiency, or it may be due to intermittent pain causing the feeling of giving way. Rest usually results in complete but temporary relief of pain. The patient may note some mild swelling when comparing this ankle to the contralateral ankle.

Physical examination reveals localized palpable tenderness at the anterolateral corner of the ankle joint. The tenderness can be over the anterior syndesmosis and can extend inferiorly around the anterior gutter over the fibula. Occasionally, there is tenderness in the sinus tarsi, but it is mild compared to the anterolateral corner. If the tenderness in the sinus tarsi is more than mild, the examiner should question the diagnosis of anterolateral soft tissue impingement. It is also important to examine the subtalar joint for decreased motion and localizing tenderness. As with any musculoskeletal examination, it is extremely important to localize the area of maximum tenderness, thereby helping to rule out other diagnoses.

Often the examiner can palpate scar tissue or a boggy fullness at the anterolateral corner compared with the normal ankle. Pain is often elicited by passive forceful dorsiflexion of the ankle. Having the patient actively dorsiflex the unloaded ankle frequently does not elicit the pain; however, asking the patient to squat from a standing position with the ankle loaded frequently localizes the impingement-induced pain.

Most patients have no positive findings on plain radiographs, but it is obviously important to obtain a three-view ankle series to rule out bony pathology. Rarely some dystrophic calcification or heterotopic ossification is seen in the syndesmotic ligaments,[8] and often a bony spur is seen on the anterior tibia or neck of the talus predisposing the patient to impingement symptoms. Bony pathology is discussed in Chapter 7.

Radionuclide studies are usually normal and are not required when radiography is normal. A magnetic resonance imaging (MRI) scan can be useful to help confirm the diagnosis in the atypical patient. MRI scans have highly variable accuracy depending on the availability of a high-resolution scanner with extremity coil and the experience of the radiologist. MRI is not required to diagnose anterolateral soft tissue impingement in the typical patient.

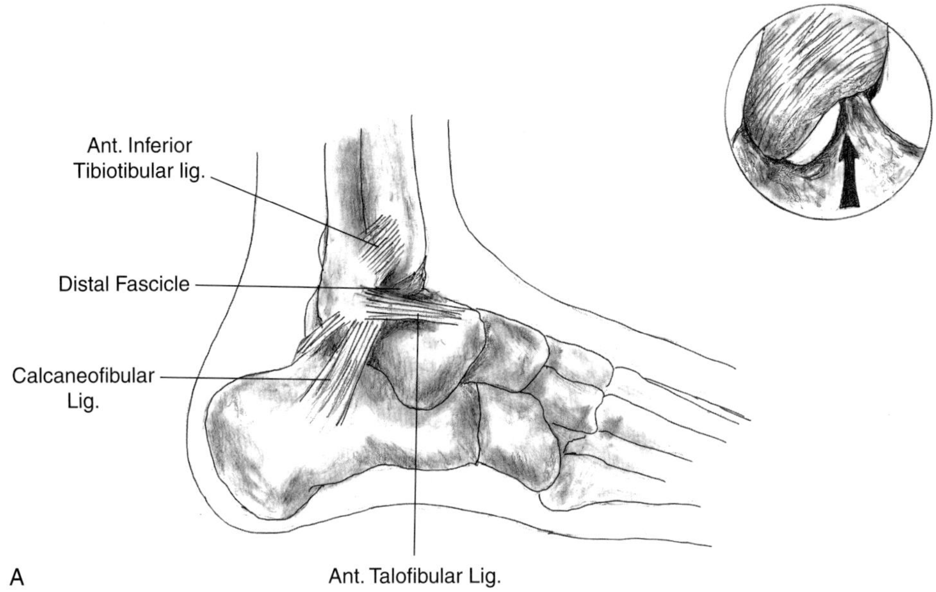

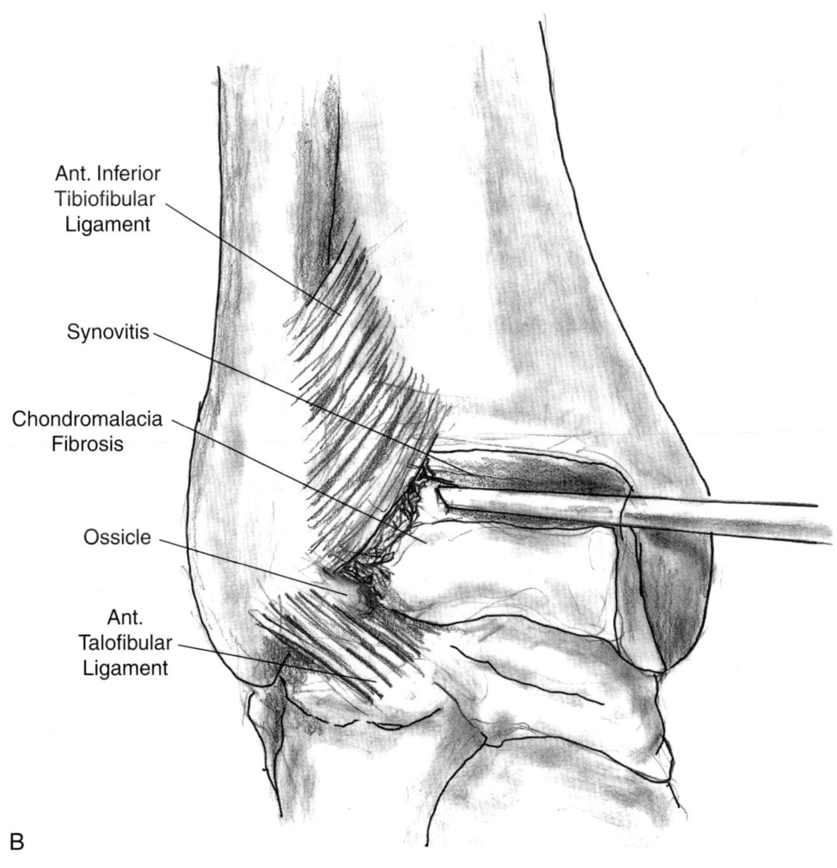

FIGURE 6.2. A: Bassett's ligament, showing the lateral aspect of the ankle joint. The distal fascicle of the anteroinferior tibiofibular ligament is parallel and distal to the anterior tibiofibular ligament proper; it is separated from it by a fibrofatty septum. **Inset.** With dorsiflexion, the distal fascicle of the anteroinferior tibiofibular ligament may impinge on the anterolateral aspect of the talus. **B:** Anteroinferior tibiofibular ligament impingement on the neck of the talus.

An important diagnostic test in patients with soft tissue impingement syndromes is a local anesthetic injection. After sterile preparation of the skin, lidocaine is injected in the area of maximal tenderness around the ankle joint. The local anesthetic can be combined with a corticosteroid preparation. Excellent pain relief is expected with an accurately placed injection, confirming the diagnosis of soft tissue impingement. Occasionally, the steroid decreases the mass of the hypertrophied synovium and obviates the need for arthroscopy. There is some controversy about the safety of an intraarticular cortisone injection, but we believe the risk of a single steroid injection is probably less than the risk of ankle arthroscopy.

Anteromedial or Medial Impingement

Localized anteromedial soft tissue impingement of the ankle can occur, although it seems to be rare. Eversion injury of the ankle can injure the deltoid ligament and anteromedial capsule. Injury to the deltoid ligament or capsule can result in scarring and hyalinization or hypertrophy synovium causing symptoms on the medial side of the ankle.[9] The history and physical findings are similar to those of anterolateral impingement, except the pain, local swelling, and tenderness is medial (Fig. 6.3).

Posterior Impingement

There are four potential posterior soft tissue impingement lesions. First, hypertrophy of the transverse tibia fibular ligament can occur. The ligament is variable in both size and shape.[10] Occasionally the transverse tibiofibular ligament tears, and the subsequent formation of hypertrophic scar tissue can result in painful posterior impingement. A secondary tibial slip of the transverse tibial fibular ligament has been described that, when present, may predispose the ankle to posterior impingement symptoms (Figs. 6.4–6.6).

Second, ballet dancers, who chronically place their ankles in hyperplantar flexion, can develop significant posterior impingement symptoms. It is important to recognize that these symptoms may be due not only to soft tissue impingement but to impingement or injury to an os trigonum.[11,12] Hamilton described a hypertrophied posterior labral structure that he termed the "meniscus of the ankle." He found tears of this hypertrophied posterior tibial labrum in ballet dancers.[13]

Third, kicking athletes, such as football or soccer players, can have violent posterior impaction of the soft tissues between the talus and the tibia. This violent posterior contact occurs intermittently and may result in synovitis. The impaction is exacerbated if the ankle has laxity secondary to injury of the anterior talofibular ligament. With insufficiency of the anterior talofibular ligament, the talus can

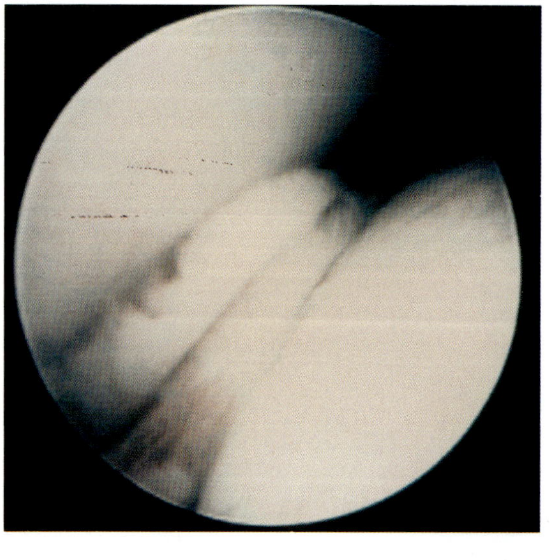

FIGURE 6.3. Ruptured deltoid ligament in medial gutter enfolded on itself. Pain resolved after arthroscopic excision.

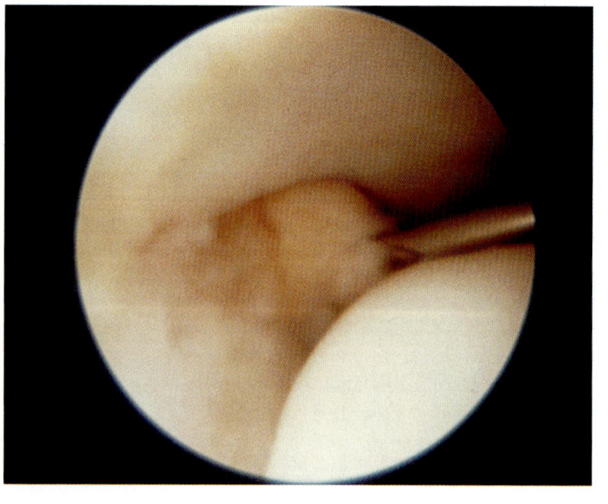

FIGURE 6.4. Typical soft tissue impingement lesion located in the posterolateral corner of the right ankle. The patient had long-standing localized pain and tenderness. Complete relief was obtained after excision.

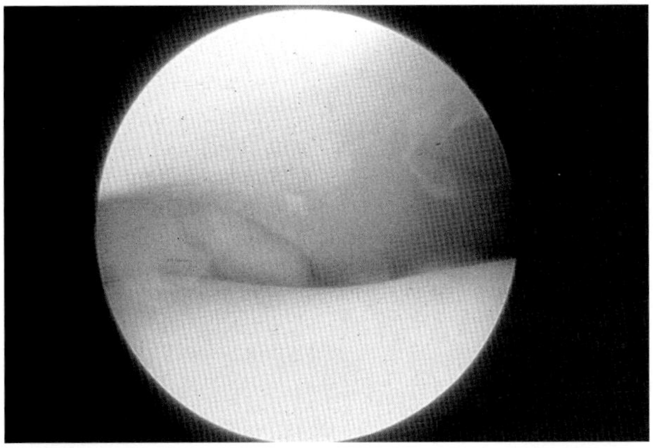

FIGURE 6.5. Soft tissue impingement lesion in the posterolateral aspect of the right ankle joint. It is typical of this pathologic entity. The patient's debilitating pain was completely relieved after excision.

sublux anteriorly during hyperplantar flexion activities. Chronic reactive synovitis may form in the posterior gutter of the ankle joint, causing significant pain and disability. This chronic reactive posterior synovitis is often due to other pathology, such as small, loose chondral debris or postfracture chondral degeneration.

Fourth, a syndesmotic impingement lesion emanating from the intraarticular portion of the distal tibiofibular joint can sit in the posterolateral corner of the ankle and cause posterior impingement symptoms. We have seen cases in which a large piece of synovial tissue is on a pedicle attached at the distal syndesmosis and sits in the posterior recess, causing posterior soft tissue impingement symptoms.

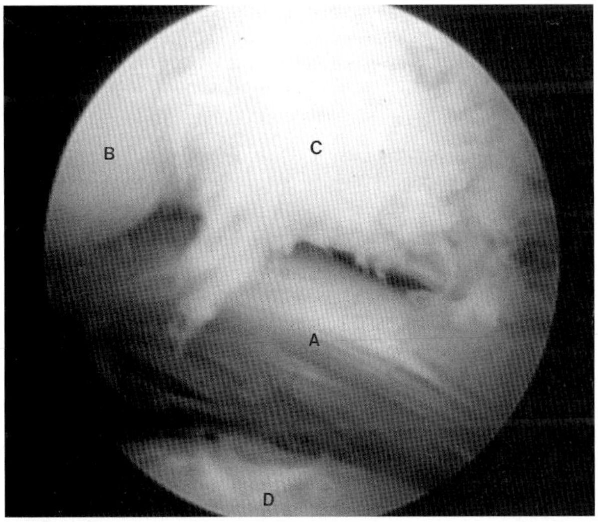

FIGURE 6.6. Enlarged transverse tibiofibular ligament (A) in the posterior compartment of the left ankle joint seen arthroscopically. It may be considered pathologic when other lesions are ruled out and the symptoms are directly related to this structure. Arthroscopic débridement should then be considered. B, plafond; C, synovitis; D, talus.

The clinical complaint with posterior soft tissue impingement is typically pain with any activity that involves forced plantar flexion. It is rare that these patients have pain with walking. If the patient is a ballet dancer, going en pointe causes significant posterior pain. If the patient is a kicking athlete, striking the ball with the foot plantar-flexed results in pain.

On physical examination, localized tenderness posterolaterally and sometimes posteromedially about the ankle joint is typical. Pain with forced plantar flexion posteriorly is typical as well. It is, however, extremely important to consider extraarticular lesions around the ankle when examining for posterior soft tissue impingement. It is our experience that extraarticular diagnoses are a more common cause of posterior pain than is intraarticular soft tissue impingement. It is important to examine the peroneal tendons for tendinitis or subluxation as well as posteromedially for posterior tibial tendon pathology, tarsal tunnel syndrome, and flexor hallucis longus tendinitis (dancers' tendinitis).[14] Flexor hallucis longus tendinitis may result in triggering the great toe (hallux saltans). It is also important to evaluate for a talocalcaneal coalition and Achilles tendinitis. A stress fracture of the calcaneus or instability of the calcaneal cuboid joint can cause confusion when attempting to make a diagnosis of posterior soft tissue impingement.[15]

Radiographs are important to rule out an os trigonum or ossified loose bodies in the posterior recess. A stress plantar flexion radiograph may show impingement, anterior ligamentous laxity, or both. If the patient has an os trigonum, a bone scan is useful for evaluating the possibility of injury to the os trigonum resulting in the posterior pain. We currently obtain a preoperative MRI scan to evaluate for intraarticular versus extraarticular pathology in patients with refractory posterior ankle symptoms because of the complexity of the diagnosis.

Lidocaine and a corticosteroid preparation are injected into the posterior recess of the ankle joint to confirm the diagnosis of posterior ankle impingement. A corticosteroid is never included in the preparation if the injection is into a tendon sheath to evaluate for tendonitis, as it may result in atrophic tendon rupture.[16,17]

Syndesmotic Impingement

Syndesmosis injuries are probably more common than is usually recognized. Severe syndesmotic disruptions are usually recognized, especially if the deltoid ligament is also injured, allowing subluxation of the talus in the mortise. However, subtle syndesmotic injuries can result in chronic intraarticular ankle symptoms without obvious clinical instability. Syndesmotic injuries should be suspected and examined for all ankle sprains. They should be especially considered when the mechanism of injury involves external rotation or hyperdorsiflexion.[18,19] Skiers,[20] soccer players, and wrestlers frequently have syndesmotic injuries. With a syndesmotic injury the anteroinferior tibiofibular ligament can become scarred and hypertrophied as described for anterolateral impingement. Chronic reactive synovitis and synovial nodules can occur at the distal tibiofibular joint and result in soft tissue lesions that are impinged on by the talus in the ankle mortise (Figs. 6.7–6.13). These lesions could not be visualized prior to the use of arthroscopy. Arthroscopy has allowed increased understanding of the existence of these lesions and provides simple treatment as well. A lesion emanating into the articular space from the distal tibiofibular joint can mimic anterolateral or posterolateral soft tissue impingement.

The clinical complaints emanating from syndesmotic impingement lesions are similar to those for anterolateral impingement. The major complaint is pain while standing or walking. Occasionally, the patient has a feeling of catching or locking secondary to a mass effect in the ankle.

On physical examination, these patients typically have localizing tenderness over the distal portion of the anterior syndesmosis. It is often difficult to elicit pain from an intraarticular synovial lesion of the distal tibiofibular joint. When examining for syndesmosis disruption, the squeeze test and external rotation test are usually positive (see Chapter 3); however, in a chronic setting these tests may not be positive. When considering surgery for a patient with syndesmosis impingement, it is im-

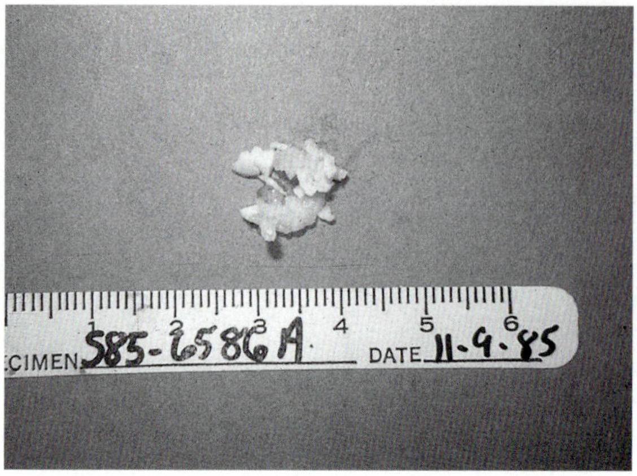

FIGURE 6.8. Aggregate of soft tissue removed from a symptomatic ankle with the diagnosis of a soft tissue impingement lesion.

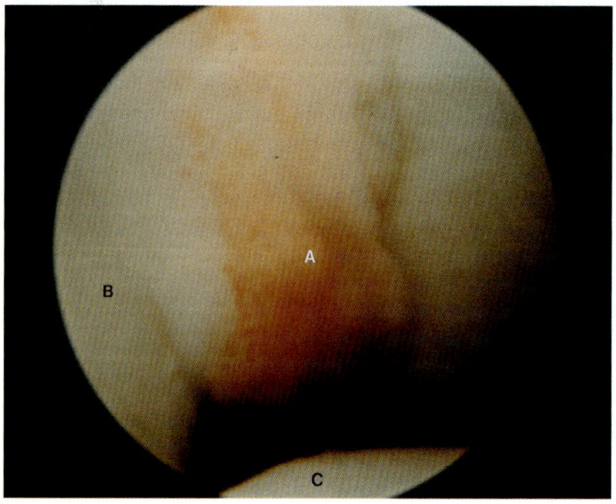

FIGURE 6.7. Typical synovial impingement lesion of the lateral aspect of the right ankle. It arises from the synovial recess of the superior portion of the lateral talomalleolar joint and extends from the anterior to the posterior aspect of the joint. Note the hemosiderin pigment. A, soft tissue impingement; B, fibula; C, talus.

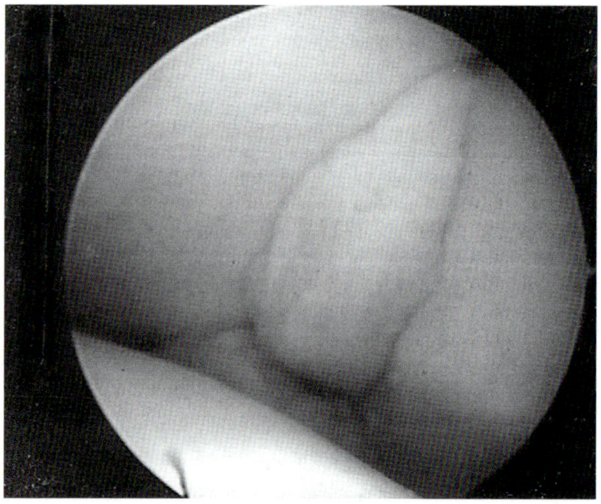

FIGURE 6.9. Anterior-third lateral soft tissue impingement lesion.

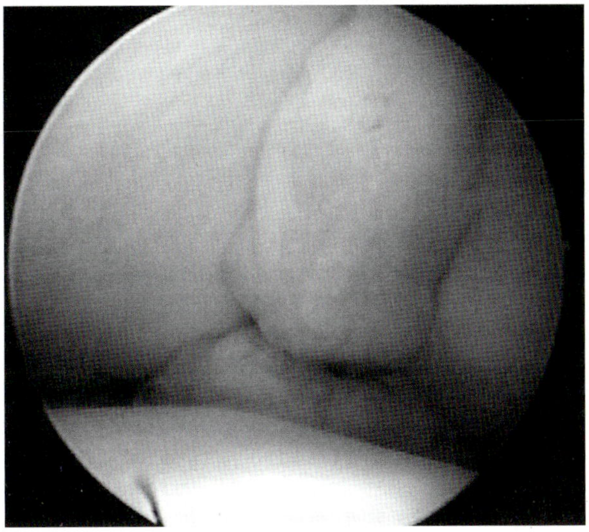

FIGURE 6.10. Middle-third lateral soft tissue impingement lesion.

portant to consider the possibility of chronic syndesmotic instability.

Radiographs are required before considering treatment to rule out bony pathology.[8] It is our experience that an MRI scan is typically not helpful for true syndesmotic impingement lesions. If there is concern about chronic syndesmotic instability at surgery, fluoroscopy is used to determine syndesmotic laxity by obtaining a mortise view with the foot in internal rotation and then a similar mortise view with the foot forcefully rotated externally. If there is significant widening of the mortise, a syndesmotic screw is placed after arthroscopic

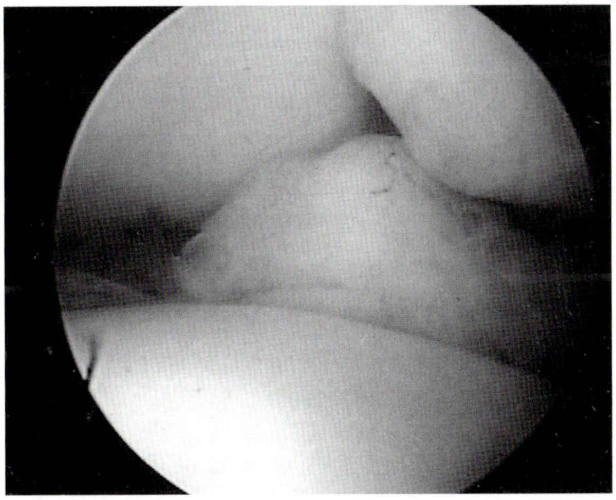

FIGURE 6.11. Posterior-third lateral soft tissue impingement lesion.

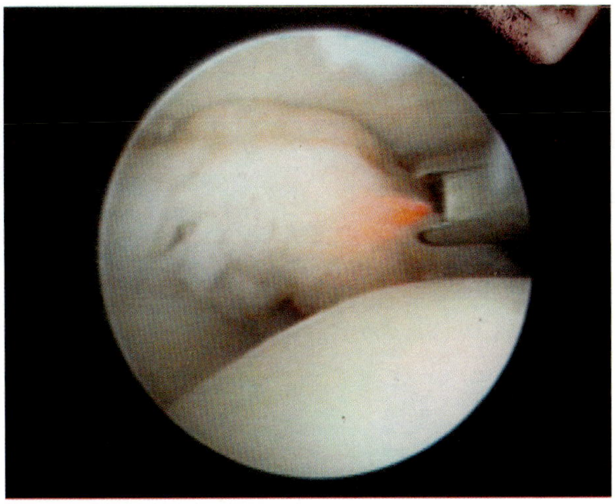

FIGURE 6.12. Arthroscopic view shows laser beam just before ablation of a posterior lateral soft tissue lesion.

débridement is performed. Consideration is also given to an open repair of the syndesmotic ligaments anteriorly.

Arthrofibrosis/Posttraumatic Adhesions

Arthrofibrosis and posttraumatic adhesions can occur after a fracture or after surgery. Treatment of these problems after an ankle fracture is described in Chapter 8. Arthroscopy is valuable for excising adhesions that occasionally occur following a mild to moderate ankle sprain or undisplaced fracture of the distal fibula or medial malleolus. It appears that fractures or ligament disruptions requiring open or closed reduction or surgical repair are not followed by adhesions or soft tissue impingement as often as the less severe injuries. With displaced fractures or ligament tears, intraarticular blood escapes into the surrounding tissue. It also escapes during open reduction/internal fixation. With sprains and undisplaced fractures, there is often a hemarthrosis that is not aspirated and is ultimately absorbed by the synovial joint lining. In some cases a marked cellular response, fibrous tissue reaction, hyalinization, and ultimately chronic synovitis with adhesion formation occurs (Figs. 6.14–6.16).

The symptoms are often more dramatic and less localized then those seen from other soft tissue entities discussed earlier. Occasionally, locking is a major complaint. The feeling of instability can be misinterpreted as a ligament disruption. The patients often experience loud clicking.

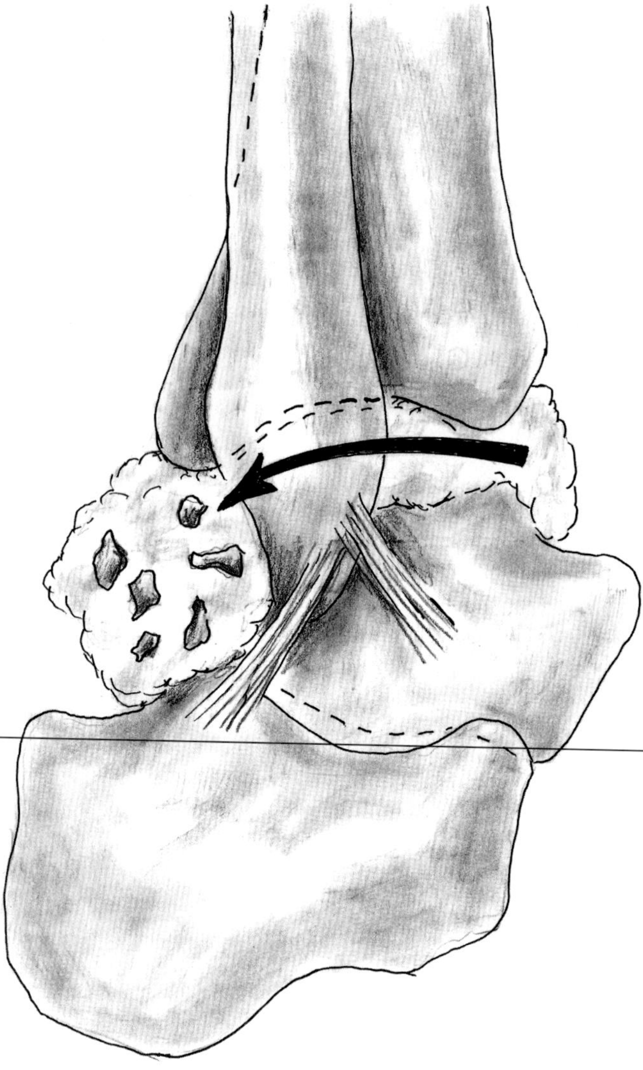

FIGURE 6.13. Chondral loose fragments often migrate to the posterior recess, as the posterior recess is 1.5–2.0 cm larger than the anterior recess.

On physical examination, mild generalized swelling is often seen with variable areas of localized tenderness. Motion is limited. The remaining motion is frequently painful and results in crepitus.

At the time of surgery, multiple fibrous bands or intraarticular adhesions are often seen. Adhesions may form between the tibia and the talus and between the fibula and the talus. The adhesions can range from small minor filaments of tissue to large bands of tissue to severe adhesions with concomitant capsulitis. This type of surgery is difficult, as there is often little room in the articular space at the beginning of the procedure. Extreme care must be taken to avoid further damage to the already friable articular cartilage. The postsurgical prognosis for the more severely affected ankle with adhesions and arthrofibrosis is limited.

ARTHROSCOPIC TREATMENT OF SOFT TISSUE IMPINGEMENT LESIONS

Surgical Technique

Anesthesia is given according to the preferences of the patient, surgeon, and anesthesiologist. Intravenous prophylactic antibiotics are prescribed—usually cefazolin (1 g IV) unless the patient has an allergy. A tourniquet is placed on the thigh. The position of the patient on the operating table is variable. We prefer the patient supine with the thigh supported by a thigh holder. Noninvasive distraction is applied using a sterile clamp attached to the operating room (OR) table. Prior to applying distraction, the skin undergoes routine preparation and sterile draping. Anatomic landmarks are outlined on the skin using a sterile skin marker. Such structures

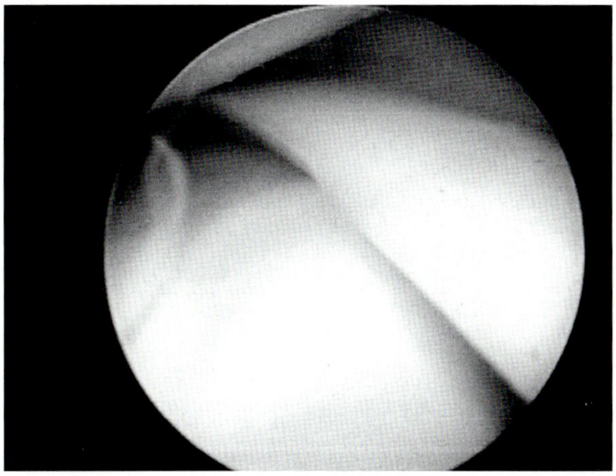

FIGURE 6.14. Arthroscopic view of an adhesion coursing its way over the mid-talus.

include the lateral and medial malleoli, anterior tibialis tendon, dorsalis pedis artery, peroneus tertius tendon, and the visible branches of the superficial peroneal nerve. By placing the foot into plantar flexion and eversion, one can often see the cutaneous branches of the superficial peroneal nerve about the ankle traveling to the foot.

The ankle joint is distended with lactated Ringer's solution using an 18-gauge needle. The ankle joint typically is maximally inflated with 15 ml of solution. The needle is inserted into the ankle joint just medial to the anterior tibialis tendon. Next, the anteromedial portal is created. We use a no. 11 blade scalpel to make a vertical skin incision. Care is taken to cut only the skin. Blunt dissection through the subcutaneous tissues to the joint capsule is carefully performed to avoid injuring the superficial nerves. The joint capsule is then entered

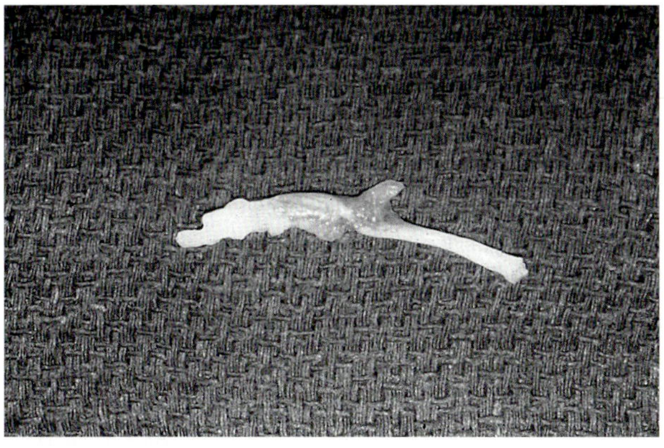

FIGURE 6.15. Gross specimen from the patient in Figure 6.14 after excision.

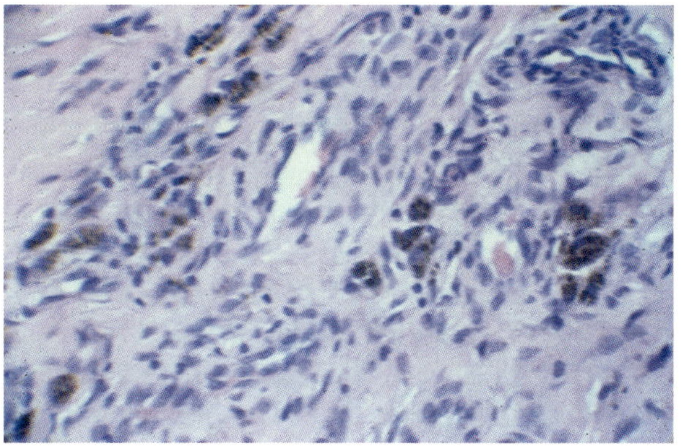

FIGURE 6.16. Histology of the lesion in Figure 6.15. Note the fibrosis, minimal vascularity, hemosiderin, and a few giant cells.

with an obturator in the arthroscopic sheath. The anterolateral portal is created under arthroscopic control using an 18-gauge needle. The needle is placed in the desired location of the portal just lateral to the peroneus tertius tendon at the level of the joint line. After confirming the location with the needle, the portal is created with the same careful technique used to create the anteromedial portal, avoiding injury to the superficial peroneal nerve branches.

After the two anterior portals are created, the arthroscope is maintained in the anteromedial portal and instruments are placed through the anterolateral portal. Inflow is initially placed through the arthroscopic sheath around the arthroscope. A posterolateral portal is created if there is difficulty with visualization or if posterior surgery is needed or expected to be performed. The posterolateral portal is created by distracting the joint. The arthroscope is inserted through the anteromedial portal through the medial notch of Harty to visualize the posterior capsule. An 18-gauge spinal needle is inserted posterolaterally. The spinal needle is started in the skin just lateral to the Achilles tendon approximately 2 cm proximal to the tip of the lateral malleolus. Once the needle is visualized, it is then removed, with care being taken by the operating surgeon to remember the needle's exact three-dimensional position. An arthroscope sheath with an obturator in place is then inserted in the same three-dimensional location and is used to puncture the capsule just distal to the transverse tibial fibular ligament. The cannula is left in place, and the obturator is removed. The posterolateral portal is used for inflow during anterior surgery and for instrumentation and visualization during posterior surgery. Care must be taken with creation and use of the posterolateral portal to avoid injury to the sural nerve or short saphenous vein.

Gentle distraction or occasionally no distraction is required for anterolateral isolated soft tissue impingement lesions. Lesions of the anterolateral corner can easily be identified with the arthroscope in the anteromedial portal. Often early in the procedure hypertrophic synovial tissue must be excised using a small-joint, motorized, full-radius soft tissue resector. Placing the ankle into slight dorsiflexion helps with visualization and makes more room for working on anterior lesions. If the foot is placed in plantar flexion, the anterior space may be closed down, making it difficult to resect hypertrophic synovial tissue safely from the anterior capsular recesses. Anterolateral impingement lesions can be resected in any of the described arthroscopic positions, but we prefer to have the patient supine using a thigh holder. The 70-degree arthroscope can be helpful for viewing and resecting anterolateral lesions as well.

After resecting some of the anterolateral lesion, complete diagnostic arthroscopy of the ankle is performed. This requires switching the arthroscope to the anterolateral portal and occasionally placing the arthroscope in the posterolateral portal. It is common to have coexisting pathologies with any soft tissue impingement syndrome; therefore complete diagnostic arthroscopy of the entire ankle joint is critically important. To complete the excision of the anterolateral impingement lesion, hand instruments may be required to excise the more distal fascicle of the anteroinferior tibiofibular ligament. Care should be taken to avoid injury to the anterior talofibular ligament. Care must also be taken when working anterolaterally or anteromedially to avoid débridement through the anterior capsule. Anterior débridement should always be carried out under direct visualization to avoid injuring the normal anterior capsule or going through the anterior capsule into the dorsal neurovascular bundle.

Often a syndesmotic lesion can be excised with the arthroscope in the anteromedial portal and instruments being placed through the anterolateral portal. The syndesmotic lesion emanating from the distal tibiofibular articulation is simply shaved down to the level of the chondral surface, leaving no soft tissue prominence. If the lesion cannot be excised adequately with the shaver in the anterolateral portal, the arthroscope can be placed in the anterolateral portal and the motorized shaver resector in the posterolateral portal. Alternatively, the arthroscope and shaver can be reversed. Posterior lesions are treated arthroscopically in a similar fashion, often requiring the arthroscope and hand instrument portals to be switched frequently. The portals are closed using 3.0 nylon suture in the skin.

Postoperatively, a bulky compression dressing is used with a splint, which keeps the ankle out of the equinus position. It is left in place for 5–7 days. The patient remains on crutches during this time. At 5–7 days the splint, bulky compression dressing, and sutures are removed; and motion is encouraged. Weight-bearing is permitted as tolerated if no osteochondral pathology is found at surgery. These patients often benefit from an aggressive physical therapy regimen involving active range of motion exercises until normal range of motion is achieved. This is followed by a strengthening program for ankle dorsal flexion, plantar flexion, inversion, and eversion. The program also includes proprioceptive retraining exercises. Patients are told that their symptoms may persist for 3–4 months. Return to activities, including sports, is variable but can be expected by 6–12 weeks after operation.

Results

Arthroscopic excision of anterolateral soft tissue impingement lesions is 80–90% successful in significantly alleviating or eliminating symptoms.[5,21–25] Most patients in published series had localized symptoms secondary to an inversion injury. It is our experience that patients with localized symptoms and a palpable lesion that responds to a local injection and no instability has the best outcome after arthroscopic excision. The literature regarding excision of syndesmotic or posterior lesions is not as plentiful or helpful in predicting postoperative outcomes.

The results of arthroscopic treatment of soft tissue impingement in atheletes has been reported by three investigators.[26–28] DeBerardino et al.[26] reported 85% excellent results in 60 cases of anterolateral impingement in athletes with an average 2-year follow-up, similar to the results of Guhl and Stone.[28] Synovial hyperplasia was universally found in these series along with occasional fibrous bands. They noted that the location of the impinging soft tissues correlated with the clinical examination. They also noted that many athletes had a diffuse pattern of synovitis that seemed to impinge in the anterior and anteromedial compartments. DeBerardino et al. suggested an ankle rating score for surgeons to review the outcome of their patients or compare their patients with those from other series.[26] Although the scoring system has subjective and objective radiographic and functional criteria, it has not yet been truly validated for use as a universal score. Ogilvie-Harris et al. reported similar results for anterior and anterolateral impingement lesions in athletes who underwent arthroscopic treatment.[27]

The overall complication rate for recently reported arthroscopic treatment of soft tissue impingement lesions is about 3%.[24,26,27] The complications in recent series included transient superficial perineal nerve neuropraxia, local numbness around the medial arthroscopic portal, and superficial wound infections that responded to antibiotics and did not progress to septic arthritis. It is possible that the complication rates in reported series are less than might be seen by the occasional ankle arthroscopist. It is reassuring that the reported complications in the large series are for the most part transient and minor, although major complications such as septic arthritis and permanent nerve injuries can occur.[22]

INFLAMMATORY DISORDERS/SYNOVITIS

Rheumatoid Arthritis

Rheumatoid arthritis is a disorder of the immune system that affects the joints. The exact etiology is unknown. Rheumatoid arthritis is known to affect any joint with articular cartilage and synovium. Pain with decreased range of motion in the subtalar joint can be an early finding of rheumatoid arthritis. Any joint in the body can be affected including the ankle. In most cases there is synovial hyperplasia with villous and papillary formation with necrosis. Areas of articular cartilage necrosis may be a late feature of the disease. Disease-related symptoms may be due to reactive inflammatory synovitis or the loss of articular cartilage (Fig. 6.17).

Arthroscopy can be useful for complete synovectomy in the ankle joint affected by rheumatoid arthritis. A more complete synovectomy can be performed in the ankle joint arthroscopically than can be performed with open techniques. The other advantage of arthroscopic synovectomy is that there is less scarring than occurs with an open procedure and therefore less stiffness. With rheumatoid arthritis, at arthroscopy the synovial lining is typically proliferative and thickened. "Rice bodies" can be seen in the synovium that are thought to result from areas

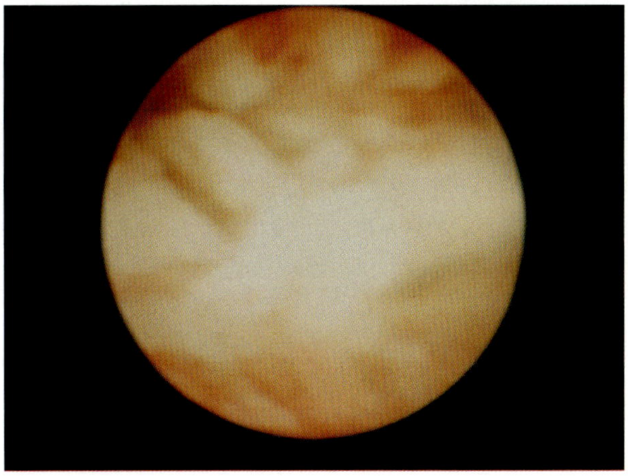

FIGURE 6.17. Arthroscopic view of rheumatoid synovitis (and arthritis) of the right ankle. Note the villous formation. (Courtesy of J.S. Parisien.)

of surface necrosis in the synovial villae. Treatment of a rheumatoid joint by synovectomy is controversial, and there are no reported series regarding the procedure on the ankle. Some state that early synovectomy provides better results in the knee joint than later synovectomy and that early synovectomy may provide increased joint function for several years.[29] Others believe that the risks of the procedure do not outweigh the benefits.[30]

Crystalline Synovitis

Pseudogout or gout can occur in the ankle, as in the knee, if nonoperative treatments have been exhausted and the joint remains inflamed, extensive lavage with the arthroscope can result in a marked decrease in symptoms. Arthroscopic lavage is less traumatic and more efficacious than open lavage (Fig. 6.18).

Infectious Synovitis

Infectious synovitis or septic arthritis of the ankle is amenable to arthroscopic treatment. The purulent effusion can be evacuated arthroscopically. The fibrin clot, containing bacteria, can be completely débrided from the joint arthroscopically as well. Occasionally, repeat arthroscopic irrigation and débridement is required for the treatment of septic arthritis. When treating an ankle joint or subtalar joint for septic arthritis, it is important to be aware of the possibility of a coexisting septic tenosynovitis around the ankle that cannot be treated by arthro-

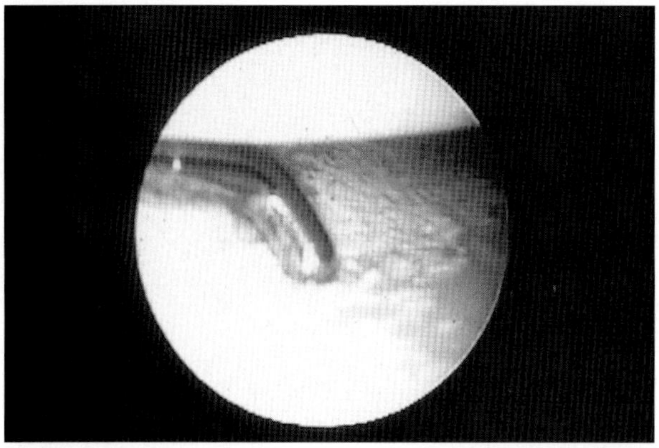

FIGURE 6.18. Crystalline synovitis. Note the probe with crystals on the talar dome.

scopic lavage and débridement of the ankle joint. Open débridement of the infected tendon sheath is required. We have seen septic arthritis of the subtalar joint and septic tenosynovitis of the flexor hallucis longus together.

Hemophilic Arthropathy

The ankle is a common joint for a hemophilic hemarthrosis. Frequently the ankle is said to be a "target joint." Once hemarthrosis occurs, the synovium begins to hypertrophy. As the synovium hypertrophies further, the joint is at increased risk for recurrent hemarthrosis. With each subsequent bleed, there is synovial proliferation. This continued proliferation predisposes the ankle to further hemarthrosis. The hypertrophic synovium secretes enzymes that degrade articular cartilage. These enzymes and the enzymes released with the hemarthrosis, damage the articular cartilage and can result in hemophilic arthropathy, which may require fusion.

Arthroscopic synovectomy can be used to decrease the frequency of hemarthroses. The assistance of the patient's hematologist to correct deficient factor levels prior to and after surgery is required for arthroscopic synovectomy just as it is for an open procedure. The patient is usually hospitalized for the procedure to allow monitoring and treatment of clotting factor deficiencies. Radioactive synovectomy can be performed in place of arthroscopic synovectomy with good early results. For radioactive synovectomy a radioactive isotope is injected into the ankle and is taken up by the synovium, subsequently resulting in synovial necrosis.[31]

Degenerative Synovitis

Posttraumatic degenerative conditions are occasionally amenable to arthroscopic treatment (see Chapter 8). An ankle with posttraumatic degeneration or primary osteoarthritic degeneration is typically unlikely to respond to arthroscopic débridement unless there are highly localized focal anterior impingement symptoms.[32] If the symptoms are severe and not responsive to nonoperative measures such as medications and bracing, arthroscopic ankle arthrodesis is most often the appropriate treatment (see Chapter 10).

Miscellaneous Disorders

Congenital Plicae

Plicae are common in the knee but rarely symptomatic. They are rarely seen in the ankle and even more rarely are symptomatic. Occasionally a congenital band is seen in the ankle, but there are few data regarding symptomatology from these congenital bends. It is seemingly harmless to excise the congenital band arthroscopically when it is an incidental finding during arthroscopy for another purpose (Fig. 6.19).

Neoplastic Disorders

Several benign neoplastic processes that occur in the ankle can be well treated arthroscopically. Presently, there is no role for arthroscopy when dealing with malignant neoplasms of the foot or ankle.

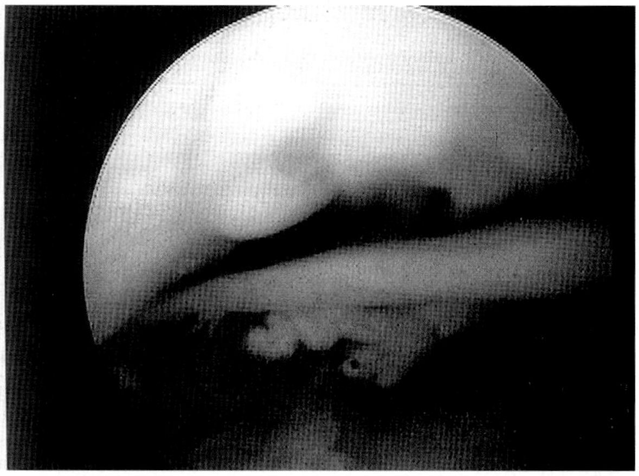

FIGURE 6.19. Congenital plica, posterior recess adjacent or close to transverse tibiofibular ligament.

Pigmented Villonodular Synovitis

Because pigmented villonodular synovitis (PVNS) can recur after excision, we consider it a benign neoplastic process. It is seen in two forms: a localized circumscribed lesion and generalized synovitis. Clinically, the ankle joint shows evidence of chronic synovitis with generalized swelling, aching, and pain aggravated by activity. Radiographs are usually negative. MRI scans often reveal swollen synovial tissue and evidence of hemosiderin deposits (Figs. 6.20, 6.21).

At arthroscopy, there is synovitis with advanced papillary formation and more pigment (hemosiderin) than is seen with inflammatory synovitis. Localized pedunculated or circumscribed lesions respond well to arthroscopy with little chance of recurrence. Recurrence is common with generalized PVNS of the ankle.

Synovial Chondromatosis

Synovial chondromatosis can occur in the ankle. This disease has been described to occur in three stages.[32] Stage I is synovial involvement only, with chondral fragments in the synovial membrane but no loose bodies. Stage II comprises active synovial disease or synovitis with formation of numerous loose bodies (often hundreds) in the joint. During early stage II there is usually no osteoid involvement, and therefore the loose bodies are not seen on radiographs. Later, during the second stage, there is bone formation in the loose osteochondral fragments. The fragments are then seen on radiographs. In stage III the synovitis becomes inactive, leaving multiple osteochondral loose bodies. In addition to the loose bodies, there is often local articular cartilage damage and early degenerative arthritis due to mechanical disruption of the articular surface by the loose bodies (Figs. 6.22–6.24).

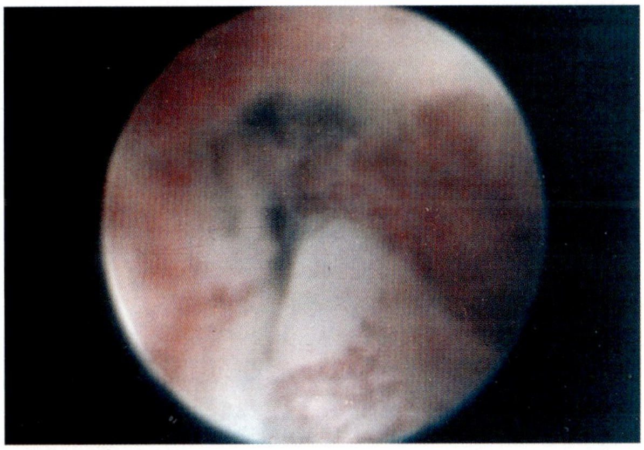

FIGURE 6.20. Arthroscopic view of pigmented villonodular synovitis (PVNS).

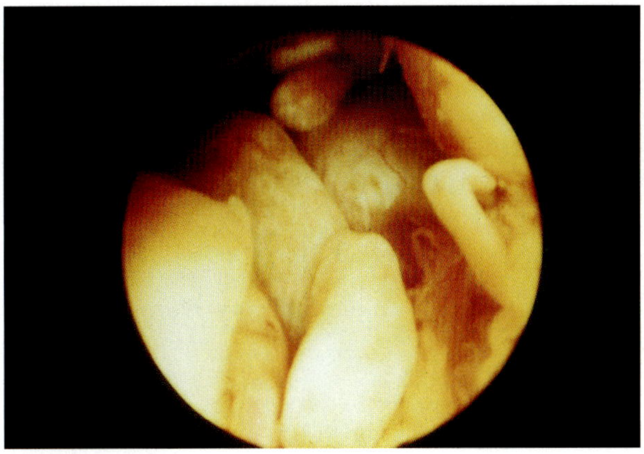

FIGURE 6.21. Another case of advanced pigmented villonodular synovitis.

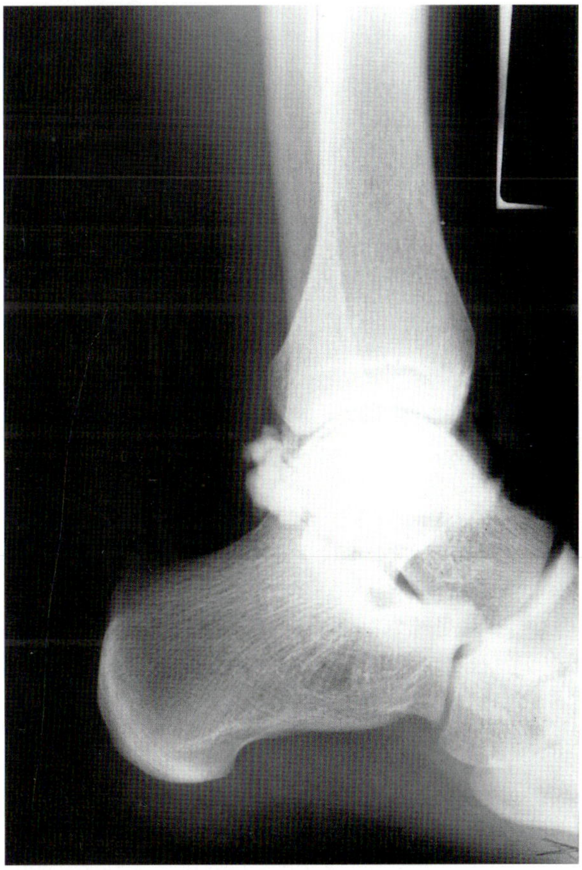

FIGURE 6.22. This lateral arthrogram shows synovial chondromatosis in the posterolateral corner.

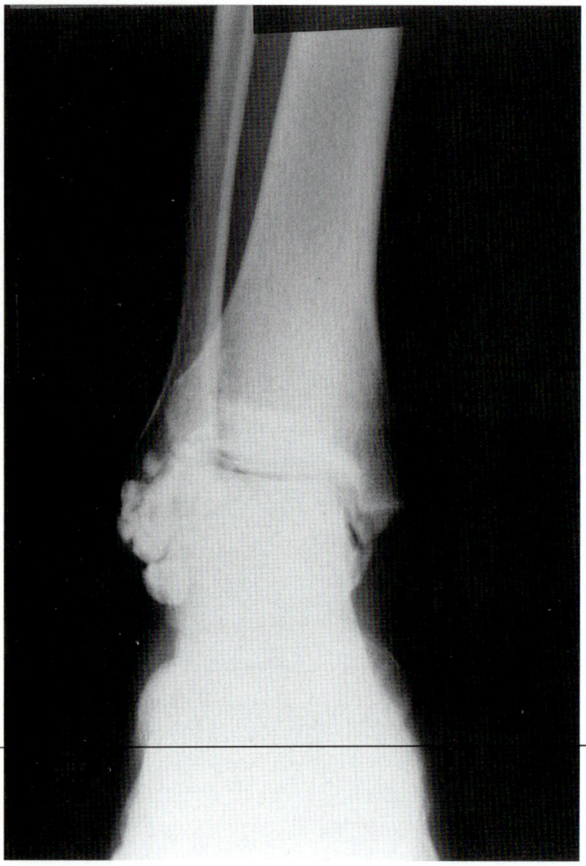

FIGURE 6.23. Anteroposterior arthrogram shows synovial chondromatosis in the posterolateral aspect of the right ankle. It was not seen on routine radiography.

The clinical findings of synovial chondromotosis depend on the stage. Typically, there is limited range of motion with mechanical locking, swelling, and palpable synovium or nodules about the ankle joint. MRI is useful for diagnosing synovial chondromatosis prior to ossification of the chondral loose bodies during stage II.

Arthroscopy is an excellent technique for diagnosing and treating synovial chondromatosis. Synovectomy must be performed during stage I or II, with loose body removal conducted during the later stage. Stage III requires arthroscopic removal of the loose bodies with no need for synovectomy. A posterolateral portal is used to examine the posterior recess for loose bodies or chondral debris in the synovium. It is important to recognize that loose bodies are frequently present in conjunction with conditions other than synovial chondromatosis, such as osteochondritis dissecans, osteochondral fractures, and degenerative joint disease. A synovial biopsy can help establish the diagnosis of synovial chondromatosis in selected cases.

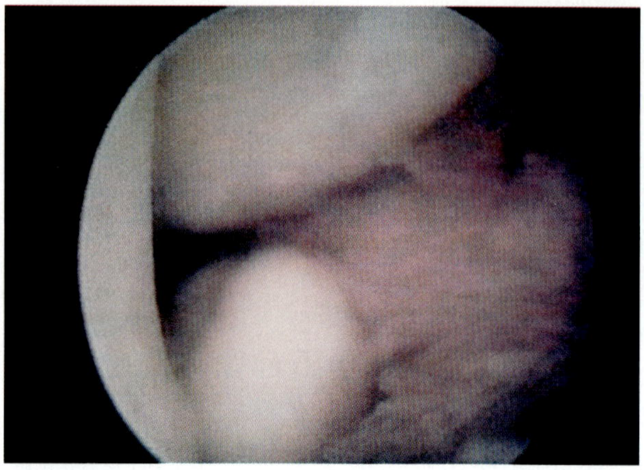

FIGURE 6.24. Same case as in Figures 6.22 and 6.23. Note the loose body in the medial talomalleolar joint and the inflamed synovium.

The recurrence rate for synovial chondromatosis after open surgery (arthrotomy) is about 5%. No series of arthroscopically treated cases has been reported.

ARTHROSCOPIC ANKLE SYNOVECTOMY: TECHNIQUE

Total or near-total synovectomy of the ankle can be performed arthroscopically.[33] Although there are no reported studies regarding the efficacy of arthroscopic total synovectomy or the ability to perform a total synovectomy, we suspect that arthroscopic synovectomy can be performed that would leave less than 5% of the synovium remaining. To perform near-total synovectomy, a posterolateral portal and two anterior portals are required. Functional distraction is essential. Both 30- and 70-degree 2.7-mm arthroscopes are used. The procedure is tedious. When excising synovium from the anterior capsule extreme care must be taken to avoid injury to the neurovascular bundle. Similarly, when excising the synovium from the posteromedial capsule, one must be careful to avoid injuring the posteromedial neurovascular bundle. Attention to detail must be applied to the inflow/outflow system to maintain good visualization without distending the extraarticular soft tissues. As with nearly all ankle arthroscopy in our center, gravity inflow is suitable for arthroscopic synovectomy. The arthroscope and instruments are switched from portal to portal frequently during synovectomy. An interchangeable cannula system is helpful to avoid loss of the portals, particularly posteriorly, and to avoid injury to the soft tissues around the portals.

Arthroscopic synovectomy of the ankle is a difficult procedure and is best performed by a surgeon with significant experience with ankle arthroscopy. The procedure is clearly efficacious in terms of infection. Most crystalline arthropathies are likely to respond to conservative measures and so do not require ankle arthroscopy. It is important to realize that synovectomy in patients with rheumatoid arthritis is controversial; and at present no studies have demonstrated that arthroscopic synovectomy in the presence of rheumatoid arthritis is the optimal treatment. Chronic synovitis in those with hemophilia can be treated with radioactive synovectomy, thereby avoiding or decreasing the need for arthroscopy. The most common arthroscopic procedure performed on the hemophiliac ankle at our center is arthroscopic ankle arthrodesis (see Chapter 9).

BIBLIOGRAPHY

1. Garrick JG. The frequency of injury, mechanism of injury, and epidemiology of ankle sprains. *Am J Sports Med* 1977;5:241–242.
2. Moseley JB, Chimenti BT. Foot and ankle injuries in the professional athlete. In: Baxter DE (ed) *The foot and ankle in sport.* St. Louis: Mosby-Year Book, 1995;321–325.
3. Freeman M. Instability of the foot after injuries to the lateral ligament of the ankle. *J Bone Joint Surg Br* 1965;47:669.
4. Smith RW, Reischl SF. Treatment of ankle sprains in young athletes. *Am J Sports Med* 1986;14:465–471.
5. Ferkel RD, Karzel RP, Del Pizzo W, et al. Arthroscopic treatment of anterolateral impingement of the ankle. *Am J Sports Med* 1991;19:440–446.
6. Wolin I, Glassman F, Sideman S. Internal derangement of the talofibular component of the ankle. *Surg Gynecol Obstet* 1950;91:193–200.
7. Bassett FH, Gates HS, Billys JB, et al. Talar impingement by the anteroinferior tibiofibular ligament: a cause of chronic pain in the ankle after inversion sprain. *J Bone Joint Surg Am* 1990;72:55.
8. Taylor DC, Englehardt DL, Bassett FH III. Syndesmosis sprains of the ankle: the influence of heterotopic ossification. *Am J Sports Med* 1992;20:147–150.
9. Egol KA, Parisien JS. Impingement syndrome of the ankle caused by a medial meniscoid lesion of the ankle. *Arthroscopy* 1997;13:522–525.
10. Chen Y. Arthroscopy of the ankle joint. In: Watanabe M (ed) *Arthroscopy of small joints.* New York: Igaku-Shoin, 1985.
11. Hamilton WG. Stenosing tenosynovitis of the flexor hallucis longus tendon and posterior impingement upon the os trigonum in ballet dancers. *Foot Ankle* 1982;3:74.
12. Quirk R. Talar compression syndrome in dancers. *Foot Ankle* 1982;3:65–68.
13. Hamilton WG. Foot and ankle injuries in dancers. *Clin Sports Med* 1988;7:160.
14. Hamilton WG. Tendonitis about the ankle joint in classical ballet dancers. *Am J Sports Med* 1977;5:84–88.
15. Marshall P, Hamilton WG. Cuboid subluxation in ballet dancers. *Am J Sports Med* 1992;20:170–175.
16. Ford LT, DeBender J. Tendon rupture after local steroid injection. *South Med J* 1979;72:827.
17. Sammarco GJ. Injuries to the tibialis anterior, peroneal tendons, and long flexors and extensors of the toes. In: Baxter DE (ed) *The foot and ankle in sport.* St. Louis: Mosby-Year Book, 1995;58.
18. Edwards GS, DeLee JC. Ankle diastasis without fracture. *Foot Ankle* 1984;4:305.
19. Hopkinson WJ, et al. Syndesmosis sprains of the ankle. *Foot Ankle* 1990;10:325.
20. Fristchy D. An unusual ankle injury in top skiers. *Am J Sports Med* 1989;17:282.
21. Liu SH, Raskin BS, Osti L, et al. Arthroscopic treatment of anterolateral ankle impingement. *Arthroscopy* 1994;10:215–218.
22. Martin DF, Baker CL, Curl WW, et al. Operative ankle arthroscopy: long-term follow-up. *Am J Sports Med* 1989;17:16–23.
23. Meislin RJ, Rose DJ, Parisien S, Springer S. Arthroscopic treatment of synovial impingement of the ankle. *Am J Sports Med* 1993;21:186–189.
24. Amendola A, Petrik J, Webster-Bogaert S. Ankle arthroscopy: outcome in 79 consecutive patients. *Arthroscopy* 1996;12:565–573.
25. Cerulli G, Caraffa A, Buompadre V, Bensi G. Operative arthroscopy of the ankle. *Arthroscopy* 1992;8:537–540.
26. DeBerardino TM, Arciero RA, Taylor DC. Arthroscopic treatment of soft-tissue impingement of the ankle in athletes. Arthroscopy 1997;13:492–498.
27. Ogilvie-Harris DJ, Gilbart MK, Chorney K. Chronic pain following ankle sprains in atheletes: the role of arthroscopic surgery. *Arthroscopy* 1997;13:564–574.
28. Guhl JF, Stone JW. Lateral soft tissue impingement lesions in the ankle joint. *Clin Sports Med* 1991;4:677–687.
29. Goldie IF. Synovectomy in rheumatoid arthritis: the-

oretical aspects and a 14-year follow-up in the knee joint. *Reconstr Surg Traumatol* 1981;18:2.

30. McEwen C. Multicenter evaluation of synovectomy in the treatment of rheumatoid arthritis: report of results at the end of 5 years. *J Rheumatol* 1988;15:765.
31. Rivard GE, Girard M, Belanger R, et al. Synoviorthesis with colloidal 32-P chromic phosphate for the treatment of hemophilic arthropathy. *J Bone Joint Surg Am* 1994;76:482–488.
32. Milgram JW. Synovial osteochondromatosis. *J Bone Joint Surg Am* 1977;59:792.
33. Martin DF, Curl WW, Baker CL. Arthroscopic treatment of chronic synovitis of the ankle. *Arthroscopy* 1989;5:110–114.

CHAPTER 7

Osteochondral Pathology

James F. Guhl and J. Serge Parisien

SECTION 1: Defects of the Talar Dome

Some defects of the talar dome are better appreciated when evaluated arthroscopically (Figs. 7.1–7.3). They should be suspected in the presence of soft tissue pathology, where they may coexist because of the mechanism of injury. Therefore these defects should be kept in mind when evaluating any form of synovial impingement syndrome, adhesions, or chronic nonspecific synovitis.

The surface of the articular cartilage should be scrutinized for irregularities. The smallest amount of fibrous tissue protruding from any linear defect, the least movement or loosening, or the loss of resilience or luster should arouse suspicion. Such areas can then be easily dissected from the surrounding normal healthy cartilage using a probe. More obvious stellate defects, linear cracks, and fibrillated necrotic areas may be seen. There also are clear-cut distinct craters with or without cartilaginous loose bodies; they appear to be more common in the talar dome than in the plafond. These lesions may be symptomatic and require treatment.

Radiographic evaluation begins with routine films followed by the usual positional views for osteochondritis dissecans. Stress films may help predict the existence of these defects and their location by the areas of contact between the talus and plafond. Bone scans are negative because there is only chondral involvement. Contrast studies can define these defects and identify chondral loose bodies. Although the computed tomography (CT) scan is not likely to be of help, a CT arthrogram may reveal subtle osteochondral lesions.

Beltran et al.[1] originally described magnetic resonance imaging (MRI) of the ankle. They suggested that this technique can demonstrate irregularities of the articular cartilage surface. Kerr et al.[2] found that MRI was useful for diagnosing osteochondral defects. The coronal and sagittal planes are most useful for evaluating the talus by employing combinations of T1- and T2-weighted images. Chondral fractures, fragments, or lesions may be overlooked as the cause of persistent ankle pain. Radiographs are negative in most of these cases. MRI is a sensitive means for demonstrating these lesions and may also be used for staging. A bone scan can be negative in the presence of these lesions.

In addition to detecting subtle osteochondral lesions, MRI has been of value for assessing the overlying cartilage. MRI can show focal defects, disruption, thinning, swelling, and signal changes within hyaline cartilage. Mild surface changes such as fibrillation may be difficult to demonstrate. However, improved visualization of cartilage is possible with several recently developed techniques or with the use of intraarticular contrast media. CT or CT arthrography is probably more accurate than MRI for demonstrating intraarticular fragments, although gradient echo images have improved MRI performance. The advantage of MRI over CT when evaluating the talus is that adjacent ligaments, tendons, and marrow space may be evaluated as well. One must consider the cost-effectiveness when using these studies. A good ankle arthroscopist can make essentially the same diagnosis based on the history and physical examination and proceed directly to treatment in many cases.

Some chondral lesions of the talar dome found at arthroscopy are actually small or shallow osteochondral fractures. In this case, the bone scan may be weakly positive or negative owing to limited bone involvement or early minimal arthritic changes. Such entities may not have been recognized on radiographs.

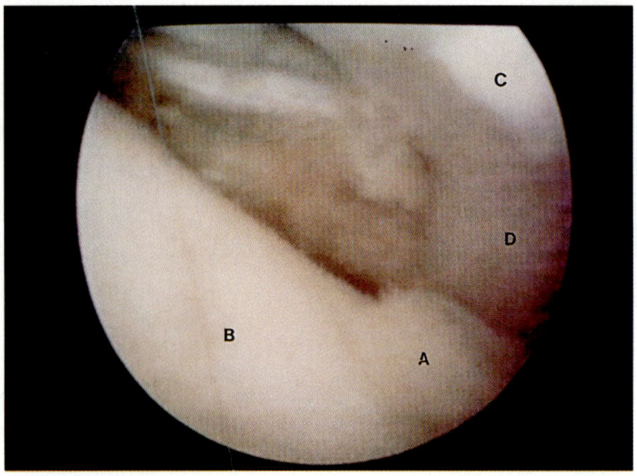

FIGURE 7.1. Video-arthroscopic view of a partially separated chondral lesion (A) of the medial talar dome (B) in the right ankle. C, plafond; D, medial malleolus.

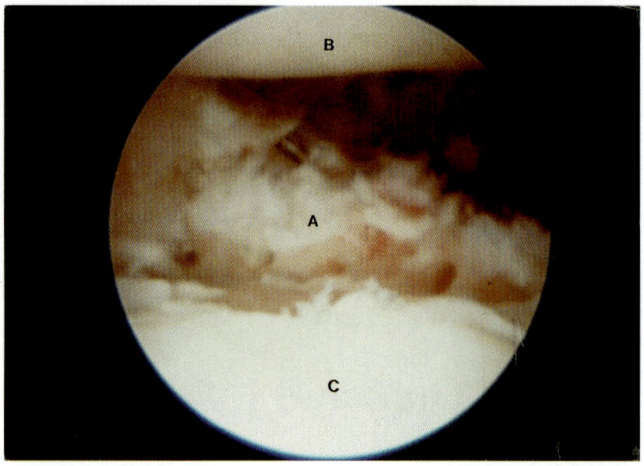

FIGURE 7.3. Arthroscopic view shows another case of a chondral lesion of the talar dome after débridement. A, débrided lesion; B, plafond; C, dome of the talus.

Treatment requires complete débridement of all necrotic or diseased articular cartilage, abrasion of the base, and drilling. Drilling is done with a 0.062 inch Kirschner wire.

A complete set of small joint instruments was designed by Ferkel and introduced by Acufex Microsurgical (now Smith/Nephew). The holmium-YAG laser can be utilized to trim the margin, as is done for osteochondritis dissecans. This practice appears to reduce the rate of destruction (i.e., further peeling or flaking of the articular cartilage) with continued use and time. Any combination of approaches that best suits the location may be used.

The posterolateral portal is of value when studying lesions located in the posterolateral aspect of the dome as well as the anterior recess and remaining joint. Posterior defects are usually located medially, but posterolateral lesions have been encountered. Viewing from the posterolateral portal is often far superior when confirming the diagnosis or for chondral bone defects.

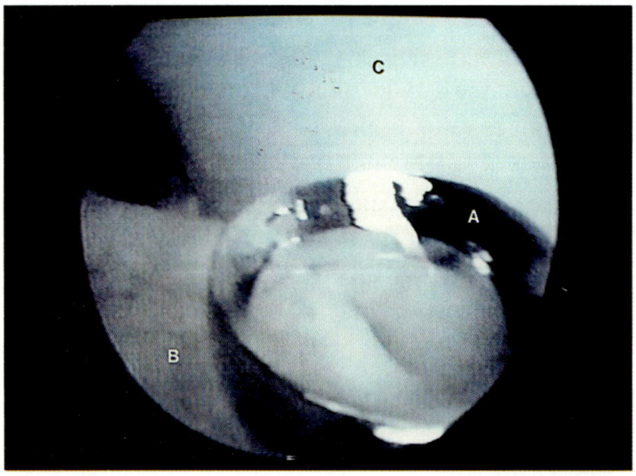

FIGURE 7.2. Video-arthroscopic view of the same lesion as in Figure 7.1 after débridement. Curette (A) is shown removing the fibrous tissue from the base. B, lesion; C, medial malleolus.

LESIONS OF THE PLAFOND

Chondral defects of the plafond are probably the most difficult lesions in the ankle joint to diagnose preoperatively. They are rarely detected on routine radiographs, and the bone scan is negative because there is only chondral involvement. These lesions may result from compression or twisting injuries in which the talus is driven up or impacted against the plafond. They may occur in the presence of more extensive fractures of the extremity and be overlooked or not considered at the time of injury. Such defects can be the source of chondral loose bodies, and they can also set the stage for future arthritic changes in the ankle joint. Theoretically, a CT arthrogram can delineate these defects, but often the studies have not proved to have practical application. MRI may be helpful.

Suspected chondral defects may be one of the best indications to proceed directly to arthroscopy for a diagnosis and then to arthroscopic surgery of the ankle (Figs. 7.4–7.6). The lesions may appear as large stellate or irregular defects with resultant sources of loose necrotic cartilage. At times a clear-cut defect with or without a separated loose body is noted. On other occasions chondromalacia or fib-

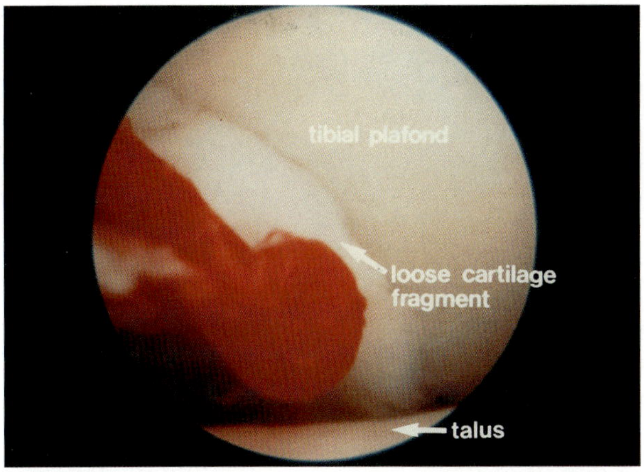

FIGURE 7.4. Arthroscopic view of a lesion of the lateral tibial plafond with a loose body in the right ankle.

rillation may be present, making the diagnosis more difficult. After the chondromalacia is débrided, the defect becomes apparent in contrast to the surrounding normal articular cartilage.

Large osteochondral defects of the plafond can also occur. They can be discovered and distinguished from lesions of the talar dome by a bone scan. Better evaluation is by pinhole columnation or single photon emission CT (SPECT) when the lesions are not visible on routine radiographic views. Further definition or confirmation can be accomplished with tomography, CT scans, or MRI.

Treatment requires complete débridement and abrasion, with drilling necessary at times. When drilling, the defect is trimmed back to healthy articular cartilage with a perpendicular margin.

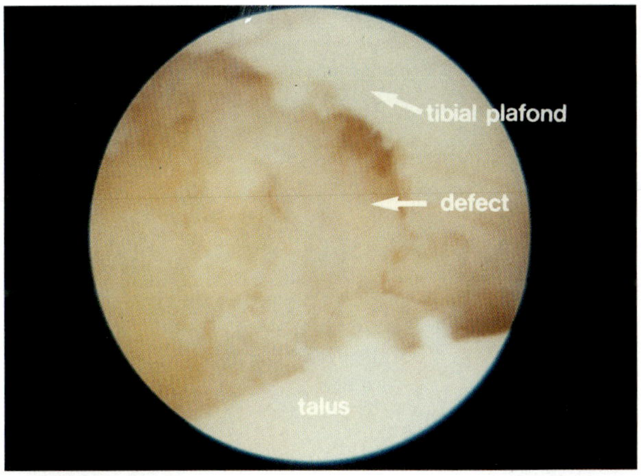

FIGURE 7.5. Arthroscopic view of the lesion in Figure 7.4 after the loose fragment was removed and the crater was débrided, abraded, and drilled.

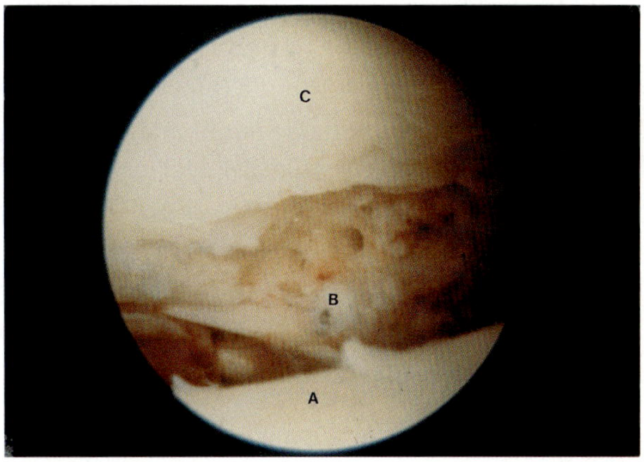

FIGURE 7.6. Arthroscopic view of another chondral lesion of the lateral tibial plafond after reconstruction, débridement, abrasion, and drilling. A, talus; B, drilled lesion; C, tibial plafond.

The open-drilling technique has long been recommended for osteochondritis dissecans and such other lesions. According to Cheung et al.[3] more stage II fibrocartilage consisting of a higher percentage of hyaline material is found when drilling is used. These lesions can be approached for surgery and drilled from the anterior portals with noninvasive distraction. The posterior approaches are of no use because of the anatomic configuration of the talocrural joint. Articular lesions of the tibial plafond can be débrided from the anterior approach. If drilling is thought necessary by the surgeon, it can be done from above. A 2- or 3-mm hole is drilled through the anteromedial tibial cortex with the use of a 0.062 inch Kirschner wire directed by the Ferkel microvector guide. Autograft resurfacing, as described for osteochondral lesions of the talar dome, is not possible for local lesions of the plafond.

Postoperative rehabilitation requires early active motion plus stretching and strengthening exercises. A period of approximately 6–8 weeks of no weightbearing is important in these cases. Continuous passive motion (CPM) is used at the discretion of the surgeon, followed by active motion.

One second-look arthroscopic procedure was performed on a patient who had undergone débridement and drilling of a plafond lesion 4 months earlier. Although the articular surface improved, maturation of the fibrocartilage was not complete. More time may have been required. Other cases treated in the same fashion had good clinical results at long-term follow-up (2 years or more).

COMBINED LESIONS OF THE DOME AND PLAFOND

Chondral lesions of the talar dome and tibial plafond may occur, causing intraarticular pain, swelling, crepitus, and limited motion (Figs. 7.7, 7.8). The etiology may be presumed to be a twisting injury, a forceful valgus or varus stress injury, compression, or multiple instances of overuse.

The treatment selected must be appropriate for the individual components of the pathologic entity. Extensive clean-up (débridement) and lavage are required, including curettage, abrasion, and drilling of all chondral surfaces as described above. The same criteria are utilized depending on the surface, depth, and position of the lesion. *Extensive abrasion arthroplasties are to be avoided.* The prognosis is generally bleak, and the end result may be an arthrodesis. Because arthroscopic ankle arthrodesis is associated with less morbidity, faster healing time, superior duration of union, better cosmesis, and, above all, fewer complications, it should be considered, although in some cases the above surgery may suffice.

CHONDROMALACIA

Chondromalcia lesions may be chondral defects of the dome or tibial plafond, or they may be combined lesions of the dome and tibial plafond. Usually they coexist with soft tissue pathology, loose bodies, and osteophytes (Figs. 7.9, 7.10).

The treatment is the same as that described for chondral defects. If extensive or advanced pathol-

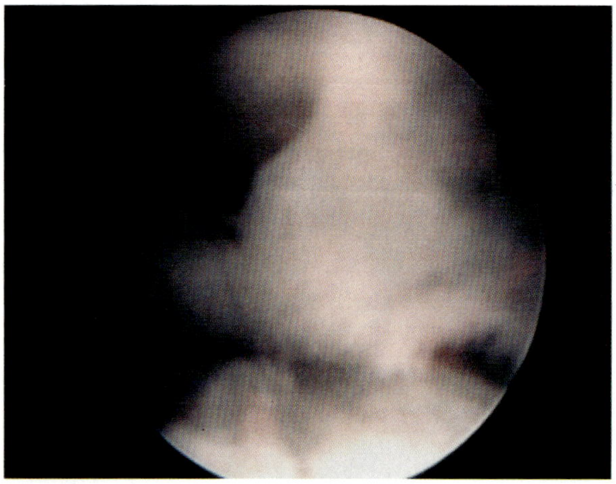

FIGURE 7.7. Combined chondral lesion of the dome and plafond.

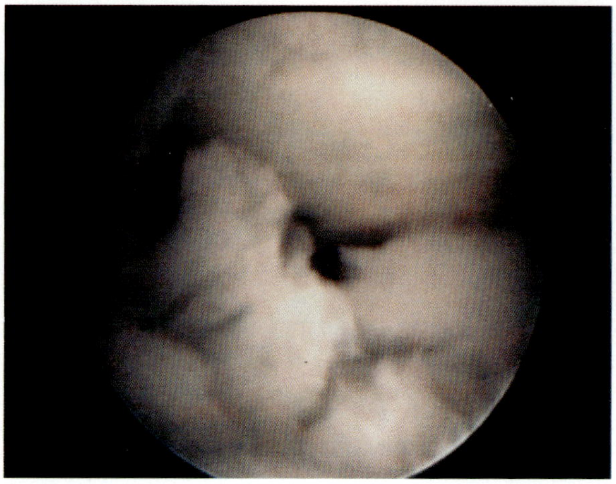

FIGURE 7.8. Another view of the combined chondral lesion of the dome and plafond shown in Figure 7.7.

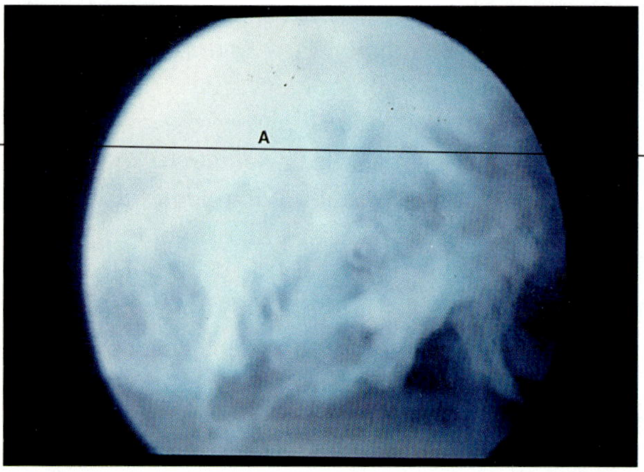

FIGURE 7.9. Video-arthroscopic view of (A) chondromalacia of the plafond.

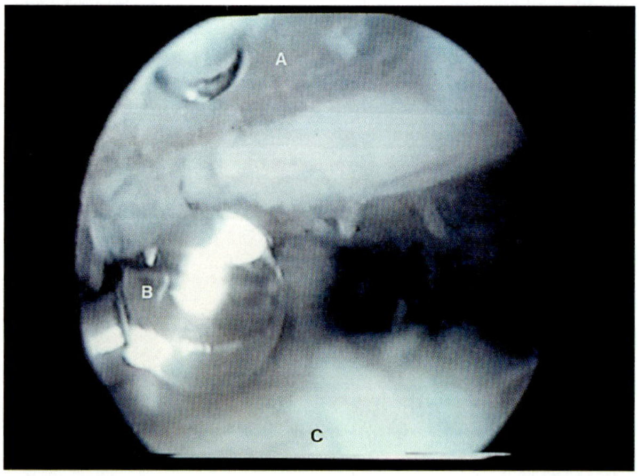

FIGURE 7.10. Video-arthroscopic view after the chondromalacia was probed and débrided. A chondral defect (A) was then apparent. B, abrader; C, dome of the talus.

ogy is present, the prognosis may be grim and is to some degree the same as that for combined chondral defects. If the lesions are small, however, a much better result can be expected.

Awareness of the pathology described above, early recognition, confirmation, and aggressive treatment are of the greatest importance. Conservative measures (i.e., antiinflammatory drugs, nonsteroidal antiinflammatory drugs (N.S.A.I.D.), physical therapy, orthotics) should be considered before advocating surgery.

CHONDRAL DEBRIS

Chondral debris requires awareness on the clinician's part. It usually is found in the anteromedial corner or posterior recess (impingement) (Fig. 7.11) and often coexists with local chronic reactive synovitis. Awareness and experience aid in early recognition. The clinical examination (and history) is most important; radiography and imaging are not especially helpful. Injection of a local anesthetic or a steroid may be diagnostic or therapeutic. Should symptoms persist, ankle arthroscopy is reasonable. Removal by débridement and lavage is employed, followed by early active exercise. A period of no weight-bearing follows for a number of weeks at the discretion of the surgeon.

MEDIAL IMPINGEMENT

Medial impingement results after a severe lateral ankle sprain that subsequently causes pain on the medial and lateral sides of the ankle joint. This was not fully understood until a series of cases were presented (unpublished data) by van Dijk.

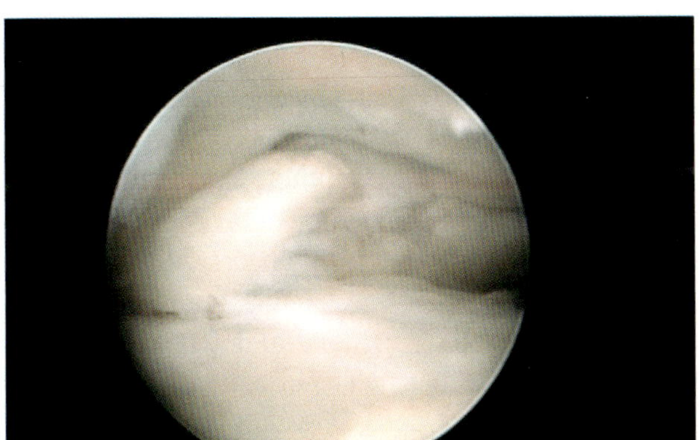

FIGURE 7.11. Iatrogenic adhesion impingement from drill hole to place graft in the dome of the talus.

The highest frequency of residual complaints occurs after plaster immobilization for 6 weeks or more. When this is preceeded by surgery, the percentage drops from 40–50% to 25–35%. If medially located problems are not included in the statistics of lateral ankle ligament treatment results, the numbers of residual complaints are substantially lower.

Basically, the mechanism is rupture or sprain of the lateral ligaments causing the superomedial corner of the talus to abut against the medial malleolus. Chondral and osteochondral fragments shear off from these surfaces, causing debris and reactive chronic synovitis in the anteromedial corner.

Van Dijk observed this at intervals following the date of injury. He documented the arthroscopic findings and treatment, especially lavage and, as necessary, ligament repair. During a 1.5-year period he treated and recorded the progress of 30 patients, subsequently documenting his findings. The combined arthroscopic views and sketches in Figures 7.12–7.20 show what the foot and ankle arthroscopist may expect to see in the anteromedial corner and the rest of the ankle joint prior to planning treatment.

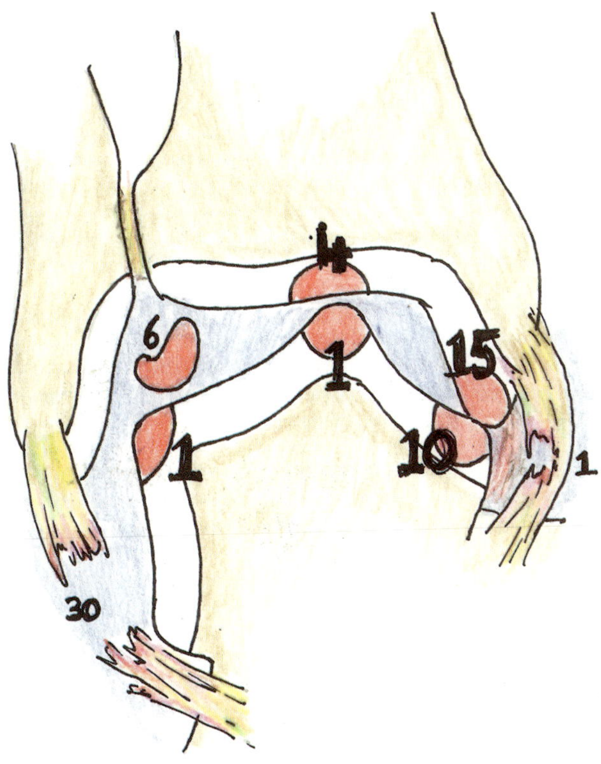

FIGURE 7.12. Localization and number of chondral lesions found at arthroscopy in a series of 30 consecutive patients with rupture of the lateral ankle ligaments after acute supination trauma. The arthroscopic procedures were all performed 4–7 days after the trauma. (Van Dijk 1996)

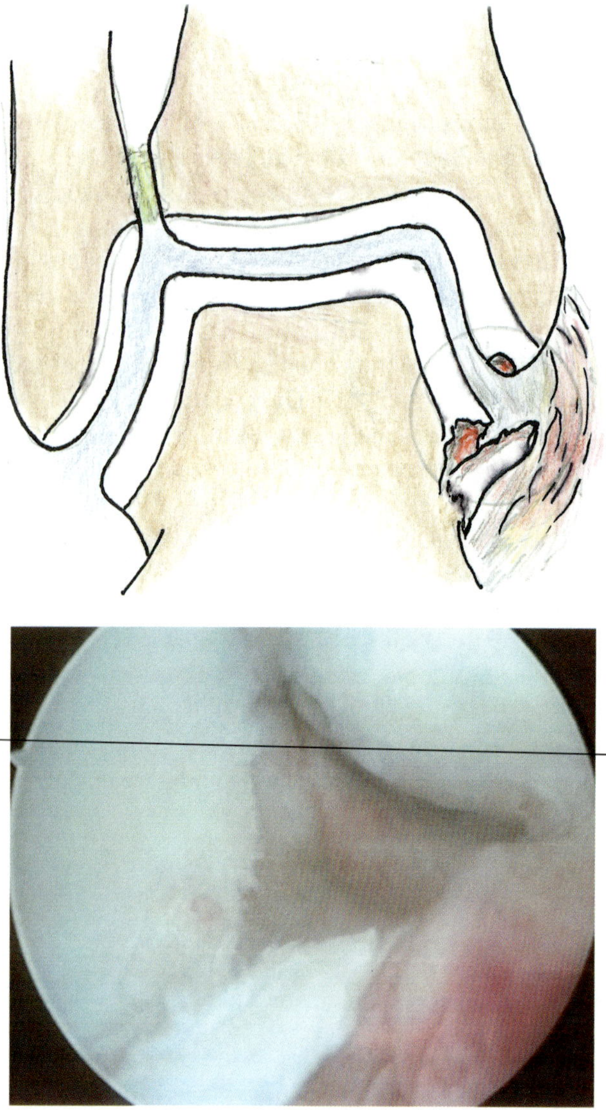

FIGURE 7.13. A 21-year-old man sustained a rupture of the anterior talofibular ligament. This arthroscopic view 5 days after trauma shows an osteochondral flake at the medial talar facet and a small, round cartilage impression on the tip of the medial malleolus.

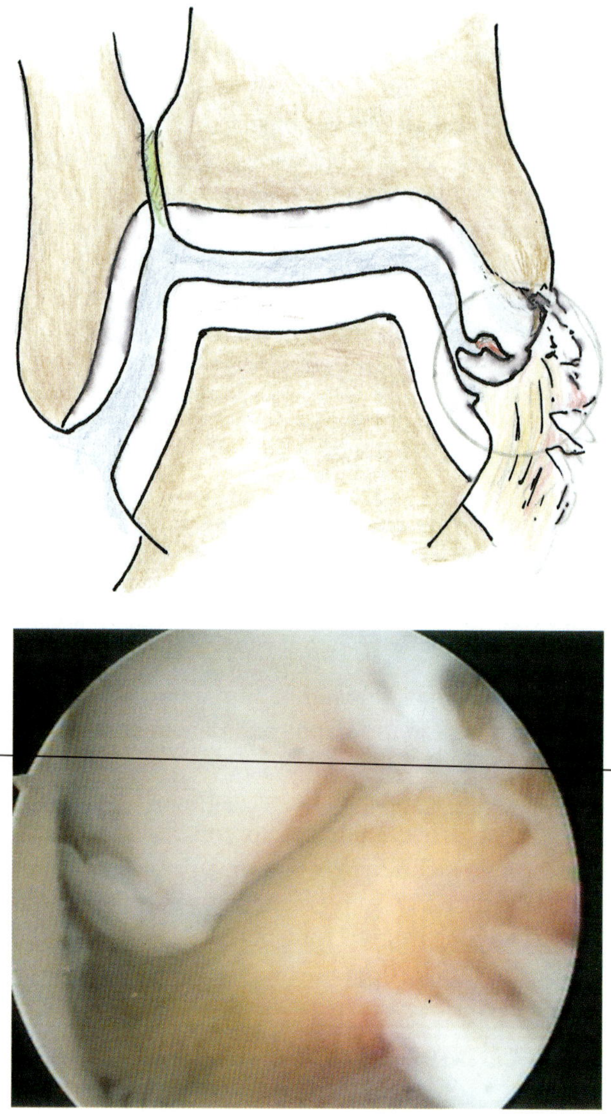

FIGURE 7.14. A 22-year-old woman had an anterior talofibular ligament lesion and a fibulocalcaneal ligament lesion. The tip of the medial malleolus demonstrates a chondral flake fracture. The fragment was left in place. There were no complaints at the 6-month or 1-year follow-up.

LOOSE BODIES

Loose bodies can be free or entrapped. Their removal is the best reason for ankle arthroscopy. The origin, development and fate of free loose bodies must be kept in mind when reviewing the history and clinical findings and then, when planning treatment. The clinical picture of loose bodies in the ankle depends on the number, size, stage of development, and associated pathology. Periodic episodes of locking, pain, and a feeling of instability are typical. The clinical examination varies depending on the factors discussed above. In advanced cases, swelling may accompany any one of these episodes. Routine radiographs often suffice, although occasionally CT scanning or CT arthrography is necessary.

According to Milgram,[4] loose bodies originate from chondral and osteochondral defects such as osteochondritis dissecans, osteochondral fractures, intraarticular fracture defects, osteophytes, degenerative arthritis, and synovial chondromatosis. They may enlarge via osteoblastic formation or decrease

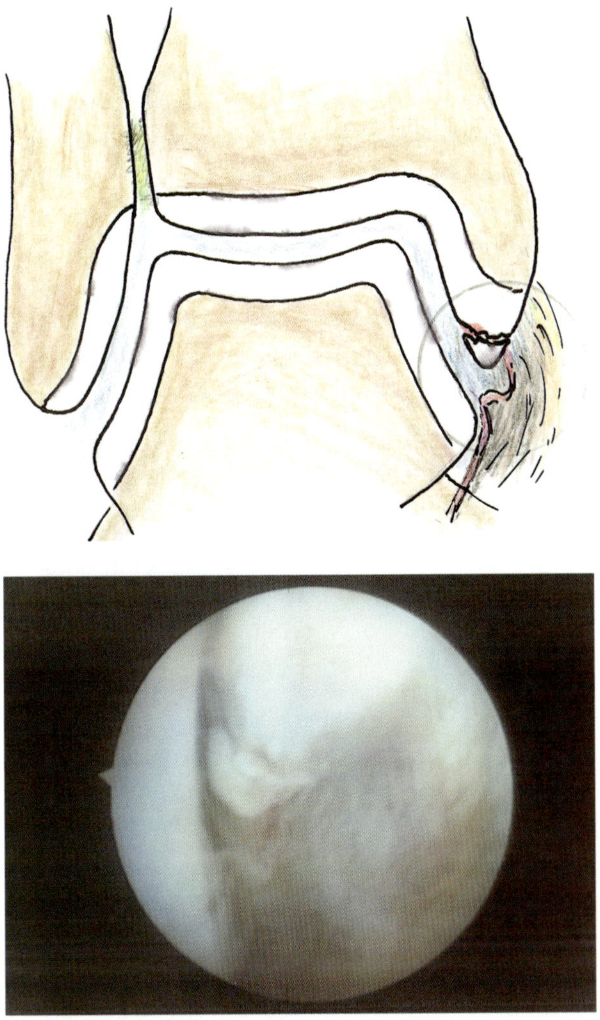

FIGURE 7.15. After a faulty landing on stage, a 26-year-old professional female ballet dancer sustained combined ruptures of the anterior talofibular ligament and calcaneofibular ligament. At 5 days after trauma this arthroscopic view demonstrates a chondral flake fracture of the tip of the medial malleolus. The fragment was left in place. After the 1-year follow-up there was stiffness after ballet performances and pain after strenuous activities.

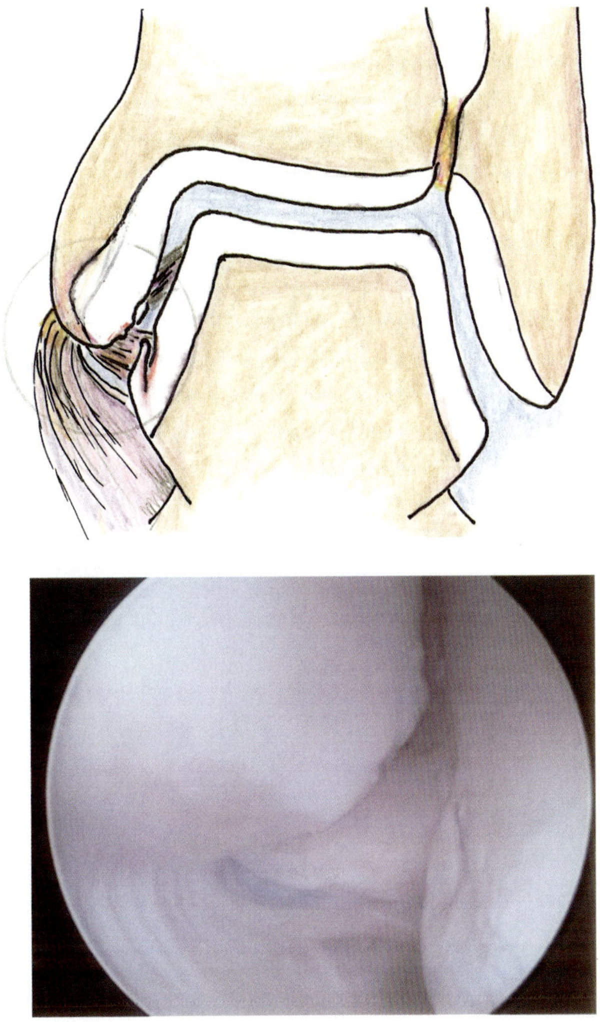

FIGURE 7.16. A 39-year-old woman made a faulty landing after a jump, thereby sustaining a rupture of the anterior talofibular ligament. This arthroscopic view 4 days after trauma shows a small cartilage flake fracture on the medial talar facet and some irregularity on the tip of the medial malleolus.

in size via osteoclastic activity. They also may become attached to the synovium and remain untreated. Arthroscopic loose body removal provides a significant advantage over open techniques (Figs. 7.21, 7.22). The limited access provided by open arthrotomy makes complete removal of a loose body subject to some guesswork. Complete arthroscopic search for a single or a few remaining loose bodies affords a much greater possibility of success. Distraction with full distension and use of any of the available approaches is employed.

During arthroscopy loose bodies may be found with equal incidence in the anterior and posterior recesses of the ankle joint, both lateral and medial gutters, with minimal room to lodge elsewhere. They can be hidden in those locations by numerous synovial folds, chronic synovitis, or adhesions. While they remain loose (i.e., do not become entrapped), they continue to migrate about the joint owing to the patient's activity. Triangulation via the anterior approach is done at first. Often loose bodies are mobilized from other areas in the joint and cause more damage.

The posterolateral portals are often necessary if the loose body is lodged in the posterior recess. A

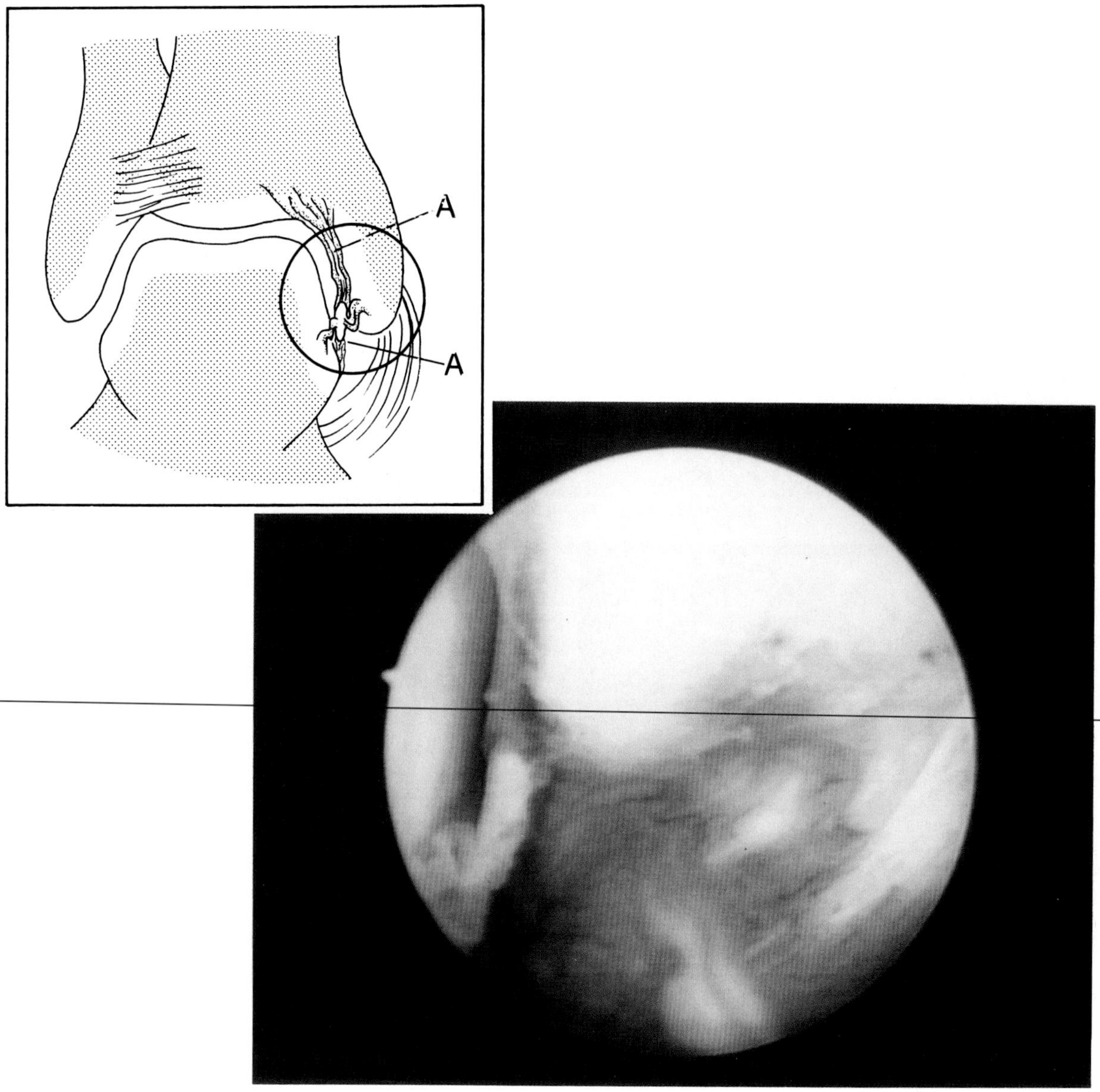

FIGURE 7.17. A 26-year-old man twisted his ankle while running and sustained an anterior talofibular ligament lesion. Arthroscopic view 6 days after trauma shows adhesion and fibrous tissue. No complaints were reported at the 6-month and 1-year follow-ups. (A) Adhesion and fibrous tissue.

large hypodermic needle, probe, or obturator can be inserted posterolaterally and is used to push the lesions forward so they can be removed from the anterior approaches. Occasionally, two stacked posterolateral portals are necessary. Triangulation can be accomplished in many combinations or approaches.

As when treating osteochondritis dissecans and chondral defects, use of the posterolateral approach for viewing has proved to be highly effective when inserting the operating instruments from anterior portals. Often a loose body hidden in the extreme anterior recess can be seen and removed best using this technique. On occasion, tapping an area around the portal with one's finger helps remove a tight loose body. Carefully twisting the grasper may result in the fragment gradually becoming dislodged. Enlarging the incision by a few millimeters may aid in removing a large loose body as well. Another technique is to insert the grasping forceps and cannula together. When the loose body is captured, the entire assembly can be extracted together, giving a bit more control. Enlarging the incision may be avoided by reducing the size of the loose body.

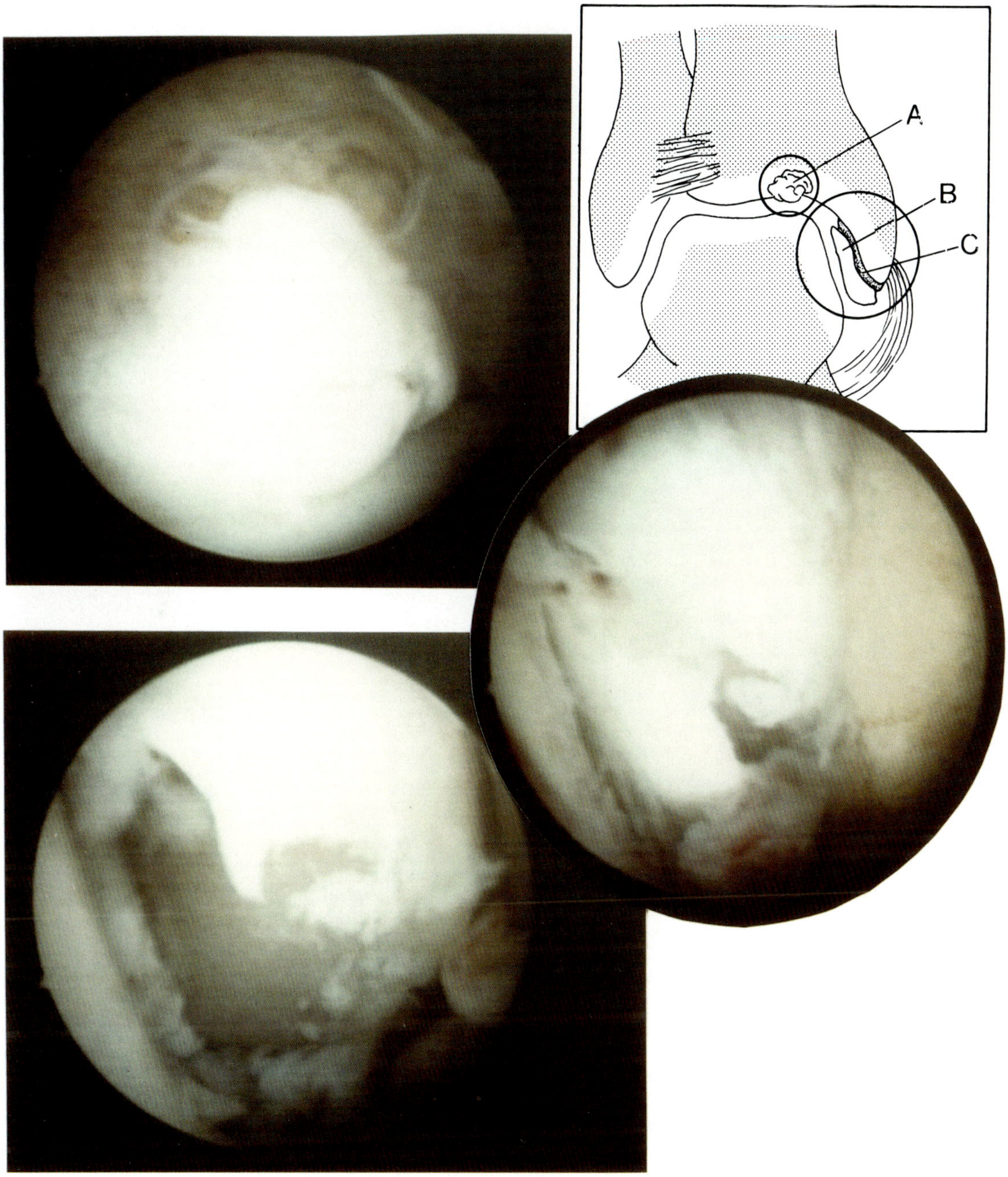

FIGURE 7.18. A 30-year-old man made a faulty landing after a jump playing soccer and sustained combined ruptures of the talar fibular ligament and calcaneofibular ligament. Arthroscopic view shows cartilage damage on the anterior aspect of the medial malleolus (A). The large chondral fragment (B) was irrigated out of the joint. At the 1-year and 2-year follow-ups, complaints about the medial side of the joint prevented him from returning to competitive soccer. (C) Defect of medial malleolus.

ENTRAPPED LOOSE BODIES

Entrapped loose bodies are found in the anterior or posterior recess or in the medial or lateral talar malleolar joint. They become firmly attached or fixed in position over long periods of time by soft tissue interposition or osteochondral attachment. They differ from "ossicles" (described below).

The diagnosis is established by a combination of clinical, radiographic, and imaging findings. Confirmation is by response to injection of a local anesthetic agent. Removal is more challenging, as they must initially be freed by a variety of mechanical

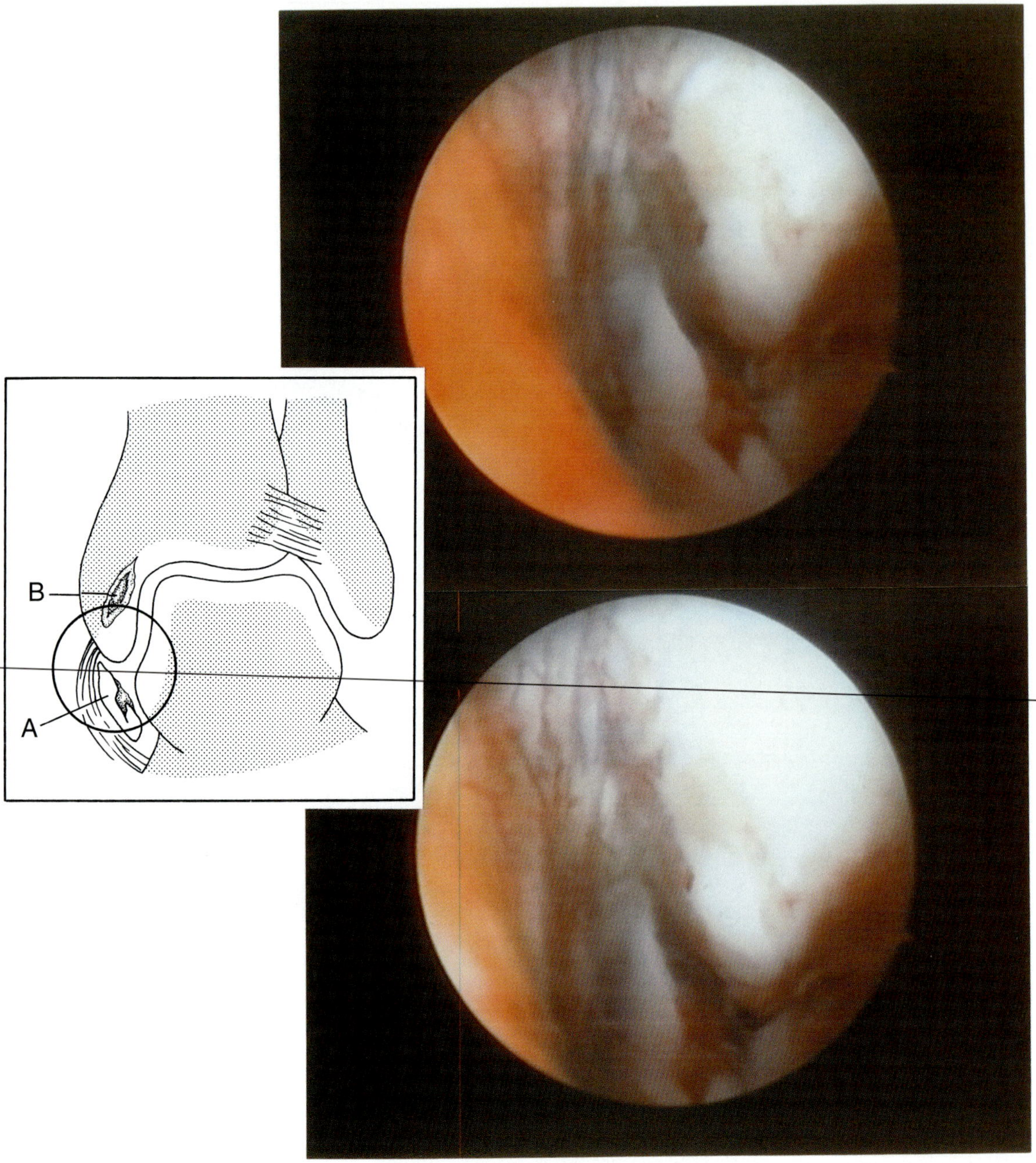

FIGURE 7.19. A 21-year-old man twisted his ankle while playing basketball and suffered combined ruptures of the anterior middle and posterior talofibular ligaments. This arthroscopic view 5 days after trauma demonstrates a loose cartilage fragment (A). The fragment was irrigated out of the joint. (B) Donor site defect.

instruments. The holmium-YAG laser can be used to great advantage during ankle arthroscopy, reducing the risk of damage to surrounding collateral soft tissue or osteochondral structures (see Chapter 19). Entrapped loose bodies may be asymptomatic, or they may become symptomatic. If left in place, they may cause further damage to the joint with continued motion. For these reasons, thorough removal is required (Figs. 7.23–7.26).

OSSICLES

Ossicles are defined as intraarticular or periarticular osteochondral fragments enmeshed in a soft tissue envelope. These fragments are often avulsed from the tips of the lateral or medial malleoli and lodge in their respective gutters as well as in the anterior recess (Figs. 7.27–7.31). Among more than 600 ankle arthroscopies, no fragments were seen in

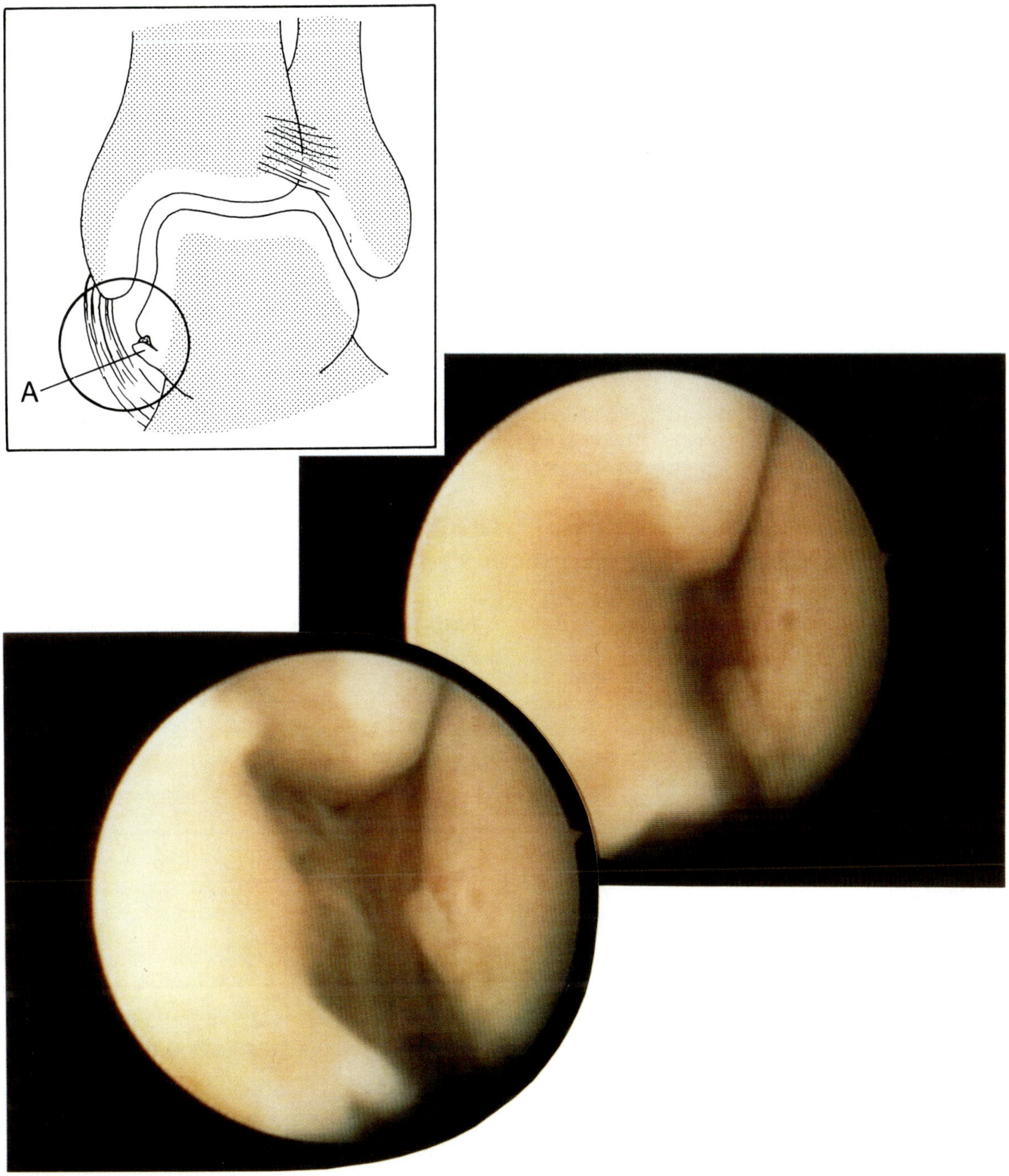

FIGURE 7.20. A 24-year-old man made a misstep during walking on uneven ground, resulting in an anterior talofibular ligament lesion and calcaneofibular ligament lesion. This arthroscopic view 4 days after trauma demonstrates a small chondral flake fragment on the medial talar facet. At the 1-year follow-up there were no complaints. (A) Chondral flake fragment from the medial talar facet.

the posterior recess. On routine radiography they are difficult at times to differentiate from free or entrapped loose bodies or osteophytes. Often ossicles are small and asymptomatic. When they are symptomatic and remain so, injection of a local anesthetic agent combined with steroid may serve as a diagnostic test or be therapeutic. The relief may be temporary or permanent. When removal is mandatory, it must be performed by careful dissection from the encapsulating soft tissue and the surrounding articular cartilage.

The ossicle is dissected from the surrounding tissue by careful use of a banana knife, similar knives, or a Frier dissecting instrument. The final avulsion

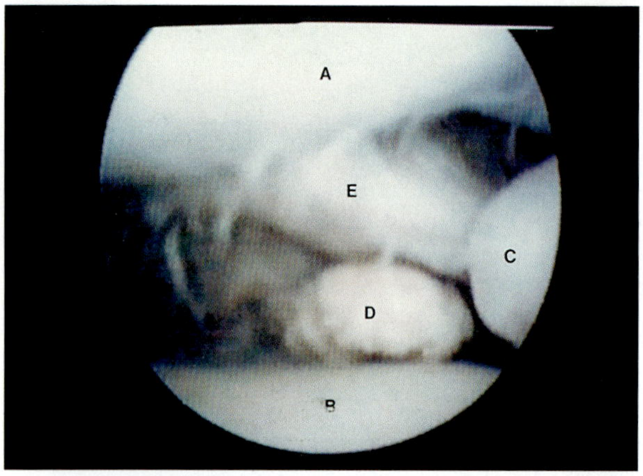

FIGURE 7.21. Video-arthroscopic view, with the plafond (A) shown above and the dome (B) below. Two osteochondral loose bodies (C,D) and the transverse ligament (E) are seen.

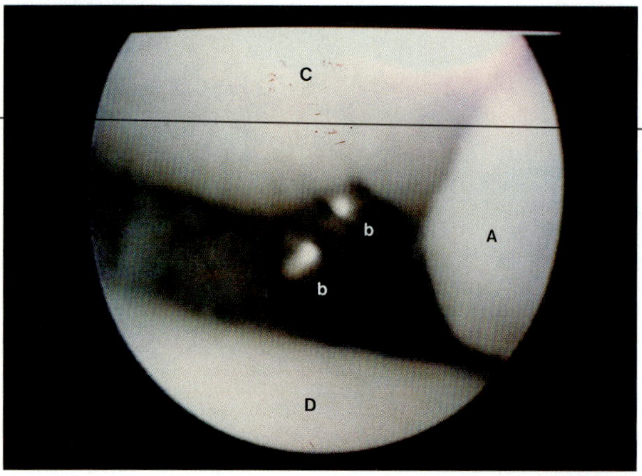

FIGURE 7.22. Video-arthroscopic view of the same case as in Figure 7.21. The loose body (A) has moved to the medial side of the ankle joint proper. The grasping forceps (b) are shown about to remove the fragment. C, plafond; D, dome of the talus.

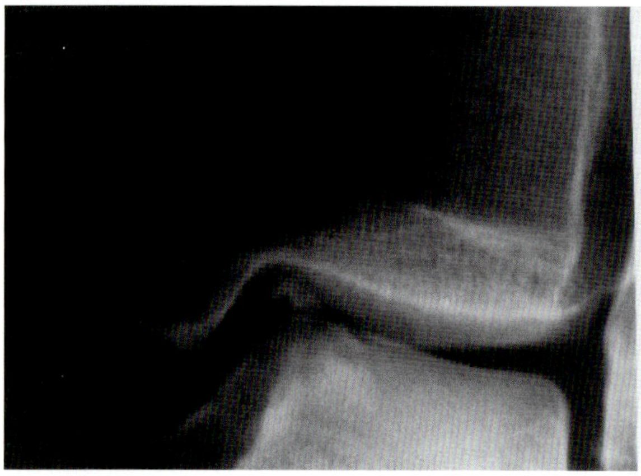

FIGURE 7.23. Radiograph of an entrapped loose body in the medial corner.

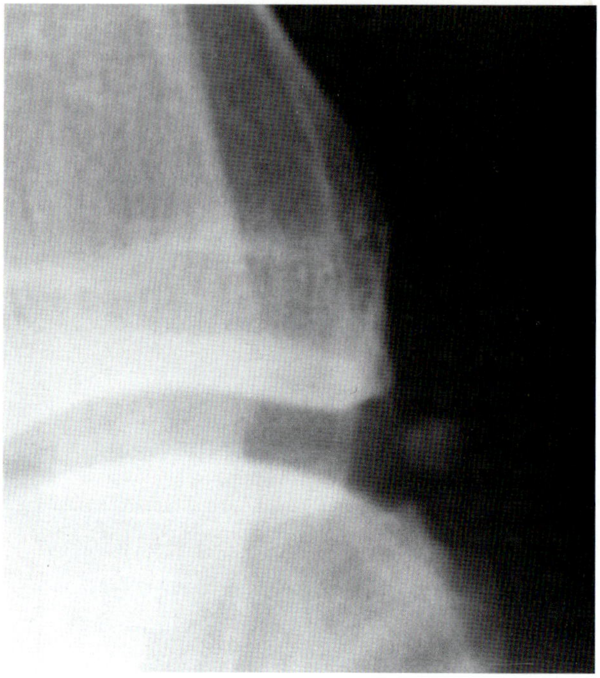

FIGURE 7.24. Loose body at the posterior aspect of the ankle.

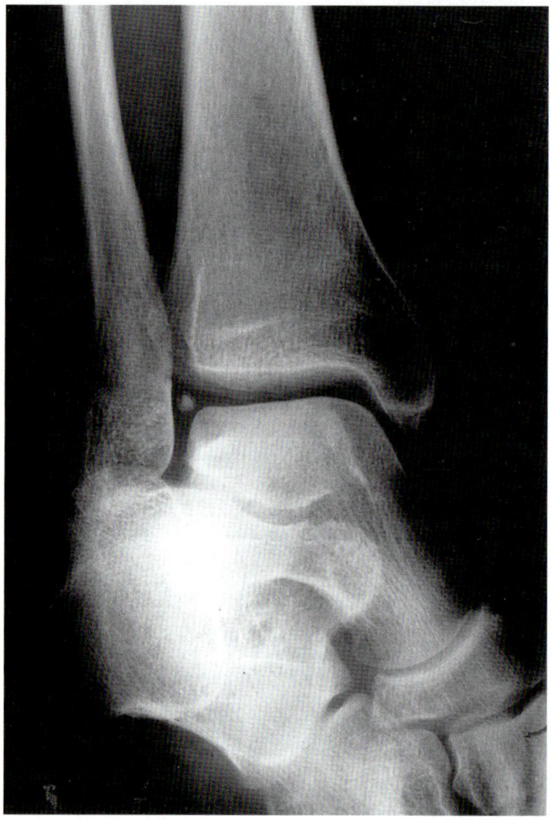

FIGURE 7.25. Radiograph shows osteochondral body at the posterolateral aspect of the ankle.

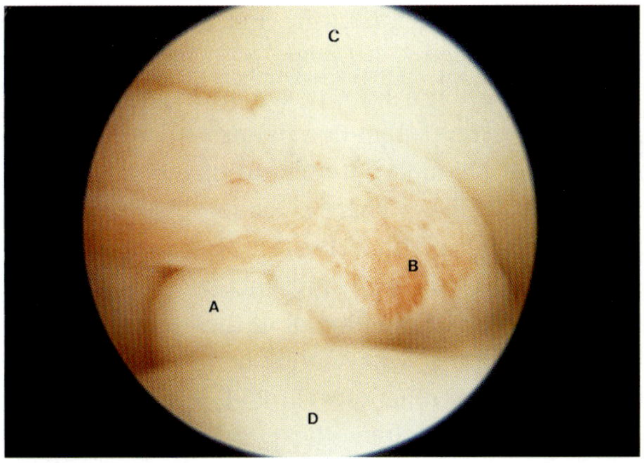

FIGURE 7.26. A 35-mm arthroscopic view of the same patient showing a loose body (A) (in the center of the illustration) held by a sling of synoidal impingement tissue (B). The loose body was easily dislodged with a probe and removed with a grasping forceps. The impingement lesion was also removed in its entirety. C, plafond; D, dome of talus.

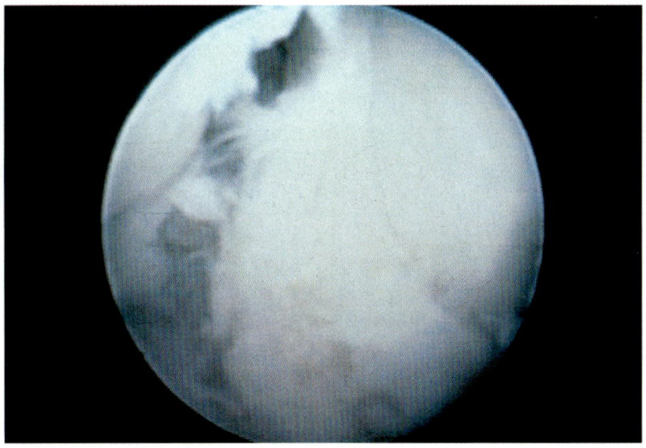

FIGURE 7.29. Arthroscopic view shows a fixed osteochondral fragment on the lower lateral talus.

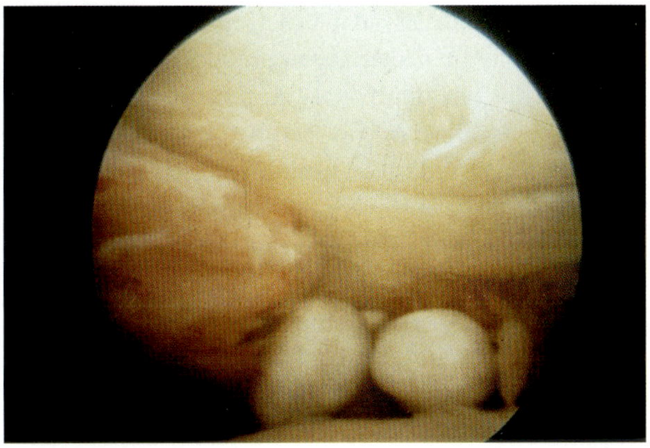

FIGURE 7.27. Arthroscopic view of two loose bodies.

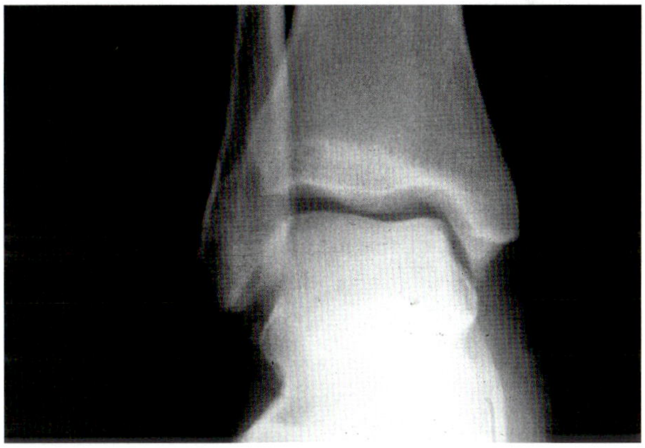

FIGURE 7.30. AP radiograph after arthroscopic surgery.

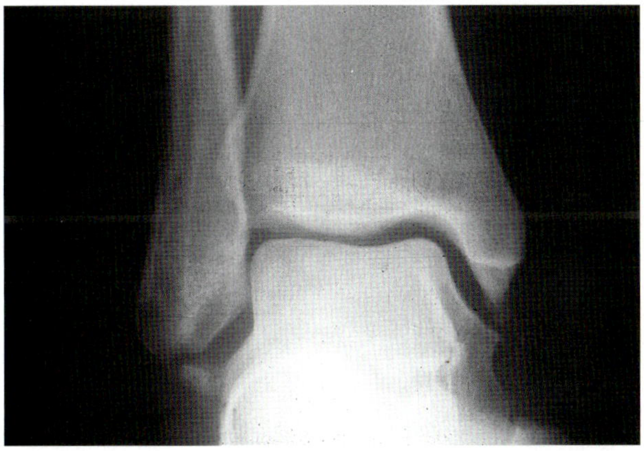

FIGURE 7.28. Anteroposterior (AP) radiograph of an ankle after trauma shows a fragment distal to the tip of the fibula.

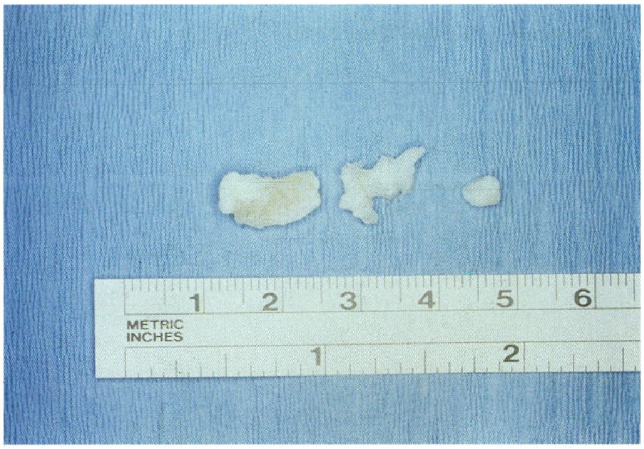

FIGURE 7.31. Specimen from the lesion seen in Figure 7.30.

can be in toto or piecemeal, similar to excision of a pathologic os trigonum. The laser can be helpful here because when dissecting away the soft tissue the fragment can be identified by its honeycomb appearance (see Chapter 19). Ossicles are the best reason for the use of laser in the ankle joint.

OSTEOPHYTES

Osteophytes are secondary to trauma or associated with a degenerative joint.[5,6] The traumatic lesions are usually due to repeated dorsiflexion injuries or may be the result of capsular traction following forced plantar flexion of the foot. A genuine traction spur situated at the attachment of the anterior capsule is rare, as most osteophytes are located well within the attachment of the joint capsule.

On the talar side, the typical osteophyte is found proximal to the talar neck notch. Both tibia and talar osteophytes can be easily detected during arthroscopy. Normally, the lower anterior tibia and the anterior part of the medial malleolus are covered with cartilage. The anterior joint capsule attaches to the tibia above the cartilage rim some 5 mm above the joint line. It is this non-weight-bearing anterior cartilage rim that undergoes osteophyte transformation. Damage to the cartilage covering the anterior surface of the distal tibia and anterior rim of the medial malleolus is known to occur with most supination injuries. Recurrent direct microtraumas to the anteriorly located cartilage rim could be an important factor.

There is often a long delay in diagnosing these conditions. The patient complains of pain with dorsiflexion of the ankle, limitation of motion, and intermittent swelling. There is tenderness to palpation along the anterior tibial tendon of the joint. Radiographic studies show the presence of an exostosis at the anterior lip of the tibia or at the anterior neck of the talus. A bone scan may be helpful for early detection of symptomatic osteophytes, and SPECT or computer tomography with contrast may be required for more accurate information. MRI is generally not necessary. Conservative treatment such as antiinflammatory drugs, injections, physical therapy, or some form of orthotics should be employed first. Arthroscopy is the procedure of choice.

The arthroscope is placed initially in the anterolateral portal and interchanged with instruments in the anterior and medial portals (Figs. 7.32–7.37). Excision can be carried out with manual distraction. Controlled noninvasive distraction with optimal positioning may be necessary to prevent damage to the closely adjacent talar dome and to carry out a detailed examination of the rest of the joint. At times, if the anterior recess is limited or extremely tight, distraction must be discontinued and the foot dorsiflexed on the ankle, which is redistended before proceeding. Small instruments may be used interchangeably here to accomplish removal. It is also necessary, as with other ankle arthroscopic proce-

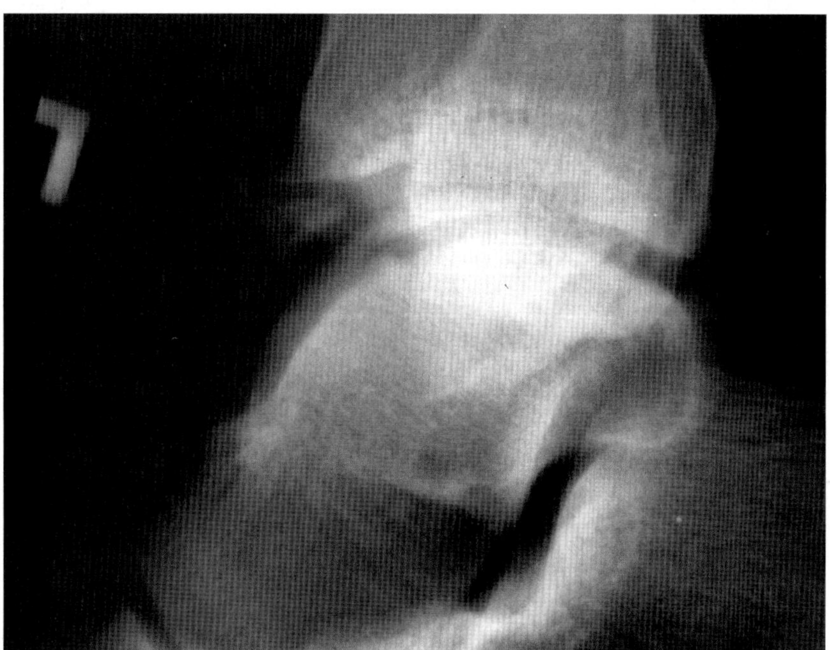

FIGURE 7.32. Lateral radiograph of the left ankle shows an interior impingement (osteophyte) in a professional football kicker.

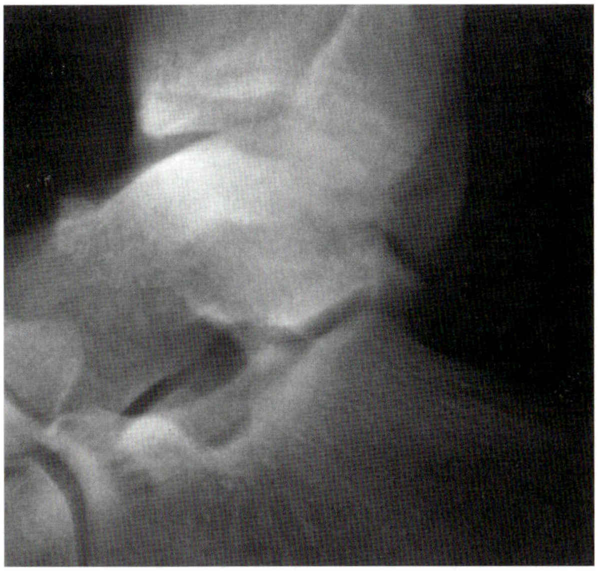

FIGURE 7.33. Same injury seen in figure 7.32 after successful arthroscopic excision.

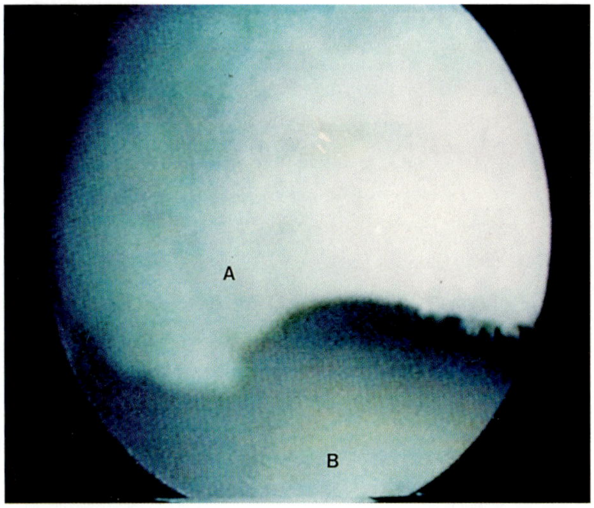

FIGURE 7.35. Video-arthroscopic view of the case seen in Figure 7.34 after a portion of the lesion has been removed. A, osteophyte; B, dome of the talus.

dures, to débride the inflamed synovial tissue often found in the anterior recess to gain adequate visualization. The usual instruments are employed (i.e., osteotome, curettes, rasps, rongeurs, power instruments, and a radiofrequency device or holmium-YAG laser.

Arthroscopic removal of osteophytes of the anterior (and posterior) tibia, medial malleolus, anterior fibula, and neck of the talus is the preferred treatment. Entrapped loose bodies or ossicles can be mistaken for anterior osteophytes and are excised. If removal of the anterior tibial and talar osteophyte (kissing lesion) is delayed, permanent tracking or destruction of articular cartilage over the talar dome and neck may result.

Postoperative management includes a soft compression dressing for a few days, early active range of motion, and strengthening exercises. Weightbearing is individualized. Intraarticular bupivacaine (Marcaine) is often helpful.

Symptomatic posterior osteophytes, as described by Schonholtz,[7] are rare. When encountered, they can be removed by any of the above-mentioned in-

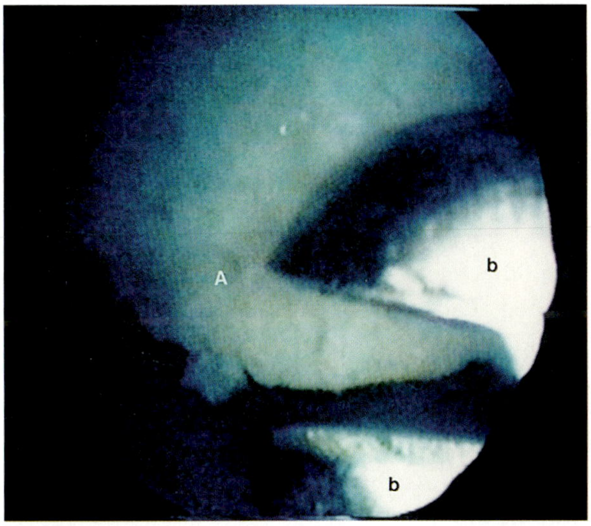

FIGURE 7.34. Video-arthroscopic view showing an osteophyte (A) being removed with a down-biting pituitary rongeur (b).

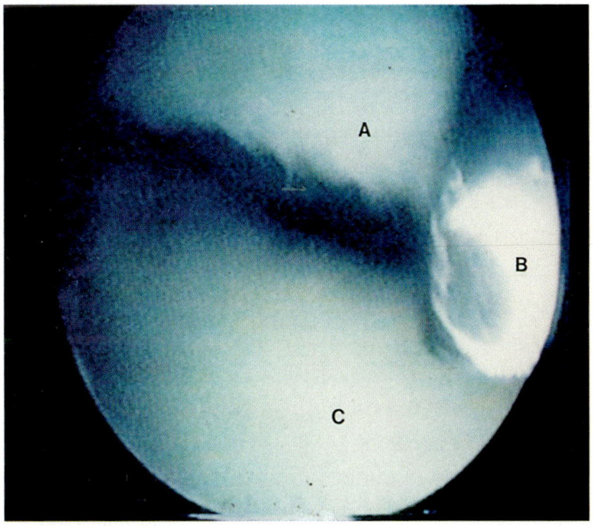

FIGURE 7.36. Another video-arthroscopic view of the case seen in Figures 7.34 and 7.35 shows the remainder of the osteophyte (A) excised with a small osteotome (B). C, dome of talus.

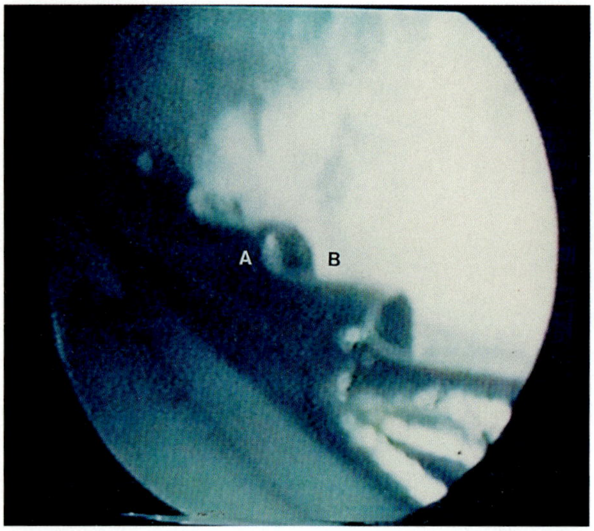

FIGURE 7.37. Final video-arthroscopic view of the case seen in Figures 7.34, 7.35, and 7.36. A rasp (A) is used to smooth the remaining margin of the anterior tibia. B, osteophyte.

struments via a posterolateral and accessory posterolateral portal. These are the same portals utilized to excise a symptomatic or pathologic os trigonum or Stieda's process.

INTEROSSEOUS BONE CYSTS

Bone cysts about the ankle are not common. They occur in the area of the plafond and in the body of the talus (juxtaarticular cyst). In the talus they are usually located in the same area as osteochondritis dissecans, which at times causes diagnostic confusion. The difference in cases we have seen is that the articular cartilage is usually intact. This is suggested by radiography, confirmed by CT scans, and further established at arthroscopy. These observations influence our choice of treatment. It is also of interest that trauma was the causative factor in these cases.

It was noted at arthroscopy that in cases of juxtaarticular cysts of the plafond the articular cartilage was intact; in a few of the cases there was a tiny dimple where impending breakthrough could be a threat. The treatment here was multiple drilling with a 0.062 inch Kirschner wire from a 2- to 3-mm hole in the tibial cortex from above using a guide. The Ferkel microvector guide is preferred for accuracy. Radiography and imaging are used as references. All healed, as did a few cases of multiple cysts located just above or adjacent to the tibial plafond. The latter lesions are related to early degenerative changes, which were thought to be the etiologic factor, rather than trauma. Bone grafting is not recommended unless the cyst is larger than 1 cm.

POSTERIOR OSTEOCHONDRAL IMPINGEMENT LESIONS

Osteochondral lesions of the posterior ankle or hindfoot must be differentiated from intraarticular soft tissue impingement lesions. Schonholtz[7] noted an osteophyte of the posterior tibial lip. Hamilton (personal communication, 1986) referred to a large posterior lip (spur) on the back of the talus that may cause posteromedial impingement. These structures are located intraarticularly. Arthroscopic surgery is now the procedure of choice.

Symptomatic nonunions of the posterior facet (attachment of the posterior talofibular ligament) can occur. Posterolateral lesions, such as those involving the os trigonum or trigonal process (Steida's process), are intraarticular and may cause symptoms in the hindfoot according to Parke.[8] If not well seen on routine radiography, they can be discovered by the bone scan and are better demonstrated by CT scans or MRI. These pathologic lesions are treated via arthroscopy by "stacked" posterolateral approaches (i.e., posterolateral and posterolateral accessory portals). They are placed in a vertical manner about 2.5–3.0 cm apart and immediately adjacent to the lateral border of the Achilles tendon.

POSTTRAUMATIC AND DEGENERATIVE ARTHRITIS

Arthroscopic treatment of the arthritic ankle was initially considered worthless by one of us (J.F.G.). Experience with abrading arthritic knees generated much initial enthusiasm, some overtreatment, and later disappointment. It then became evident that with proper selection some indications could be developed. Patients with arthritis of the ankle who should be excluded from arthroscopic consideration are those with advanced destruction, marked joint line narrowing, extensive fibrosis, and a significant degree of instability or deformity. Candidates for arthroscopic surgery include patients presenting with ankles having some limited motion due to capsulitis, a minimal to moderate degree of fibroarthrosis, osteophytes, chondral defects, loose bodies, chondromalacia, early arthritis, or only minimal instability. Also to be considered when contemplating arthroscopic treatment of degenerative arthritis of the ankle are the degree of disability, alternative forms of treatment, results of previous treatment, type of job demand, and expected result. Finally, a cooperative patient with a positive attitude and reasonable expectations can be considered a candidate for this type of surgery.

Results are sometimes highly favorable, whereas at other times there is only limited improvement. Partial recovery may be much appreciated and allow continued function and employment. The results may be further enhanced with the aid of antiinflammatory medications, aspirin, or other means of keeping these patients comfortable. Overtreatment for this condition should be carefully avoided. It should also be remembered that the radiographic picture of arthritis of the ankle does not always correlate with the symptoms. Some patients with advanced findings on radiographs and long-standing involvement are relatively asymptomatic. The ankle is sometimes a forgiving joint, whereas at other times, even with minimal involvement (especially on radiography), it is not.

When selecting patients with ankle arthritis for arthroscopic intervention, the above indications and conditions should be kept in mind. Long-standing symptoms, significant disability, and failure to respond to conservative treatment are prime indications for arthroscopic treatment. The expected results should always be clearly outlined to the patient.

The pathologic components of the arthritic ankle, as viewed from the arthroscopic standpoint, should be considered separately for treatment and the total picture assessed. These defects may be on any of the surfaces described; they include chondromalacia, osteophytes, loose bodies, and chondral and osteochondral defects. Treatment of all of the above has been discussed previously. Also to be considered are extensive chronic synovitis, synovial impingement lesions (local or general), adhesions, fibroarthrosis, and in some cases capsulitis. Initial débridement with motorized equipment and lavage is required.

Ogilvie-Harris reviewed 27 patients who had arthroscopic debridement for osteoarthritis of the ankle. The average age of the patients was 40 years, and their preoperative duration of symptoms was 4 years. The average follow-up was 45 months. Altogether, 20 patients were men, and 7 patients were women. Radiographs for arthritis were graded 1 to 3.

Arthroscopic débridement of the ankle had limited success. Two-thirds of the patients exhibited some improvement. It is clear that the goals of arthroscopy are limited. Patients can be afforded reasonable alleviation of their pain and improved function that will probably last for years.[9] The best results were in the mildest cases, and the least benefit was seen in severe cases.

CONCLUSIONS

Ankle arthroscopy has a great deal to offer patients with osteochondral pathology. For many of these entities, the results have lived up to our expectations, and the approach is rapidly becoming the standard of care. The results are limited, however, for arthroscopic débridement of the osteoarthritic ankle.

BIBLIOGRAPHY

1. Beltran J, Motor AM, Mosure JC, et al. Ankle: surface coil MR imaging at 1.5 T1. *Radiology* 1986; 161:203–209.
2. Kerr R, Forrester DM, Kingston S. Magnetic resonance imaging of foot and ankle trauma. *Orthop Clin North Am* 1990;21:591–603.
3. Cheung HS, Cottrell WH, Stephenson K, et al. In vitro collagen biosynthesis in healing and normal rabbit articular cartilage. *J Bone Joint Surg Am* 1978;60: 1076–1081.
4. Milgram JW. The classification of loose bodies in human joints. *Clin Orthop* 1977;124;282–291.
5. O'Donoghue DH. Chondral and osteochondral fractures. *J Trauma* 1966;6:469–481.
6. Stoller SM. A comparative study of the frequency of anterior impingement exostosis of the ankle in dancer and nondancer. *Foot Ankle* 1984;4:201–203.
7. Schonholtz GJ. *Arthroscopic surgery of the shoulder, elbow and ankle*. Springfield, IL: Charles C Thomas, 1986.
8. Parks JC. Injuries of the hindfoot. *Clin Orthop* 1977; 122:28–36.
9. Ogilvie-Harris DJ, Sekyiotu A. Arthroscopic debridement for the osteoarthritic ankle. *Arthroscopy* 1995;11: 433–436.

SECTION 2: Osteochondritis Dissecans

Osteochondritis dissecans is synonymous with osteochondral fracture of the dome of the talus. It is referred to as a transchondral fracture, an intraarticular fracture, or a flake fracture.

ETIOLOGY

In 1856 Alexander Munro[1] first reported the presence of loose bodies in the ankle joint. Konig[2] in 1888 classified loose bodies in other joints and suggested spontaneous necrosis as their origin. He also proposed the term *osteochondritis dissecans* to describe these lesions. Barth[3] described the same lesion in 1898 and proposed it to be an intraarticular fracture. Fisher[4] in 1920 and Phemister[5] in 1924 classified the many conditions that produced loose bodies. Kappis[6] in 1922 was the first to use the term osteochondritis dissecans of the ankle joint. In 1932 Rendu[7] described it as an intraarticular fracture of the talus. Berndt and Harty[8] reviewed the world literature in 1959 and presented their own theories. They suggested that the term *transchondral fracture* of the talus best described the etiology and pathology of this lesion. O'Donoghue[9] during the mid-1960s also stated that these lesions were intraarticular fractures.

Davidson et al[10] thought that although O'Donoghue's work referred primarily to the knee joint it also applied to any discussions of the ankle joint. In separate discussions Goldstone and Pisani[11] and Campbell and Ranawat[12] indicated that there were causes for osteochondritis dissecans of the ankle other than trauma. Campbell and Ranawat pointed out that bone infarction preceded these pathologic fractures.

The predominant theory regarding etiology, however, still appeared to be trauma. Yvars[13] in 1976 and Alexander and Lichtman[14] in 1980 emphasized that the usual etiology was trauma and the preferred treatment was operative. In Canale and Balding's[15] 1981 series 25 of 29 injuries were due to trauma. Since the days of Berndt and Harty, trauma has been considered the leading cause of osteochondritis dissecans or osteochondral fractures.

INCIDENCE

Osteochondritis dissecans of the talus comprises about 4% of all cases of osteochondritis dissecans. It occurs most commonly during the third decade. McCullough and Venugopal[16] reported an average age of 27 years in their series. Males predominate slightly in most series.

Medial dome lesions are more common than lateral lesions in most series. Yao and Weis[17] reported 56 lesions located on the medial aspect of the talar dome compared to 34 of the lateral talar dome. A review of several series found that the incidence of bilateral lesions averaged about 10%. According to Berndt and Harty,[8] 9 of 207 cases were bilateral. Blom and Strijk[18] reported that 2 of 16 were bilateral in their study. Lindholm et al.[19] stated that 3 of 17 were bilateral. There were two central lesions in Canale and Belding's series of 29 talar dome lesions.

MECHANISM OF INJURY

According to Yao and Weis,[17] lateral lesions are caused by eversion of the foot with the ankle dorsiflexed and the tibia internally rotated on the talus. These lesions are almost always secondary to trauma. The medial lesions are almost always secondary to trauma. The medial lesions are likely caused by inversion of the foot with the ankle plantar-flexed. They may occur without any antecedent trauma.

LOCATION

Lesions of the medial aspect of the dome of the talus occur in the mid or posterior third. Osteochondral fractures on the lateral side of the dome are in the mid or anterior portion, with some exceptions. On occasion they are centrally located on the talar dome. Rarely, multiple lesions are seen (Fig. 7.38).

STRUCTURAL CHARACTERISTICS

Medial dome lesions are usually asymmetric, whereas lateral dome lesions are symmetric. Also, the medial lesions appear to be deep and cup-shaped, and they usually remain in situ. Lateral lesions are more shallow. Medial lesions cause fewer symptoms, heal spontaneously at times, and do not lead to the development of arthritis according to Canale and Belding.[15] According to Roden et al.,[20] lateral lesions rarely heal with conservative treatment, cause more symptoms, and may lead to early arthritic changes after open surgery.

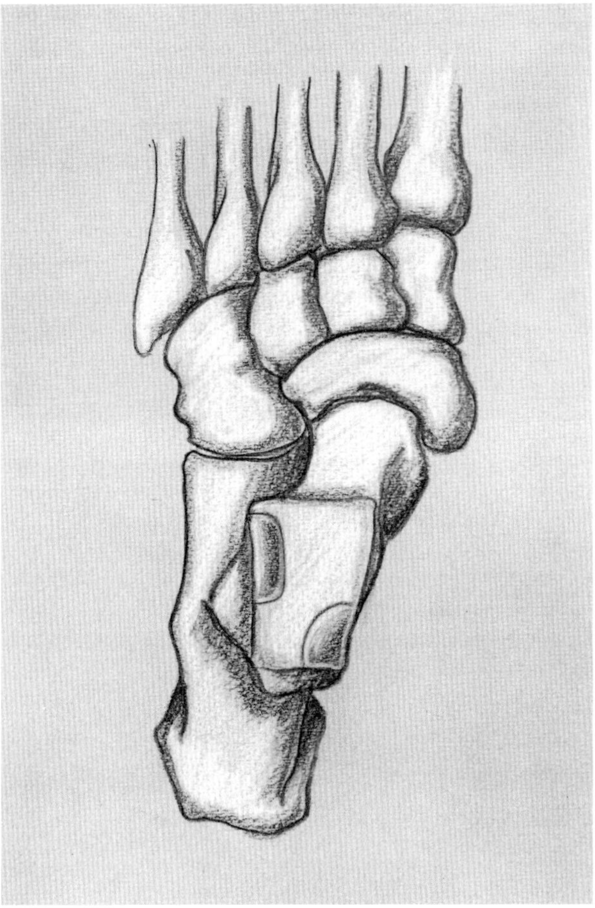

FIGURE 7.38. Location of osteochondritis dissecans in the medial and lateral aspects of the talar dome. (Courtesy of G.R. Paul.)

SYMPTOMATOLOGY

The presenting symptomatology in acute cases may include pain, swelling, ecchymosis, and limited range of motion. In chronic cases joint stiffness can be found associated with a deep aching sensation and crepitus. Swelling and joint-line tenderness can also be elicited. Joint locking is highly unusual.

RADIOGRAPHIC AND IMAGING TECHNIQUES

Radiographic examination includes anteroposterior (AP), lateral, and internal oblique views. Tomography is helpful for better defining the lesion. This particular investigation can be helpful for stage I and II osteochondral lesions. Plain computed tomography (CT) or axial CT following injection of contrast material have been used successfully for diagnosing osteochondral fractures of the talus. Coronal CT following double-contrast arthrography has been used to study the stability of the osteochondral fragments. The presence of contrast material between the osteochondral fragments and the talar bed demonstrates the absence of any bony or fibrous union between the fragments and the talar dome. The interpretation of coronal arthrotomography results is easy, as the plane of the osteochondral separation and the articular cartilage lining is at a right angle to the plane of imaging. Bone scans can be helpful for stage I lesions. Osteochondral fractures are clearly demonstrated using surface coil magnetic resonance imaging (MRI) (see Figs. 7.51 and 7.52, below).

STAGING

Berndt and Harty[8] staged lesions of the talar dome according to their appearance at surgery. Stage I was defined as a compression fracture without displacement (intact). Stage II represented an incomplete avulsion of the osteochondral fragment (early separation). Stage III was complete avulsion of an osteochondral fragment without displacement (detached). Stage IV was a completely displaced osteochondral fragment (displaced). Stage IV lesions may lie upside down in the crater or may be completely separated from the lesion. This classification applies to both medial and lateral lesions (Figs. 7.39–7.42).

Berndt and Harty[8] concluded in 1959 and Canale and Belding[15] agreed, that stage I and II medial or lateral lesions, along with stage III medial lesions, should be treated nonoperatively. Lateral stage III and medial and lateral stage IV lesions should be excised and the base of the lesion curetted. Blom and Strijk[18] found that stage II and stage III lesions were not always distinguishable by radiographic techniques. They also stated that the degree of involvement of bone and cartilage can vary from fracture of only the cartilage (i.e., chondral fracture) to fracture of only the osseous part, which leaves the articular cartilage intact (the latter was described by Berndt and Harty as a transchondral fracture).

Both medial and lateral lesions predispose to the formation of loose bodies. It occurs more so in the latter.

Arthroscopy has added a new dimension to the evaluation of ankle osteochondritis dissecans. The arthroscopic examination is frequently at odds with that predicted by radiographic evaluation. Although arthrography combined with computed tomography

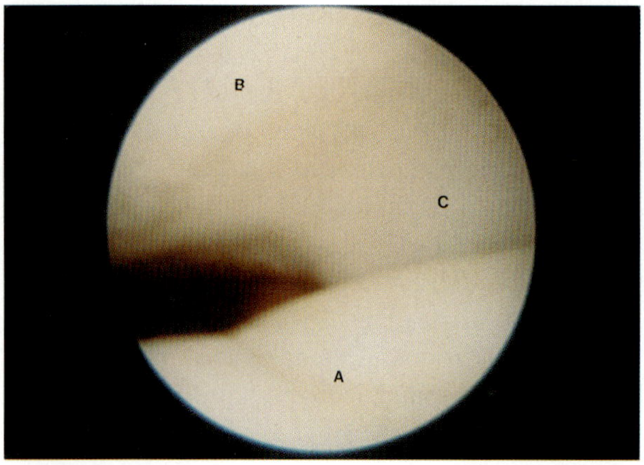

FIGURE 7.39. Arthroscopic view of an intact lesion in a young patient. There is slight bulging or elevation of the lesion, which is magnified to some degree by the arthroscope. The entire border was intact, and there was no break in the articular cartilage. The lesion was firm in its bed when probed. Transmalleolar drilling in situ is the treatment of choice, especially in young patients. A, intact osteochondritis lesion; B, plafond; C, medial malleolus. In older patients (15 years and up), if the bulging lesion is large, hard when probed, and causes incongruity with joint motion, débridement, abrasion, and drilling should be considered.

and magnetic resonance imaging techniques attempt to determine the integrity of the articular cartilage, the predictions are frequently found to be incorrect at arthroscopic examination.

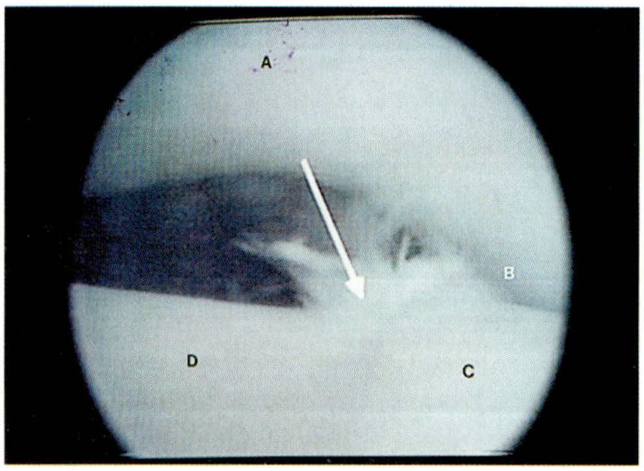

FIGURE 7.40. Video-arthroscopic view of osteochondritis dissecans of the medial dome of the talus, showing partial separation. Note the break in the articular cartilage at the border of the lesion where fibrous tissue protrudes. When probed, this lesion appears to be slightly loose, indicating early separation. The treatment in this case is complete excision, débridement, abrasion, and drilling of the base. Arrow, fibrous margin; A, plafond; B, medial malleolus; C, separated osteochondritis lesion; D, dome of talus.

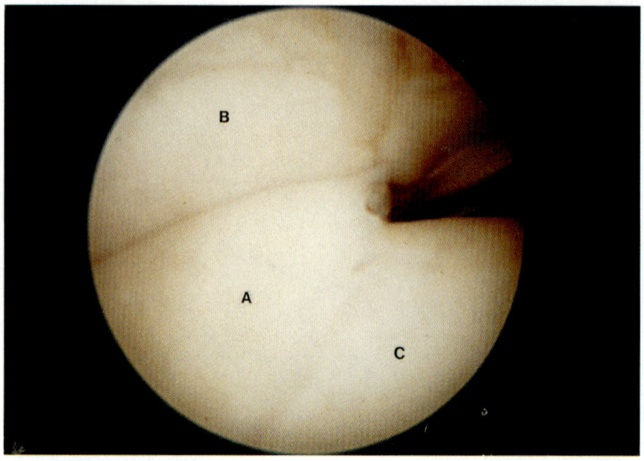

FIGURE 7.41. Arthroscopic view of a separated osteochondritis lesion. A, Break in the cartilage is complete. The fragment was easily lifted from its bed with a probe. Reconstruction (excision, débridement, abrasion, drilling) of the defect is the treatment of choice. Postoperatively, early motion within a few days and weight-bearing were employed at about 2 weeks with a good result. B, medial malleolus; C, dome of talus.

MANAGEMENT OF OSTEOCHONDRITIS DISSECANS OF THE TALUS

Osteochondral fractures of the talus can be treated nonoperatively or surgically. The nonoperative approach consists of immobilization in a plaster cast. The period of immobilization in the reported series is 8–18 weeks. According to Canale, stage I and

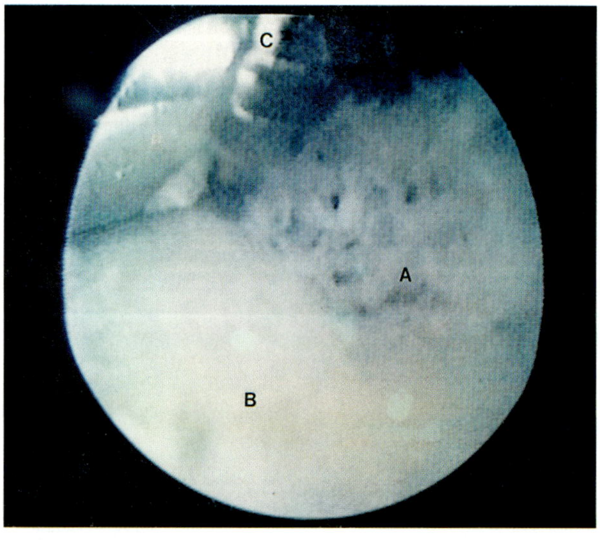

FIGURE 7.42. Video-arthroscopic view of a reconstructed crater (A) (osteochondral dissecans) in the medial dome of the talus (B). Note the arthroscopic abrader (C) in the top left corner.

some stage II lesions, medial or lateral, can heal with conservative treatment. Although stage III medial lesions can heal by nonoperative means, stage III lateral lesions often require surgical excision.

Several authors have advocated early surgery for the treatment of osteochondral lesions of one talar dome in active individuals. Surgical treatment has been shown to yield good long-term results in some reported cases. Many methods are available, such as the use of large soft tissue incisions, grooving of the distal tibia, and ostotomy of the medial malleolus.

ARTHROSCOPIC TECHNIQUES

The introduction of arthroscopy for the diagnosis and treatment of osteochondritis dissecans and dome fractures of the talus offers improved results. Distraction (invasive or noninvasive) has added another dimension to surgery performed for these lesions. Prior to ankle arthroscopy, the exact status of the health of the articular cartilage could not always be evaluated adequately. Now, however, utilizing direct viewing and probing, the articular cartilage is evaluated in a much more accurate fashion. Whereas the radiographic images may have suggested that the lesion was intact, direct observation often proves otherwise. This added dimension affects the treatment and prognosis.

Classification by arthroscopy should result in selection of the most appropriate surgical procedure. For example, intact lesions (as found on radiography) have at times been seen to be separated at arthroscopy, and lesions that appeared separated were subsequently found to be intact. Furthermore, intact lesions can now be treated in young patients by arthroscopic drilling in addition to or instead of immobilization alone.

With the use of arthroscopy and distraction, it has often been noted that the articular cartilage is a little soft or fibrillated and therefore invariably becomes loose with time. Areas of elevation or depression are often observed. Fibrous tissue may be noted protruding from the border of the lesion between the normal and abnormal articular cartilage. If these changes are present, there is no reason to try to save the cartilage or the separated osteochondral fragments. This observation indicates the presence of fibrous tissue between the necrotic bone fragment and underlying normal bone. These pathologic changes are irreversible, and healing in situ cannot be expected. Treatment of these lesions should include removing the loose cartilage or fragments, and curretting, abrading, and drilling the base to freshly bleeding bone (Figs. 7.43–7.47).

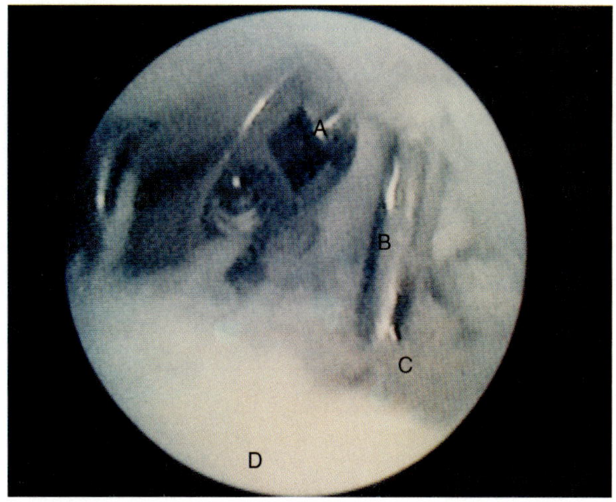

FIGURE 7.43. Anteromedial view showing the 70-degree oblique arthroscope (A) (posterolateral portal) in the top left corner and a 0.062 inch Kirschner wire (B) through the medial malleolus and into the crater (C) for drilling the base. D, dome of the talus.

The goal of treatment is to obtain good, tough fibrocartilaginous tissue to fill the defect, which yields good results. Should arthroscopic reconstruction (excision, débridement, abrading, drilling) not be done, it is likely that degenerative arthritis will occur at an early age.

At the present time, arthroscopic surgery is the rule. The status of the articular cartilage can be eval-

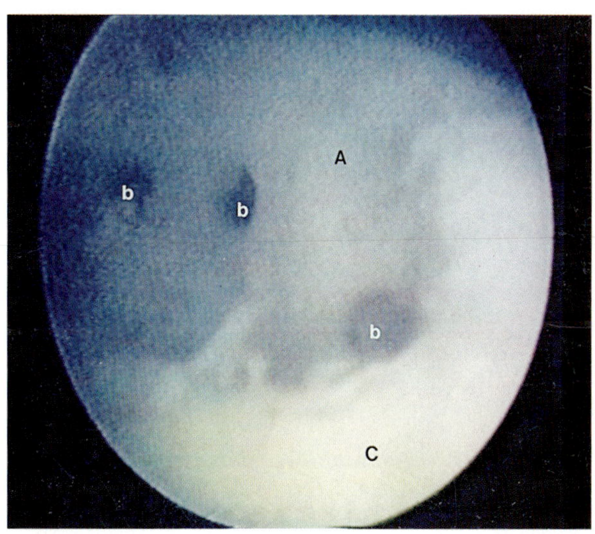

FIGURE 7.44. Arthroscopic view of the same crater as in Figure 7.43 (A) through the 70 degree oblique arthroscope inserted through the posterolateral portal. A, crater; b, drill holes; C, dome of the talus.

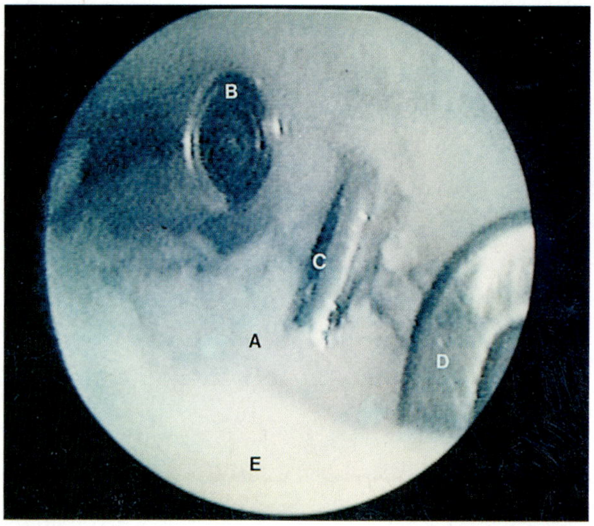

FIGURE 7.45. Video-arthroscopic view of the same crater (A) as in Figure 7.44. Note the medium-size (2.5 mm) arthroscope (B) in the upper left corner (posterolateral portal). Kirschner wire (C) is in the middle, and the probe (D) is in the lower right corner. E, dome of talus.

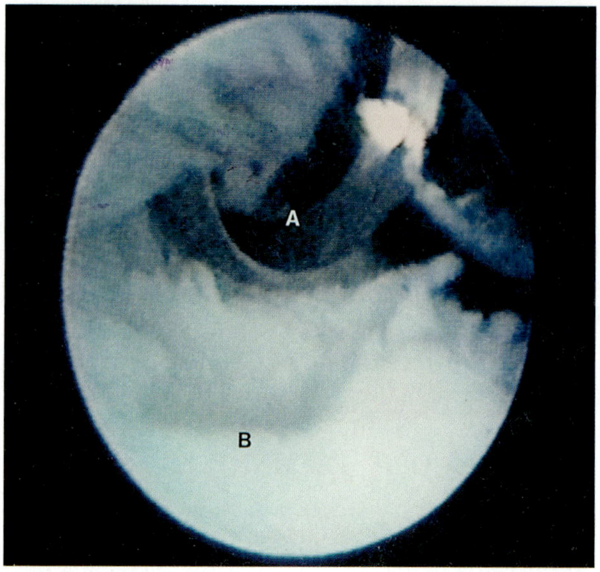

FIGURE 7.47. View through the 2.3-mm arthroscope (posterolateral probe) showing a curette (A) removing the remaining loose cartilage. B, margin of deficit.

uated and the viability of the lesion determined to decide whether the lesion can be left alone, drilled, pinned, or excised. When the articular cartilage is normal and the lesion is stable, drilling may be indicated. When the articular cartilage lining is normal with an unstable lesion (presence of dermarcation or fracture line) that has enough subchondral bone, pinning or grafting (large lesion) may be performed. If there is not enough subchondral bone, excision with drilling or abrasion is preferable.

When the articular cartilage lining is soft on palpation or is fibrillated or degenerated, although the lesion may be stable, excision is recommended followed by drilling or abrasion. When the articular cartilage is soft, fibrillated, or degenerated with an unstable lesion, excision and curettage are recommended followed by drilling or abrasion of the bed of the lesion.

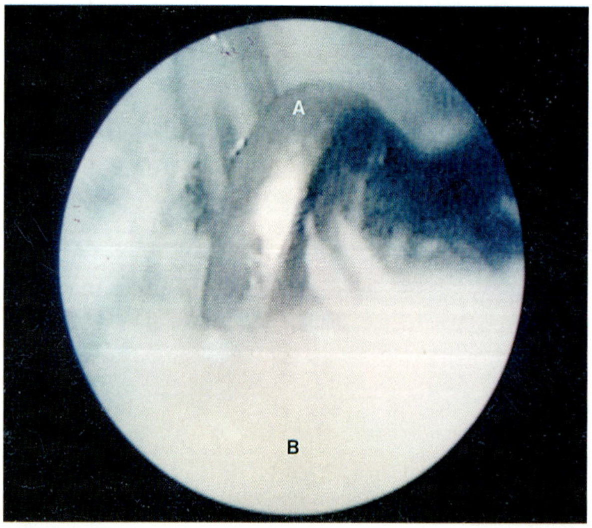

FIGURE 7.46. Video-arthroscopic view through a medium-size arthroscope (2.5 mm) from the posterolateral approach. The probe (A) is shown lifting the posterior surface of the crater, demonstrating an additional significant amount of loose diseased cartilage (B) that was not appreciated from the anterolateral approach.

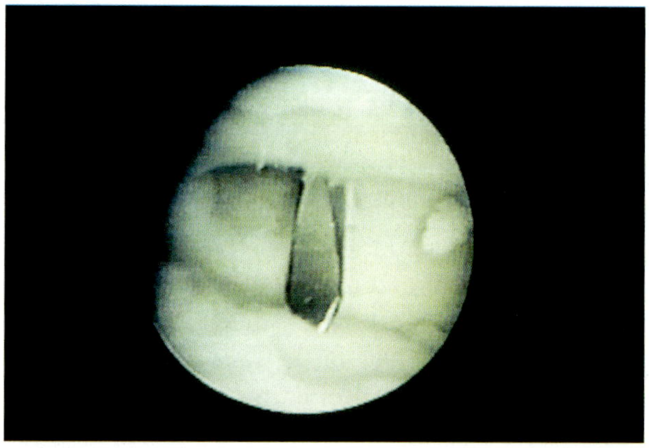

FIGURE 7.48. Video-arthroscopic view by way of the posterolateral portal of drilling with a 0.062 inch wire by way of the transmalleolar canal for intact lesion.

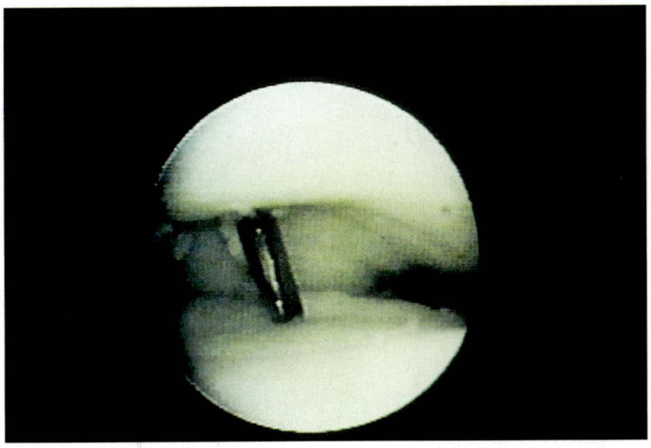

FIGURE 7.49. Another view of the area shown in Figure 7.48.

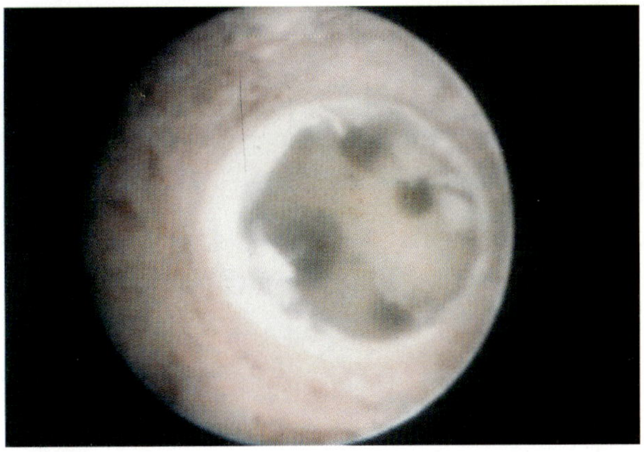

FIGURE 7.50. Video-arthroscopic view via the transmalleolar portal showing multiple holes through intact cartilage.

Drilling, Débridement, Pinning, or Bone Grafting

Osteochondral lesions located laterally are usually anterior and are easily accessible for arthroscopic drilling or pinning (Figs. 7.48–7.60). Two portals are required: one on the medial side for placing the arthroscope and the other on the lateral side for introducing the operating instrument. Kirschner wire (0.062 inch) is used for the drilling to stimulate revascularization. If the chondral fragment has underlying bone, it can be reattached with absorbable (biodegradable) pins or screws.

Because medial lesions are usually located on the posterior aspect of the ankle, they may be difficult to drill or pin using the anterior portals. The

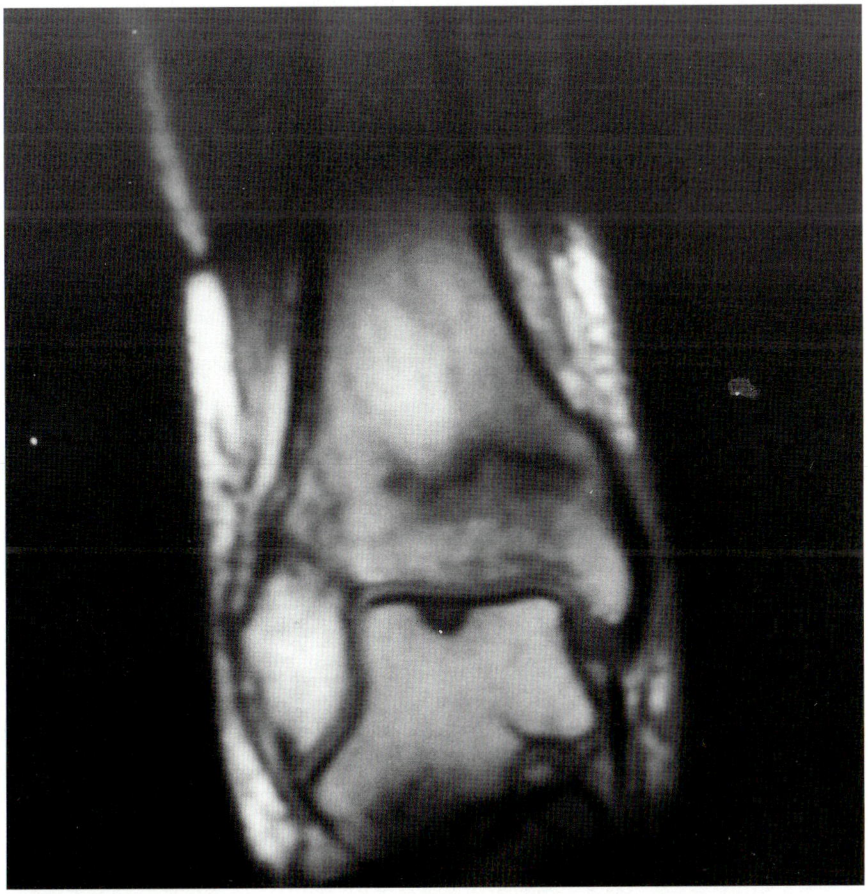

FIGURE 7.51. Anteroposterior magnetic resonance imaging (MRI) scan shows a large central osteocartilaginous defect of the central talus, which was not seen on routine films or tomograms in both planes.

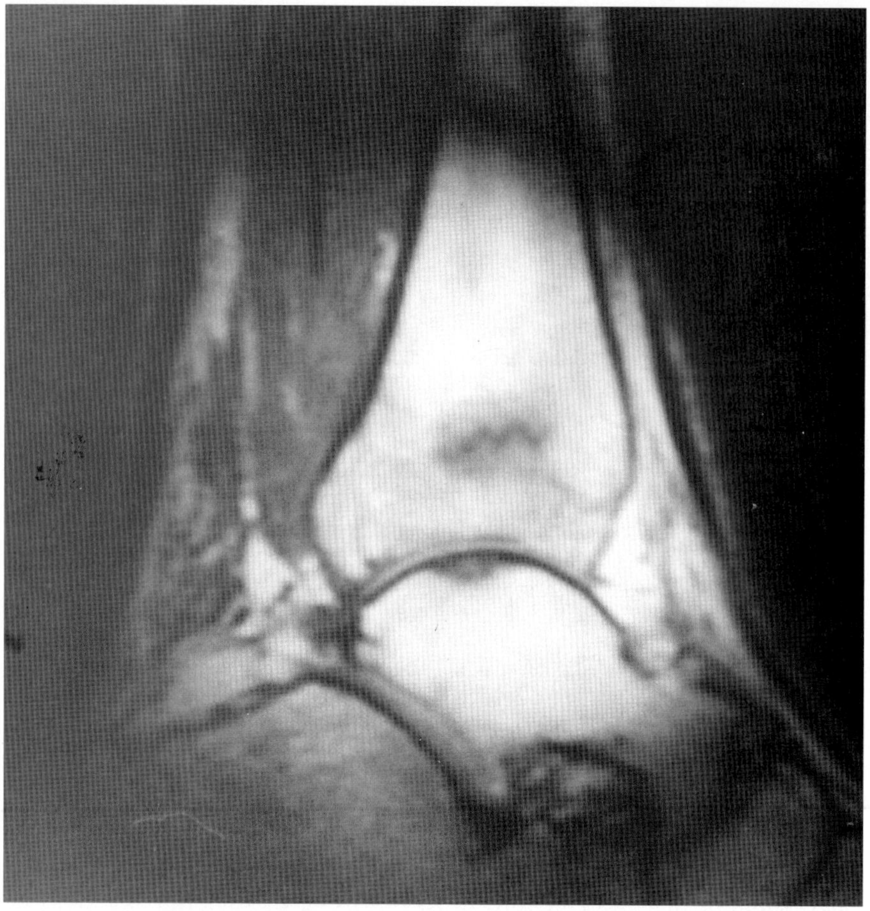

FIGURE 7.52. MRI lateral view of the defect seen in Fig. 7.51. The articular cartilage was intact at arthroscopy.

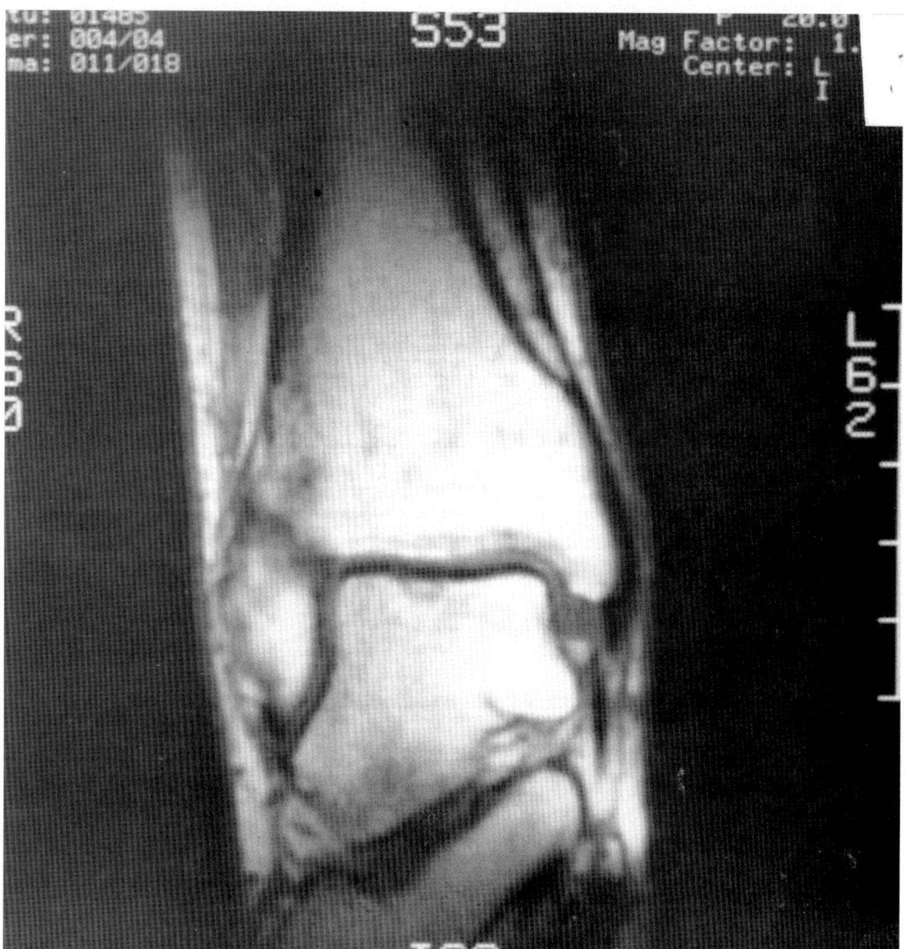

FIGURE 7.53. Anteroposterior MRI scan at 2 months after operation. The lesion was drilled arthroscopically with fine (0.062 inch) Kirschner wires, using the transmalleolar approach. The arthroscopic anterior cruciate ligament guide was used for accuracy during wire placement.

FIGURE 7.54. Lateral MRI scan demonstrates healing.

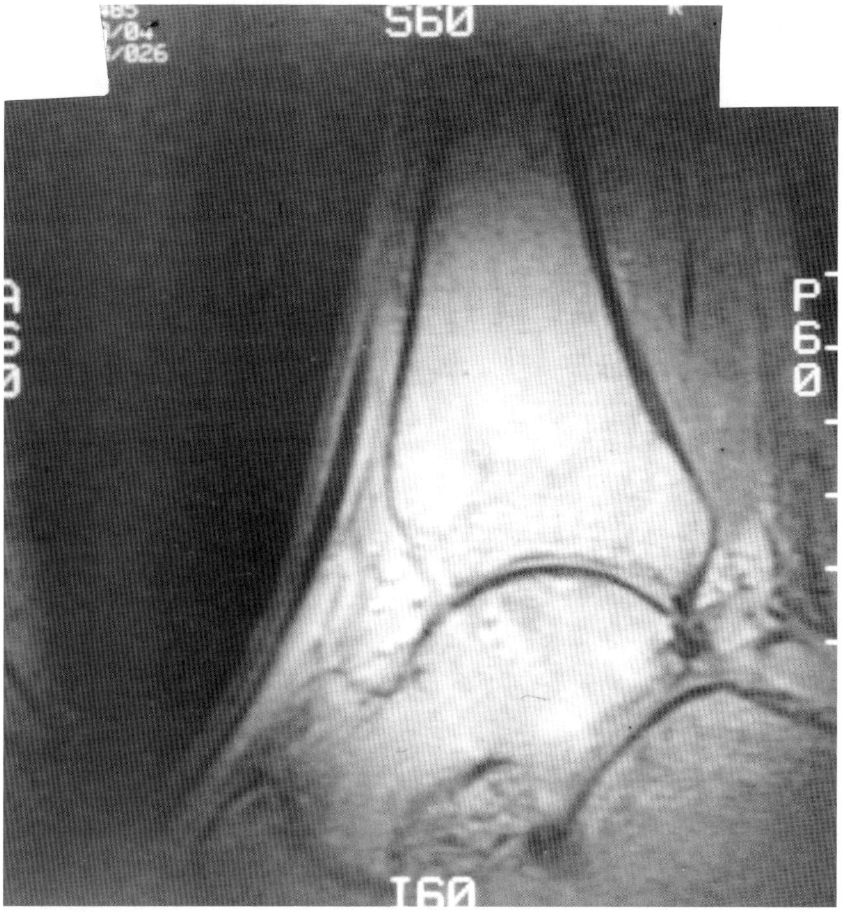

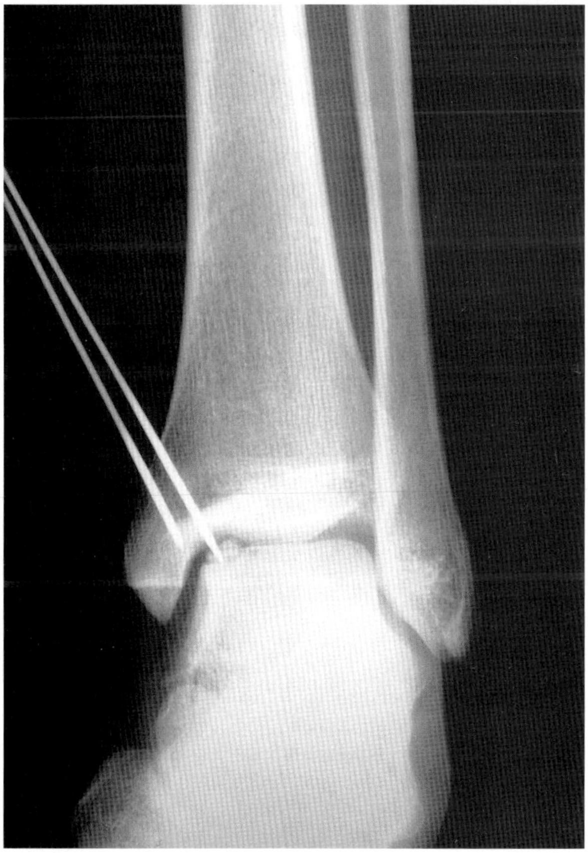

FIGURE 7.55. Anteroposterior radiographic view showing two 0.062 inch Kirschner wires drilling the lesion by the transmalleolar approach.

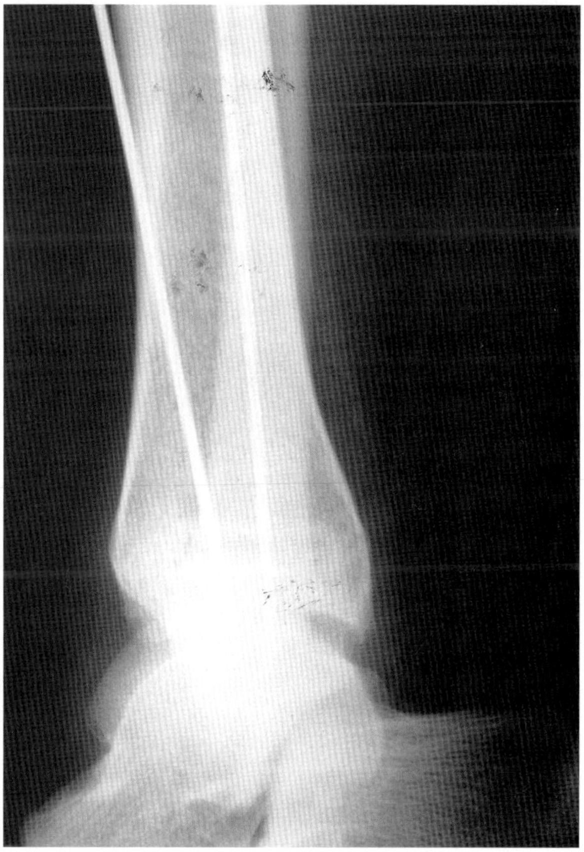

FIGURE 7.56. Lateral radiographic view shows the wire placement for transmalleolar drilling.

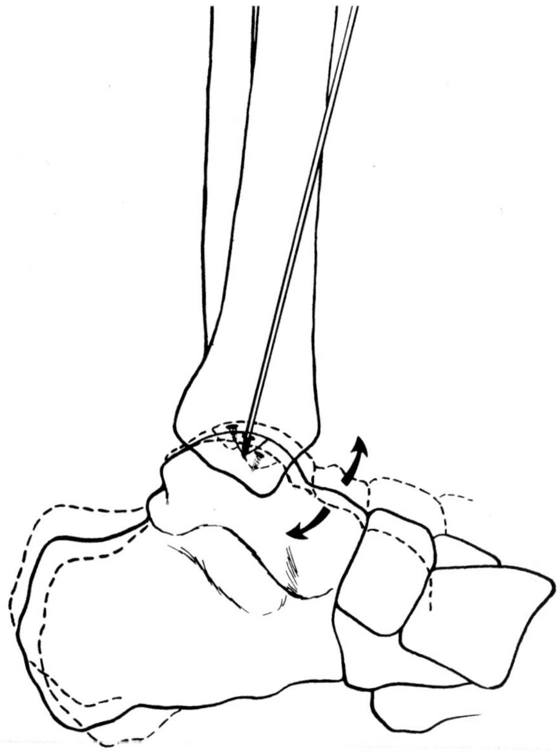

FIGURE 7.57. Two parallel wires are used for drilling. The ankle is flexed and extended. Although up to eight drill holes can be made, in this case there were six.

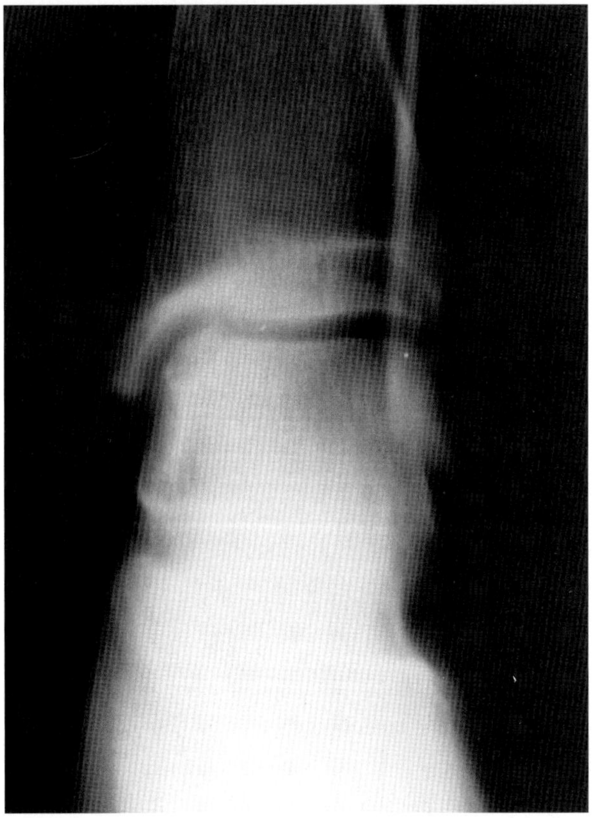

FIGURE 7.58. Anteroposterior radiographic view shows healing 2 months after drilling.

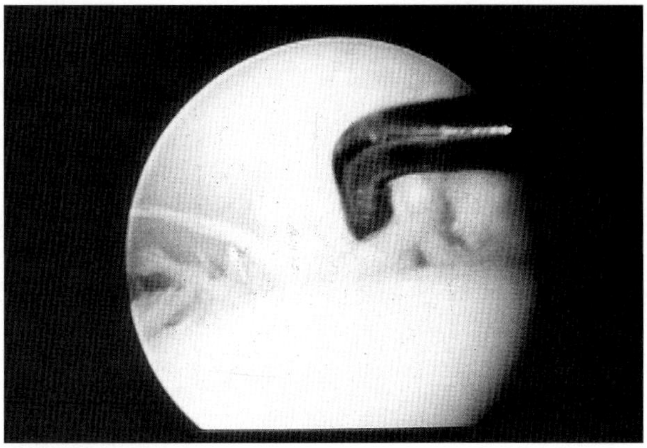

FIGURE 7.59. Arthroscopic view shows the detached lesion being lifted from its bed with a probe.

transmalleolar portal can be used with noninvasive distraction (Guhl noninvasive distraction; Smith/Nephew–Acufex). A drill guide (Ferkel guide) is recommended to facilitate drilling on the lesion. If bone grafting is contemplated, the technique requires a tunnel in the medial malleolus.

However, concerns exist regarding the use of this approach. The hole made in the malleolus represents a potential area of stress concentration and theoretically increases the risk of postoperative fracture, although this has not been a problem clinically. Placing a 4- to 5-mm hole through the articular surfaces of the talus and the tibia may contribute to the development of later degenerative changes in the ankle joint. Finally, scar tissue or adhesions may form in the area between the osteochondritis dissecans

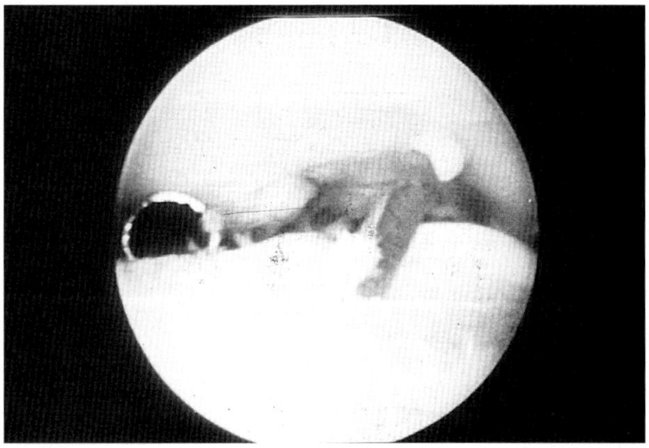

FIGURE 7.60. Arthroscopic view shows the procedure for retrograde (distal to proximal) drilling of the osteochondral defect with a 0.062 inch Kirschner wire. The procedure was performed with noninvasive distraction in this woman with relatively lax ligaments. The Kirschner wire was redirected slightly to place multiple drill holes into the lesion from the same starting point.

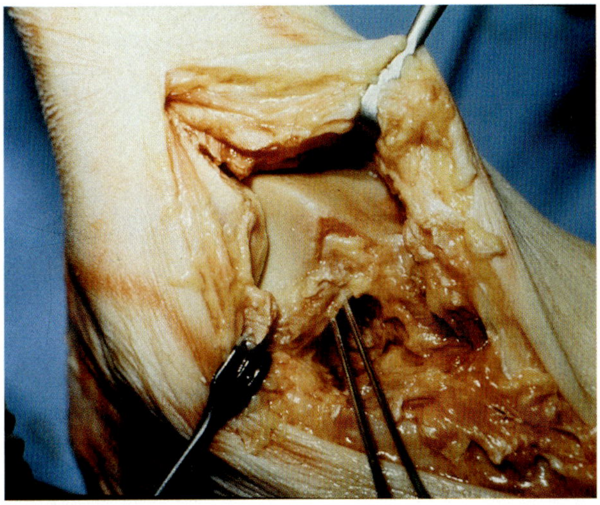

FIGURE 7.61. Cadaver dissection specimen identifies the starting point for the retrograde drilling procedure. Two guide pins were placed percutaneously under arthroscopic control for a simulated lesion of the posteromedial dome of the talus in the cadaver specimen. The pins pass through the sinus tarsi and enter the talus in its nonarticular portion distal to the articular surface of the dome of the talus and anterior to the articular surface of the lateral side of the talus. The entry point is anterior to the insertion of the anterior talofibular ligament.

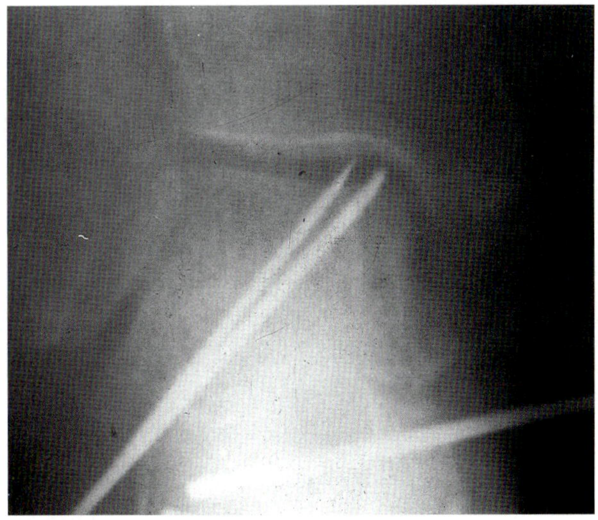

FIGURE 7.63. Anteroposterior radiograph of the ankle seen in Figures 7.61 and 7.62 demonstrates placement of the two pins into the posteromedial talar dome lesion.

lesion and the medial malleolar drill hole, which are in close proximity to each other. This complication did occur in the patient whose postoperative pain was relieved by arthroscopic resection of the adhesive band.

These potential complications have spurred the development of a new technique for drilling and bone grafting posteromedial osteochondritis dissecans lesions of the talar dome. Guhl and James W. Stone developed the technique that employs retrograde drilling of the lesion through the talus (Figs. 7.61–7.69). This approach avoids the potential complications involved with a transmalleolar approach. A guide pin is placed percutaneously in the sinus tarsi such that it enters the talus in its nonarticular portion just anterior to the insertion of the anterior talofibular ligament. This location is distal to the articular surface of the lateral aspect of the talus. The pin is angled in the direction of the posteromedial dome of the talus. Use of an anterior cruciate liga-

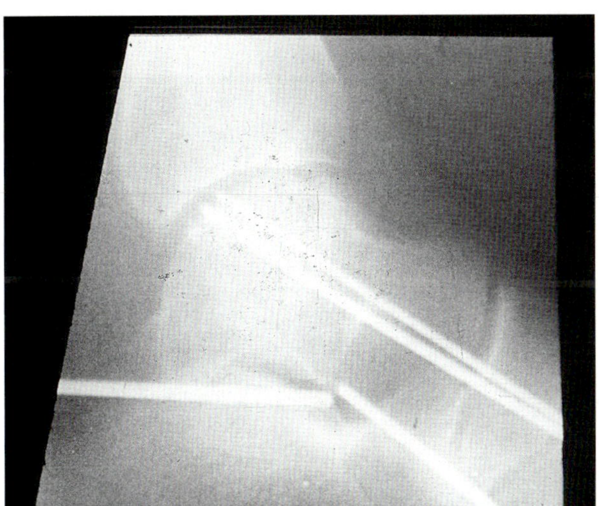

FIGURE 7.62. Lateral radiograph of the ankle seen in Figure 7.61 with two guide pins in place. (The two lower pins were placed in the subtalar joint.)

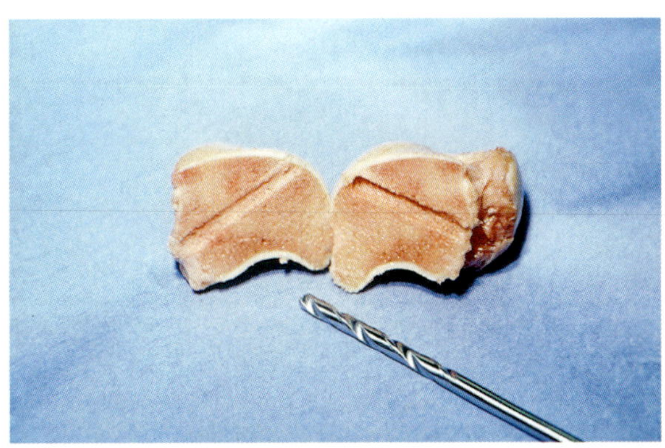

FIGURE 7.64. One of the guide pins shown in Figure 7.63 was overdrilled with a 5-mm cannulated reamer, after which the talus was disarticulated from the specimen and split in half along the path of the reamer. The path of the reamer passes through the middle of the talus and therefore is unlikely to compromise the support of the articular cartilage of the talar dome.

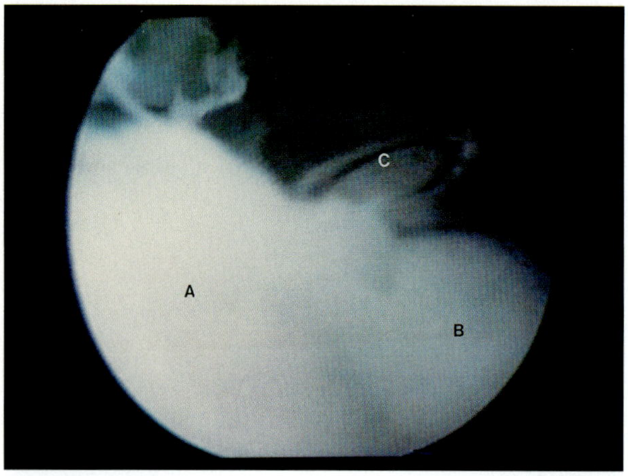

FIGURE 7.65. Video-arthroscopic view of the lesion seen in Figure 7.64. The lesion appeared intact on radiography but was not intact at arthroscopy because the articular cartilage over the lesion had a different texture and color. The lesion was easily lifted with a needle. A, separated osteochondritis lesion; B, dome of the talus; C, tip of the hypodermic needle.

ment reconstruction guide or the small ankle guide designed by Ferkel can facilitate placement of this pin. Cadaver studies have shown that pin placement in this area does not damage the articular surface, nor does it significantly undermine or weaken support of the talar dome. The pin can be repositioned to place multiple drill holes in an area that has been débrided.

The technique can also be used to bone-graft an intact posteromedial osteochondritis dissecans lesion without traversing the medial malleolus or penetrating the overlying articular cartilage. The guide pin is overdrilled with a 4- to 5-mm cannulated drill

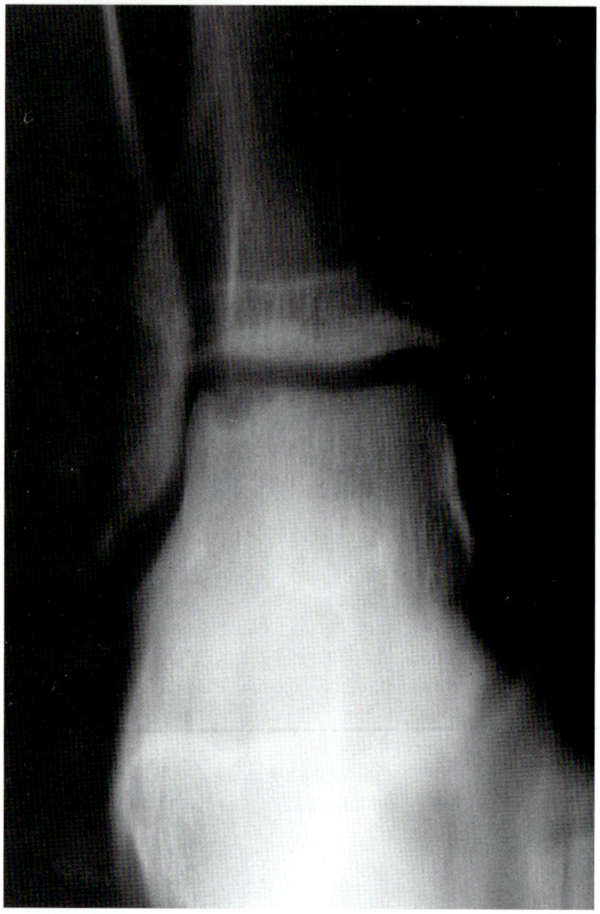

FIGURE 7.67. Anteroposterior radiographic view of an intact lesion of the medial talus.

under direct arthroscopic visualization. The pin is advanced to, but not through, the articular cartilage. Care is taken to avoid injury to the articular surface. The drilling can be motivated intraoperatively us-

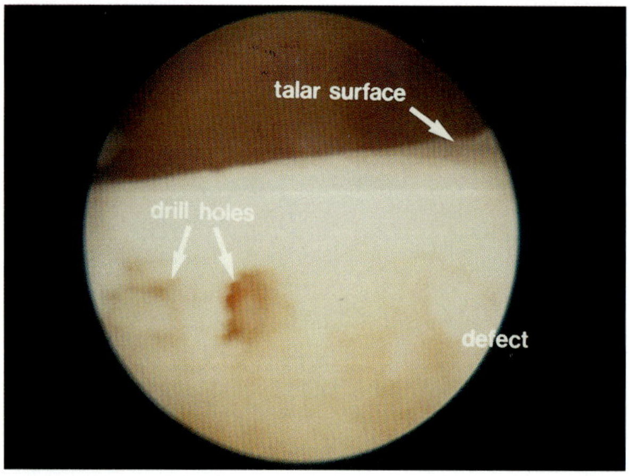

FIGURE 7.66. Postoperative arthroscopic view of the patient shown in Figure 7.65 shows a lesion in the right ankle after drilling.

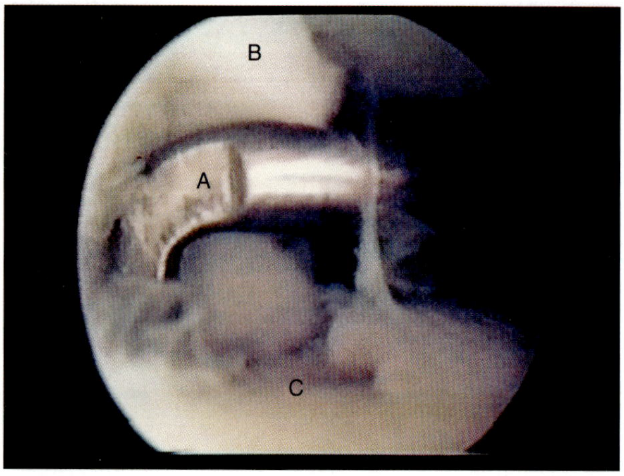

FIGURE 7.68. Video-arthroscopic view shows the probe lifting off the diseased articular cartilage at the site of the lesion. A, probe; B, flap of cartilage; C, base of the lesion.

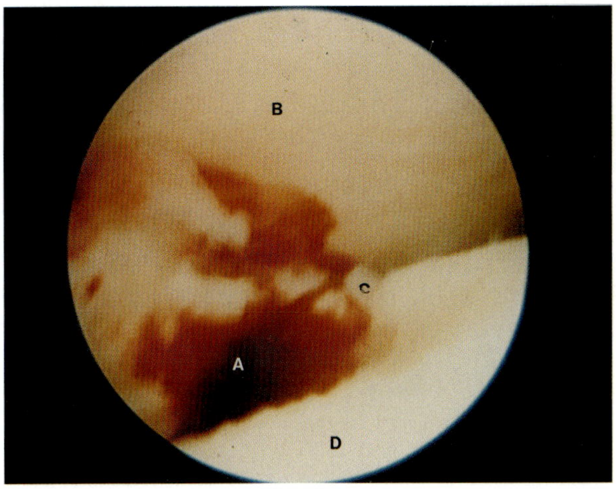

FIGURE 7.69. Arthroscopic view after reconstruction shows bleeding following release of the tourniquet, which is important for confirming that there was sufficient abrasion and drilling. A, fresh bleeding; B, plafond; C, reconstructed crater; D, dome of the talus.

ing image intensification. After drilling the hole so it is 4–5 mm in diameter, a bone graft is packed into the hole. Early postoperative motion is instituted, but weight-bearing is limited for approximately 6 weeks.

Excising Posteromedial Lesions of the Talus With Distraction

Technique

General or spinal anesthesia is used to sedate the patient for excising a posteromedial lesion of the talus with distraction. The patient is then placed in a supine position, with the ipsilateral buttock elevated on a folded sheet. The leg is immobilized in a leg holder and the ankle placed on a well padded box or a rolled sheet. A tourniquet is placed on the thigh but is usually not inflated. After localizing the two branches of the superficial peroneal nerve, anterolateral and anteromedial portals are placed. A standard 4 mm, 30 degree angled arthroscope is used as well as a 70 degree arthroscope for visualizing a posteriorly placed lesion. The small instrumentation set is necessary and consists of a small probe, small cutting instruments, basket forceps scissors, grasping forceps, and small motorized instruments. The use of a disposable cannula system with a side port that allows inflow or outflow of saline eliminates the need for an accessory portal and also prevents soft tissue damage by constantly inserting and removing the surgical instruments. After localizing the lesion, a partial synovectomy is performed to improve visualization. A small flat-ended probe is used to palpate the lesion, which is scooped out with a small, curved knife and displaced into the anterior compartment where it can be excised with a grasping forceps. Curettage and drilling or abrasion complete the procedure (see Postoperative Care). The procedure is outlined in Figures 7.70–7.86.

Postoperative Care

Patients with reconstructed lesions (excision, débridement, abrasion, drilling) should institute early motion postoperatively and begin weight-bearing as tolerated. Participation in sports should be withheld until the lesion is judged completely healed and the tissue is mature. Patients with extensive, shallow lesions of

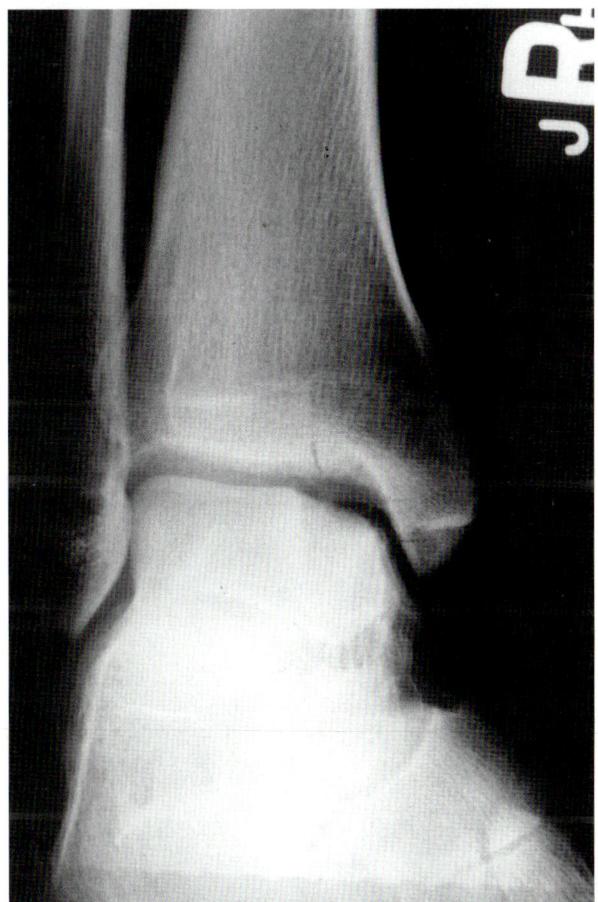

FIGURE 7.70. Anteroposterior radiograph with a large lesion of the right ankle. This 37-year-old man had osteochondritis dissecans treated by arthrotomy and curettage 3 years before being seen by one of the authors (J.F.G.). A large loose body was removed at that time. According to the operative report, drilling was not done. The patient continued to have symptoms.

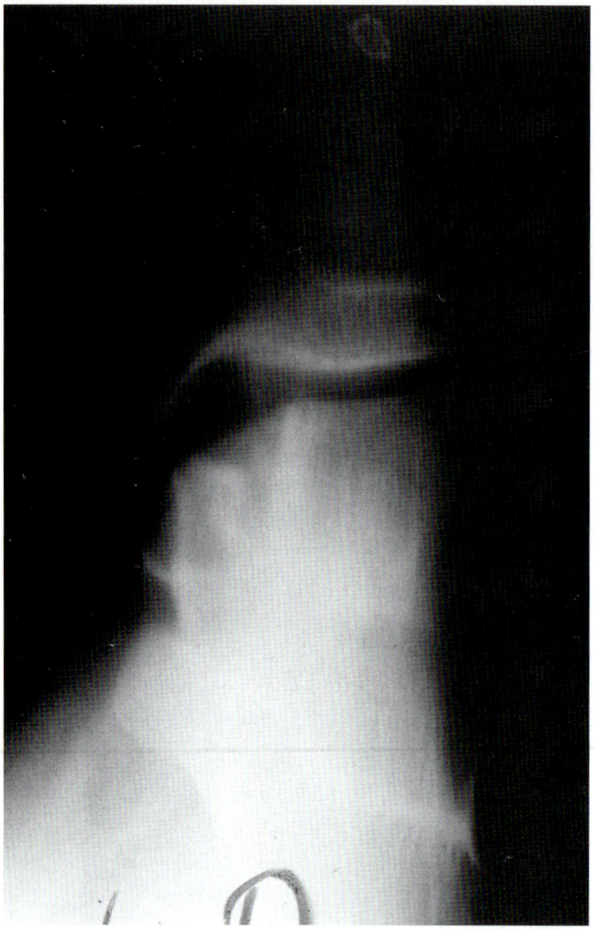

FIGURE 7.71. Tomogram shows a lesion much larger and more extensive than it appears on radiography.

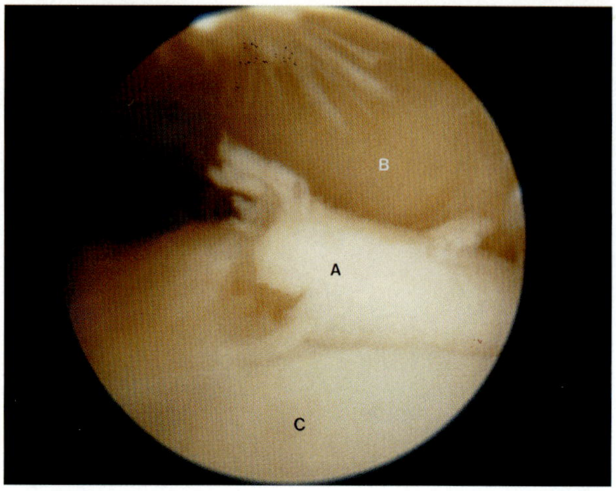

FIGURE 7.73. Arthroscopic view shows the poor quality of fibrocartilage that filled in the defect. A flap of tissue (A) was easily lifted from this lesion with a probe. B, medial malleolus; (C) dome of the talus.

the talus (more than 1.5 cm in diameter) should begin early motion but maintain non-weight-bearing following reconstruction and drilling for approximately 8–10 weeks. Return to heavy work or any demanding activity should be slow, according to the individual case. Rehabilitation may require several months to more than 1 year.

In young patients intact lesions that have been drilled should be kept non-weight-bearing with active motion for about 8–10 weeks. Return to sports is best judged independently by clinical criteria, ir-

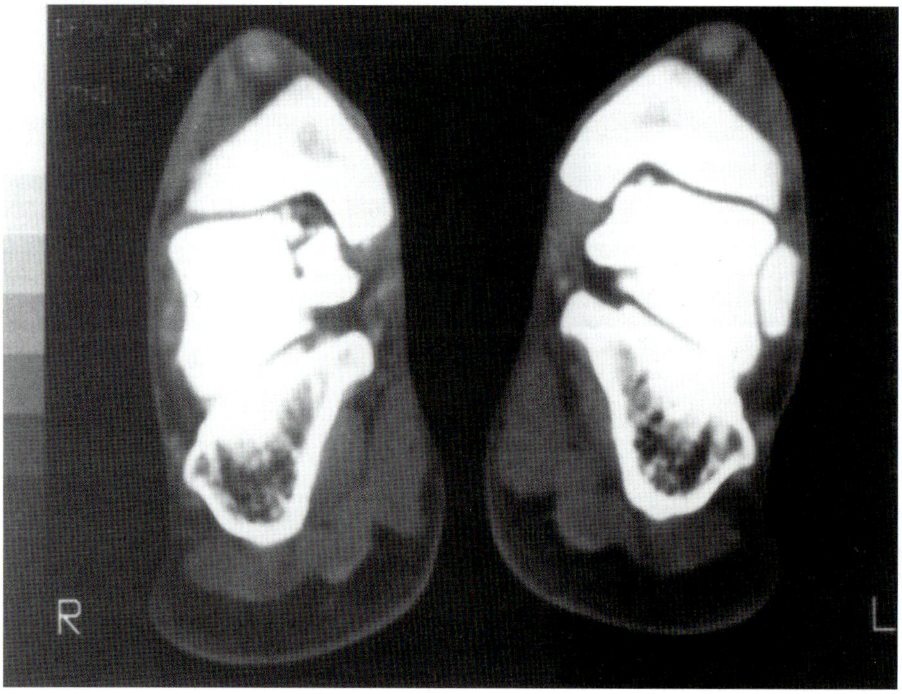

FIGURE 7.72. Same lesion as in Figure 7.71 demonstrated by a computed tomography (CT) scan. This technique is reported to be superior to the tomogram for showing the location and extent of the lesion for preoperative planning.

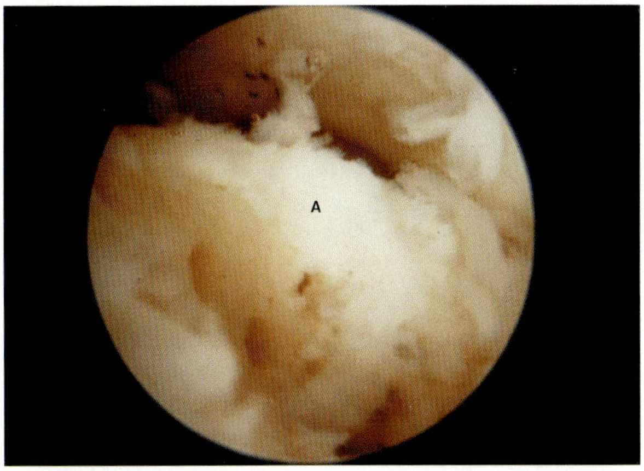

FIGURE 7.74. Arthroscopic view after excision. Note that drilling was also done in the posterior direction to get at that portion of the lesion (A) underlying good bone and articular cartilage.

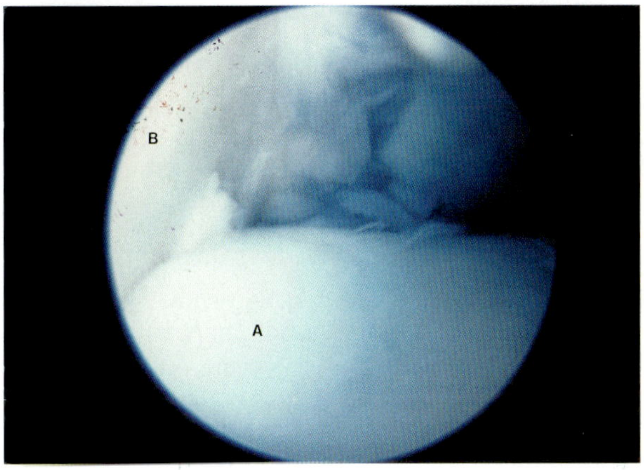

FIGURE 7.75. Arthroscopic view shows another lesion of the medial talar dome that appears intact. The diseased articular cartilage is outlined and is white after injection of the methylene blue dye. A, osteochondritis lesion; B, medial malleolus.

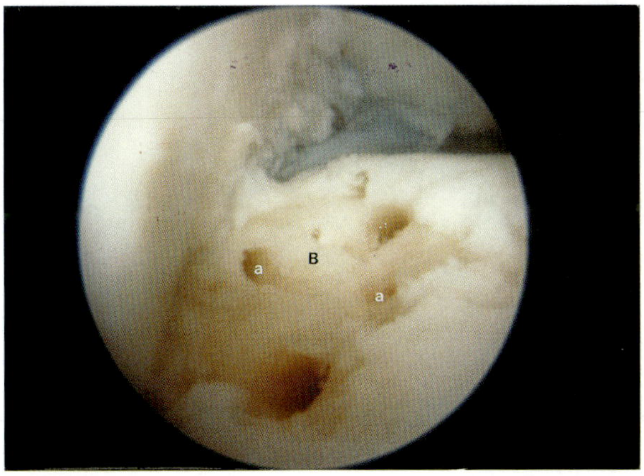

FIGURE 7.76. Arthroscopic view of the same lesion as in Fig. 7.75 after reconstruction. A, drill holes; B, lesion.

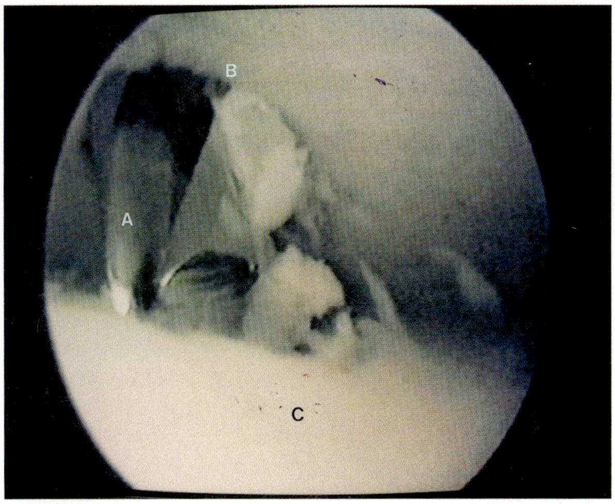

FIGURE 7.77. Arthroscopic video shows the drill tip creating an adequate channel for instrumentation in a lesion located far posteriorly. Several graduated drill sizes can be used (or a cannulated reamer as an alternate method). A, drill; B, transmalleolar canal; C, dome of the talus.

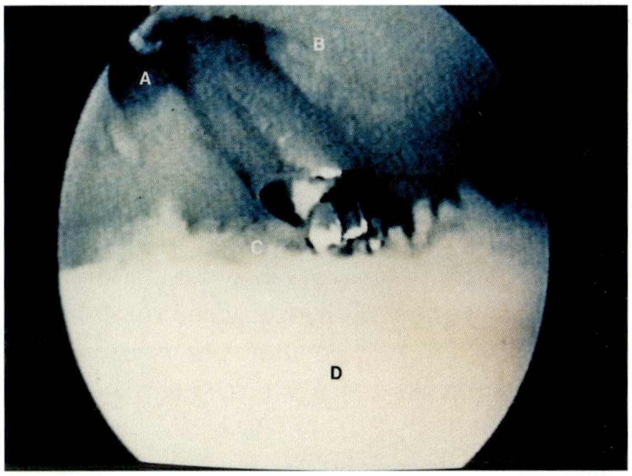

FIGURE 7.78. Arthroscopic view shows the abrader for preparing the base and trimming the margin of the lesion. A, channel through medial malleolus; B, abrader; C, defect; D, dome of the talus.

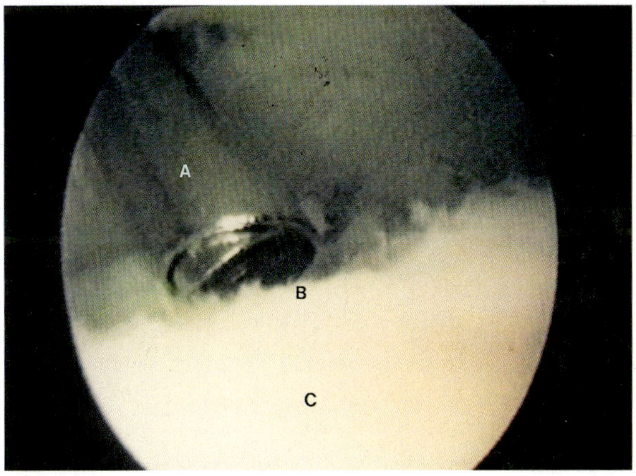

FIGURE 7.79. Same arthroscopic video view as in Figure 7.78. Note the 2.5-mm arthroscope (A) protruding through the canal. B, margin of canal; C, dome of the talus.

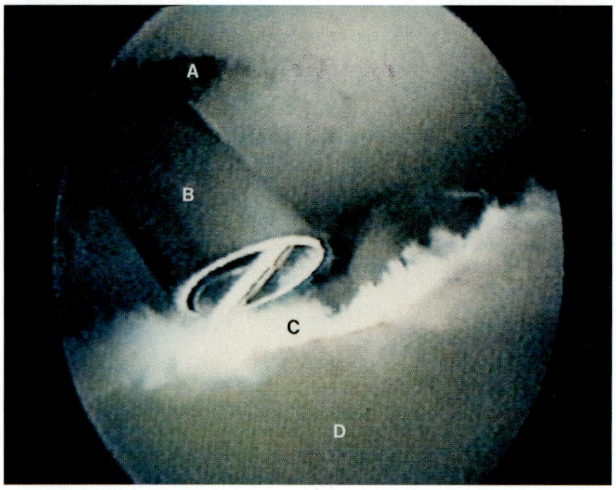

FIGURE 7.80. Same arthroscopic video view as in Figures 7.78 and 7.79. The light cable is now changed to the small arthroscope. A, canal; B, arthroscope; C, defect; D, dome of the talus.

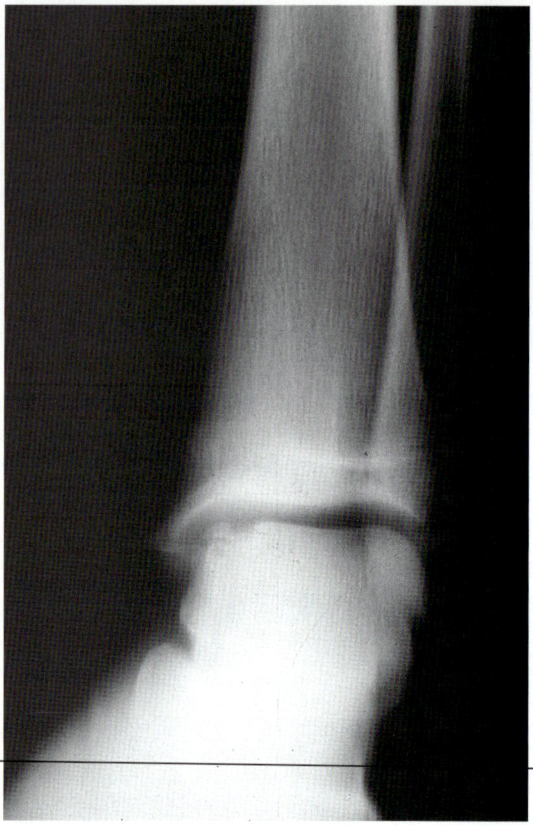

FIGURE 7.82. Anteroposterior radiograph of separated lesion of osteochondritis dissecans; separated, in a 16-year-old girl.

respective of the radiographic findings. It is best to wait until the extremity has been fully rehabilitated.

Patients who have received bone grafts should be immobilized 6–8 weeks until the graft is adequately incorporated. Weight-bearing is withheld until healing is complete clinically, radiographically, or both. Bone scans are of no practical value for following the progression of healing after surgery because the radiographic uptake remains pronounced.

Results and Conclusions

At the present time, open treatment for transchondral fractures of the talus is obsolete in most instances. Since the advent of arthroscopy, closed treatment is the rule in the hands of an experienced arthroscopist and has been associated with a more rapid recovery period, less morbidity, and increased

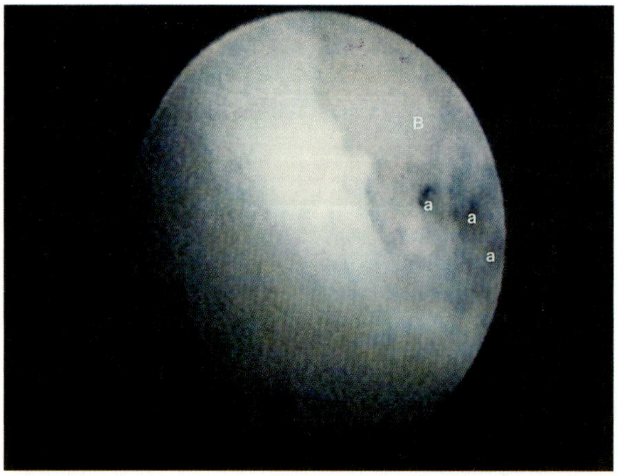

FIGURE 7.81. Same lesion as in Figures 7.78–7.80 through a 2.5-mm arthroscope by way of the transmalleolar channel. A, drill holes; B, base of lesion.

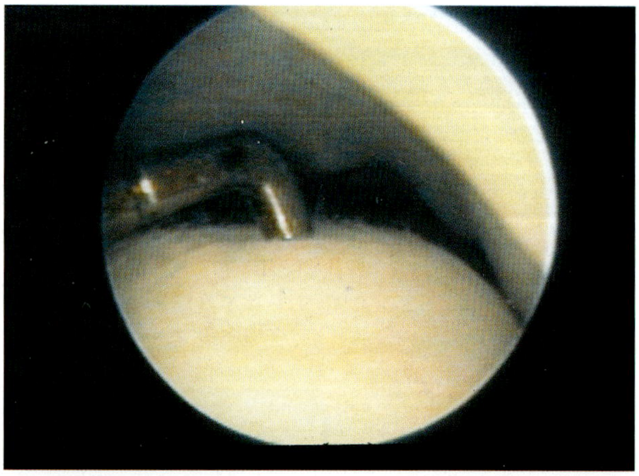

FIGURE 7.83. Arthroscopic view (Polaroid) of the probe used to evaluate a separated osteochondritis dissecans lesion.

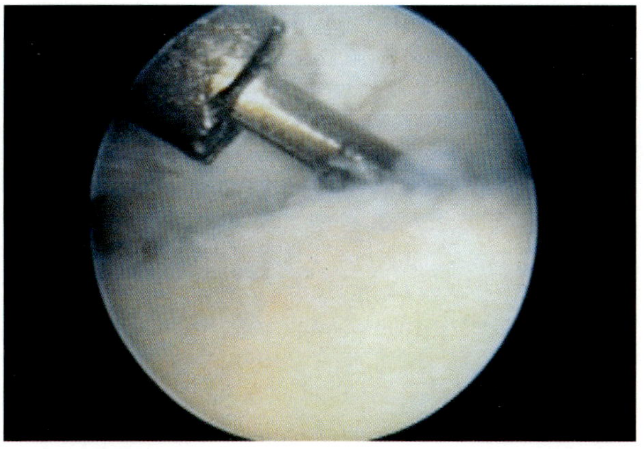

FIGURE 7.84. Biodegradable pins and driver.

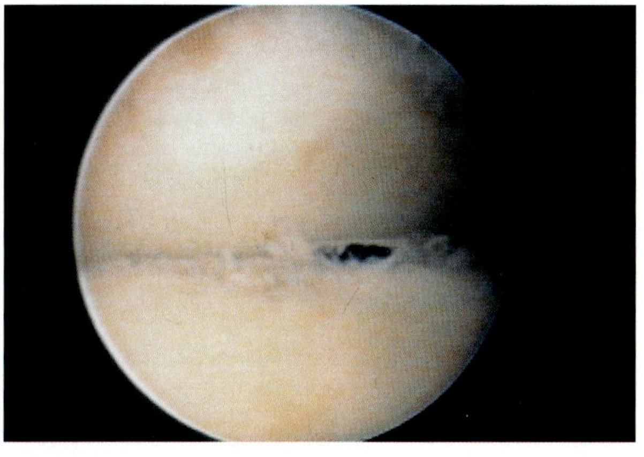

FIGURE 7.85. Arthroscopic view (Polaroid) of biodegradable pin in place.

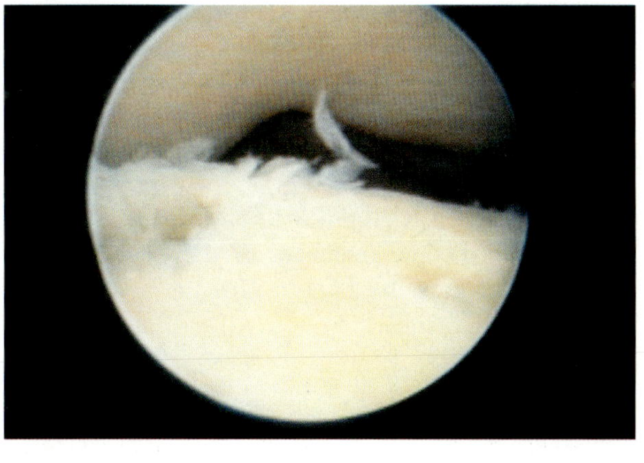

FIGURE 7.86. Arthroscopic view (Polaroid) shows two holes in the lesion where biodegradable pins were placed and properly countersunk.

acceptance by the patient. Various reports are available in the literature with some short follow-up periods and a few long follow-up periods.[21–39]

No deterioration of the results has been observed with time. Residual changes in the talus at the site of the excision have been present radiographically with no evidence of joint space narrowing. Guhl[29] and Ferkel and Fischer[26] emphasized the use of the noninvasive distractor to facilitate débridement. They also advocated the use of a posterolateral portal. Ewing[25] has successfully used a purely noninvasive distraction technique in the management of osteochondritis dissecans of the talus. Kelberine and Frank,[30] reporting 48 ankle arthroscopies performed to treat osteochondral fracture of the talus, used the posterolateral portal once and the distractor in 11 cases to gain access to the posteromedial lesion. No patient in their series developed complications from the use of the distractor. In the Parisien series,[36] arthroscopic management of osteochondritis dissecans/transchondral fractures of the talus (even when they were located posteromedially or posterolaterally) was performed successfully in 92 patients with only 2 anterior portals and no mechanical distraction. This technique was facilitated by the availability of small surgical instruments and the use of a 70-degree arthroscope.

BIBLIOGRAPHY

1. Munro A. *Mikrogeologie*. Berlin: Billroth, 1856;236. Cited by Phemister.[5]
2. Konig F. Ueberfreie Korper in Den Gelenken. *Dtsch Z Fuer Chir* 1887–1888;27:90.
3. Barth A. Die Enstchung und das Wachsthum der Frein Gelenkkor per. *Arch Klin Chir* 1898;56:507–573.
4. Fisher A. A study of loose bodies composed of cartilage or of cartilage and bone occurring in joints with special reference to their pathology and etiology. *Br J Surg* 1920–1921;8:493–523.
5. Phemister DB. The causes of and changes in loose bodies arising from the articular surfaces of the joint. *J Bone Joint Surg* 1924;6:278.
6. Kappis M. Weiter Beitrage sur Traumatisch-Mechaniscen en Tastehung der "Spontanen" Knorpelablasungen (Sogen Osteochondritis Dissecans). *Dtsch Z Chir* 1922;171:13–29. Cited by Berndt and Harty.[8]
7. Rendu A. Fracture intra-articular Parcellaire de la Poulie Astraglienne. *Lyon Med* 1932;150:220–222. Cited by Berndt and Harty.[8]
8. Berndt AL, Harty M. Transchondral fractures (osteochondritis dissecans) of the talus. *J Bone Joint Surg Am* 1959;41:988–1017.
9. O'Donoghue DH. Chondral and osteochondral fractures. *J Trauma* 1966;6:469–481.
10. Davidson AM, Steele HD, MacKenzie DA, Penny JA. A review of twenty-one cases of transchondral fracture of the talus. *J Trauma* 1967;7:378–415.

11. Goldstone RA, Pisani AJ. Osteochondritis dissecans of the talus. *NY State J Med* 1965;65:2487–2494.
12. Campbell CJ, Renawat CS. Osteochondritis dissecans: the question of etiology. *J Trauma* 1966;6:20–21.
13. Yvars MF. Osteochondral fractures of the dome of the talus. *Clin Orthop* 1976;114:185–191.
14. Alexander AH, Lichtman DM. Surgical treatment of transchondral talar dome fractures (osteochondritis dissecans). *J Bone Joint Surg Am* 1980;62:646–652.
15. Canale ST, Belding RH. Osteochondral lesions of the talus. *J Bone Joint Surg Am* 1981;62:97–102.
16. McCullough CJ, Venugopal V. Osteochondritis dissecans of the talus: the natural history. *Clin Orthop* 1979;144:264–268.
17. Yao J, Weis E. Osteochondritis dissecans. *Orthop Rev* 1985;14:190–204.
18. Blom JMH, Strijk SP. Lesions of the trochlea tali. *Radiol Clin North Am* 1975;44:387–396.
19. Lindholm TS, Osterman K, Vankka E. Osteochondritis dissecans of elbow, ankle and hip: a comparison survey. *Clin Orthop* 1980;148:245–253.
20. Roden S, Tillegaard P, Unander-Scharin I. Osteochondritis dissecans and similar lesions of the talus. *Acta Orthop Scand* 1953;23:51–66.
21. Baker CL, Andrews JR, Ryan JB. Arthroscopic treatment of transchondral talar dome fractures. *Arthroscopy* 1986;2:82–87.
22. Baker CL, Morales RW. Arthroscopic treatment of transchondral talar dome fractures: a long-term follow-up study. *Arthroscopy* 1999;2:197–202.
23. Baker CL, Parisien JS. Arthroscopic surgery in osteocartilaginous lesions of the ankle. In: McGinty JB, Caspari RB, Jackson RW, Poehling GG (eds) *Operative arthroscopy*, 2nd ed. Philadelphia: Lippincott-Raven, 1996;1157–1171.
24. Bryant DD, Siegel MG. Osteochondritis dissecans of the talus: a new technique for arthroscopic drilling. *Arthroscopy* 1993;9:238–241.
25. Ewing JW. Arthroscopic management of transchondral talar dome fractures (osteochondritis dissecans) and anterior impingement lesions of the ankle joint. *Clin Sports Med* 1991;10:677–687.
26. Ferkel RD, Fischer SP. Progress in ankle arthroscopy. *Clin Orthop* 1989;240:210–220.
27. Frank A, Cohen P, Beaufils P, Lamare JP. Traitement arthroscopique des lesions du dome astragalien. *Rev Chir Orthop* 1988;74(suppl II):233–237.
28. Frank A, Cohen P, Beaufils P, Lamare JP. Arthroscopic treatment of osteochondral lesions of the talar dome. *Arthroscopy* 1989;5:57–61.
29. Guhl JF. New concepts (distraction) in ankle arthroscopy. *Arthroscopy* 1988;4:160–167.
30. Kelberine F, Frank A. Arthroscopic treatment of osteochondral lesions of the talar dome: a retrospective study of 48 cases. *Arthroscopy* 1999;1:77–84.
31. Kristensen G, Lind T. Fracture stage 4 of the lateral talar dome treated arthroscopically using biofix for fixation. *Arthroscopy* 1990;6:242–244.
32. Loomer R, Fisher C. Osteochondral lesions of the talus. *Am J Sports Med* 1993;21:13–19.
33. Lundeen RO, Strieta JJ. Arthroscopic treatment of transchondral lesions of the talar dome. *J Am Podiatr Med Assoc* 1987;77:456–461.
34. Martin DF, Baker CL, Curl WW. Operative ankle arthroscopy. *Am J Sports Med* 1989;17:16–23.
35. Parisien JS. Arthroscopic treatment of osteochondral lesions of the talus. *Am J Sports Med* 1986;12:211–217.
36. Parisien JS. Is mechanical distraction or the use of posterolateral portal always necessary in the arthroscopic management of osteochondritis dissecans of the talus? Experience with 92 cases. Presented at the 1999 annual meeting of the Arthroscopy Association of North America, Vancouver, April 1999.
37. Pritsch M, Horoshowski H, Farine I. Arthroscopic treatment of osteochondral lesions of the talus. *J Bone Joint Surg Am* 1986;68:862–864.
38. Stone JW, Guhl JF. Ankle arthroscopy in the management of costeochondral lesions. In: Parisien JS (ed) *Current techniques in arthroscopy*. Philadelphia: Thieme, 1994;225–237.
39. Van Buecken K, Barrack RL, Alexander AH, Ertl JP. Arthroscopic treatment of transchondral talar dome fractures. *Am J Sports Med* 1989;17:350–355.

CHAPTER 8

Fracture Problems

Michael D. Feldman

The incidence of osteochondral injury due to ankle sprains has been reported to be 6.5% and could be as high as 50%.[1] The incidence of osteochondral injuries in patients with an acute ankle fracture requiring fixation is approximately 75%.[2,3] Although the long-term results of operative and nonoperative ankle fractures is generally good, there are some patients who have persistent symptoms despite minimal findings on the physical examination and unremarkable radiographs. Quite possibly these patients have unidentified intraarticular pathology caused by the initial injury that was not treated. Arthroscopic evaluation is helpful for identifying and treating these problems in patients who remain symptomatic and in those for whom the likelihood of intraarticular damage is high. The treatment of fracture problems can be divided into two categories: treatment of acute fractures and treatment of chronic fractures and postfracture pathology.

ACUTE FRACTURES

Indications

The indications for arthroscopy of acute ankle fractures include displaced intraarticular fractures and extraarticular ankle fractures that can be expected to cause significant intraarticular pathology. Intraarticular fractures, such as medial malleolar, posterior malleolar, tillaux, triplane, and mildly comminuted tibial plafond fractures, and amenable to arthroscopic or arthroscopy-assisted reduction and internal fixation. In addition to visualizing the intraarticular fracture lines seen on preoperative radiographs adequately, it is not uncommon to see additional fracture lines or osteochondral fragments at arthroscopy. It has also been reported that impaction injuries (usually to the lateral tibial plafond) are associated with bimalleolar, trimalleolar, and fracture-dislocations of the ankle.[4] Unless specifically looked for during open or arthroscopic surgery, these lesions are frequently missed.

Displaced fractures of the fibula, especially those at the level of the distal tibiofibular syndesmosis, have been reported to cause intraarticular pathology.[5] Chondral fractures of the lateral talus or a vertical fracture of the anterior border of the distal fibula (Wagstaffe's fracture[6]) can be the source of a chronic posttraumatic impingement lesion if left untreated. Finally, even though there is no intraarticular fracture line present on the preoperative radiographs, ankle fractures that displace the mortise (Fig. 8.1), such as deltoid substitution supination external rotation (SER IV D) and deltoid substitution pronation external rotation (PER IV D) fractures, or fractures that disrupt the syndesmosis, such as pronation abduction (PA II) fractures, typically cause intraarticular damage and should be considered for arthroscopy at the time of internal fixation.

Contraindications

Absolute contraindications to arthroscopy of acute ankle fractures are neurovascular injury and severe edema or swelling that precludes palpation of anatomic landmarks. Relative contraindications in-

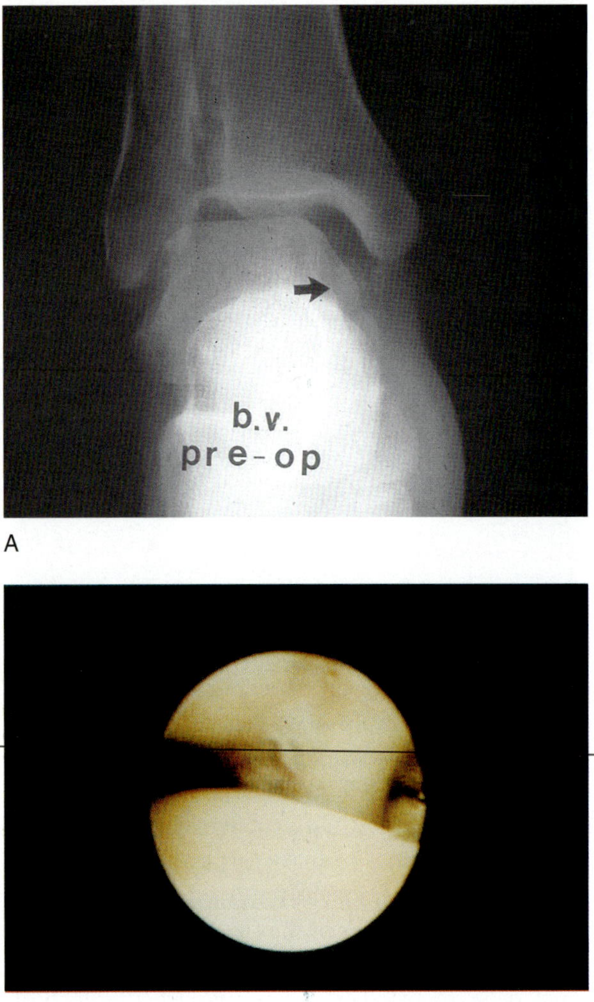

A

B

FIGURE 8.1. A: Anteroposterior (AP) radiograph of an acute supination-external rotation ankle fracture. The talus is displaced laterally out of the mortise. Note that the fibula fracture exits above the level of the syndesmosis. These fractures commonly have intraarticular pathology even though no fracture line extends into the ankle joint. The arrow points to two loose bodies that were related to a previous injury but were easily removed arthroscopically at the time of surgery. **B:** Arthroscopic view of the same fracture showing an impaction injury to the medial tibial plafond.

clude some fracture-dislocations that cause significant distortion of ankle anatomy. Additionally, complications secondary to severe localized soft tissue swelling due to fluid extravasation is possible in these cases. Some would also say that open fractures are a relative contraindication to arthroscopy, although in grade I and selected grade II open fractures arthroscopy may provide better irrigation and débridement while minimizing further soft tissue trauma than do conventional open techniques.

Surgical Technique

Thoughtful preoperative planning is essential to optimize the postoperative outcome. Anteroposterior (AP), lateral, and mortise radiographs of the ankle should be obtained and studied prior to surgery. Some fractures, such as tibial plafond and triplane fractures, may also require preoperative tomograms or computed tomography (CT) scans for better definition of the fracture configuration. Potential locations of hardware (interfragmentary screws, plates) and proposed incisions should be identified.

Under adequate anesthesia, the patient is placed supine on the operating room table. A tourniquet is placed high on the thigh, the operative extremity placed in a knee arthroscopy leg holder, and the foot of the table dropped. After the extremity is appropriately prepared and draped and the anatomic landmarks and proposed incisions are marked, the tourniquet is inflated. A sterile Mayo stand is placed nearby to support the foot when the lower extremity is not in a dependent position. A mini C-arm is also draped sterile for use.

Ankle distraction is helpful in most cases to improve arthroscopic visualization and provide ligamentotaxis, which may aid in fracture reduction. Manual (noninvasive) distraction is usually adequate; invasive distractors are not recommended. However, if the fracture configuration dictates postoperative external fixation, the fixator may be placed prior to arthroscopy and used as an invasive distractor. It may be particularly useful for selected trial plafond fractures.

Because of the risk of excessive soft tissue swelling secondary to fluid extravasation, gravity inflow rather than pump inflow is used during arthroscopy of acute fractures. Ankle arthroscopy can be performed with a 2.7- or 4.0-mm 30 degree arthroscope. I prefer the 4.0 mm arthroscope as it affords better gravity inflow through the arthroscopic cannula. Additionally, because soft tissue restraints are frequently disrupted in acute fractures, visualization of all intraarticular structures with a 4.0 mm arthroscope is usually accomplished without difficulty. If visualization is inadequate with a 4.0 mm arthroscope, a 2.7 mm arthroscope is acceptable, but the posterolateral portal is frequently required for inflow.

Anteromedial and anterolateral portals are routinely used; the posterolateral portal is used to enhance visualization of the posterior aspect of the ankle joint or to provide supplemental inflow. The anteromedial portal is usually established first. Upon entering the ankle joint, visualization may be difficult because of hemoarthrosis and fibrinous debris. A double-port arthroscopic cannula is useful at this point as it allows both inflow and outflow, which aids in irrigating the joint. The anterolateral portal is now created under direct visualization and a 3.5 mm full radius shaver is inserted to remove the remaining hematoma and fibrinous debris from the joint. If visualization is still unsatisfactory at this point, inflow is placed through the posterolateral portal.

A thorough arthroscopic examination is performed utilizing all portals for visualization. Articular surfaces are evaluated for chondral defects (Fig. 8.2) and fracture lines; recesses are checked for loose osteochondral fragments (Fig. 8.3); and ligamentous structures such as the deltoid ligament and the syndesmosis are evaluated for disruption (Fig. 8.4). In some instances the joint capsule is torn, and this is documented as well. After determining the intraarticular pathology, loose fragments are removed, chondral lesions are débrided to a stable rim, and standard treatment of the fracture is undertaken.

When intraarticular fracture fragments are present, a determination is made whether to fix or excise the fragments. Fragments that have healthy articular cartilage with adequate subchondral bone should be repaired; conversely, fragments with comminuted or damaged cartilage and little attached bone should be excised. Fracture reduction can be performed with a probe, grasper, or reduction tenaculum (Fig. 8.5). Once acceptable reduction is obtained, provisional reduction is maintained with

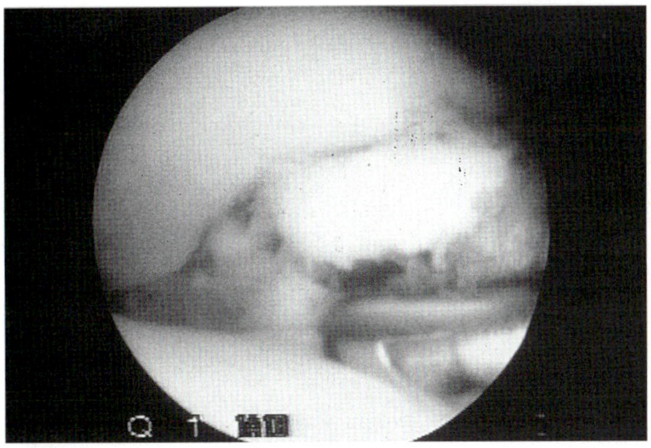

FIGURE 8.3. Untreated pathology, such as this osteochondral fragment arising from the intraarticular extension of a fibular fracture, may lead to persistent postoperative symptoms. Once identified, the fragment was easily removed arthroscopically with a grasper.

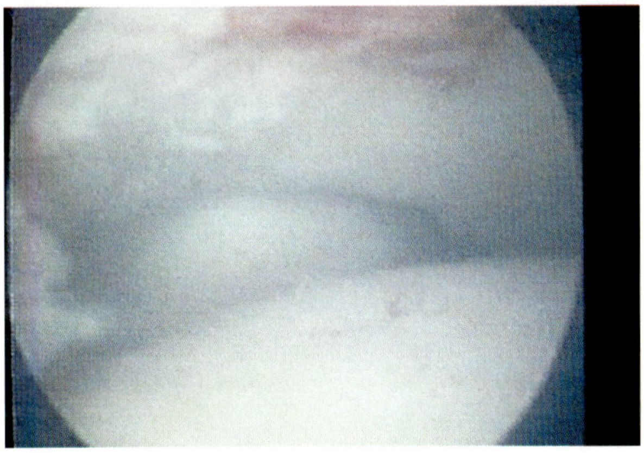

A

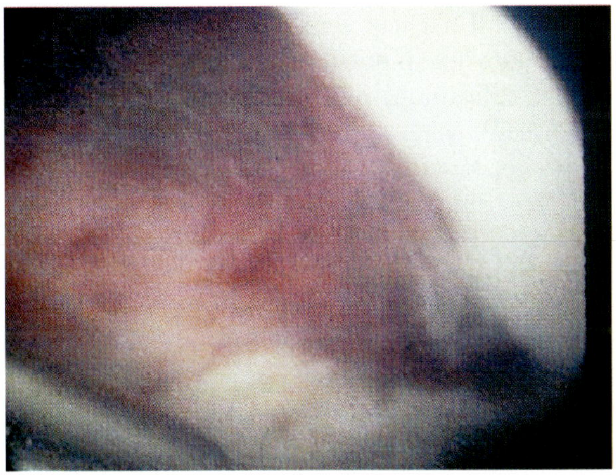

B

FIGURE 8.4. Intraarticular view of an acute injury to the syndesmosis of a right ankle viewed through the anteromedial portal. **A:** Normal syndesmosis. **B:** Injured syndesmosis with acute hemorrhage and widening of the distal tibiofibular joint.

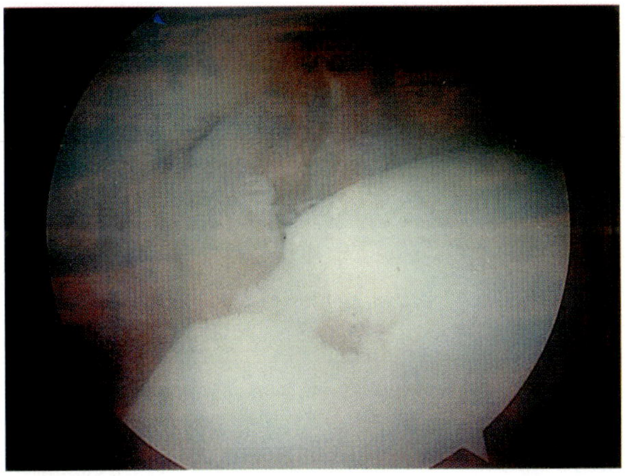

FIGURE 8.2. Arthroscopic view of an acute chondral defect in the anteromedial talus resulting from tibiotalar impaction in a displaced ankle fracture.

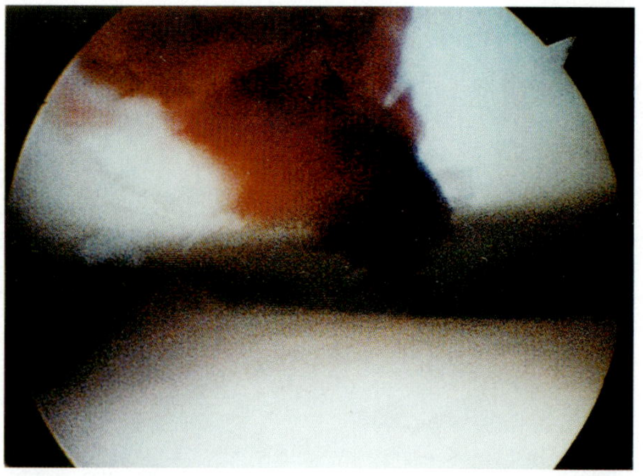

A

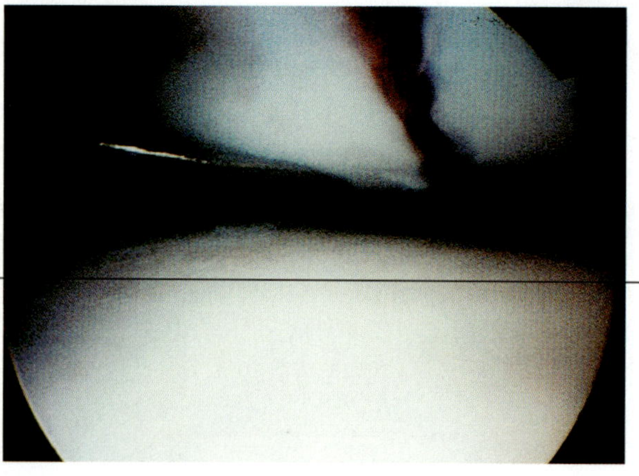

B

FIGURE 8.5. Use of a small periosteal elevator to aid in reduction of the articular surface. **A:** Before reduction. **B:** After reduction.

0.045 inch Kirschner wires placed perpendicular to the fracture line, if possible. The mini C-arm is now used to confirm the reduction, and final fixation is performed using cannulated screws, headless screws, or absorbable pins, depending on the fracture configuration.

Certain fracture patterns, such as those involving the tibial plafond, talar neck, or fibula, may require both an arthroscopic and an open approach. In these cases, the intraarticular fracture fragments are reconstructed first using the arthroscope to aid in reduction of the articular surface. Once the articular surface has been satisfactorily aligned, the extraarticular fracture fragments are reduced using conventional open techniques. Limited incisions, ligamentotaxis, and other indirect reduction maneuvers are helpful at this point to minimize further soft tissue injury. Even if the intraarticular fractures cannot be reduced arthroscopically, the arthroscope may still be used in a dry fashion to aid in visualization. This is particularly useful when evaluating posterior fracture lines in comminuted plafond fractures.

After fracture fixation has been performed, arthroscopic visualization is used to confirm satisfactory articular congruency, and fluoroscopy is used to confirm acceptable placement of the hardware (Fig. 8.6). Generally, fracture fixation should be as rigid as possible to allow early range of motion. Finally, incisions are closed, and a bulky dressing incorporating a posterior splint placing the ankle in neutral dorsiflexion is applied. At 7 days after operation the incisions are inspected, and range of motion exercises are begun. Weight-bearing status is dictated by the fracture pattern and rigidity of fixation and is individualized for each patient.

Potential Pitfalls and Complications

Pitfalls and complications can be subdivided into two categories: those related to ankle arthroscopy in general and those related specifically to arthroscopy of acute fractures. Examples of the former include neurovascular damage during portal placement, iatrogenic articular injury due to scuffing, and postoperative sinus or fistula formation at the portal sites. Most of these complications can be prevented with careful attention to anatomy and the principles of portal placement, as discussed in Chapter 2.

Because arthroscopy of acute fractures involves working on an acutely traumatized joint, the potential for complications is high. Soft tissue swelling may distort and disguise anatomic landmarks, making portal placement difficult. An 18-gauge spinal needle with or without fluoroscopy can be extremely helpful for locating proper portal position. In arthroscopy-assisted reductions, proposed incisions occasionally fall over portal sites. In these cases, the incision is made first to protect neurovascular structures and to locate the capsule prior to creating the portal.

Fluid inflow and outflow must also be monitored closely during arthroscopy of acute fractures. Although an arthroscopic pump is commonly used for ankle arthroscopy, it is not recommended for arthroscopy of acute fractures as the capsule can be torn, leading to significant fluid extravasation. Maintaining high flow and low pressure during the surgery avoids potential complications due to excessive soft tissue swelling, such as compartment

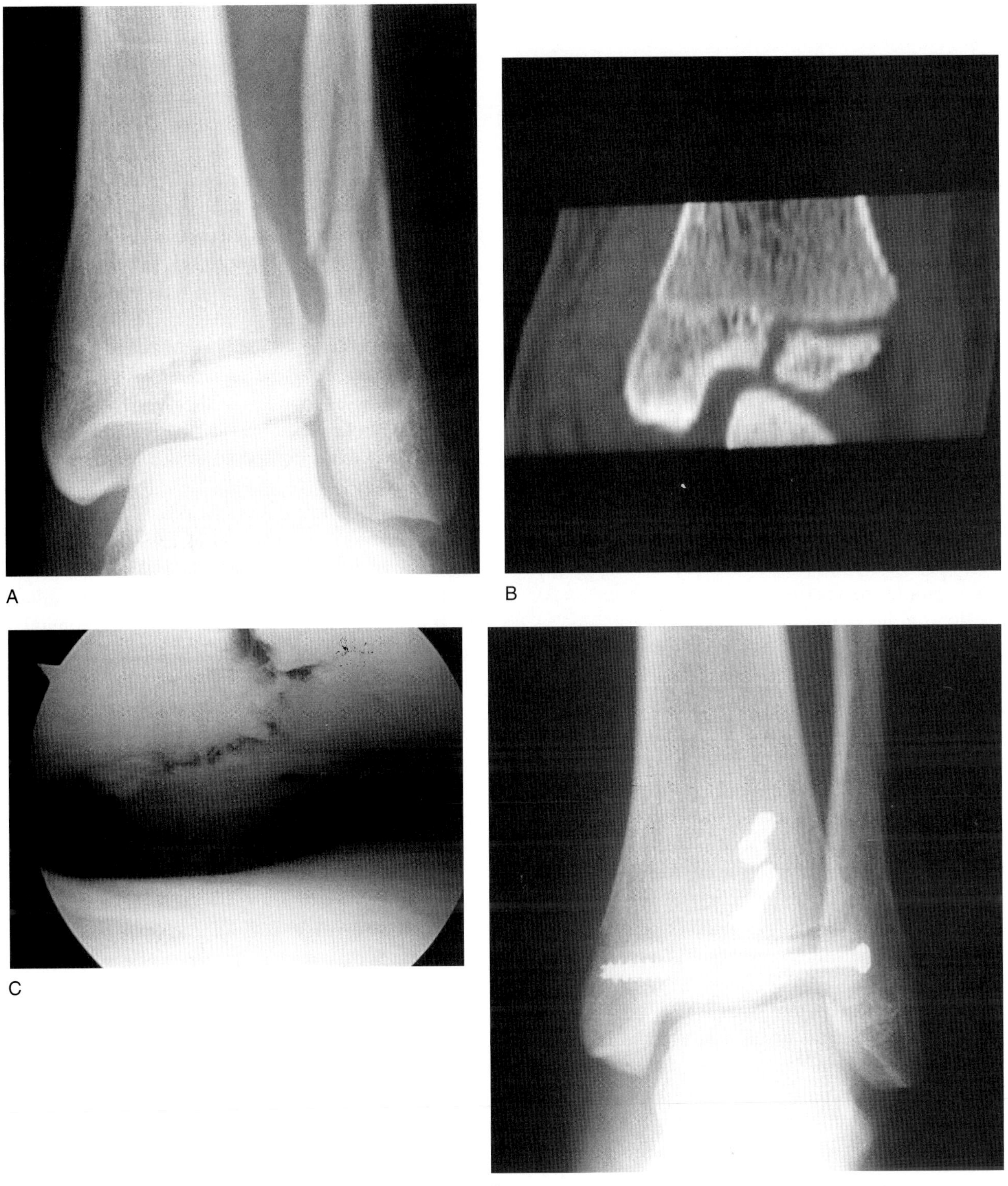

FIGURE 8.6. Arthroscopic reduction of a distal tibial triplane fracture. A: Preoperative AP radiograph. B: Preoperative coronal computed tomography (CT) scan showing displacement of the articular surface. C: Intraarticular view after reduction. D: Postoperative AP radiograph.

syndrome and vascular compromise. A posterolateral portal is occasionally used to increase inflow, thereby improving arthroscopic visualization.

Inadequate reduction or inadequate fixation are two potential pitfalls that deserve special attention. Although arthroscopy of acute fractures aids in visualization of the fracture lines, it is still a technically demanding procedure to reduce the fragments through limited incisions or indirect reduction techniques. More demanding still is the ability to provide rigid fixation through these limited incisions. In cases where the reduction or fixation is tenuous, it is better to revert to conventional open techniques so the principles of fracture treatment (i.e., anatomic reduction and rigid fixation) are maintained.

The incidence of postoperative wound complications is slightly higher with arthroscopic treatment of acute ankle fractures than with ankle arthroscopy in general owing to the traumatized soft tissue envelope and prolonged surgical time. Fracture blisters denote significant soft tissue injury, and surgery should be delayed until they resolve. Superficial and deep infections can be prevented by administering preoperative antibiotics, handling the skin and soft tissues gently, and monitoring closely for soft tissue swelling. Fistulas and sinus tracts may be prevented by suturing the portals and incisions closed. Finally, skin necrosis or breakdown can be minimized by placing portals and incisions in appropriate locations so instruments do not put excessive tension on the skin.

Results

Until recently, there has been little mention in the literature of arthroscopy of acute ankle fractures. Most reports were limited to a few cases in larger studies covering all indications of ankle arthroscopy, and recommendations were based on anecdotal experience. As more surgeons are now performing ankle arthroscopy for acute fractures, the results and technical tips are becoming more meaningful.

Whipple et al. reported two cases of arthroscopic reduction and internal fixation of triplane fractures using Steinmann pin fixation.[7] They recommended using a 2.7 mm arthroscope to decrease articular scuffing. Follow-up at 6 months after operation revealed that the fractures healed with full range of motion and without leg length discrepancy, angulation, or malalignment. The point of their article was that the "fundamental tenet of intraarticular fracture treatment is anatomic reduction of the articular surface."[7]

Saltzman et al. reported a case of arthroscopy-assisted open reduction and internal fixation of a displaced talar fracture. Their approach combined the advantages of both open and closed techniques: mainly the ability "to remove osteochondral fragments from the ankle and subtalar joints, to directly reduce the fracture, and to assess flexion stability, while causing minimal disruption of talar blood supply."[8] Technical pearls included positioning similar to that used for knee arthroscopy with the foot dangling, applying a temporary tibiocalcaneal small wire external fixator for distraction, and placing two small cannulated screws from posterior to anterior through an incision just lateral to the Achilles tendon. In the case of proximal neck or body fractures or body fractures with a large posteromedial fragment, they recommended placing the screws from anterior to posterior. Finally, they noted that using the arthroscopy-assisted technique would be "particularly helpful in cases with massive soft tissue swelling causing increased risk of developing wound problems" compared with traditional open techniques.

In 1994 Holt presented one of the first series of patients treated by arthroscopy-assisted reduction and internal fixation for acute ankle fractures.[9] He treated 14 fractures, four of which were trimalleolar fractures and 10 were minimally comminuted tibial plafond fractures. Technical recommendations included using a large uterine tenaculum for provisional fixation, extending the fibular incision posterior to the peroneal tendons, and mobilizing the peroneus brevis both anteriorly and posteriorly to allow palpation of the posterior lip fragment and free passage of reduction instruments. He also advocated reducing the posterior lip fragment with cannulated screws prior to fixing the fibula fracture. Postoperative evaluation of the four trimalleolar fractures at 15 months revealed that all fractures had healed without arthrosis. Range of motion was within 5 degrees of the uninjured ankle in three patients and lacked 10 degrees of dorsiflexion and plantar flexion in one patient. One patient was also noted to have transient neuropraxia of the deep peroneal nerve secondary to screw placement.

In addition to aiding fracture reduction and fixation, arthroscopy of acute fractures is valuable for identifying and treating intraarticular pathology caused at the time of injury. Prior to arthroscopy, the true incidence of occult intraarticular lesions due to acute ankle fractures was unknown. Ferkel and Orwin presented the largest series to date, consisting of 33 patients.[3] Osteochondral lesions were identified in 26 of 33 cases (79%); 9 lesions were found on the tibia, 16 on the talus, and 1 on the fibula. Of the talar lesions, 13 were located medially and 3 laterally. Loose bodies were present in

18 of 33 cases (55%). Unfortunately, fracture classification was not discussed in their series, which could have been helpful for predicting which fractures were likely to have intraarticular involvement.

It stands to reason that if a fracture line extends into the articular surface on preoperative radiographs intraarticular damage will be noted at the time of arthroscopy. However, what about fracture patterns that have forces that pass through the joint but do not have an intraarticular fracture line present? Such examples are deltoid substitution supination-external rotation and pronation-external rotation injuries (Lauge-Hansen classification).[10] With these displaced extraarticular fractures the fracture forces start at the fibula fracture, travel down the syndesmosis through the ankle joint, and exit through the deltoid ligament rupture. Are the fracture forces significant enough to cause intraarticular damage even in the absence of an intraarticular fracture line?

In a personal review of ankle fractures treated during 1989–1996, a group of 15 were classified as displaced extraarticular fractures: 14 supination-external rotation injuries and 1 pronation-external rotation injury.[2] Although type II pronation-abduction injuries also satisfy this criterion, none was treated during this time. At the time of arthroscopy, 11 of the 15 patients (73%) were noted to have intraarticular damage not predicted by the preoperative radiographs. Seven patients (47%) had talar lesions, four (27%) had tibial lesions, and four (27%) had extension of the fibular fracture into the ankle joint. Five patients (33%) had combined lesions. Three patients (20%) were noted to have the deltoid ligament infolded into the medial gutter. Free osteochondral fragments were seen in two patients (13%). Tourniquet time for the entire operation averaged 89 minutes (range 39–170 minutes), and no complications were directly or indirectly related to the arthroscopy.

The results of the previous two studies are remarkably similar (Table 8.1). The percentages of patients with intraarticular pathology, talar lesions, and tibial lesions were almost identical. The differences regarding the presence of loose bodies and fibular lesions are most likely explained by the difference in fracture patterns. In Ferkel and Orwin's study, intraarticular fracture lines were probably responsible for the development of small osteochondral fragments that broke off and became loose bodies.[3] The increased percentage of fibular lesions identified in my review was due to the increased number of fractures where the fracture forces extended through the fibula instead of the syndesmosis and into the joint. In both studies, though, the results demonstrate an extraordinarily high incidence of intraarticular pathology that would otherwise not be expected.

In summary, arthroscopy of acute ankle fractures is gaining acceptance as a valuable tool for identifying, treating, and preventing intraarticular pathology. Arthroscopy allows minimally invasive surgical exposures while providing superior visualization of fracture fragments. Although technically demanding, decreased soft tissue dissection and improved articular reductions should minimize postoperative complications. Thorough arthroscopic débridement of organized hematoma and fibrinous tissue from the joint may also decrease postoperative adhesions and improve ankle range of motion. Identification of intraarticular pathology may be valuable in providing a more accurate prognosis re-

TABLE 8.1. *Arthroscopic findings of acute ankle fractures*

Parameter	*Ferkel*[3]	*Feldman*[2]
No. of fractures	33	15
Fracture pattern	N/A	14 SER/1 PER
Tourniquet time (avg.)	81 min	89 min
Intraarticular lesions	26 (79%)	11 (73%)
Talar lesions	16 (48%)	7 (47%)
Tibial lesions	9 (27%)	4 (27%)
Fibular lesions	1 (3%)	4 (27%)
Loose bodies	18 (55%)	2 (13%)
Infolded deltoid ligament	N/A	3 (20%)
Arthroscopic complications	N/A	0

SER, type IV supination-external rotation deltoid substitution; PER, type IV pronation-external rotation deltoid substitution; N/A, not available.

garding the outcome of these fractures. In the case of displaced extraarticular ankle fractures, arthroscopic examination at the time of open reduction and internal fixation allows the diagnosis and treatment of otherwise unrecognized intraarticular pathology, which may decrease early postoperative complications and improve long-term results. With many potential benefits and minimally increased risks, arthroscopy of acute ankle fractures should be seriously considered in operative cases.

CHRONIC FRACTURES AND POSTFRACTURE PATHOLOGY

Indications

Chronic fractures are defined as those that have been present more than 3 months since the time of injury. Postfracture pathology includes nonunions, syndesmosis disruptions, medial or lateral talomalleolar diastases, intraarticular loose bodies, and reduction incongruities causing impingement or early degenerative changes (Fig. 8.7). The main indication for arthroscopy of chronic ankle fractures and postfracture pathology is persistent pain unresponsive to conservative measures, such as immobilization, bracing, or physical therapy. Resultant ligamentous instability and posttraumatic arthritis requiring fusion are also indications for arthroscopy; these subjects are discussed in Chapters 9 and 10.

Contraindications

The absolute contraindications to arthroscopy of chronic fractures and postfracture pathology are bony ankylosis and acute infection of the tibiotalar joint. Relative contraindications include previous septic arthritis, vascular insufficiency, extensive arthrofibrosis, and severe joint destruction or narrowing that may make entering the joint difficult.

Surgical Treatment

Arthroscopy of chronic fractures and postfracture pathology is generally more difficult than arthroscopy of acute fractures because of the presence of multiple adhesions and a contracted joint space. Even with distraction, entering the tibiotalar joint can be difficult. Initial visualization is also usually compromised because of abundant scar tissue in the anterior aspect of the joint. Adherence to sound

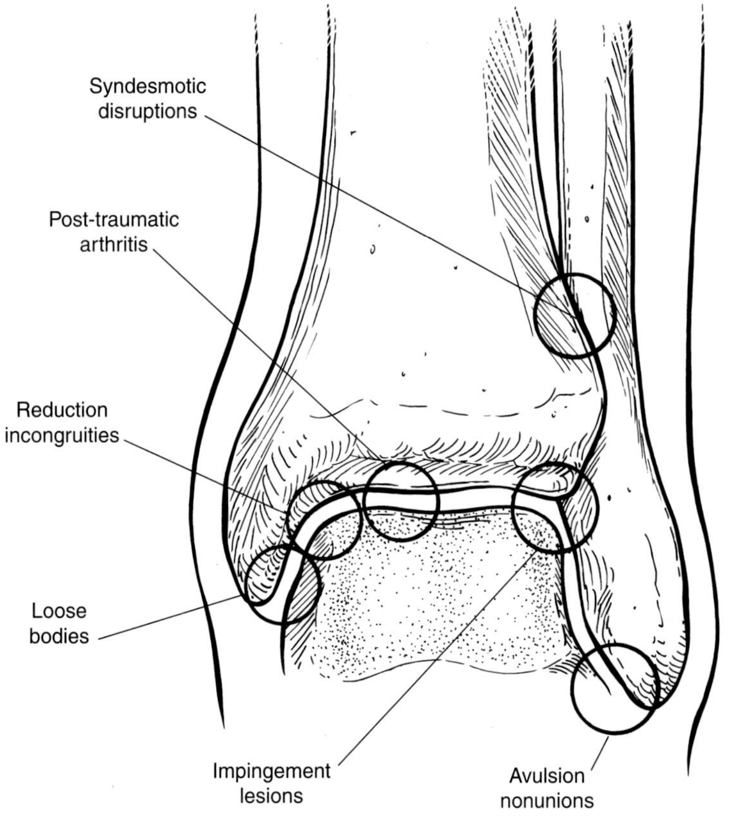

FIGURE 8.7. Common areas of postfracture pathology.

arthroscopic principles is mandatory to avoid iatrogenic neurovascular injury or scuffing on the articular surface.

Positioning for arthroscopy of chronic fractures and fracture defects is similar to arthroscopy of acute fractures. After adequate anesthesia has been administered, the patient is placed supine on the operating room table and the ankle is examined. Passive range of motion, ligamentous stability, and neurovascular status are documented. A tourniquet is placed on the thigh, and the operative extremity is placed in a knee arthroscopy leg holder with the foot of the table dropped. After preparing the area and draping it, anatomic landmarks are located. Specifically, the anterior tibial artery, the course of the superficial peroneal nerve, and the tibialis anterior, extensor hallucis longus, and extensor digitorum communis are identified and marked on the skin with a marking pen. Knowledge of the position of these anatomic structures is paramount prior to arthroscopy to minimize the risk of injury during débridement of the anterior scar tissue that is usually present. The lower extremity is exsanguinated and the tourniquet inflated. If an arthroscopic pump is used, the tourniquet is usually not necessary, but careful attention for fluid extravasation is maintained.

Noninvasive ankle distraction is almost always required during arthroscopy of chronic fractures and postfracture defects to allow access into the joint. Ten to fifteen pounds is usually sufficient, although up to 25 pounds may be used. Whereas for acute fractures a 2.7 mm or 4.0 mm arthroscope may be used, chronic fractures almost always require a 2.7 mm arthroscope to visualize the entire joint without scuffing the articular surfaces.

Anteromedial, anterolateral, and posterolateral portals are routinely used. Anterior portals may be more difficult to establish here than when treating acute fractures because of anterior capsular scar tissue. It is recommended that proposed portal sites be identified with an 18-gauge spinal needle prior to incising the skin and that a mosquito clamp be used for blunt penetration of the soft tissues and capsule. Occasionally, upon entering the joint the anterior scar tissue is so dense that visualization is impossible. In these cases it is helpful to place blunt obturators in the anteromedial and anterolateral portals and triangulate them until you can feel the tips of the obturators touching. Once this is accomplished, the obturators are swept horizontally to "create" a space in the anterior aspect of the joint (Fig. 8.8). The arthroscope and shaver are now placed in this "space," and the anterior scar can be débrided under direct vision. Under no circumstances should the anterior capsular tissues be débrided without unequivocal visualization

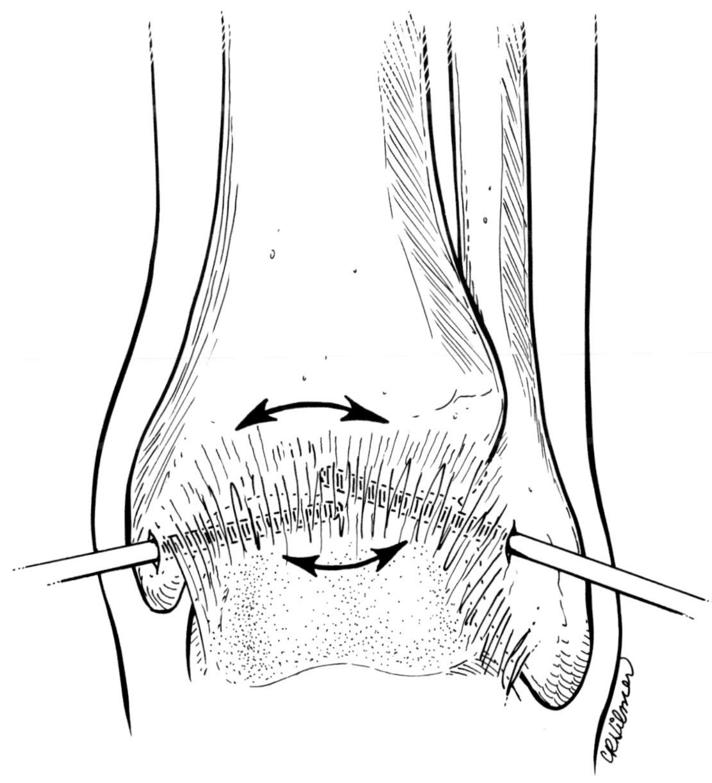

FIGURE 8.8. Technique for creating a "space" to allow initial visualization of the anterior aspect of the ankle joint in patients with arthrofibrosis after ankle fractures. Obturators are placed in the anteromedial and anterolateral portals and triangulated so they touch. The obturators are then swept in a horizontal motion to break the dense adhesions and create an area for visualization. Once this is accomplished, débridement can be performed under direct visualization using standard principles.

of the mouth of the shaver at all times. Identification of fatty tissues in the anterior scar is important, as it signals that the capsule has been violated and neurovascular structures are close by.

After débriding the anterior scar tissue, the joint is thoroughly examined with specific attention to the medial and lateral gutters. Loose bodies (Fig. 8.9), avulsion fracture nonunions (Fig. 8.10), and impingement lesions are commonly found. The articular surfaces are carefully inspected for chondral lesions and posttraumatic degenerative changes. If posttraumatic degenerative changes are more severe than initially expected, arthroscopy-assisted ankle fusion may be performed at this time. Finally, the syndesmosis should be inspected as it occasionally shows evidence of chronic injury, which can be missed on preoperative radiographs.

At the completion of the procedure, the portal sites are reapproximated with 4-0 nylon; 10 cc of 0.5% bupivacaine with epinephrine (1:200,000) is then injected intraarticularly to decrease bleeding and provide postoperative pain relief. A sterile dressing is applied. Patients are instructed to ambulate with crutches, bearing weight as tolerated. Sutures are removed 1 week after operation, and physical therapy is started.

Potential Pitfalls and Complications

Pitfalls and complications for arthroscopy of chronic fractures and postfracture defects parallel those for ankle arthroscopy in general. They include neurovascular damage, damage to articular surfaces, infection, and incisional problems. The surgeon should always be aware of the anterior neurovascular structures, as they can easily be injured during débridement of anterior scar tissue. Constant visualization of the mouth of the motorized shaver and identification of anterior fatty tissue are useful tips for minimizing this disastrous complication.

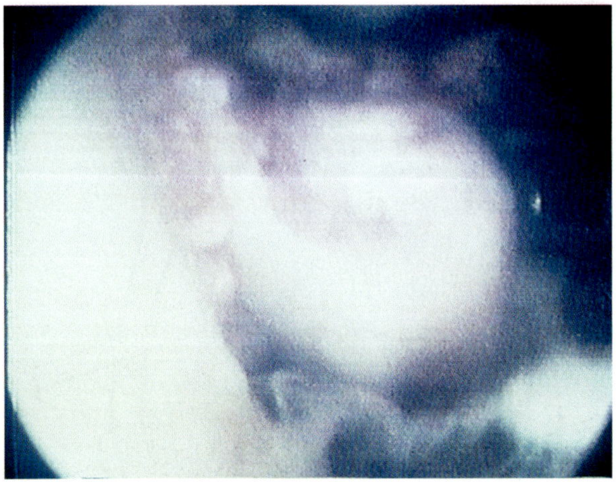

FIGURE 8.9. Loose body identified and easily removed from the medial gutter in a patient with persistent pain 1 year after a nondisplaced ankle fracture.

Because of the frequently decreased joint space seen with chronic fractures and postfracture defects, iatrogenic scuffing of the articular surface is relatively common. Accurate portal placement, adequate distraction of the joint, and the use of a 2.7 mm arthroscope is essential for minimizing this problem. Even with meticulous technique, it is not uncommon to note some damage to the articular surface caused by probing instruments due to the soft, friable nature of the articular cartilage.

Lastly, postoperative hematoma can be a problem secondary to aggressive débridement of abundant scar tissue. Although rarely necessary during ankle arthroscopy, careful hemostasis with arthroscopic electrocautery may help minimize this problem. An intraarticular injection of 0.5% bupivicaine with 1:200,000 epinephrine is given at the completion of the case, as it helps decrease postoperative bleeding. It is important to minimize this complication, as it can lead to prolonged decreased range of motion and a recurrence of intraarticular adhesions.

Results

Although more is written about arthroscopy of chronic fractures and postfracture defects than arthroscopy of acute fractures, much of the information is hidden within broader studies discussing the results of ankle arthroscopy in general.[11–14] There are, though, a few studies entirely devoted to arthroscopy of chronic fractures and postfracture defects.[3,15,16] Because these studies are retrospective reviews and include many types of postfracture pathology, however, it is impossible to compare these studies to each other, although useful information leading to outcome trends and treatment recommendations can be obtained by reviewing them.

In all the studies reviewed, the indication for arthroscopy was pain uncontrolled by conservative measures for at least 6 months after fracture or syndesmosis disruption. Although every study listed the postoperative arthroscopic findings and clinical results, there were significant disparities regarding the details and classification of the arthroscopic findings and the postoperative outcome. One fact, though, was obvious. The postoperative clinical out-

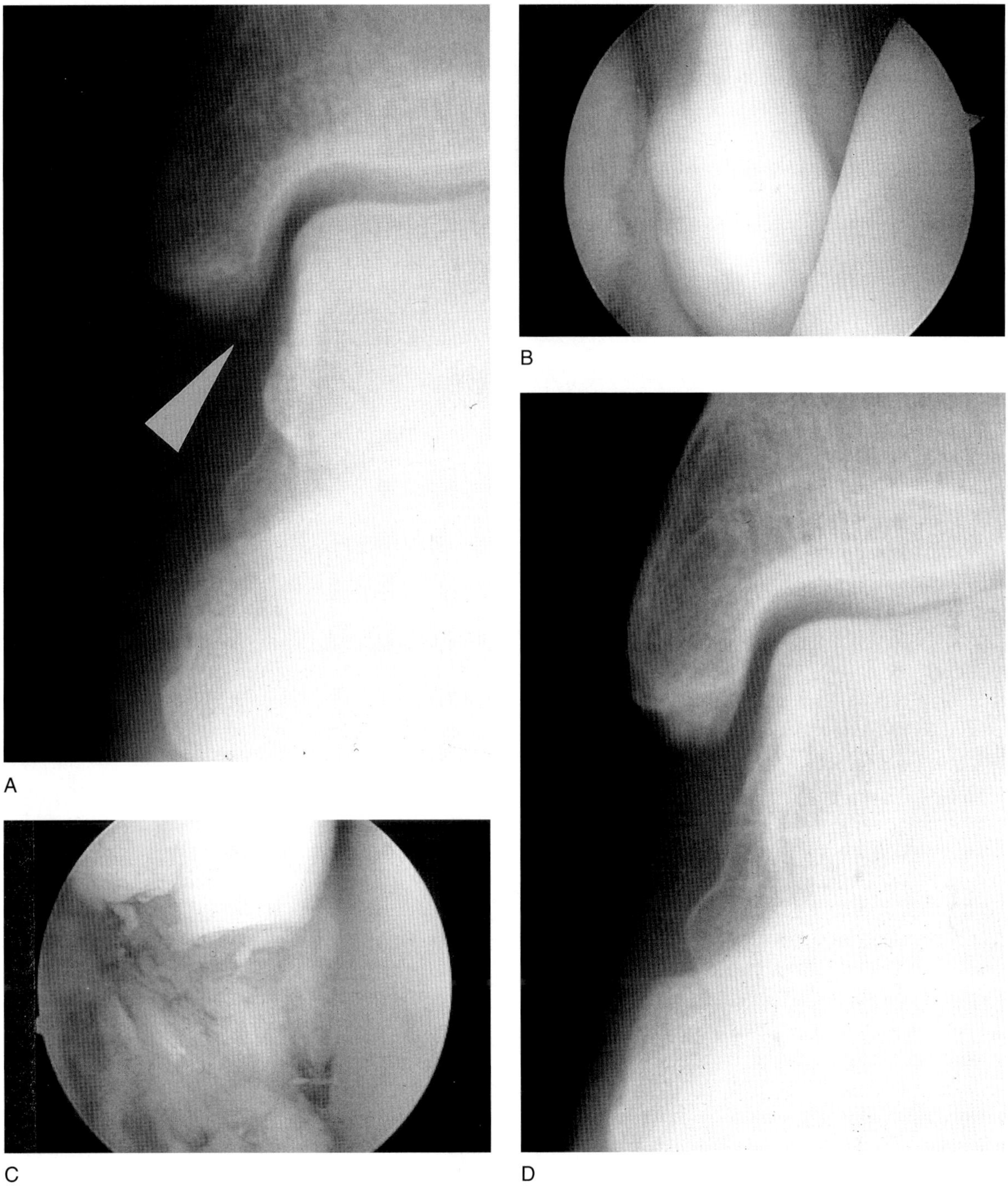

FIGURE 8.10. This patient had a 6-month history of persistent pain following a "severe ankle sprain." **A:** AP radiograph demonstrating a small avulsion fracture of the distal medial malleolus. **B:** Arthroscopic view of the medial gutter revealing fibrous nonunion of the avulsion fracture. **C:** View of the medial gutter after arthroscopic excision of the fibrous nonunion. **D:** Postoperative AP radiograph after excision of the avulsion nonunion. The patient experienced complete relief of symptoms within 8 weeks after operation.

come was highly dependent on the arthroscopic findings at surgery. Amendola et al. noted that patients who had localized pathology, such as osteochondritis dissecans of the talus, fared much better than those who had diffuse conditions such as posttraumatic scarring or osteoarthritis.[11] Similarly, Pritsch et al. discovered that patients who had localized adhesions at the tibiofibular syndesmosis had great pain relief, and those who had talar dome chondral lesions had some pain relief.[16] Patients who had a normal arthroscopic examination often had no pain relief, as symptoms appeared to be subjective and pathology was either minimal or nonexistent.

Arthroscopy for the treatment of chronic syndesmosis disruptions also produced good results. In a retrospective review of 19 patients treated an average of 24 months after injury, 14 of 17 (82%) returned to their preinjury level of activity.[15] A triad of findings were always noted at arthroscopy: disruption of the deep portion of the posterior tibiofibular ligament, rupture of the interosseous ligament with a syndesmotic gap of more than 2 mm, and a chondral fracture of the posterolateral portion of the tibial plafond in the area of insertion of the deep posteroinferior tibiofibular ligament. These authors also noted that the "external rotation stress test" was positive in all patients preoperative and negative in all patients postoperatively.[17] They concluded that the test does not measure instability but, instead, measures irritation or mechanical disruption of the syndesmosis.

Arthrofibrosis, on the other hand, was a more difficult problem to treat. Objective criteria, such as range of motion, were poorly evaluated, if at all, in these studies. Ferkel and Orwin reviewed 25 patients who underwent arthroscopy for postfracture problems; 8 of those patients had arthrofibrosis preoperatively.[3] For all patients, an average increase in dorsiflexion of 4 degrees and an average increase in plantar flexion of 11 degrees was noted after arthroscopic débridement. Of the 25 patients, 5 (20%) regained motion equivalent to that on the nonoperated side. One patient developed loss of motion postoperatively and subsequently underwent successful ankle fusion to relieve persistent symptoms. Two patients redeveloped arthrofibrosis and required repeat arthroscopic débridement. Although 19 of 25 (76%) patients reported a decrease in ankle pain and an increase in activity, fewer than 50% of the patients with preoperative arthrofibrosis showed improvement (Table 8.2).

In summary, arthroscopy of chronic fractures and postfracture defects is useful for diagnosing and treating persistent pain unresponsive to conservative measures such as antiinflammatory medications, immobilization, and bracing. Pathology not identified by radiologic studies, such as chondral lesions, postfracture adhesions, and chronic ligament injuries, are easily identified and treated with arthroscopy. Because of the increased fibrosis and scarring found in these patients, following the basic arthroscopic principles regarding portal development and use of motorized shavers is essential to avoid neurovascular complications. The postoperative outcome depends on the pathology found. Localized injuries and soft tissue pathology clearly did better than diffuse articular injuries and bony pathology.

CONCLUSIONS AND FUTURE DEVELOPMENTS

For treatment of acute ankle fractures arthroscopy has the advantage of providing better visualization of the articular surface to improve fracture reductions while at the same time minimizing soft tissue dissection. Arthroscopy also allows the surgeon to remove small osteochondral fragments and other debris from the joint more easily, which may help decrease the formation of postoperative adhesions and other late complications. Recent improvements in support equipment, such as the mini C-arm fluoroscopic unit, cannulated screws for fixation, and small wire external fixators have expanded the indications of arthroscopy-assisted reduction and fixation of many fractures previously thought to require extensive soft tissue exposures.

In addition to treating intraarticular fractures, arthroscopy of acute fractures helps identify associated intraarticular pathology not usually seen on pre-

TABLE 8.2. *Arthroscopic findings of postfracture pathology*

	No. of cases		*No. of lesions*		*Results*	
Study	*Total*	*With postfracture pathology*	*Soft tissue*	*Articular*	*E/G*	*F/P*
Amendola[11]	79	20	14 (70%)	6 (30%)	15 (75%)	5 (25%)
Pritsch[16]	19	19	11 (58%)	2 (11%)	13 (68%)	6 (32%)
Ogilvie-Harris[15]	17	17	17 (100%)	0 (0%)	14 (82%)	3 (18%)
Liu[13]	68	4	N/A	N/A	N/A	N/A
Ferkel[3]	25	25	25 (100%)	20 (80%)	19 (76%)	6 (24%)

E/G, excellent or good; F/P, fair or poor.

operative radiographs or at the time of surgery. Chondral lesions, syndesmotic injuries, and loose bodies are frequently found in displaced fractures. Although most patients fully recover after appropriate treatment for displaced ankle fractures, some remain in persistent pain secondary to associated intraarticular injuries. It is these patients in whom acute arthroscopic evaluation and débridement may be beneficial for preventing a poor outcome. Larger numbers and longer follow-up are needed to determine if acute arthroscopy of ankle fractures statistically alters the outcome.

In the case of chronic fractures and postfracture pathology, arthroscopy has provided a minimally invasive yet accurate method of diagnosing and treating the intraarticular pathology that causes chronic pain. As for arthroscopy of other joints with chronic symptoms, the results of ankle arthroscopy are much better for localized injuries and soft tissue pathology than for diffuse articular injuries. Even in cases of extensive posttraumatic arthritis, arthroscopy helps determine which patients are candidates for ankle fusion or other salvage procedures. So long as the principles of portal placement and the use of motorized instruments are maintained, the risk of complications is small.

Some have advocated the use of holmium: YAG lasers to treat ankle pathology.[18] Advantages include easier accessibility to confined spaces, decreased iatrogenic injury (articular scuffing), and increased intraarticular hemostasis. Common applications have been synovectomy, chondoplasty, and ablation of impingement lesions. Although there have been no complications reported in the literature regarding laser use in the ankle, the cost of the equipment and the risk of developing localized osteonecrosis (as seen after laser-assisted partial meniscectomy in the knee) have limited its use.[19] Additionally, one study demonstrated that damage to meniscal tissue caused by a laser is much greater than is evident intraoperatively and is much greater than the damage caused by mechanical instruments.[20] Because the articular surface and soft tissues are already traumatized owing to the injury, lasers are not recommended for treating acute ankle fractures. Further study is also indicated to determine the true efficacy and safety of lasers in the treatment of chronic fractures and postfracture pathology.

Finally, although arthroscopic treatment of acute fractures has been limited to treating the ankle joint, future consideration should be given to treatment of subtalar fractures and dislocations. Studies have shown that intraarticular fractures or osteochondral fragments in the subtalar joint lead to an increased chance of posttraumatic arthritis and may result in persistent stiffness of the subtalar joint.[21,22] It has been shown that plain radiographs do not always reliably identify osteochondral or intraarticular pathology after these injuries, and CT scans or tomograms are recommended.[21,23] Arthroscopic evaluation and treatment of the subtalar joint may prove to be helpful in minimizing posttraumatic arthritis, chronic pain, and stiffness in these cases.

BIBLIOGRAPHY

1. Renström PAFH. Persistently painful sprained ankle. *J AAOS* 1994;2:270–280.
2. Feldman MD, Campbell ED Jr, Collins HR. The role of arthroscopy in the treatment of displaced extra-articular ankle fractures [scientific exhibit]. Presented in part at the annual meeting of the American Academy of Orthopaedic Surgeons, Orlando, 1995.
3. Ferkel RD, Orwin JF. Arthroscopic treatment of acute ankle fractures and postfracture defects. In: Ferkel RD (ed) *Arthroscopic surgery: the foot and ankle*. Philadelphia: Lippincott-Raven, 1995.
4. Coonrad RW. Fracture-dislocations of the ankle joint with impaction injury of the lateral weight-bearing surface of the tibia. *J Bone Joint Surg Am* 1970;52: 1337–1344.
5. Pankovich AM. Fractures of the fibula at the distal tibiofibular syndesmosis. *CORR* 1979;143:138–147.
6. Wagstaffe WW. An unusual form of fracture of the fibula. *St Thomas Hosp Rep* 1875;6:43.
7. Whipple TL, Martin DR, McIntyre LF, et al. Arthroscopic treatment of triplane fractures of the ankle. *Arthroscopy* 1993;9:456–463.
8. Saltzman CL, Marsh JL, Tearse DS. Treatment of displaced talus fractures: an arthroscopically assisted approach. *Foot Ankle Int* 1994;15:630–633.
9. Holt ES. Arthroscopic visualization of the tibial plafond during posterior malleolar fracture fixation. *Foot Ankle Int* 1994;15:206–208.
10. Lauge-Hansen N. Fractures of the ankle. II. Combined experimental-surgical and experimental-roentgenologic investigations. *Arch Surg* 1950;957–985.
11. Amendola A, Petrik J, Webster-Bogaert S. Ankle arthroscopy outcome in 79 patients. *Arthroscopy* 1996; 12:565–573.
12. Stetson WB, Ferkel RD. Ankle arthroscopy. II. Indications and results. *J AAOS* 1996;4:24–33.
13. Liu SH, Raskin A, Osti L, et al. Arthroscopic treatment of anterolateral ankle impingement. *Arthroscopy* 1994;10:215–218.

14. Ferkel RD, Fischer SP. Progress in ankle arthroscopy. *CORR* 1989;240:210–220.
15. Ogilvie-Harris DJ, Reed SC. Disruption of the ankle syndesmosis: diagnosis and treatment by arthroscopic surgery. *Arthroscopy* 1994;10:561–568.
16. Pritsch M, Lokiec F, Sali M, et al. Adhesions of the distal tibiofibular syndesmosis. *CORR* 1993;289: 220–222.
17. Boytim MJ, Fischer DA, Neumann L. Syndesmotic ankle sprains. *Am J Sports Med* 1991;19:294–298.
18. Smith C, Dillingham M, Fanton G. The use of laser in ankle arthroscopy. In: Guhl JF (ed) *Foot and ankle arthroscopy*, 2nd ed. Thorofare, NJ: Slack, 1993: 189–196.
19. Fink B, Schneider T, Braunstein S, et al. Holmium:YAG laser-induced aseptic bone necroses of the femoral condyle. *Arthroscopy* 1996;12:217–223.
20. Bernard M, Grothues-Spork M, Hertel P, et al. Reactions of meniscal tissue after arthroscopic laser application: an in vivo study using five different laser systems. *Arthroscopy* 1996;12:441–451.
21. DeLee JC, Curtis R. Subtalar dislocation of the foot. *J Bone Joint Surg Am* 1982;64:433–437.
22. Merchan ECR. Subtalar dislocations: long-term follow-up of 39 cases. Injury 1992;23:97–100.
23. Bohay DR, Manoli II A. Occult fractures following subtalar joint injuries. *Foot Ankle Int* 1996;17:164–169.

CHAPTER 9

Arthroscopic Ankle Arthrodesis

James M. Glick

More than 40 surgical techniques for performing an ankle arthrodesis were described during the twentieth century.[1–13] As these and other studies indicated, this procedure has been plagued with complications, slow time to fusion, and nonunion. Nonunion rates as high as 41% and overall complication rates of 31–60% have been reported.[14–18] In contrast, a 1985 study by Morgan et al. reported a 96% fusion rate and few complications among 101 ankle fusions.[8] Morgan et al.'s fusion technique maintained the bony contour of the ankle mortise and used two crossed transmalleolar screws for internal fixation. Schneider was the first to report ankle fusion using arthroscopy.[10] The patient in that case experienced little pain and was able to ambulate shortly after the procedure. In addition, the ankle fused quite rapidly.

The purpose of the present chapter is to describe the operative technique of ankle arthrodesis and to show the advantages of the procedure. Arthroscopic ankle arthrodesis is indicated to relieve intractable disabling pain at the tibiotalar joint. Because visualization through the arthroscope is two-dimensional, it is difficult to correct deformities, so it cannot be used when there is significant malalignment (varus or valgus of more than 15 degrees) or when there is extensive bone loss, such as with avascular necrosis of the talus or after a failed total joint replacement. The indications I use include traumatic arthritis, hemophilic arthropathy, congenital deformity, rheumatoid arthritis, old osteochondritis dissecans, and previous ankle infection now eradicated.

OPERATIVE TECHNIQUE

Similar to open methods for ankle fusion, the arthroscopic procedure consists of three main steps: (1) removal of all hyaline cartilage and subchondral bone; (2) reduction of the ankle in the neutral position; and (3) internal fixation with two transmalleolar screws.

The arthroscopic equipment necessary to perform this procedure includes a 30 degree fore-oblique 4 mm arthroscope with camera and appropriate video equipment, high-speed motorized suction abraders and shavers, arthroscopic graspers, 15 degree angle curettes, an image intensifier, and large-diameter cannulated compression screws (6.5, 7.0, or 7.3 mm).

After a general or spinal anesthetic is administered, position the patient supine toward the foot end of a standard operating table. Place the thigh of the operative leg in a leg holder just above the knee and flex the knee over the end of the table, so the sole of the foot is parallel with the floor (Fig. 9.1A). Space should be allowed for placing the image intensifier at the end of the case. Next, make sure that the ankle can be easily dorsiflexed to neutral. Inability to obtain the neutral position may be due to a contracted Achilles tendon and posterior capsule, bony impingement between the talar neck and anterior tibia, or a combination of the two. If radiographs do not show evidence of bony impingement (anterior spurs), percutaneous Achilles tendon lengthening should be performed prior to arthroscopy (Fig. 9.2).[19] This step not only allows

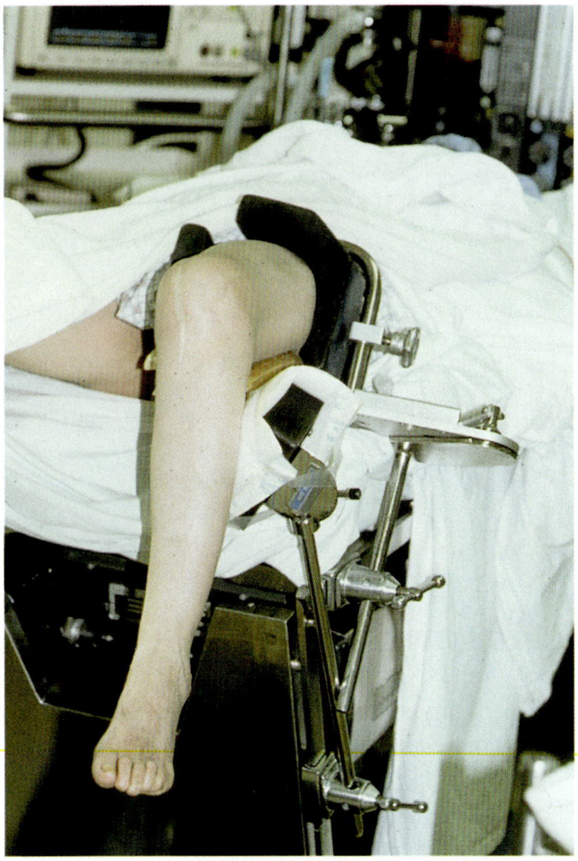

A

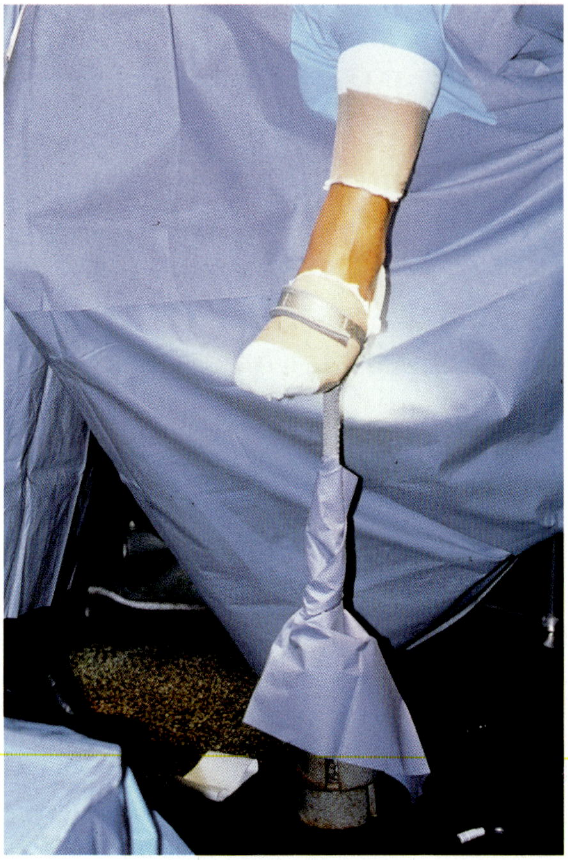

B

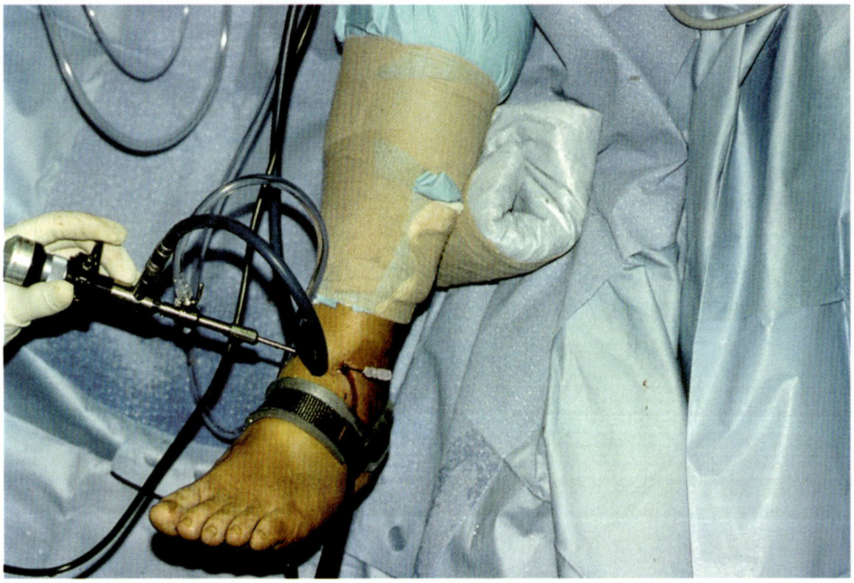

C

FIGURE 9.1. Setup for left ankle arthrodesis using noninvasive (strap) distraction. When the image intensifier is brought in, the knee is extended and the foot is placed on its flat portion. **A:** Thigh is supported in a standard thigh holder, and the knee is flexed over the end of the table so the sole of the foot is parallel to the floor. **B:** Leg is draped with the distraction strap and weights in place. **C:** A sterile rolled towel in back of the calf keeps the back of the ankle away from the drapes.

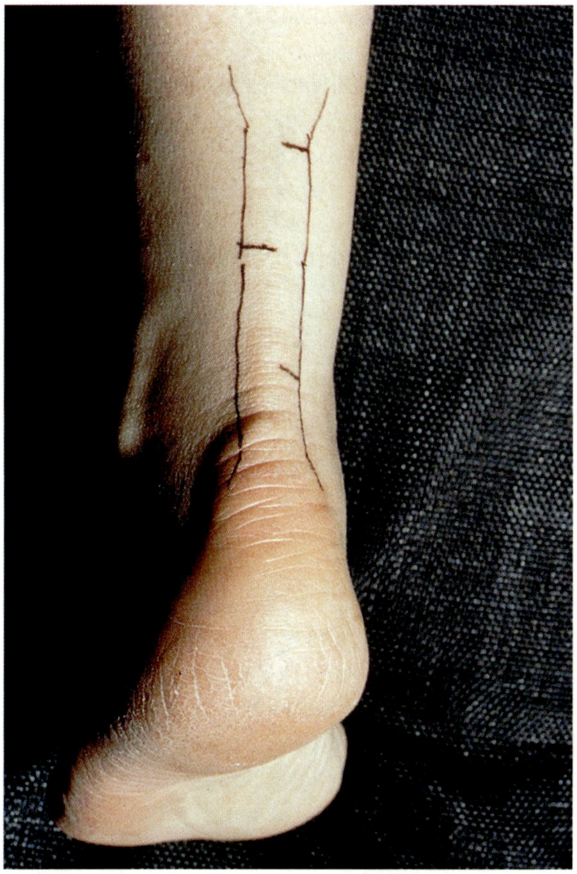

FIGURE 9.2. Position of the three subcutaneous incisions used for lengthening the Achilles tendon.

reduction to a neutral position for fusion but facilitates distraction of the ankle during the procedure. If radiographs show bony impingement, the anterior spur should first be arthroscopically removed. If the ankle still cannot be brought to the neutral position, Achilles tendon lengthening should be performed after the arthroscopic part of the procedure and before reduction. Now, prepare and drape the operative leg from the proximal tibia to the toes to allow intraoperative assessment of ankle alignment.

If desired, apply a traction device to distract the ankle. I use a soft strap, rather than skeletal traction, to distract the ankle joint. This method eliminates the need for two incisions and provides adequate distraction to accomplish the fusion (Fig. 9.1B). To keep the heel from pressing back against the drapes, insert sterile rolled towels between the upper calf and the drapes (Fig. 9.1C).

Establish standard anterolateral and anteromedial arthroscopic portals. Then débride all hypertrophic synovium and loose osteochondral fragments that block the view of the joint. A posterolateral portal can now be established for fluid outflow (Fig. 9.3). Next, débride the articular surfaces of the tibial plafond, talar dome, and medial and lateral talomalleolar surfaces of all remaining hyaline cartilage and subchondral bone in a systematic fashion. This step is performed with a motorized arthroscopic abrader (burr) to expose cancellous bone on all joint surfaces (Fig. 9.4). During the débridement, care is taken to maintain the normal bony contours of the talar dome and tibial plafond. Attempting to reshape the surfaces of the talar dome and tibial plafond to planar surfaces (known as "squaring off" the mortise) should be avoided, as it may leave a bony gap when the ankle is reduced and prolong the time to fusion (Fig. 9.5).

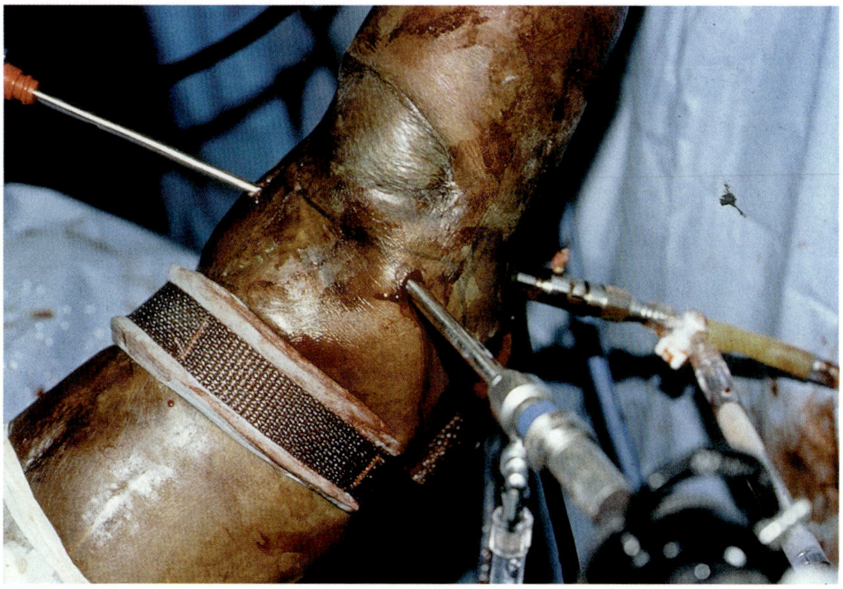

FIGURE 9.3. Three portals used for left ankle arthrodesis. The arthroscope is in the anterolateral portal, a shaver is in the anteromedial portal, and a combined outflow pressure-sensing cannula for a fluid pump is in the posterolateral portal. The bulge on the front of the ankle is an old soft tissue graft in the patient whose case is shown in Figure 9.13.

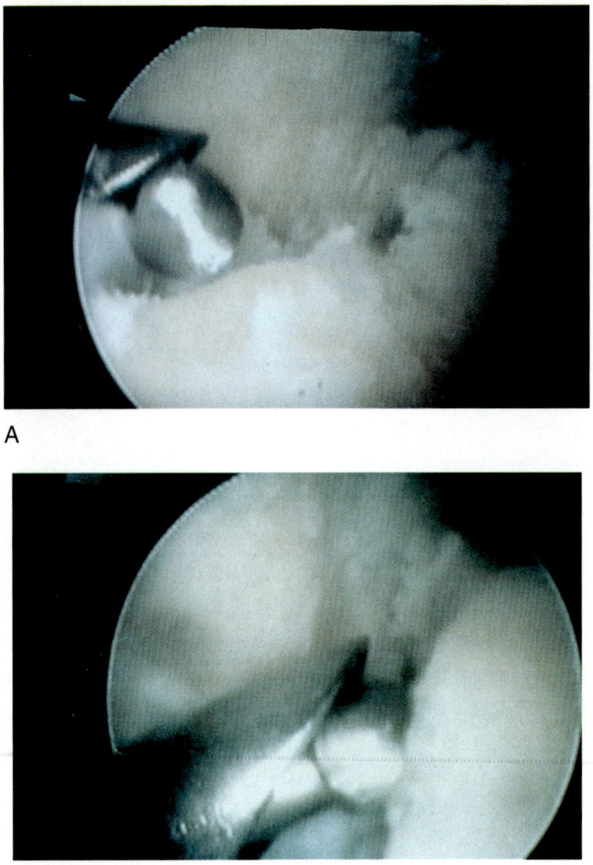

A

B

FIGURE 9.4. Abrasion of the articular surfaces, exposing bleeding bone while maintaining the normal contour of the joint. **A:** Abrasion of the talus (bottom). The tibia is shown at the top. **B:** Abrasion of the talus adjacent to the medial malleolus (medial gutter).

In general, débridement of the medial half of the joint is done with the arthroscope placed anterolaterally and the abrader placed anteromedially. Conversely, débridement of the lateral half of the joint is done with the arthroscope placed anteromedially and the abrader placed anterolaterally. The posterior aspect of the joint can be débrided sufficiently through the anterior portals, with the joint distracted. Removal of extremely sclerotic bone or subchondral cysts may be facilitated by using 15 degree angled curettes (Fig. 9.6). A large anterior osteophyte on the tibia that blocks dorsiflexion of the ankle is removed with an arthroscopic burr through one anterior portal while visualizing the bony protuberance through the other anterior portal. Alternatively, a 0.25 inch osteotome can be used in place of the burr.[20]

Once viable cancellous bone is visualized on all surfaces of the talus and tibia, secure the ankle joint with two crossed cannulated screws. At the anterior aspect of the medial malleolus and above the joint line, percutaneously drill one guide pin through the tibia, directing it posteriorly and laterally toward the talus (Fig. 9.7). Repeat the same procedure on the lateral side, but start the guide pin through the lateral malleolus and aim it anteromedially into the neck of the talus. If the bone is osteopenic or if concomitant Achilles tendon lengthening was performed, a third screw may be needed for additional stability. This additional guide pin for the third screw is begun laterally in the tibia, anterior to the fibula, pointed toward the talus and at the same time

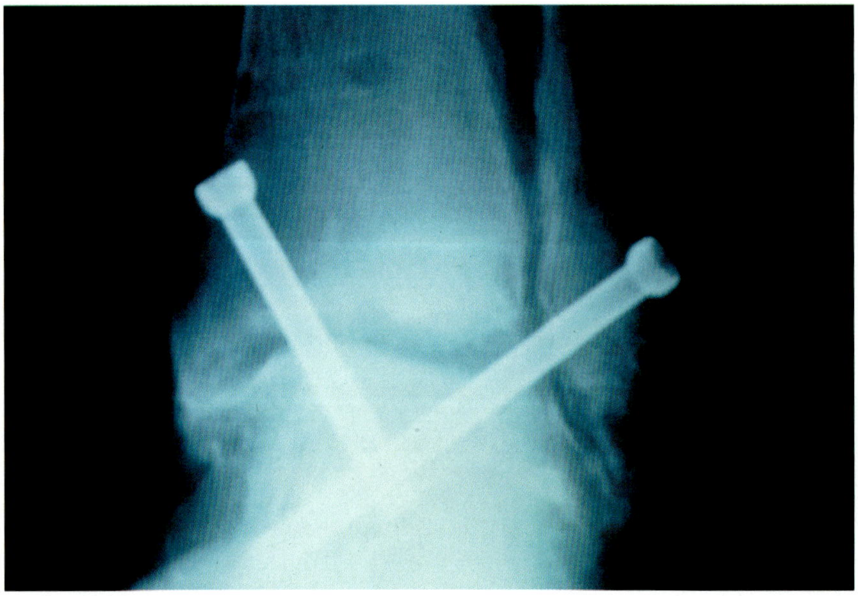

FIGURE 9.5. Ankle in which an attempt was made to reshape (square off) the talar surface. Note the wide space and the lack of congruity. This ankle went on to delayed union.

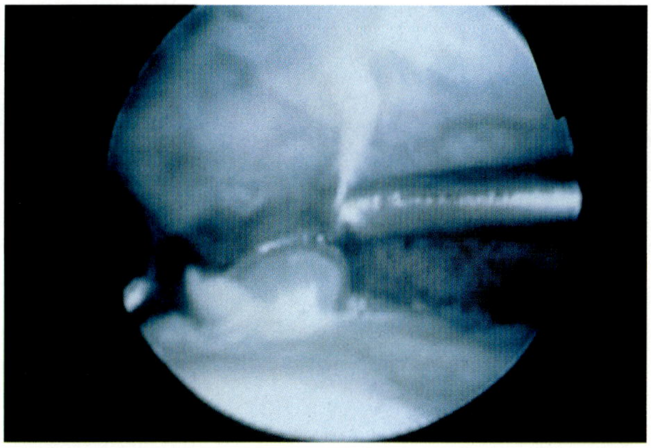

FIGURE 9.6. Removing a cyst in the talus with an angled curette.

aimed as far anteriorly as possible. Through the arthroscope visualize the precise location of the pins crossing the joint and entering the talus. If necessary, they can be redirected (Fig. 9.8A). Then back the guide pins out so the tips are level with the denuded surfaces of the tibial plafond and lateral malleolus. Next, removal all arthroscopic equipment from the joint, release the distraction (Fig. 9.8B), and reduce the fusion surfaces under fluoroscopic guidance. Hold the talus in the position of fusion. The correct position for fusion is neutral dorsiflexion, 0–5 degrees of valgus, and 0–5 degrees of external rotation. With this position for fusion carefully held, drill the guide pins into the talus (Fig. 9.9), determining the precise depth by image intensification (Fig. 9.10A). Then insert the corresponding screws over the guide pins and screw them into place (Fig. 9.10B). Confirm the reduction and screw placement with permanent radiographs (Fig. 9.11).

Close the wounds with single nylon sutures and apply a well-padded sterile dressing that allows absorption of extravasated fluid. Immobilize the ankle in a posterior splint. At the first postoperative visit, convert the splint to a walking cast or removable walking fracture boot (Fig. 9.12). The patient may bear as much weight as he or she can tolerate. The fracture boot may be removed when lying in bed so long as the patient reapplies it for weight-bearing. Obtain radiograms every 3–4 weeks until the joint is solidly fused.

RESULTS

The final method of arthroscopic ankle fusion, described above, was gained from the experience of 78 cases performed by four surgeons in three centers: I and my partner Thomas G. Sampson from San Francisco, California; Craig D. Morgan from Wilmington, Delaware; and Mark S. Myerson from Baltimore, Maryland. All of the surgeons performed the procedure in a similar manner and added to the refinement of the operation. Various débridement and fixation techniques were tried, with the safest, most reliable ones incorporated into the final procedure. Sampson and I,[21–24] Morgan et al.,[24–26] and Myerson et al.[24,27,28] have published on the topic.

The ages of the patients ranged from 18 to 83 years (average 46 years). Follow-up ranged from 16 months to 10 years (average 44 months). The final

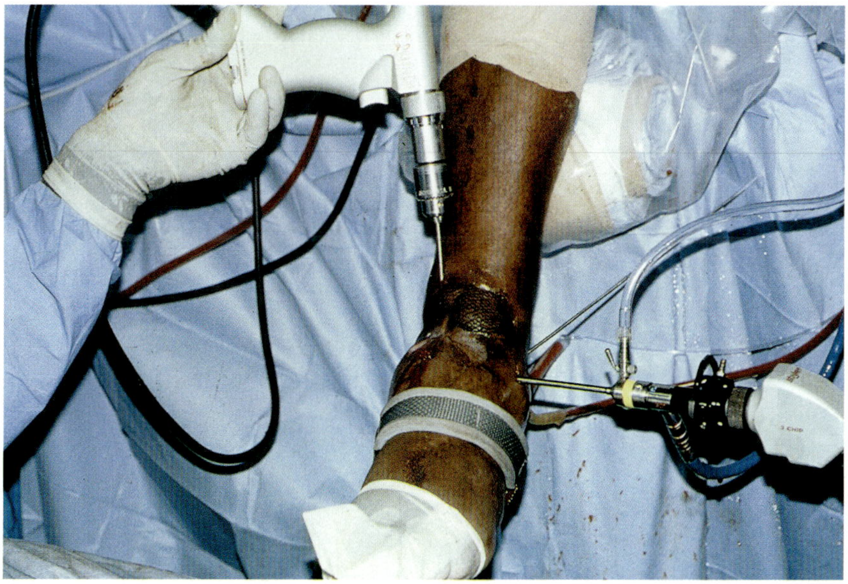

FIGURE 9.7. Inserting a guide pin for a cannulated screw, starting above the medial malleolus. This is the same patient described in Figure 9.13.

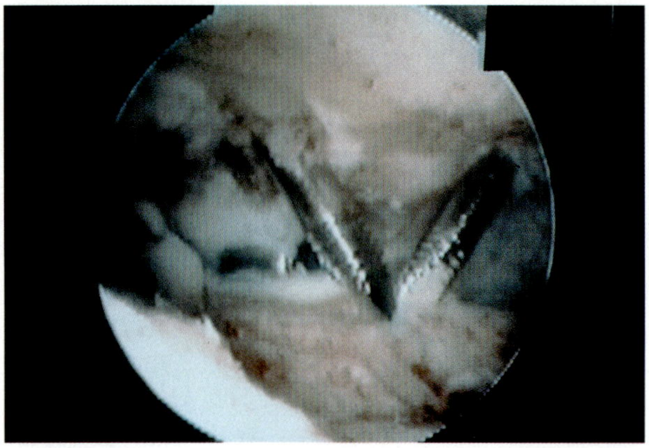

A

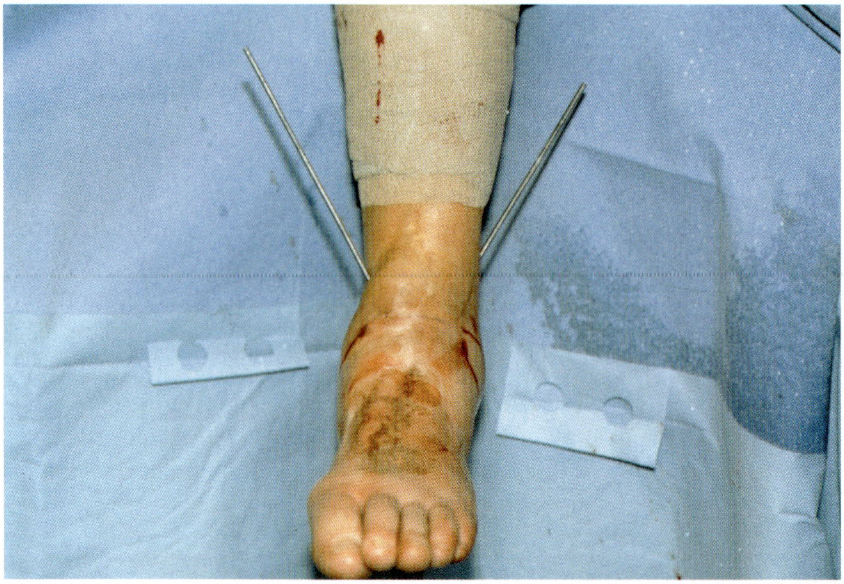

B

FIGURE 9.8. Guide pins for the cannulated screws have been placed from the medial and lateral aspects of the ankle. **A:** Arthroscopic view of the tips of the guide pins penetrating the joint surface of the tibial plafond. **B:** Outside view with the guide pins in place and the ankle ready to be reduced.

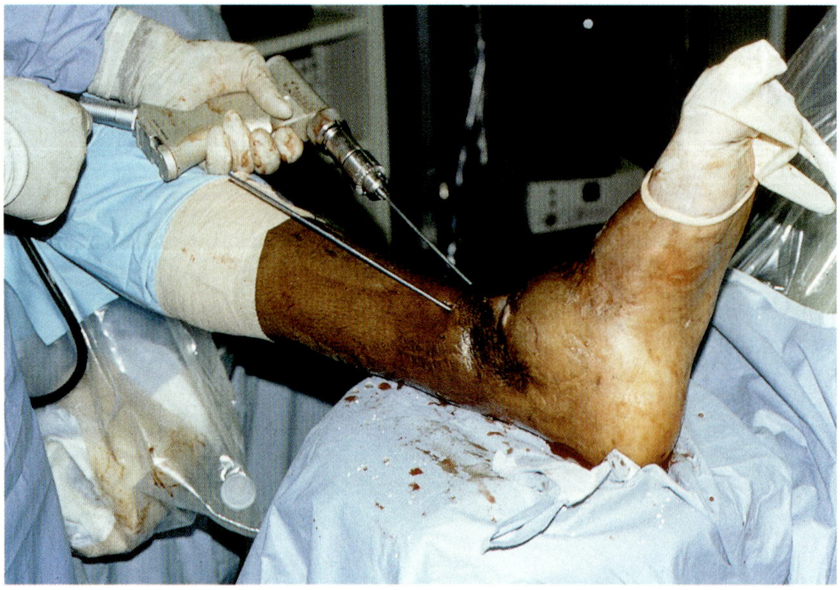

FIGURE 9.9. Ankle reduced on an image intensifier. This is the patient shown in Figure 9.13. The ankle has been placed on the flat surface of the image intensifier. One of the guide pins is being drilled into the talus.

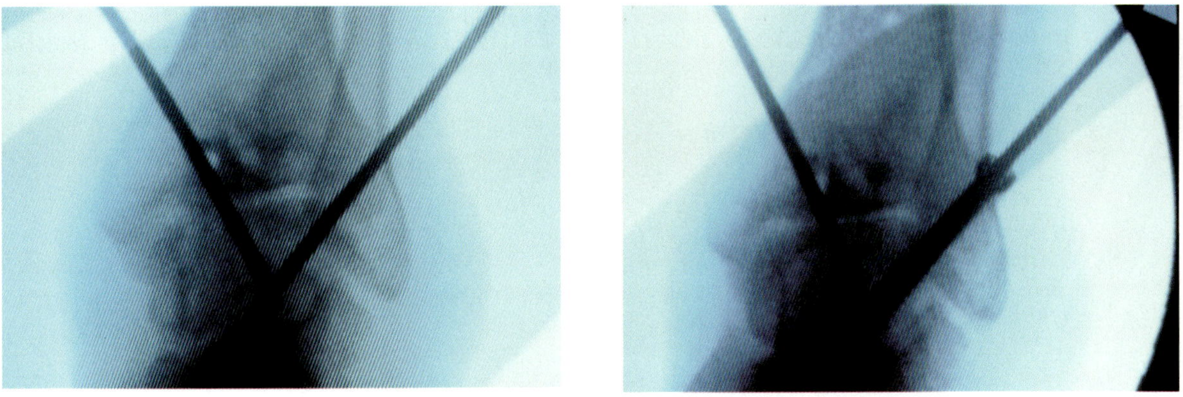

A B

FIGURE 9.10. Fluoroscopic views of the progression of fixation. **A:** Two guide pins have been inserted to the correct depth on this anteroposterior (AP) view. **B:** View of the lateral cannulated screw in place.

results were based on a rating scale developed by Morgan et al.[8] (Table 9.1). Of the 78 ankles, 71 (91%) fused solidly. Four of the seven nonunions resulted from a surgical technique no longer used. Two nonunions developed after using a Charnley compression device for fixation. The other two occurred after holmium:YAG laser was used for débridement, which induced osteolysis. These four went on to successful fusion after a conventional arthrodesis.

The three other nonunions were attributed to technical errors and were part of the learning curve for this technique. In one case a central portal was used for the arthroscope, causing damage to the dorsalis pedis artery. In the same case, fixation was not secure, so when the artery was repaired 1 week after operation the fixation was lost and the fusion subsequently did not unite the fracture. Later, a fusion performed through a conventional incision went on to unite the fracture successfully. For the first eight cases performed by me, fixation was accomplished with either threaded or smooth Steinmann pins. Another nonunion occurred in a case in which the lateral and medial gutters were not débrided of articular cartilage. We no longer use a central portal and carefully débride the gutters in all of our ankle arthrodeses (Fig. 9.4B). The third

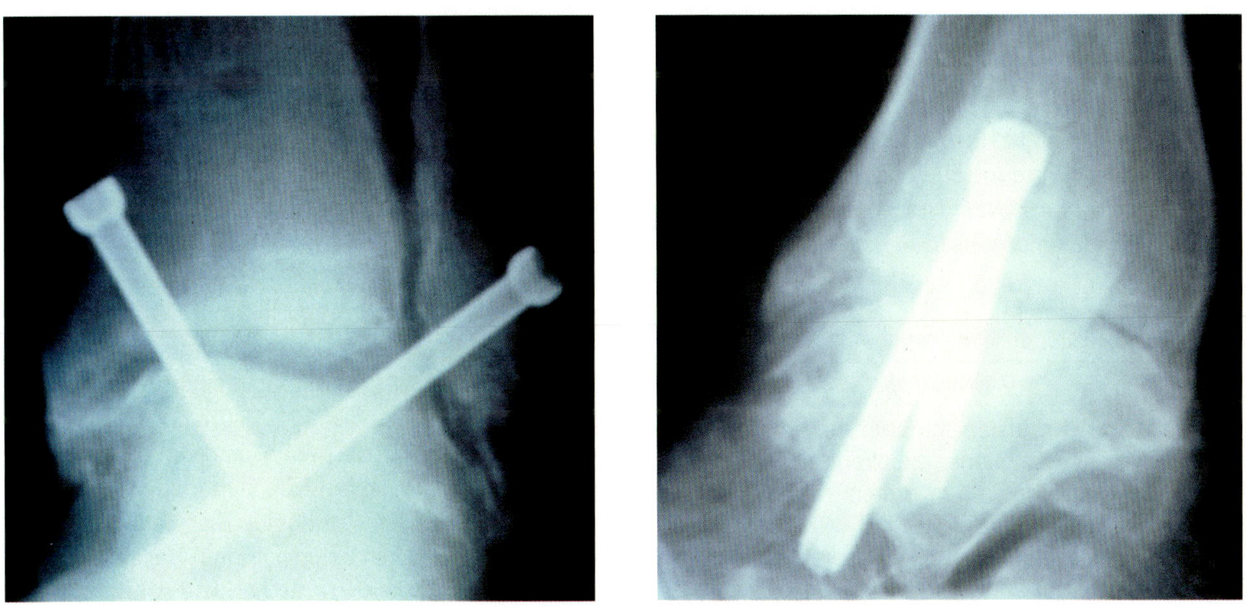

A B

FIGURE 9.11. Final intraoperative radiographs with cannulated screws in place. **A:** AP view. **B:** Lateral view.

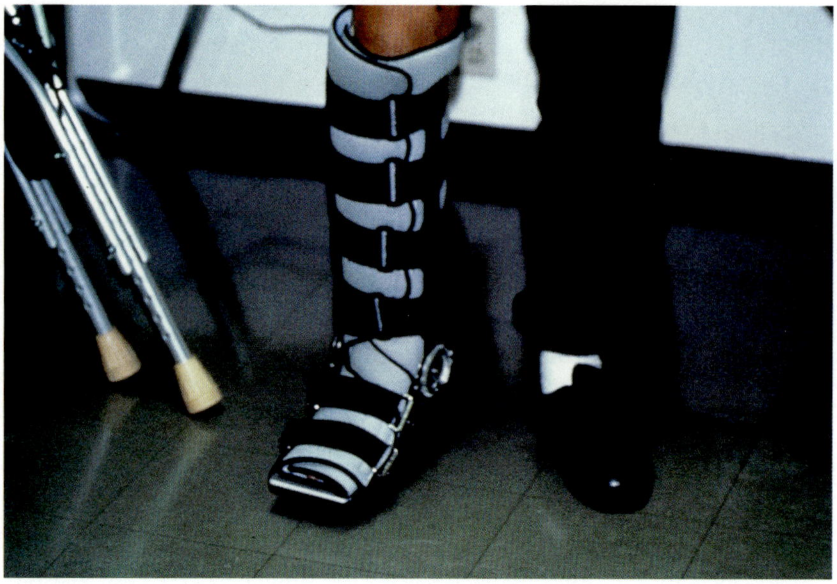

FIGURE 9.12. Walking fracture boot used for postoperative immobilization.

nonunion was a case of noncompliance. The patient was obese and a heavy smoker, and he removed his cast several weeks prematurely to return to work as a truck driver. He failed subsequent follow-up appointments.

The average time to arthrodesis was just over 8 weeks (58 days), with a range of 4–14 weeks. Bony fusion was determined mainly from a lateral radiographic view (Fig. 9.13). There were three delayed unions: two following Achilles tendon lengthening and one after two screws were used to fixate an unstable ankle. There were no deep wound infections and only one superficial wound infection. There were 85% excellent and good results, 5% fair results, and 10% poor results. Two ankles were rated as fair because of moderate to severe subtalar pain. Of the eight poor results, seven were nonunions, and the other was a malunion, fused in excessive equinus.

TABLE 9.1. *Clinical rating scale*

Rating	*Clinical characteristics*
Excellent	Solid fusion, no pain, no limp, no job restrictions, excellent appearance
Good	Solid fusion, mild pain, mild inconstant limp, same job but with some restriction and acceptable appearance
Fair	Solid fusion, moderate pain, constant limp, job change, poor appearance
Poor	Any ankle with fusion failure or severe pain

Other than the nonunions, there was one major and one minor complication. The major complication was in the patient who underwent fusion in 20 degrees of equinus. It required revision of the fusion. The minor complication was a wound infection over prominent hardware well after the patient had achieved a solid arthrodesis. The problem resolved with hardware removal and local wound care.

DISCUSSION

I have been performing arthroscopy-assisted ankle arthrodeses since February 1984, and several key points have been established from the mistakes made over the years: (1) A central portal should never be used because of its close proximity to the dorsalis pedis artery and the deep branch of the peroneal nerve. (2) The Charnley apparatus does not work when the arthroscope is used because the fusion surfaces must be flat to provide a stable construct. It is almost impossible to shape the joint surfaces so they are perfectly flat with arthroscopic visualization. (3) The medial and lateral tibiotalar surfaces (gutters) should be denuded of all cartilage. (4) At this time, a device that ablates by heat (e.g., laser, electric current) should not be used for débriding the joint surfaces because it kills the underlying bone cells. (5) Finally, three screws should be used for fixation when Achilles tendon lengthening is performed or when an unstable situation exists.

There are several advantages of the arthroscopic technique of the ankle fusion over open methods of ankle fusion. Morbidity of the arthroscopic procedure is significantly less. The surgery requires only a few small incisions and minimal soft tissue dissection. For this reason, the surgery can usually be done as an outpatient procedure or occasionally with hospitalization overnight. In addition, the minimal soft tissue disruption makes arthroscopic ankle fusion ideal for patients with compromised healing potential, such as patients with vascular disease, diabetes, rheumatoid arthritis, a history of corticosteroid use, or prior skin or soft tissue grafts.

A case of poor healing potential is shown in Figure 9.13. The patient sustained a severe open fracture-dislocation of the ankle that included loss of the soft tissue covering the anterior aspect of the ankle. Extensive skin grafting was required. Two problems occurred during the fusion procedure. First, a wide gap was created between the faces of the tibia and talus because extensive débridement was required to obtain bleeding surfaces. Second, optimal placement of the two screws was difficult

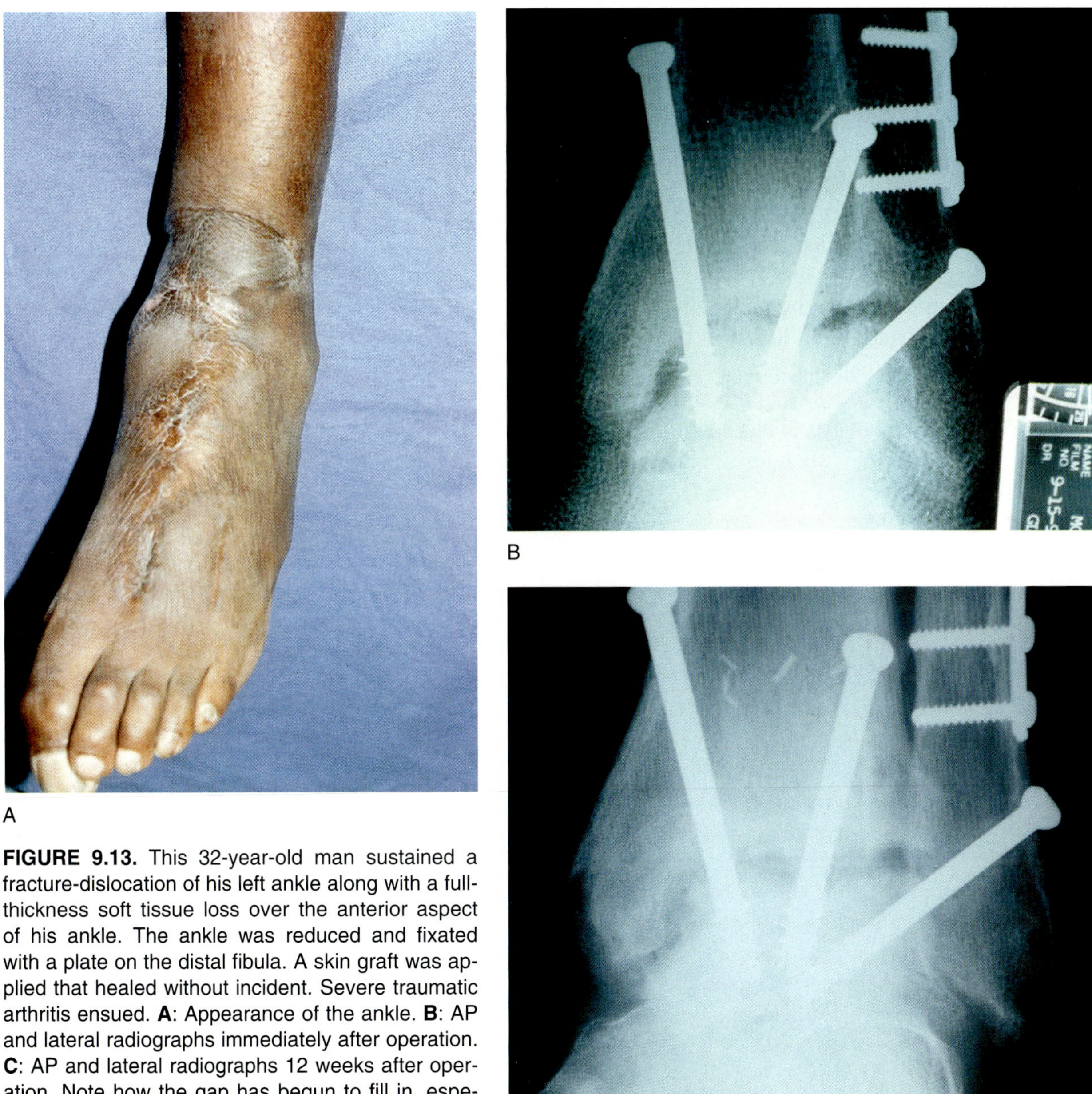

FIGURE 9.13. This 32-year-old man sustained a fracture-dislocation of his left ankle along with a full-thickness soft tissue loss over the anterior aspect of his ankle. The ankle was reduced and fixated with a plate on the distal fibula. A skin graft was applied that healed without incident. Severe traumatic arthritis ensued. **A**: Appearance of the ankle. **B**: AP and lateral radiographs immediately after operation. **C**: AP and lateral radiographs 12 weeks after operation. Note how the gap has begun to fill in, especially on the lateral view. The patient did not experience pain or swelling on weight-bearing, so immobilization was discontinued.

because of the need to position the incision for the anterior screw outside the skin graft and to keep the lateral screw from striking the plate on the fibula. To offset these problems, three screws were inserted that increased the security of the fixation, and a short leg walking cast was applied rather than a fracture boot for further postoperative stability. A fracture boot was applied after 6 weeks, and the ankle fused at 12 weeks. The gap that was left between the tibia and talus could not be helped in this case because of the need for extensive débridement. In our reported series, exact placement of the screws did not appear to be paramount for fusion to occur. In this case all three screws were in the posterior aspect of the talus, and the ankle fused without incident.

The time until fusion and thus the immobilization time is, on average, 4–8 weeks less than with open methods of arthrodesis. This is a distinct advantage in many respects. It allows patients to return to their previous level of independence much more quickly, and it cuts down on the time out of work for those whose jobs require ambulation. The significantly shorter time to fusion is a distinct advantage to certain physically disabled patients, such as those with rheumatoid arthritis, who have difficulty ambulating with upper extremity walking aids.

The reason for the shorter time to fusion is speculative. The most likely basis is that minimal interruption of the soft tissue structures around the ankle preserves the blood supply to the bones and soft tissue envelope. An intact blood supply enhances the fusion process. It is also possible that the original contour of the bony surfaces is better maintained with the arthroscopic technique, given the precise removal of bone using an arthroscopic burr. This may lend added stability to the fusion construct and leave a larger surface area of bony contact, allowing more rapid fusion.

The arthroscope is an excellent device to help with arthrodesis of an ankle. We have found that this method of fusing ankles is reliable and delivers results comparable to those seen with open techniques. The time to fusion is rapid, and morbidity is low. Arthroscopic ankle arthrodesis is a viable choice in a patient with minimal or mild deformity of the ankle joint and may be the preferred method for fusion in patients with compromised healing potential.

BIBLIOGRAPHY

1. Baciu CC. A simple technique for arthrodesis of the ankle. *J Bone Joint Surg Br* 1986;68:266–267.
2. Campbell P. Arthrodesis of the ankle with modified distraction-compression and bone-grafting. *J Bone Joint Surg Am* 1990;72:552–556.
3. Johnson EE, Weltmer J, Lian GJ, Cracchiolo A. Ilizarov ankle arthrodesis. *Clin Orthop* 1992;280: 160–169.
4. Malarkey RF, Binski JC. Ankle arthrodesis with the Calandruccio frame and bimalleolar onlay grafting. *Clin Orthop* 1991;268:44–48.
5. Mann RA, Van Manen JW, Wapner K, Martin J. Ankle fusion. *Clin Orthop* 1991;268:49–55.
6. Marcus RE, Balourdas GM, Heiple KG. Ankle arthrodesis by chevron fusion with internal fixation and bone-grafting. *J Bone Joint Surg Am* 1983;65: 833–838.
7. Mears DC, Gordaon RG, Kann SF, Kann JN. Ankle arthrodesis with an anterior tension plate. *Clin Orthop* 1991;268:70–77.
8. Morgan CD, Henke JA, Bailey RW, Kaufer H. Long-term results of tibiotalar arthrodesis. *J Bone Joint Surg Am* 1985;67:546–549.
9. Partio EK, Hirvensalo E, Partio E, et al. Talocrural arthrodesis with absorbable screws: 12 cases followed for 1 year. *Acta Orthop Scand* 1992;63:170–172.
10. Schneider D. Arthroscopic ankle fusion. *Arthroscopic Video Journal* 1983;3.
11. Scranton PE. Use of internal compression in arthrodesis of the ankle. *J Bone Joint Surg Am* 1985;67: 550–555.
12. Sowa DT, Krackow KA. Ankle fusion: a new technique of internal fixation using a compression blade plate. *Foot Ankle* 1989;9:232–239.
13. White AA. A precision posterior ankle fusion. *Clin Orthop* 1974;98:239–249.
14. Campbell CJ, Rinehart WT, Kalenak A. Arthrodesis of the ankle: deep autogenous graft with maximum cancellous bone apposition. *J Bone Joint Surg Am* 1974;56:63–70.
15. Frey C, Halikus NM, Vu-Rose T, Ebramzadeh E. A review of ankle arthrodesis: predisposing factors to nonunion. *Foot Ankle* 1994;15:581–584.
16. Johnson EW, Boseker EH. Arthrodesis of the ankle. *Arch Surg* 1968;97:766–773.
17. Morrey BF, Wiedeman GP. Complications and long-term results of ankle arthrodeses following trauma. *J Bone Joint Surg Am* 1980;62:777–784.
18. Scranton PE, Fu FH, Brown TD. Ankle arthrodesis: a comparative clinical and biomechanical evaluation. *Clin Orthop* 1980;151:234–243.
19. Hatt RN, Lamphier TA. Triple hemisection: a simplified procedure for lengthening the Achilles tendon. *N Engl J Med* 1947;236:166–170.
20. Scranton PE, McDermott JE. Anterior tibiotalar spurs: a comparison of open versus arthroscopic débridement. *Foot Ankle* 1992;13:124–129.

21. Glick JM, Parisien JS. Arthroscopic ankle arthrodesis. In: Parisien JS (ed) *Techniques in therapeutic arthroscopy*. New York: Raven, 1993;19.1–19.5.
22. Glick JM, Ferkel RD. Arthroscopic ankle arthrodesis. In: Ferkel RD (ed). *Arthroscopic surgery: the foot and ankle*. Lippincott-Raven, 1996;215–229.
23. Glick JM, Mann JA. Ankle arthrodesis using an arthroscopic method. *Foot Ankle Clin* 1996;1:163–175.
24. Glick JM, Morgan CD, Myerson MS, et al. Ankle arthrodesis using an arthroscopic method: long-term follow-up of 34 cases. *Arthroscopy* 1996;12:428–434.
25. Morgan CD. Arthroscopic tibio-talar arthrodesis. *Jefferson Orthop J* 1987;16:50–52.
26. Morgan CD. Arthroscopic tibiotalar arthrodesis. In: McGinty JB (ed) *Operative arthroscopy*, 2nd ed. Philadelphia: Lippincott-Raven, 1996;1133–1139.
27. Myerson MS, Allon SM. Arthroscopic ankle arthrodesis. *Contemp Orthop* 1989;19:21–27.
28. Myerson MS, Quill G. Ankle arthrodesis: a comparison of an arthroscopic and an open method of treatment. *Clin Orthop* 1991;268:84–95.

CHAPTER 10

Posterior Subtalar Joint Arthroscopy

J. Serge Parisien

At the present time, accurate assessment of the subtalar joint is possible through the use of some investigative procedures such as contrast arthrography, special radiographic projections, computed tomography (CT) scanning, and magnetic resonance imaging (MRI).[1–5] Direct visualization of the posterior subtalar joint via the arthroscope is also possible.[6] With the availability of miniature surgical instruments, some selected surgical procedures can also be performed. The relevant regional anatomy, arthroscopic portals, arthroscopic anatomy, the technique for diagnosis and surgery, and the possible indications for subtalar joint arthroscopy are reviewed in this chapter.

ANATOMY

Three joints form the hind part of the foot: posterior subtalar joint, talocalcaneal-navicular joint (or anterior subtalar joint), and calcaneocuboid joint. Two grooves form the tarsal canal: one on the inferior surface of the talus and one on the superior surface of the os calcis. Its lateral opening is called the sinus tarsi. The tarsal canal and sinus tarsi divide the subtalar joint into the anterior talocalcaneal-navicular joint and posterior talocalcaneal joint. Cahill[7] studied the contents of the tarsal canal and found that it contains the cervical and talocalcaneal interosseous ligaments, the medial root of the inferior extensor retinaculum, a large fat pad, and blood vessels. Whereas the interosseous ligament has no role in the limitation of inversions and eversion of the subtalar joint, the cervical ligament is important for the limitation of inversion.

Harper[8] described the supporting ligaments of the subtalar joint and divided them into superficial, intermediate, and deep layers. The superficial layer is formed by the lateral talocalcaneal ligament, posterior talocalcaneal ligament, medial talocalcaneal ligament, lateral root of the inferior extensor retinaculum, and calcaneofibular ligament. The intermediate layer is composed of the intermediate root of the inferior extensor retinaculum and the cervical ligament. The deep layer is formed by the medial root of the inferior extensor retinaculum and the interosseous talocalcaneal ligament.

The anterior portion of the subtalar joint is complex, consisting of the convex head of the talus, the concave posterior part of the navicular, the anterior part of the superior surface of the os calcis, and the short plantar calcaneonavicular (spring) ligament. Posteriorly located behind the tarsal canal is the posterior part of the subtalar joint formed by the convex superior facet of the os calcis and the concave facet of the talus. The joint line is oblique (Figs. 10.1, 10.2) and is directed upward with a convex orientation. A part of the joint is hidden by the peroneal tendons, located behind the lateral malleolus. The joint capsule has a posterior pouch and is reinforced laterally by the talocalcaneal and calcaneofibular ligaments. The small saphenous vein and sural nerve are superficially located posterior to the peroneal tendons.

PORTALS

Two arthroscopic portals, one anterior and one posterior to the lateral malleolus, can be used for arthro-

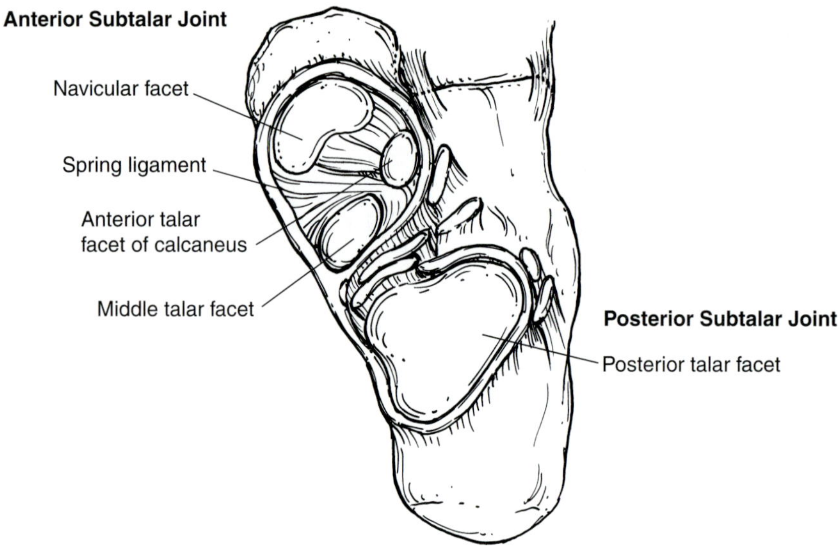

FIGURE 10.1. Posterior subtalar joint. (From Ferkel,[12] with permission.)

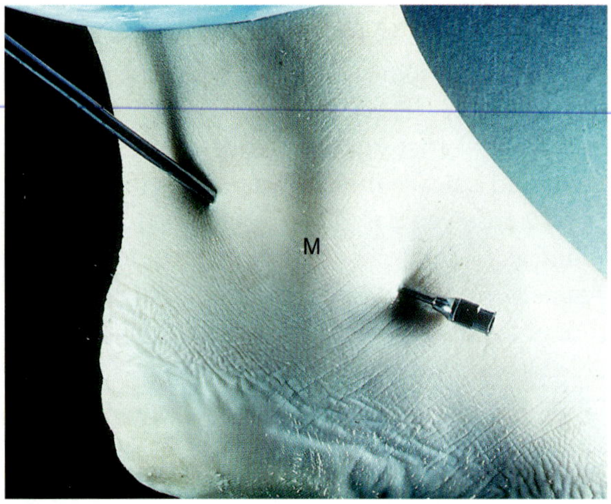

A

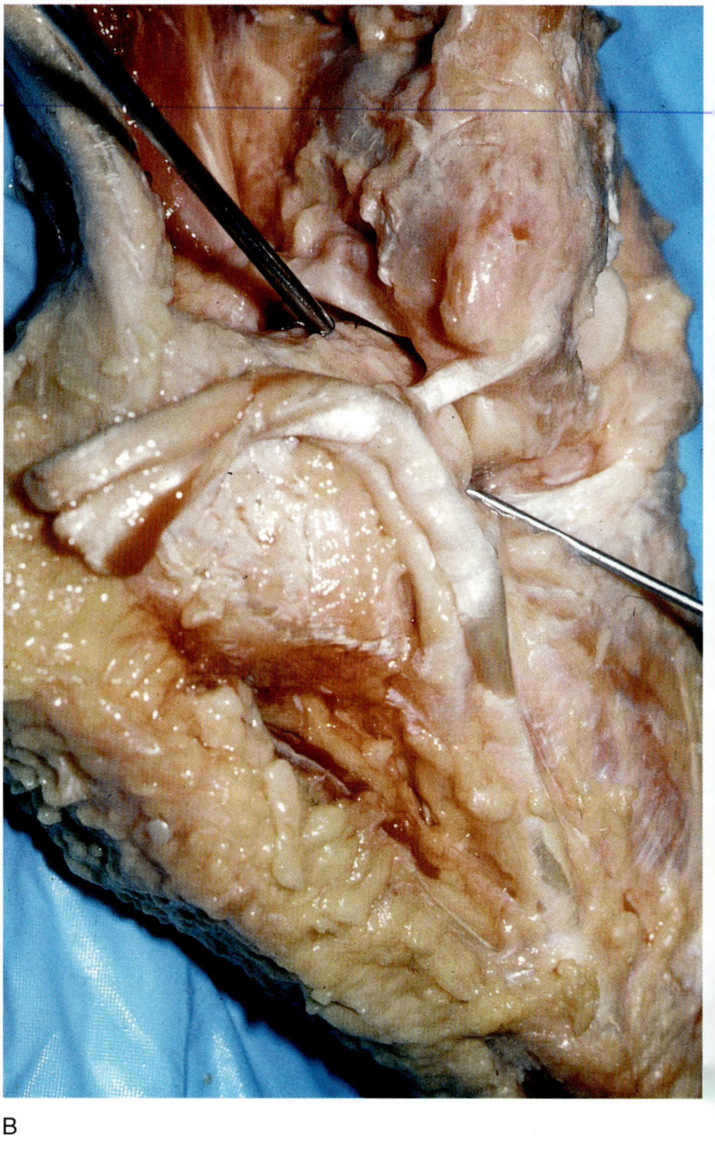

B

FIGURE 10.2. A: This cadaver specimen shows the position of the anterior and posterior portals with the foot in plantar flexion. (M) lateral malleolus. The anterior portal is 10 mm anterior and inferior from tip of fibula. **B:** Amputation specimen showing posterior subtalar joint, with peroneal tendons retracted.

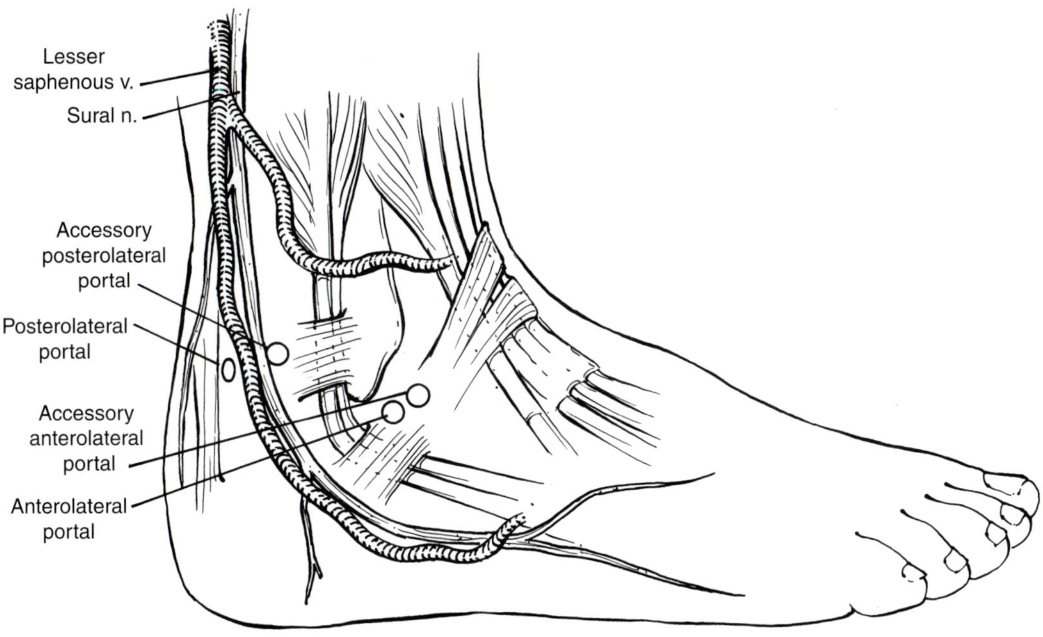

FIGURE 10.3. Subtalar portals with neurovascular structures. (From Ferkel,[12] with permission.)

scopy of the posterior subtalar joint (Figs. 10.3, 10.4). The anterior portal is placed 2 cm anterior and 1 cm distal to the tip of the fibula. The posterior portal is located at the level of the tip of the fibula or slightly proximal to it, close to the Achilles tendon, to avoid injury to the sural nerve. Two accessory anterior and posterior portals can be developed anterior to the main, previously described portals. However, the accessory posterior portal puts the sural nerve at risk. When a 2.2 mm or 2.7 mm 10 degree arthroscope is used through the anterior portal, there is good visualization of the anterior aspect of the joint. Visualization of the extremely posterior aspect of the articulation with 10 degree angulation usually requires a posterior position for the arthroscope; however, with a 25 degree angle arthroscope, either portal can be used for adequate joint visualization. Concomitant use of the two portals is necessary for an outflow needle or for triangulation of surgical instruments.

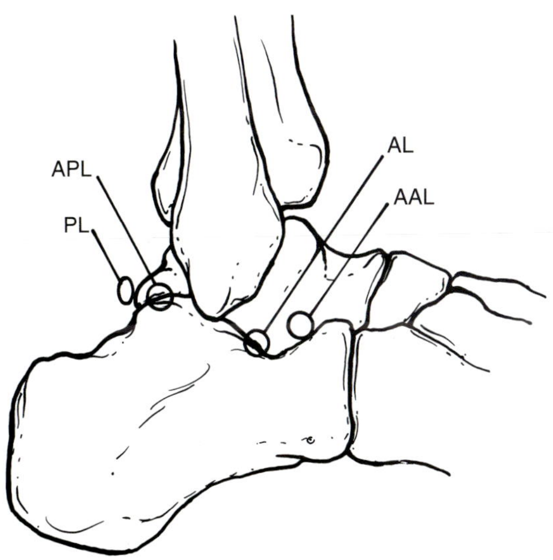

FIGURE 10.4. Subtalar portals with soft tissues removed. (From Ferkel,[12] with permission.)

INSTRUMENTATION

The posterior subtalar joint is a small joint, and its visualization requires the use of small instrumentation (Figs. 10.5, 10.6). Most diagnostic arthroscopic procedures can be performed with the 2.2 mm or

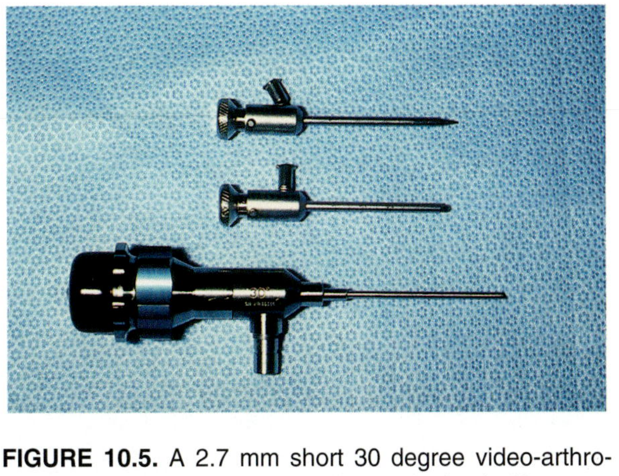

FIGURE 10.5. A 2.7 mm short 30 degree video-arthroscope (bottom) with trocar and cannula (top). (Courtesy of Smith & Nephew Inc./Arthroscopy—Andover, MA.)

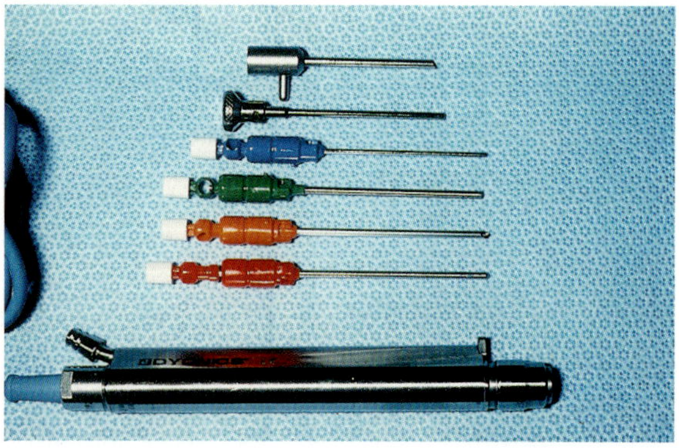

FIGURE 10.6. Motorized shaver with various surgical blades. (Courtesy of Smith & Nephew Inc./Arthroscopy—Andover, MA.)

2.7 mm 10 degree arthroscope. We prefer the increased field of view afforded by the 2.7 mm 25 degree arthroscope. Diagnostic arthroscopy can be performed by establishing only an anterior portal. In addition to the arthroscope, a spinal needle and 60 cc syringe with small plastic tubing are needed. When surgical arthroscopy is contemplated, surgical tools such as small grasping forceps, small motorized instruments, and a disposable plastic cannula are needed. Joint distension is by the gravity system. Distraction is done manually by an assistant.

TECHNIQUE

Arthroscopy of the posterior subtalar joint is carried out in the operating room under spinal or general anesthesia. The patient is placed in supine position with a sand bag under the buttocks to allow internal rotation of the lower extremity, providing better access to the posterior lateral aspect of the foot (Fig. 10.7). A leg holder is optional, and a tourniquet can be placed high over the thigh to be inflated when necessary. From the beginning of the examination, careful planning for the arthroscopic portal should be done by outlining the important landmarks. The posterior subtalar joint is a superficial structure, and the key to anatomy is definition of the tarsal canal and the sinus tarsi. Behind these structures, the joint line is oblique and directed upward with a convex orientation. Other important landmarks are the lateral malleolus and the peroneal tubercle. The tubercle can be palpated as a small protuberance on the lateral aspect of the os calcis between the tendons of the peroneus longus and brevis. A vertical line drawn from this tubercle passes anterior to the tip of the lateral malleolus and crosses the sinus tarsi area. No neurovascular bundle exists in this region. Posteriorly, the peroneal tendons, which partially overlie the posterior part of the subtalar joint, curve around the posterior aspect of the lateral malleolus. The sural nerve is located behind the lateral malleolus along with the small saphenous vein.

By inverting and everting the foot, the sinus tarsi can be palpated in front of the lateral malleolus. Approximately 2 cm anterior and 1 cm distal to the tip of the lateral malleolus, a spinal needle is placed in the joint to inflate the joint cavity with approximately 5–8 mm of normal saline or Ringer's lactate. The needle is removed, and a

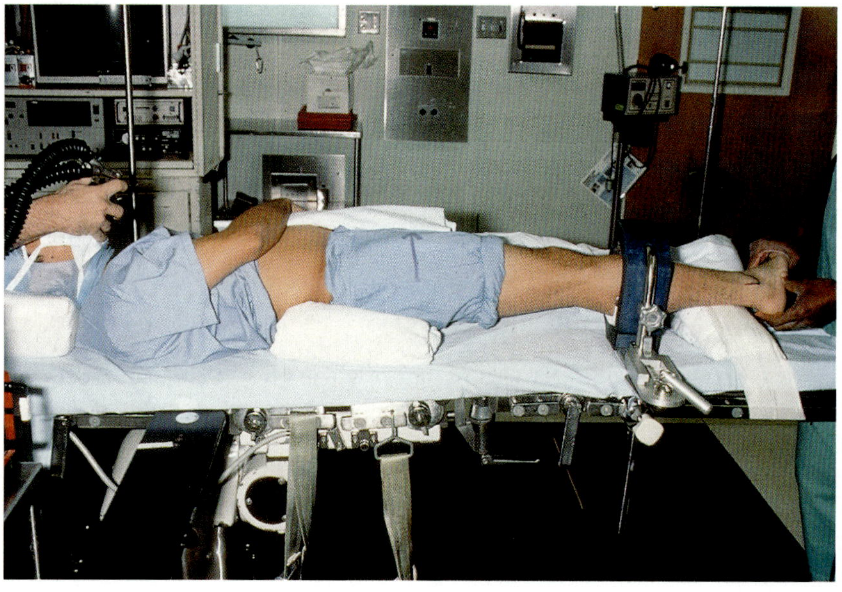

FIGURE 10.7. Patient positioning for ankle and subtalar arthroscopy.

small skin incision is made at the same site. An arthroscopy cannula with a blunt obturator is introduced into the joint in a slightly upward direction with a firm, twisting motion. The trocar is exchanged for the 2.7 mm 25 degree arthroscope, and the foot is held in slight inversion. If only diagnostic arthroscopy is contemplated, the examination can be performed through an anterior portal with a 25 degree arthroscope. Joint distension is obtained with a 50 cc syringe filled with normal saline or Ringer's lactate attached to the sleeve of the arthroscope by means of small plastic tubing. However, if an outflow needle or surgical instruments are needed, a posterior portal is necessary. This portal is slightly proximal to the tip of the lateral malleolus anterior to the Achilles tendon. Too-proximal placement of the portal may inadvertently enter the posterior aspect of the ankle joint. A spinal needle can be used posteriorly to develop a posterior portal while the joint is being visualized through an anterior portal. The posterior portal can also be found by palpating the tip of the anteriorly placed arthroscopic obturator. When surgical instruments are used, an overhead irrigation system should be used.

With the outflow in place, examination of the posterior subtalar joint is begun. The synovial lining of the posterior aspect of the interosseous talocalcaneal ligament is seen; then the articular cartilage of the anterior aspect of the subtalar joint is visualized, as is the lateral aspect of the capsule and the small lateral recess of the joint. Field-of-view angulation allows visualization of the posterior aspect of the talus and os calcis. The posterior pouch of the joint with its synovial lining can be visualized by further advancing the arthroscope posteriorly. While the scope is being maneuvered and the field of view changed, an assistant can invert and evert the foot. Even for diagnostic arthroscopy it is sometimes desirable to switch portals. Before introducing the arthroscope posteriorly, a small skin incision is made and a hemostat is used to move the neurovascular structures. A disposable cannula can be used to avoid repeated penetration through the skin posteriorly. If arthroscopic surgery is required, the same two portals just outlined can be used for visualizing and triangulating surgical instruments. After completing the procedure, the portals are closed with sutures. When there is extravasation of fluid into the subcutaneous tissue, the portals are sometimes left open so the irrigating solution can escape.

POSTOPERATIVE CARE

At the end of the procedure, a compression dressing is applied from the toes to the mid-calf. This dressing is removed the following day, and ice is applied, with the leg elevated for 2–3 days. The patient is allowed to ambulate with the use of crutches, and weight-bearing is permitted as tolerated. The sutures are removed approximately 1 week after the procedure, and the patient is encouraged to start range-of-motion exercises of the foot and ankle immediately after surgery. Once the joint swelling has completely subsided, if indicated the patient is referred to a physical therapist for rehabilitation under supervision.

INDICATIONS

The indications for arthroscopic examination and surgery of the subtalar joint are not common. From a review of the literature and my own experience, the indications may fall into the following groups.[9–17]

- Persistent posttraumatic symptoms with intraarticular adhesions.
- Chondral or osteochondral fractures with loose fragments
- Degenerative or inflammatory arthritis
- Assessing the status of the articular surface prior to some procedures for subtalar instability
- Excision of painful os trigonum
- Arthrodesis of the subtalar joint
- Evaluation and treatment of chronic pain in the sinus tarsi

Posttraumatic Conditions

Patients with a history of injuries to the hindfoot who continue to have pain and swelling in the subtalar joint and for whom radiographs have failed to demonstrate any abnormalities can benefit from arthroscopic exploration of the joint. The presence of chondromalacia of the articular surface of a chondral fracture can be ruled out. The appropriate surgical procedures, whether chondroplasty or excision of a cartilage flap or a loose body, can be performed using the triangulation technique (Fig. 10.8).

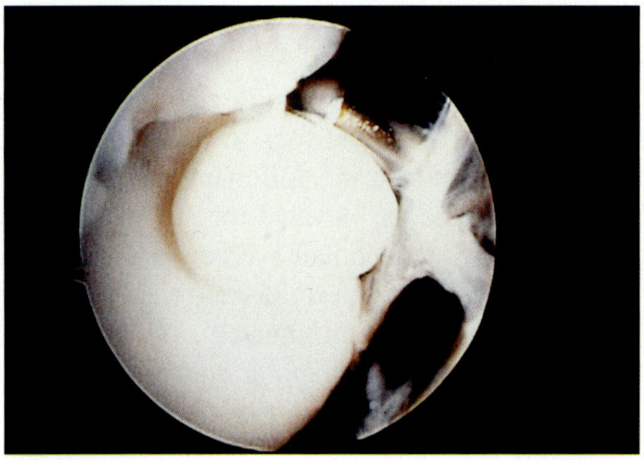

A

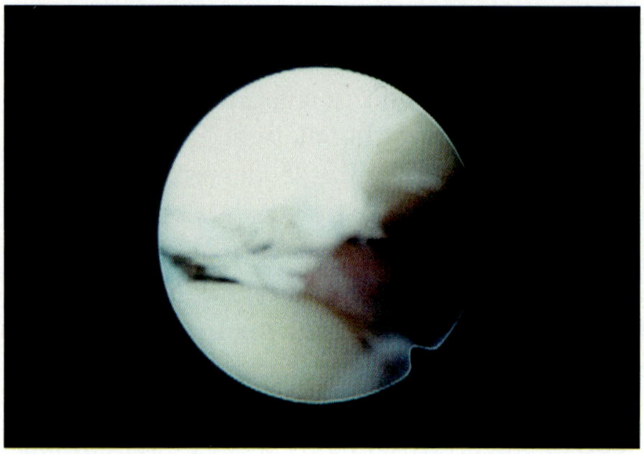

B

FIGURE 10.8. A: Loose body in the posterior subtalar joint. **B:** Chondral lesion articular surface in the posterior subtalar joint.

Chondral or Osteochondral Fractures

Some fractures of the os calcis or the talus involve the articular surfaces of the posterior talocalcaneal joint. An assessment of articular damage is necessary at times. Loose chondral fragments, if present, can be removed arthroscopically (Fig. 10.9).

Degenerative or Inflammatory Conditions

In patients in whom degenerative or inflammatory arthritis is suspected (Fig. 10.10), an arthroscopic evaluation can provide information on the condition of the articular surfaces. These patients may be helped temporarily by joint lavage. In some situations, débridement of osteophytes and hypertrophic synovium temporarily relieves the symptoms. In suspected cases of rheumatoid arthritis, in addition to establishing the precise diagnosis by means of direct biopsy of the synovium, arthroscopy can confirm the presence of a chondral defect. In cases of infection of the subtalar joint, the arthroscopic technique allows joint débridement followed by drainage tube placement.

Arthrofibrosis

Experience has shown that in cases of arthrofibrosis of the subtalar joint dramatic relief of pain and improved range of motion can be obtained after arthroscopic excision of adhesions (Fig. 10.11). Although some fine adhesive bands can be broken by manipulating a small obturator through the joint, surgical instruments such as motorized shavers or small retrograde knives are necessary to excise thick adhesive bands. Holmium: YAG laser or radiofrequency may also be used if available.

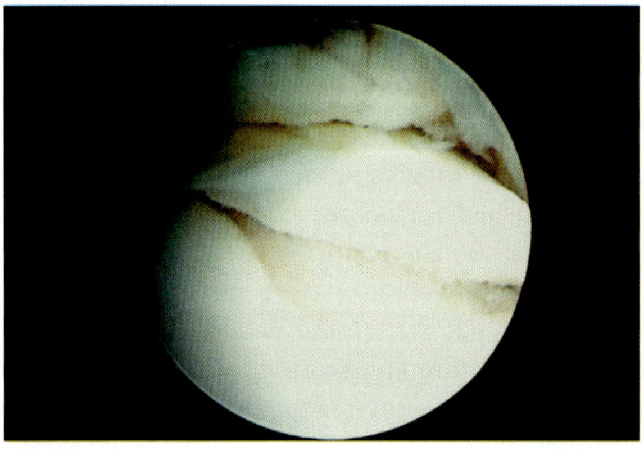

FIGURE 10.9. Osteochondral fracture of the posterior subtalar joint.

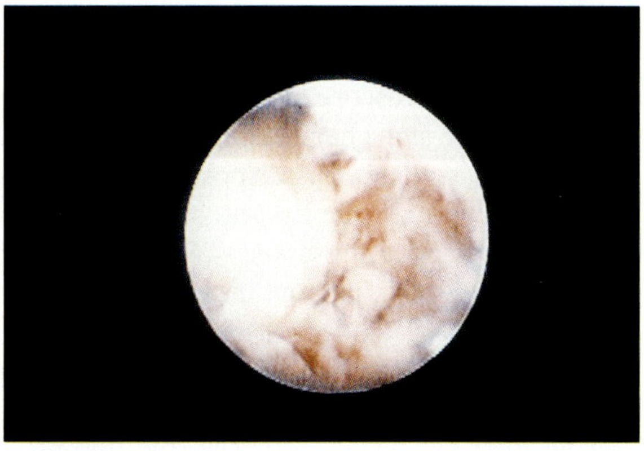

FIGURE 10.10. Rheumatoid arthritis in the posterior subtalar joint.

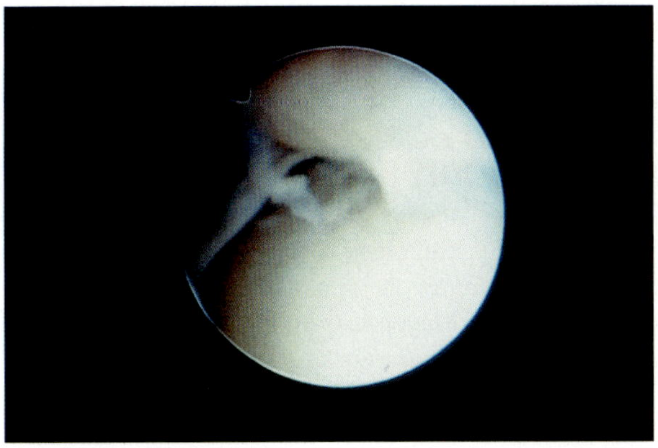

FIGURE 10.11. Adhesions in the posterior subtalar joint.

Chronic Instability

Patients with chronic instability of the subtalar joint or posttraumatic arthritis, for whom open procedures such as ligamentous reconstruction or arthrodesis are contemplated, may benefit from direct evaluation of the articular surface afforded by arthroscopy. The information obtained helps the physician decide on the procedure of choice.

Painful Os Trigonum

Ferkel[12] reported successful use of the arthroscope in the management of symptomatic os trigonum. The nonunited fragment of the posterior aspect of the talus can be excised through a posterolateral portal, and visualization is achieved through the anterolateral portal or by stacked posterior portals, immediately adjacent to the Achilles tendon and 2 cm apart or more for alternating visualization and instrumentation. During excision of the fragment, the flexor hallucis longus and posteromedial neurovascular bundle are at risk. Visualizing the tip of the surgical instruments is required at all times to avoid injury to these structures.

Subtalar Arthrodesis

Tasto[16] described a technique of arthroscopy-assisted subtalar joint arthrodesis in patients with subtalar pain secondary to posttraumatic arthritis, rheumatoid arthritis, and osteoarthritis without gross malalignment or significant bone loss (see Chapter 11).

SINUS TARSI SYNDROME

Sinus tarsi syndrome has been historically described as pain in the sinus tarsi area secondary to trauma. The pain, relieved by injecting the sinus area, is associated with complaints of instability in the subtalar region. According to Frey et al.,[15] it is an inaccurate term, as it can include many other pathologies such as interosseous ligament tears, arthrofibrosis, and joint degeneration. A more accurate diagnosis can be obtained using arthroscopy, with the appropriate treatment applied in most situations (Fig. 10.12).

COMPLICATIONS

Possible complications include infection, instrument breakage, and scuffing of the articular cartilage. Knowledge of the anatomy and proper technique can avoid injury to the neurovascular structures at risk (i.e., the lesser saphenous vein, the sural nerve, and branches of the superficial peroneal nerve).

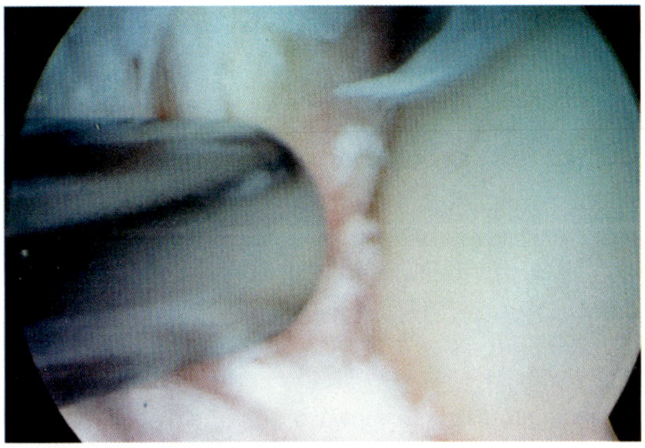

A

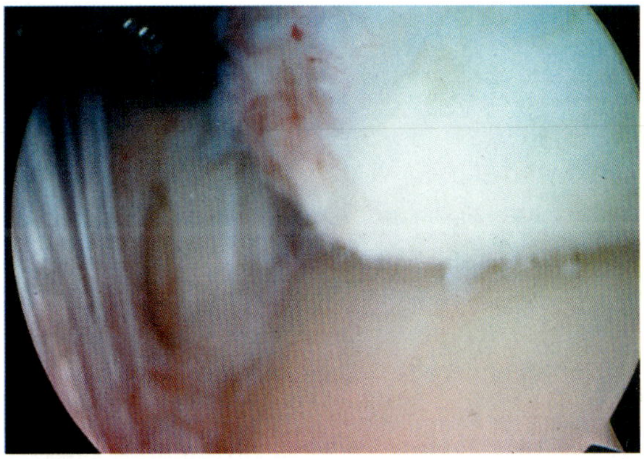

B

FIGURE 10.12. Interosseous ligament area in a patient with sinus tarsi syndrome before and after arthroscopic débridement.

RESULTS

Subtalar arthroscopy has been shown to be beneficial by many orthopedic surgeons over the past several years. Williams and Ferkel[13] reported overall good to excellent results in 86% of 50 patients. In their study 21 patients underwent diagnostic arthroscopy alone; and 29 underwent various procedures performed for synovitis, degenerative joint disease, chondromalacia, loose bodies, arthrofibrosis, and symptomatic os trigonum. Frey et al.[14] reported a success rate of 94% good and excellent results with arthroscopic treatment of various subtalar pathologic conditions in 49 patients. The complication rate was extremely low, with the most common complication being transient neuropraxia involving branches of the superficial peroneal nerve. Parisien[11] reported similar results for 20 patients who underwent subtalar joint arthroscopic procedures for various conditions (e.g., arthrofibrosis, chondromalacia, osteochondral lesions, synovitis, and sinus tarsi dysfunction). Fourteen other patients underwent only diagnostic procedures. There were no complications in either group. In another series of 22 patients who underwent arthroscopic subtalar arthrodesis, Tasto[16] reported successful complete bony union in all patients, with an average follow-up of 22 months. Among his 22 patients, 9 had posttraumatic changes, 8 had osteoarthritis, 2 had rheumatoid arthritis, 2 had chronic posterior tibial tendon disruption, and 1 had a tarsal coalition. The time until union was 8–9 weeks. There were no major complications in his series. Scranton,[17] in a retrospective review, compared the results of arthroscopic subtalar arthrodesis (5 patients) with open procedures (12 patients). He concluded that both techniques, when properly performed, yielded satisfactory results.

CONCLUSIONS

Direct arthroscopic visualization of the posterior subtalar joint is possible with the use of small arthroscopes (ranging in size from 2.2 to 2.7 mm). Valuable information can be obtained regarding the status of the articular cartilage and synovial lining in cases of degenerative and inflammatory arthritis. Posttraumatic pain syndrome of the hindfoot can be assessed, and limited surgical procedures, such as biopsy, breakage or excision of adhesions, joint lavage, or removal of loose chondral or osteochondral bodies, can be performed with less morbidity for the patient. With proper technique, excision of symptomatic os trigonum and subtalar arthrodesis can be achieved with success.

BIBLIOGRAPHY

1. Resnick D. Radiology of the talocalcaneal articulations. *Radiology* 1974;3:581–586.
2. Taillard W, Meyer J, Garcia J, Blanc Y. The sinus tarsi syndrome. *Int Orthop* 1981;5:117–130.
3. Isherwood I. A radiographic approach to the subtalar joint. *J Bone Joint Surg Br* 1961;43:566–574.
4. Smith RW, Staple TW. Computerized tomography (CT) scanning technique of the hindfoot. *Clin Orthop* 1983;177:34–38.
5. Beltran J, Munchow AM, Khabiri H, Magee D, et al. Ligaments of the lateral aspect of the ankle and sinus tarsi: an MR imaging study. *Radiology* 1990; 177:455–458.
6. Parisien JS, Vangsness T. Arthroscopy of the subtalar joint: an experimental approach. *Arthroscopy* 1985;1:53–57.
7. Cahill DR. The anatomy and function of the contents of the human tarsal sinus and canal. *Anat Rec* 1965; 153:1–18.
8. Harper MC. The lateral ligamentous support of the subtalar joint. *Foot Ankle* 1991;12:354.
9. Parisien JS. Arthroscopy of the posterior subtalar joint: a preliminary report. *Foot Ankle* 1986;6:219–224.
10. Parisien JS. Arthroscopy of the posterior subtalar joint and great toe. In: Parisien JS (ed) *Techniques in therapeutic arthroscopy*. New York: Raven, 1993; 20.1–20.10.
11. Parisien JS. Arthroscopy of the posterior subtalar joint. In: Parisien JS (ed) *Current techniques in arthroscopy*. Philadelphia: Thieme, 1998;161–168.
12. Ferkel RD. Subtalar arthroscopy. In: Ferkel R (ed) *Arthroscopic surgery: the foot and ankle*. Philadelphia: Lippincott-Raven, 1996;231.
13. Williams M, Ferkel R. Subtalar arthroscopy; indications, techniques and results. *Arthroscopy* 1998;4: 373–381.
14. Frey C, Gasser S, Feder K. Arthroscopy of the subtalar joint. *Foot Ankle* 1994;15:424–428.
15. Frey C, Feder K, Digiovanni C. Arthroscopic evaluation of the subtalar joint: does sinus tarsi syndrome exist? *Foot Ankle* 1999;20:185–191.
16. Tasto JP. Arthroscopic subtalar arthrodesis. In: *Proceedings of the 18th annual meeting, Arthroscopy Association of North America*, April 1999, Vancouver, p 41.
17. Scranton PE. Comparison of open isolated subtalar arthrodesis with autogenous bone graft versus outpatient arthroscopic subtalar arthrodesis using injectable bone morphogenic protein-enhanced graft. *Foot Ankle* 1999;20:162–165.

CHAPTER 11

Arthroscopic Subtalar Arthrodesis

James P. Tasto

Operative procedures designed for subtalar fusion have been in existence for nearly 100 years. Nieny performed the first subtalar arthrodesis in 1905. Since then numerous techniques have been reported in the literature that have utilized both intraarticular and extraarticular methods.[1–9] Results have generally been favorable, with a variety of complications reported.[10–12] Data on the rate of union, time until union, complications, and long-term follow-up are noticeably missing in the early and more recent literature. A number of other procedures for subtalar pathology have been described, including arthroscopy, arthroplasty, triple arthrodesis, and sinus tarsi exploration. Surgical open reduction of calcaneal fractures to restore the normal anatomic alignment of the joint surfaces has gained acceptance. This is an effort to avoid the sequelae of posttraumatic degenerative arthritis of the subtalar joint. Operative and conservative care of calcaneal fractures, however, continues to be plagued with long-term symptomatic degenerative changes in the subtalar joint.

Arthroscopic subtalar arthrodesis (ASTA) as a surgical procedure was developed in 1992 and was first reported at the 1994 annual meeting of the Arthroscopy Association of North America (AANA) as a preliminary review. The procedure was designed to improve traditional methods by using a microinvasive technique. The decision to proceed with this surgical technique grew out of the success with arthroscopic ankle arthrodesis.[13] Subtalar arthroscopy has been described by a number of authors, but no reported cases or attempts at arthroscopic subtalar fusion have been published.[14] Work by Solis has paralleled some of our earlier work (V.H. Solis, personal communication, 1996).

The development of an arthroscopic technique was intended to yield less morbidity if it could be performed using the same techniques and principles as for arthroscopic ankle fusion. It was hypothesized that perioperative morbidity could be reduced, the blood supply preserved, and proprioceptive and neurosensory input enhanced. A prospective study was initiated to document the effectiveness of the procedure and determine the time until complete fusion, the incidence of delayed union and nonunion, and the prevalence of complications.

The subtalar joint is comprised of three articulations: posterior, middle, and anterior joints or facets (Figs. 11.1, 11.2). Numerous extraarticular ligaments stabilize the subtalar joint. The major ligaments encountered during subtalar arthroscopy are the intraarticular components, which consist of the interosseous talocalcaneal ligament, the lateral talocalcaneal ligament, and the anterior talocalcaneal ligament (Fig. 11.3). These ligaments coalesce to form the division between the posterior and middle facets of the subtalar joint. The interosseous ligament is a broad, stout structure measuring approximately 2.5 cm in breadth from medial to lateral. It is an important landmark and marks the arthroscopic boundary for posterior subtalar arthroscopy.

The subtalar joint is a single-axis joint that acts like a mitered hinge connecting the talus and calcaneus.[15,16] The direction of the axis of movement

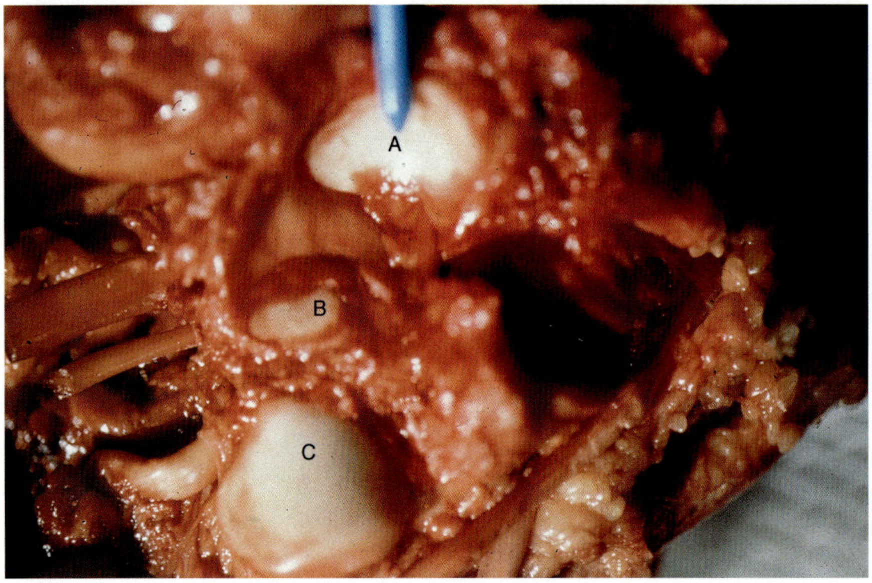

FIGURE 11.1. Topographic view of a prosected anatomic specimen of the posterior subtalar joint. A, Undersurface of talus; B, middle facet of talus; C, superior surface of calcaneus.

about this joint is backward, downward, and lateral, running from the dorsal medial talus to the posterolateral calcaneus. It is a determinative joint that influences the biomechanics of the distal portion of the midfoot and forefoot. The more horizontal the hinge, the greater is the influence of torque and rotation on the midfoot and forefoot. Various researchers performing anatomic cadaver studies have related the range of motion of the subtalar joint to be 20–60 degrees of combined inversion and eversion.[15–17]

The three articulations of the subtalar joint are able to provide rotation simultaneously between the talus and calcaneus about a common axis of rotation.[15–17] At the end of its normal range of motion, the curves of the three articulations suddenly become incongruous, no longer providing motion about a common axis of rotation. Further motion disarticulates the subtalar joint. This force must be rotational and must exceed the compressive forces holding the talus and calcaneus together.[15,17]

At the end of its normal range of motion, the subtalar joint stops and the ligaments continue to be relaxed. Only when the transverse rotational force is increased to the extent that it exceeds the compressive force do the ligaments tighten. The ligaments therefore become taut only at the beginning of an imminent dislocation or subluxation.[15,17]

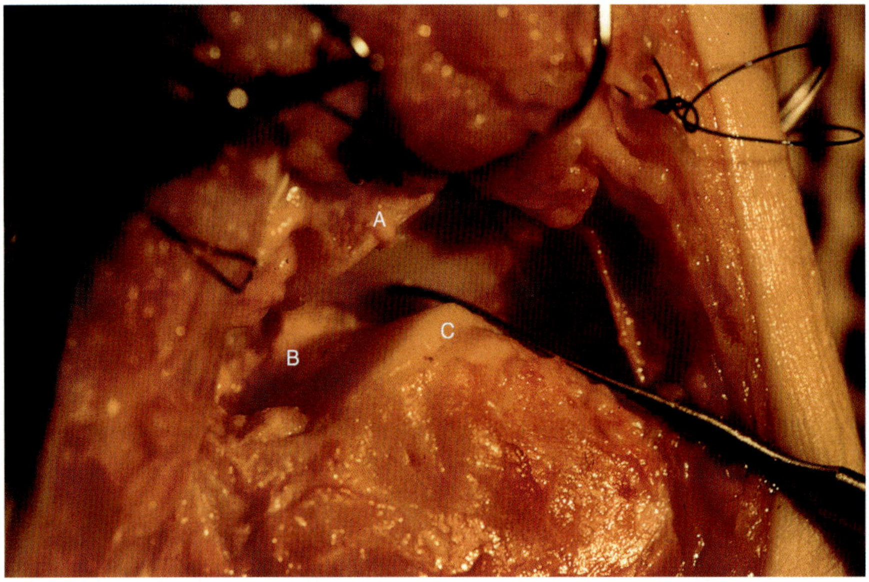

FIGURE 11.2. Anatomic dissection of lateral posterior subtalar joint. A, talus; B, calcaneus; C, resected interosseous ligament; D, subtalar joint.

FIGURE 11.3. A, Interosseus talocalcaneal ligament; B, lateral talocalcaneal ligament; C, anterior talocalcaneal ligament; D, calcaneus.

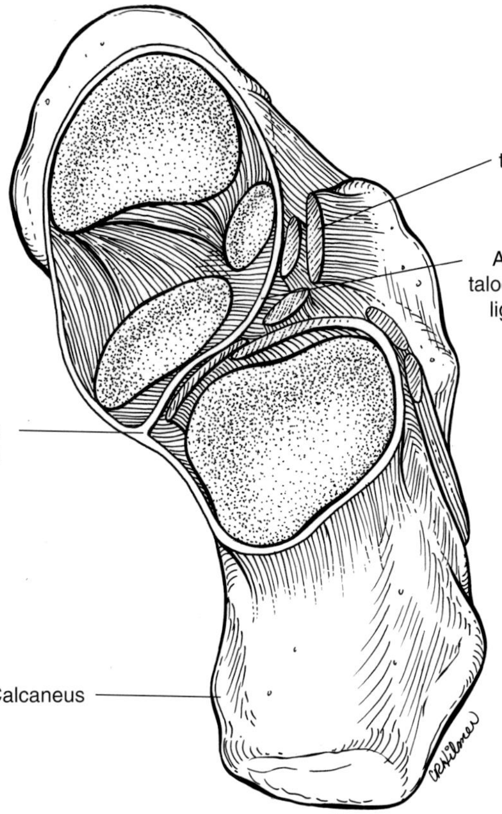

INDICATIONS

The major indication for arthroscopic subtalar arthrodesis is intractable subtalar pain secondary to rheumatoid arthritis, osteoarthritis, or posttraumatic arthritis. Other indications include neuropathic conditions, gross instability, paralytic conditions, and posterior tibial tendon rupture. Most of the early literature on subtalar surgery focused on stabilization of paralytic deformities secondary to poliomyelitis. Most patients encountered in today's medical environment who require this procedure have posttraumatic or arthritic disorders.

Patients must have failed conservative management to qualify for arthroscopic subtalar fusion. Conservative treatment includes a variety of modalities, including orthotics, nonsteroidal antiinflammatory drugs, activity modification, and occasional cortisone injections into the subtalar joint. Patients must also be apprised of the possibility of requiring an open procedure should this technique not be technically feasible.

The patient's history is usually one of lateral hindfoot pain, which can be confused quite easily with ankle pathology. Increased symptoms with weight-bearing on uneven ground is a classic complaint. History of a previous calcaneal fracture should immediately alert one to the possibility of subtalar pathology. The clinical findings consist of pain over the sinus tarsi and the posterolateral subtalar joint. They also report reproduction of the symptoms on inversion and eversion of the subtalar joint with the ankle locked in dorsiflexion.

The clinical workup for this patient profile is simple. Often a good history and physical examination, with the results confirmed by plain radiographs, are sufficient to confirm the diagnosis. On occasion, computed tomography (CT) or plain tomography is necessary.[18] There is little need for magnetic resonance imaging (MRI) or arthrography.[19] Differential injections continue to be a valuable diagnostic aid to confirm the diagnosis as well as distinguish ankle pain from subtalar pain. Radiographic changes do not have to show profound degenerative changes, as only small alterations in the biomechanics of this joint can produce significant symptoms.

CONTRAINDICATIONS

The contraindications to this procedure are previously failed subtalar fusions, gross malalignment requiring correction, infection, and significant bone loss. On occasion, a patient with gross malalignment is a candidate for in situ stabilization. Although significant bone loss is not frequently encountered, when it does occur it has not presented a serious problem in a series of arthroscopic ankle arthrodeses.[13]

SURGICAL TECHNIQUE

Each patient was treated in an ambulatory surgery center environment and discharged the same day. The only exception was the occasional patient treated at the Veterans Administration (VA) hospital affiliated with our teaching institution.[20] Patients were given preoperative, intraoperative, and postoperative antibiotics for a total of three doses because of the use of internal fixation. General anesthesia was used in most cases.

Patients were placed in the lateral decubitus position with the patient lying on the unaffected side. Two pillows were placed between the legs and the affected ankle and subtalar joint were allowed to hang over a blanket roll in a natural position of plantar flexion and inversion. After thoroughly preparing and draping the patient, anatomic landmarks and portal sites were identified and marked with a surgical pen. The tourniquet was then elevated. In general, the operative procedure was completed within one tourniquet time (1 hour 45 minutes).

Establishing the portal sites is one of the more difficult parts of the procedure. To determine an accurate location for the anterolateral portal, the surgeon places his or her thumb in the sinus tarsi while attempting to invert and evert the subtalar joint. The portal is in line with the tip of the fibula, approximately 1 cm distal to the anterior border of the fibula (Fig. 11.4). The needle is placed slightly posterior to the sinus tarsi and angled cephalad 20–30 degrees and posteromedially approximately 45 degrees. The posterior portal is approximately 1 cm superior to the tip and 1 cm posterior to the border of the fibula. It may be established at this time but can also be established under direct vision once the arthroscope is placed in the anterolateral portal via transillumination. It is critical to predetermine the angles of the subtalar joint because its unique geometry and limited access leave little room for error (Figs. 11.5, 11.6). Do not hesitate to use fluoroscopy to confirm the portal location, if necessary.

These are the two conventional portals. If necessary, an accessory portal may be established approximately 1 cm posterior to the anterolateral portal. This portal can be used for débridement or for flow or drainage enhancement. It cannot be used for visualization. Both anterolateral and posterolateral portals are used in an alternating fashion during the surgery for viewing and for instrumentation. Occasionally, significant arthrofibrosis is present, making entry and visualization difficult. The accessory anterolateral portal is quite useful in these cases.

The arthroscope used for this procedure should be a 2.7 mm, wide-angled, shortened small-joint arthroscope. It should be equipped with a choice of sheaths to accommodate limited or increased flow. The blunt trocar and sheath is introduced through the anterolateral portal, and the posterolateral portal can be established at this time. In the initial cases,

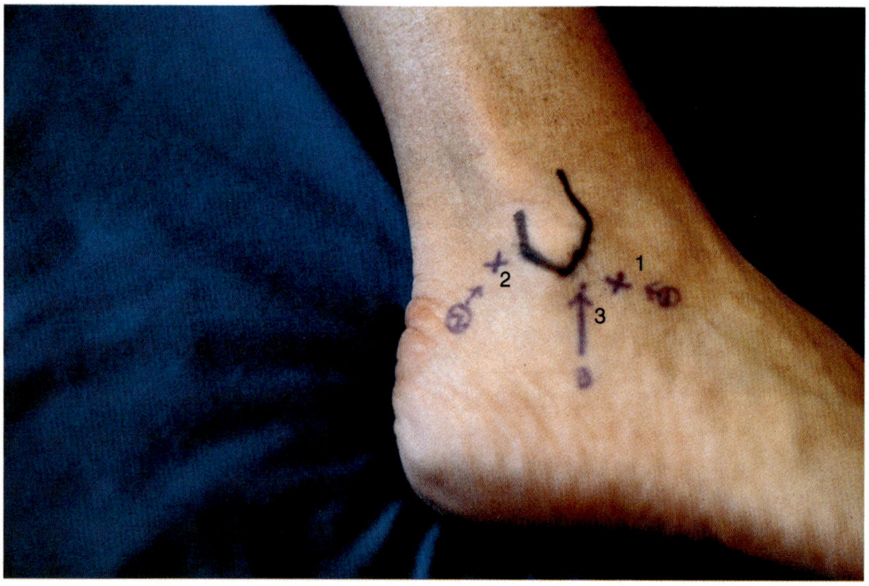

FIGURE 11.4. Portal sites for subtalar arthrodesis. 1, anterolateral portal; 2, posterolateral portal; 3, accessory lateral portal.

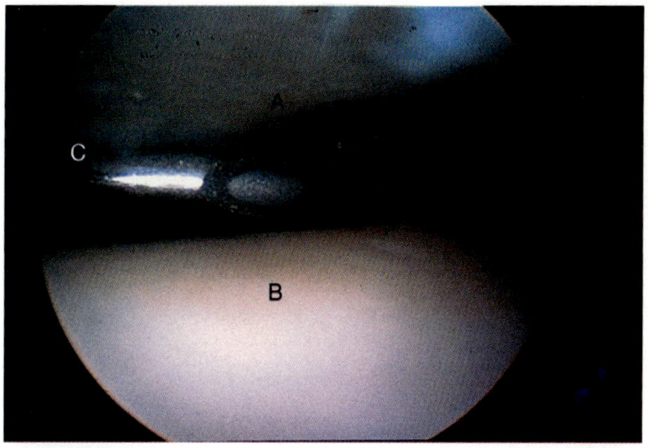

FIGURE 11.5. Arthroscopic view of a right posterior subtalar joint. A, talus; B, calcaneus; C, posteromedial corner.

a small laminar spreader was used in the anterolateral portal to increase access. This was later abandoned as routine but may still be utilized if distraction is a significant problem. Arthroscopic resection of the interosseous ligament may also be used for additional distraction, but I have not used it to date.

It is important to be absolutely certain the arthroscope is in the subtalar joint and that the ankle joint or the fibular talar recess has not been entered inadvertently. All débridement and decortication is done posterior to the interosseous ligament, as only the posterior facet is fused. The middle and anterior facets are not visualized under normal circumstances unless the interosseous ligament is absent. Most of the procedure is done with the arthroscope in the anterolateral portal and the instruments in the posterolateral portal. The remaining and final débridement is accomplished alternating these two portals.

Primary synovectomy and débridement are necessary for visualization, as with other joints. The articular surface is débrided, which makes the joint more capacious and makes instrumentation easier. Complete removal of the articular surface down to subchondral bone is the next phase of the procedure (Fig. 11.7). The talocalcaneal geometry is unique and requires a variety of instruments. In general, multiangular currettes and a complete set of burrs suffice.

Once the articular cartilage has been resected, approximately 1–2 mm of subchondral bone is removed to expose the highly vascular cancellous bone. Care must be taken not to alter the geometry and not to remove excessive bone, as it would lead to poor coaptation of the joint surfaces. Once the subchondral plate is removed, small "spot-weld" holes measuring approximately 2 mm in depth are created on the surfaces of the calcaneus and talus to create vascular channels (Fig. 11.8).

The posteromedial corner must be carefully assessed, as residual bone and cartilage may be left there, which can interfere with coaptation. Often the currette safely breaks down this corner and provides the surgeon with additional tactile feedback. The neurovascular bundle is directly posteromedially and must be taken into consideration at all times and protected.

After viewing from both portals to ensure complete débridement and decortication, the tourniquet is released and the vascularity of the calcaneus and talus is carefully assessed. The joint is then thoroughly irrigated of bone fragments and debris. No autogenous bone graft or bone substitute is needed for this procedure.

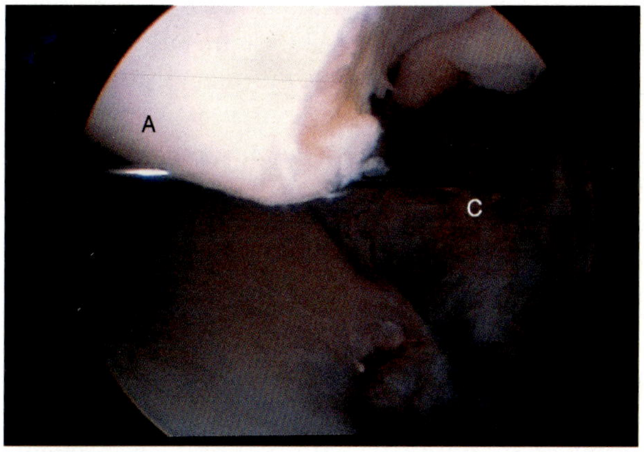

FIGURE 11.6. Arthroscopic view of a left posterior subtalar joint. A, talus; B, calcaneus; C, posterolateral portal.

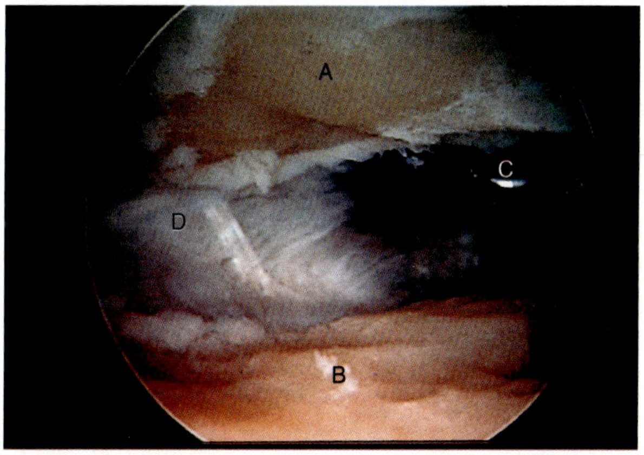

FIGURE 11.7. Posterior subtalar joint, viewing from the posterolateral portal. A, talus; B, calcaneus; C, sinus tarsi; D, interosseus ligament.

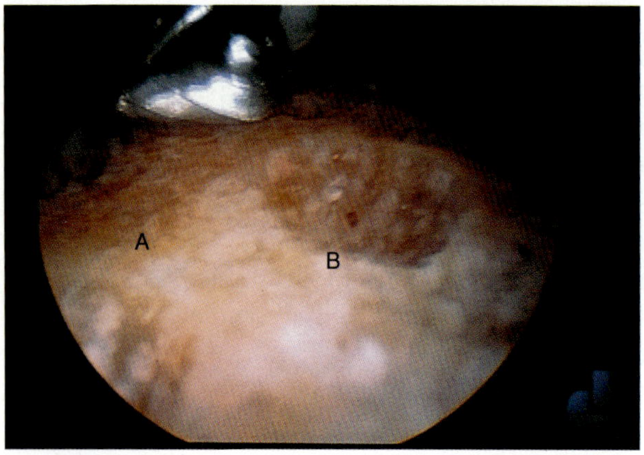

FIGURE 11.8. Superior surface of the calcaneus following removal of the articular surface, decortication, and "spot-welding." A, calcaneus; B, "spot-weld."

Fixation of the fusion is accomplished with a large cannulated 7.0 screw. The guide pin is started at the dorsal anteromedial talus and angled posterior and inferior to the posterolateral calcaneus, but it does not violate the calcaneal cortical surface. Under fluoroscopy, the guidewire is placed with the ankle in maximum dorsiflexion to avoid any possible screw head encroachment or impingement on the anterior lip of the tibia. Once the guidewire is placed under these conditions, the ankle can then be relaxed, the screw inserted under fluoroscopic control, and the fusion site compressed. The screw runs along the natural axis of rotation of the subtalar joint using this technique. Starting the screw from the dorsal and medial aspect of the talus avoids painful screw head prominence over the calcaneus and avoids the need for a second procedure to remove the screw. To date, there have been no fractures or complications with this fixation technique (Figs. 11.9, 11.10).

Steri-Strips are used instead of sutures to allow adequate drainage. A bulky dressing and a short leg bivalve cast is applied. The patient is discharged home after appropriate circulatory checks in the recovery room. The first clinical evaluation takes place in the office within 48 hours. At approximately 1 week, the cast is removed and the patient is fitted immediately with an AFO ankle brace if the swelling is minimal. Full weight-bearing is allowed as tolerated at any time following surgery. In general, patients can tolerate full weight-bearing without crutch support within 7–14 days after surgery. Although patients wear the AFO brace almost 24 hours a day, they are able to bathe and take the ankle and foot through a range of motion exercise without the brace. It is removed when full union has been achieved. The standard three views of the ankle plus a Broden view are the radiographs of choice for follow-up assessments.

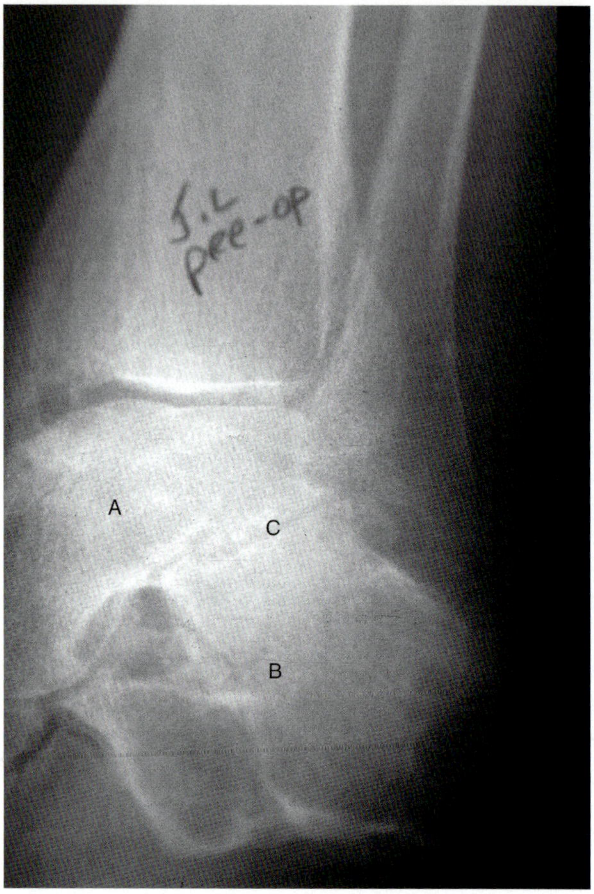

FIGURE 11.9. Broden view of an arthritic posterior subtalar joint. A, talus; B, calcaneus; C, subtalar joint.

RESULTS

Since September 1992 a total of 25 patients have undergone arthroscopic subtalar fusion with sufficient follow-up to determine the effectiveness of this procedure. Fusion rate, time until complete union, surgical technique, and complications were analyzed. Only one procedure was used, and the method of internal fixation was not altered during this entire series. The posterior subtalar joint was the only joint fused during this procedure. Of the 25 patients, 3 underwent combined arthroscopic ankle and subtalar fusion. There were eight patients with osteoarthritis, 10 with posttraumatic arthritis, two with rheumatoid arthritis, 4 with posterior tibial tendon tears and 1 with a talocalcaneal coalition.

Every patient underwent a radiographic evalua-

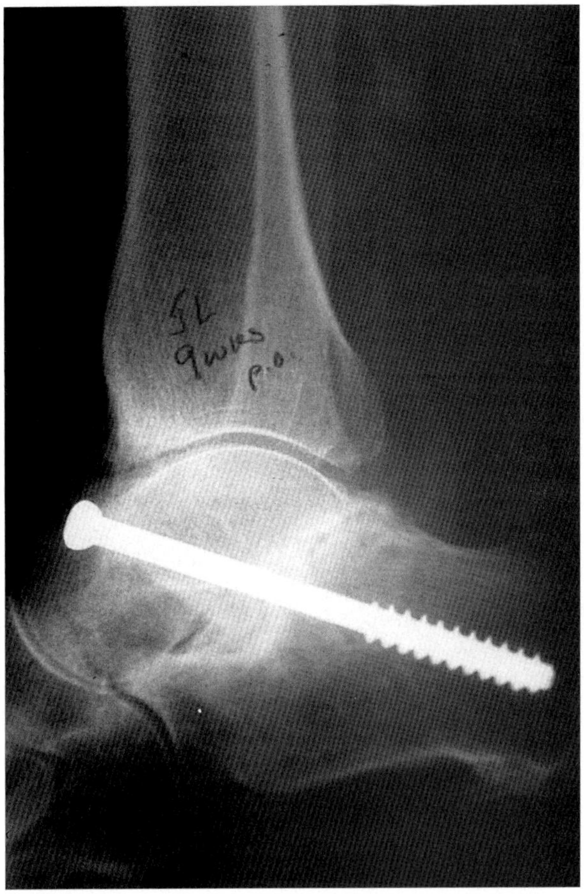

FIGURE 11.10. Lateral radiograph of a fused subtalar joint with a single cancellous screw across the posterior facet.

tion at 2-week intervals to determine the rate and quality of fusion. Determining that an arthrodesis is completely fused requires both clinical and radiographic support. The parameters required for a successful arthrodesis are the following: evidence of bone consolidation across the subtalar joint, no motion at the screw, clinical absence of pain with weight-bearing, and pain-free forced inversion and eversion. The average mean follow-up was 29 months (range 6–120 months). All fusions were successfully united clinically and radiographically, with the average time to complete fusion being 8.9 weeks (range 6–16 weeks).

There are considerable advantages to this technique when compared to open procedures. It is a minimally invasive technique that theoretically preserves the blood supply of the calcaneus and talus. This is especially important considering the fact that many of these patients have had previous invasive surgery. By definition, conventional open procedures interrupt the blood supply and compromise vascular ingrowth and eventual fusion. Avoidance of incisions coupled with early range of motion and weight-bearing helps avoid stress deprivation and enhances proprioception, thereby reducing the devastating effects of reflex sympathetic dystrophy.

COMPLICATIONS

There have been no reoperations, with the exception of one screw removal. This patient had a painful screw at the calcaneus where the screw penetrated the cortex, and the possibility of a stress fracture was entertained. Symptoms resolved after screw removal. Two patients had some residual anterolateral pain with some radiographic changes and clinical evidence of minor degenerative joint disease in the ankle. Both patients responded with complete relief to a diagnostic lidocaine (Xylocaine) injection into the ankle joint. Valgus tilting of the ankle joint following subtalar arthrodesis has been reported, but it is unclear if it is secondary to the fusion or merely a natural progression of the disease.[21] Two cases (not included in this series) could not be completed arthroscopically because of significant malformation of the calcaneus and arthrofibrosis of the subtalar joint. These patients underwent modified mini open posterior subtalar arthrodesis. The identical screw fixation and postoperative protocol were used in these two patients.

Skin problems about the hindfoot can be catastrophic and are obviously avoided using this technique. All arthroscopic procedures have been reported to be associated with a lower incidence of infection, and one hopes that this procedure will fall into that same category. There have not been sufficient cases, however, to validate this hypothesis.

Most open surgery series show a longer time until union, with some prevalence of nonunion. Although too early to validate, preliminary observations indicate a more rapid time until union and an increased rate of union. There has been a paucity of literature on isolated subtalar arthrodeses with adequate follow-up statistics over the past 25 years.

CONCLUSIONS

The obvious socioeconomic advantages are quite dramatic, with early weight-bearing and AFO immobilization, allowing patients an early return to work. Outpatient surgery is a cost-effective benefit. Patient satisfaction and comfort are greatly enhanced, with only oral pain medication being required. All patients have tolerated their postoperative regimen and same-day discharge.

Arthroscopic subtalar arthrodesis is a technically demanding procedure that requires the surgeon to have some rather advanced arthroscopic skills. Joint access is tight and restricted, and the procedure requires small instrumentation. Deformities cannot be corrected; therefore at this stage, the procedure must be considered fusion in situ. The learning curve is steep because of the small number of patients available to enhance the physician's surgical skills.

Overall, this procedure has stood the test of time and follow-up. The results appear to be excellent in terms of patient satisfaction, fusion rate, time until union, and postoperative morbidity. The recognition and enhancement of this technique and the development of more advanced technology will certainly allow arthroscopic subtalar arthrodesis to mature even more over time.

BIBLIOGRAPHY

1. Thomas FB. Arthrodesis of the subtalar joint. *J Bone Joint Surg* 1967;1:93–97.
2. Dick IL. Primary fusion and the posterior subtalar joint and the treatment of fractures of the calcaneus. *J Bone Joint Surg Br* 1953;35:375.
3. Gallie WE. Subastragalar arthrodesis and fractures of the os calcis. *J Bone Joint Surg* 1943;25:731–736.
4. Grice DS. An extra-articular arthrodesis of the subastragalar joint for correction of paralytic flat feet in children. *J Bone Joint Surg Am* 1952;34:927.
5. Grice DS. Further experience with extra-articular arthrodesis of the subtalar joint. *J Bone Joint Surg Am* 1955;37:246.
6. Hall MC, Pennal GF. Primary subtalar arthrodesis in the treatment of severe fractures of the calcaneus. *J Bone Joint Surg Br* 1960;42:336.
7. Geckler EO. Comminuted fractures of the os calcis. *Arch Surg* 1943;61:469.
8. Harris RI. Fractures of the os calcis. *Ann Surg* 1946;124:1082.
9. Wilson PD. Treatment of fractures of the os calcis by arthrodesis of the subtalar joint. *JAMA* 1927; 89:1676.
10. Gross RH. A clinical study of bachelor subtalar arthrodesis. *J Bone Joint Surg* 1976;58:343–349.
11. Mallon WJ, Nunley JA. The Grice procedure, extra-articular subtalar arthrodesis. *Orthop Clin North Am* 1989;20:649–654.
12. Moreland JR, Westin GW. Further experience with Grice subtalar arthrodesis. *Clin Orthop* 1986;207: 113–121.
13. Tasto JP. Arthroscopic ankle arthrodesis, a seven year follow-up. *JAAOS* February 1997.
14. Ferkel RA. *Arthroscopic surgery: the foot and ankle*. Philadelphia: Lippincott-Raven, 1996.
15. Inman VT, Mann RA, Du Vries HL. *Surgery of the foot*. St. Louis: Mosby, 1973;17–19.
16. Root M, Orien WP, Weld J. Normal and abnormal function of the foot. *Clin Biomechanics* 1977;2:79.
17. Hicks JH. The mechanics of the foot: the joints. *J Anat* 1953;87:345–357.
18. Seltzer SE, Weisman B. CT of the hindfoot with rheumatoid arthritis. *J Arthritis Rheumatol* 1985; 28(11):12–42.
19. Goossens MD, N. DeStoop, et al. Posterior subtalar joint arthrography: a useful tool in the diagnosis of hindfoot disorders. *Clin Orthop* 1989;249:248–255.
20. Thomas FB. Arthrodesis of the subtalar joint. *J Bone Joint Surg* 1967;1:93–97.
21. Fitzgibbons, TC. Valgus tilting of the ankle joint following subtalar arthrodesis. Presented to the International Society of Foot and Ankle Surgery, Dublin, August 1995.

CHAPTER 12

Arthroscopic Excision of the Os Trigonum

Richard O. Lundeen

The biomechanical secrets of the subtalar joint have long been unlocked by anatomists. Yet because of its size and relative unimportance compared to larger joints, little attention has been given to it by arthroscopic surgeons. Other than fusion, resection of the symptomatic os trigonum is perhaps the most common surgical procedure performed on the subtalar joint.

The os trigonum is an often confusing structure in that it occupies the most posterior aspect of the talus. This portion of the talus has a prominence with two tubercles between which lies a groove for passage of the flexor hallucis longus tendon. The medial tubercle is small and wide, whereas the lateral tubercle is large and often presents a secondary ossification center that may or may not form a bony bridge to the talar body. A process that appears separate from the talus is termed an "os trigonum" (Fig. 12.1). If there is no break in the continuity of the lateral talar process with the talar body, the posterior process appears elongated and is termed "Stieda's process" (Fig. 12.2), named after German anatomist Ludwig Stieda.

Specifically, the os trigonum is part of the subtalar joint, located in the posterior aspect of the posterior calcaneal facet of the subtalar joint (Fig. 12.3). It occupies the superior portion of that joint, forming the roof of the talar component; but it frequently has its own articular surface with the underlying posterior calcaneal facet (Fig. 12.4). Its shape and size vary, and it may appear attached or unattached to the talus (observations that are not directly related to symptomatology).

On the lateral posterior aspect of the talus is a more prominent area that contains two tubercles. The medial tubercle is small and wide with a lateral groove for passage of the flexor hallucis longus tendon. The posterior tibiotalar ligament attaches to this tubercle. Adjacent to the groove for the flexor hallucis longus tendon is a larger lateral tubercle referred to as the lateral talar process or trigonal process. It has the origin of the posterior talocalcaneal ligament, which is a short, strong ligament that anchors the lateral talar process. The lateral tubercle of the talus can be attached directly to the talus or appear as a visible secondary ossification center attached with a synchondrosis. It can also appear as a free ossicle unattached to the talus.

The flexor hallucis longus tendon encroaches on the lateral talar process and is separated by a fibrous "tunnel" that is attached to the medial surface of the process. Adjacent to the origin of the lateral talar process is the trochlear surface of the talus, which takes the insertion of the posterior talofibular ligament. Familiarity of the anatomic area between the attachment of these ligaments is of utmost importance, as it is where the process is resected.

The talus sits on the calcaneus at an angle of approximately 30 degrees internally rotated in the transverse plane. This places the posterior process quite medially along with the entire posterior talar border. Perhaps this is why some surgeons risk a medial surgical approach when excising the os trigonum. Even though this practice places the process deeper to the lateral cutaneous structures of

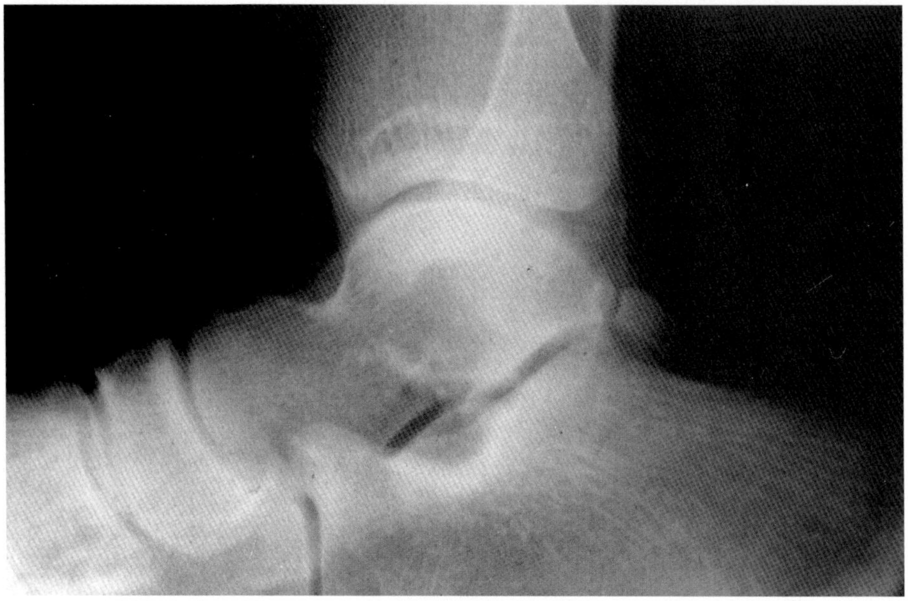

FIGURE 12.1. Lateral radiograph showing an os trigonum.

the foot, it creates a unique situation, allowing the talar process to be not only the most posterior talar component but to have its access perpendicular to a point located at the junction of the superior surface of the calcaneus and the posterior surface of the peroneal tendons. A portal placed at this level is perpendicular to the long axis of the trigonal process, allowing an osteotome to be inserted to excise the process from the body of the talus.

SYMPTOMATIC OS TRIGONUM

Posterior ankle pain, discussed frequently in the literature, is often described as being difficult to diagnose. Perhaps this is due to a traumatic injury healing spontaneously or to the fact that patients often put up with residual pain as acknowledgment of having sustained the injury. Often lifestyle modifications are required to prevent exacerbating the condition.

DIAGNOSIS OF A SYMPTOMATIC TRIGONAL PROCESS

Diagnosis of a symptomatic os trigonum is difficult, as it may be due to acute or chronic pathologies. Acute injuries may not appear any different from chronic ones. Pain often appears in other anatomic

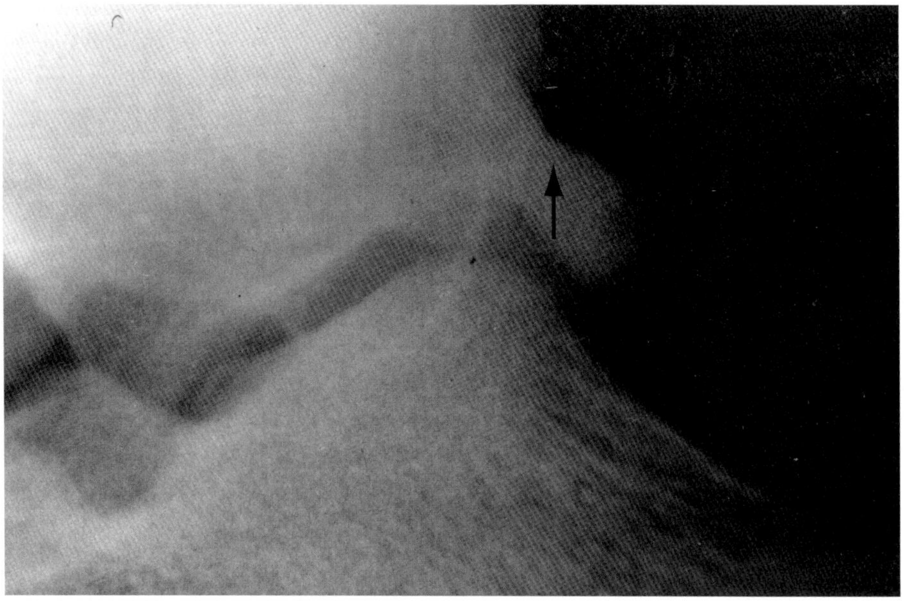

FIGURE 12.2. Lateral radiograph showing Stieda's process.

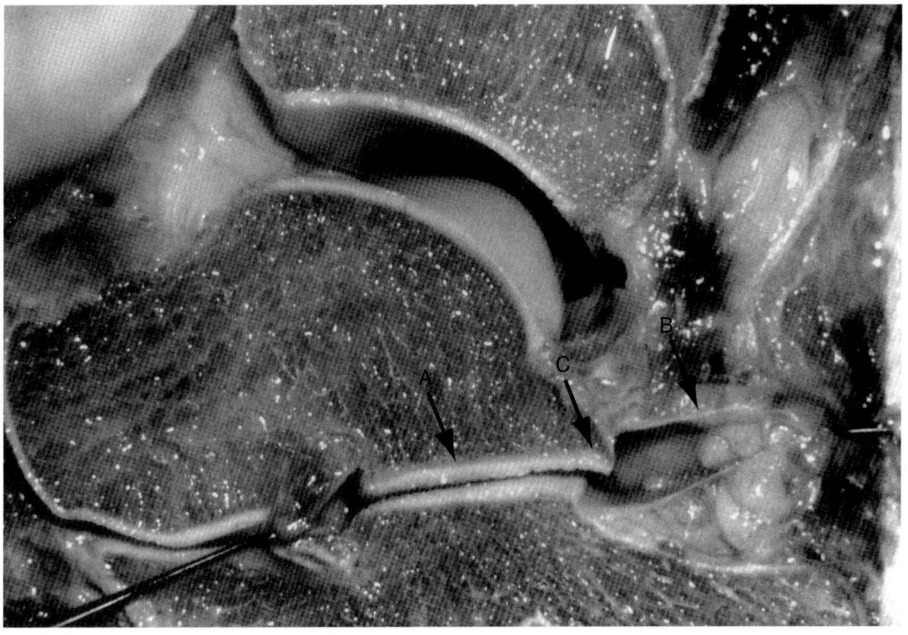

FIGURE 12.3. Sectioned specimen showing the posterior subtalar facet (A), joint pouch (B), and lateral talar process (C). (Courtesy of G. Bauer, Pennsylvania College of Podiatric Medicine.)

areas secondary to compensation. In addition, pain may be present in the absence of trauma, and radiographs may show an identical "lesion" in the opposite ankle. Most surgeons agree that the os trigonum occasionally causes a distinct set of symptoms that can be alleviated by excising this accessory bone.[1] This "set of symptoms" varies and has been called talar compression syndrome,[2] os trigonum syndrome,[3] or posterior ankle impingement.[4]

Diagnostic pitfalls for symptomatic os trigonum vary. Often considerable peroneal tendon problems result from the subtalar pathology, inciting spasticity or compensation from other muscle groups. Pro-

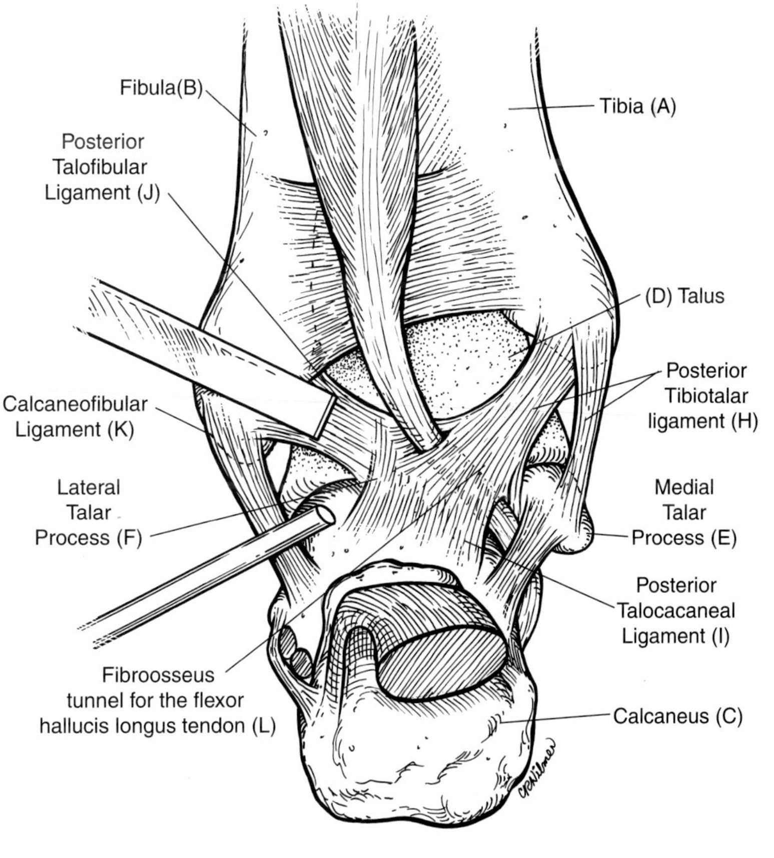

FIGURE 12.4. Anatomy of the posterior aspect of the subtalar joint. A, tibia; B, fibula; C, calcaneus; D, talus; E, medial talar process; F, lateral talar process; H, posterior tibiotalar ligament; I, posterior tibiotalar ligament; J, posterior talofibular ligament; K, calcaneofibular ligament; L, fibrous tunnel for passage of the flexor hallucis longus tendon. Watch for inadvertent contact with the flexor hallucis longus tendon or the calcaneal facet. The posterior tibiotalar ligament and the fibrous sheath of the long flexor tendons must also be released.

tective splinting of the foot in a supinated position prevents compression of the ossicle by the tibia. Traumatic fractures more than 3 months old begin to present radiographically with rounding of the fracture line, making the trigonal process appear as an accessory ossicle. In addition, there are no special radiographic views to aid in the diagnosis. Bone scans can be helpful but are not consistently positive for pathology in symptomatic feet.[5]

Consistent symptoms have been reported including a decreased amount of plantar flexion of the foot on the affected leg compared to the unaffected side, pain on palpation posterior to the talus and anterior to the Achilles tendon, increased pain with ankle joint plantar flexion, and pain with passive dorsiflexion of the hallux.[6] These symptoms are brought on by the "nutcracker" effect of the trigonal process being compressed between the tibia and calcaneus with plantar flexion of the talus and from the close relation between the lateral talar process and the flexor hallucis longus tendon.

MECHANISM OF TRIGONAL PROCESS INJURY

The trigonal process can become a source of pain in two situations: trauma or repetitive stress. Trauma is perhaps the most common cause, evidenced by an acute onset of ecchymosis, edema, and a fracture line if the trigonal process has been separated from the talar body. A separate, or free, os trigonum would not show a fracture line owing to the synchondrosis, and it is not usually displaced, although with a severe enough injury this can occur. The mechanism of the injury that causes fracture of the trigonal process is a triplanar supinator injury or a severe plantar flexor force. Therefore inversion ankle sprains are the most common cause of the symptomatic os trigonum.

Repetitive stress is caused by overuse or faulty biomechanics. Overuse can be precluded by an unusually large Stieda's process or os trigonum. A large, degenerated calcaneal component under the talar process is frequently observed. Biomechanical considerations are important, as excessive subtalar pronation causes the talus to adduct, plantar-flex, and move anteriorly relative to the calcaneus, moving it in the opposite direction. The trigonal process is caught in the middle but is strongly anchored by the posterior talocalcaneal ligament. A synchondrosis creates a stress riser that can induce fracture. A long trigonal process or free os trigonum is pulled in opposite directions by the two ligaments attaching the posterior trochlear surface of the talus and talar process. In the talar process, concentrating forces can lead to fracture at the small osseus area in between. Injuries caused by repetitive stress can occur with normal activities at home or at work, during sports such as running and soccer, or during dance, especially ballet.

With cases of fracture or repetitive stress, symptoms are initiated by movement of the trigonal process in the posterior facet of the subtalar joint. Typical inflammatory changes occur, including hypertrophy of the synovial villi, injection of the central vessel of villous formation, production of a fibrin exudate, or gradual necrosis of the villi and fragmentation of the villous tips (Fig. 12.5). Hyalinization can occur, forming a meniscoid lesion; or there may be adhesive capsulitis due to trauma or severe inflammatory changes.

CONSERVATIVE TREATMENT

Acutely inflamed trigonal lesions are treated usually with rest, ice, elevation, and a compression dressing. Recent fractures require casting for 6–8 weeks. The use of an Unna's boot, cast brace, or crutches may also be helpful. Chronic or acute injuries that do not respond to conservative methods after a 3-month period are subjected to a local injection that is of both diagnostic and therapeutic value.[7] Often this is done with 1 cc of an equal combination of 2% lidocaine and dexamethasone phosphate placed in the posterior aspect of the subtalar joint. For diagnostic purposes, a small amount of local anesthetic can be injected directly into the area of the trigonal process. After several minutes the patient can walk on the affected foot with the pain significantly reduced, confirming the diagnosis. A nonrepository steroid can then be injected into the area and the patient followed up a week later. Because of the close correlation between the trigonal process and function of the subtalar joint, a biomechanical foot strapping (i.e., plantar rest strap, low dye with a longitudinal and medial pad) or an orthotic device can be prescribed as a conservative form of treatment.

SURGICAL TECHNIQUES

Traditional Surgical Procedures

Traditional surgical approaches for the symptomatic trigonal process are a linear incision or a combination of linear and curvilinear longitudinal incisions lateral or medial to the Achilles tendon. The lateral approach is more common, as the posteromedial

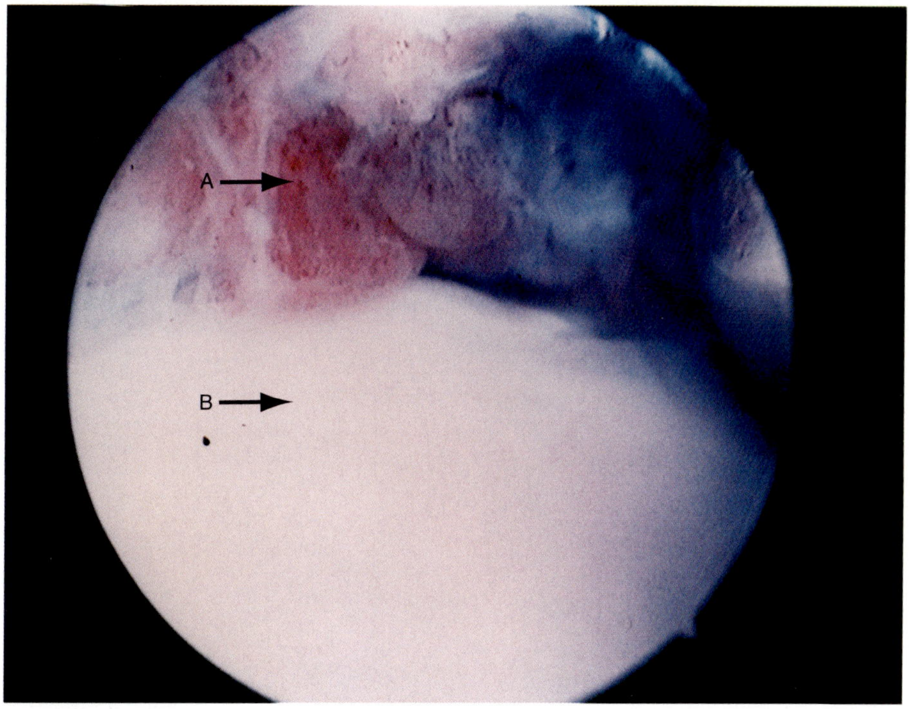

FIGURE 12.5. Acute hypertrophic hemorrhage synovitis (A) above the calcaneal component of the posterior talar facet (B).

neurovascular bundle is then not at risk. The incision is deepened to the level of the posterior calcaneal facet, which is then opened to expose the trigonal process. This is more difficult with a lateral approach because of the depth at which the process lies: It rests more medially, making the medial approach easier for some surgeons. Once identified, the process is sharply dissected, resected from the body of the talus, and removed through the incision.

Arthroscopic Surgical Procedure

Instrumentation

The instruments used to resect the trigonal process are similar to those used for ankle arthroscopy. A 4.0 mm 25 degree oblique arthroscope can be used, although smaller ones may be considered depending on the surgeon's preference. Along with the arthroscope, a compatible light source, light guide, camera, monitor, and shaver are required. A 4.0 mm full-radius blade is used in the shaver. In addition to this equipment, the usual probes, graspers, and so on are needed. A small Lambotte osteotome is required along with a small nylon-headed mallet.

Portals of Entry

The patient is placed in a lateral recumbent (decubitus) position. A leg holder is not required. The leg is elevated for exsanguination, and a thigh tourniquet is inflated to an appropriate pressure. Once the patient is secured, the foot can be prepared and draped at the discretion of the surgeon. The lateral side of the foot is exposed, and superficial anatomic structures of the ankle and heel are marked or observed. The posterior aspect of the ankle and subtalar joint are palpated to locate the fibula and adjacent peroneal tendons and the superior surface of the calcaneus. At the juncture of the superior calcaneal surface and posterior aspect of the peroneal tendons, a small cutdown portal incision is made, and a hemostat is used to retract any underlying vital structures. A second portal is made 2.5–3.0 cm above the first portal, directly behind the peroneal tendons (Fig. 12.6). Following the incision, a hemostat is used to retract any soft tissue structures.

Access to the Posterior Facet

Using an obturator, such as the one used to place the arthroscopic cannula, the incisions are deepened; and the posterior recess of the posterior facet of the subtalar joint is identified and palpated. Using the obturator as a probe, the foot is inverted and everted to locate the joint. Care must be exercised not to access the ankle inadvertently. The ankle is detected through dorsiflexion and plantar flexion, whereas the subtalar joint is detected by pronation and supination of the foot. Once a channel has been made to the posterior aspect of the joint in both portals, the obturator is removed, inserted into the

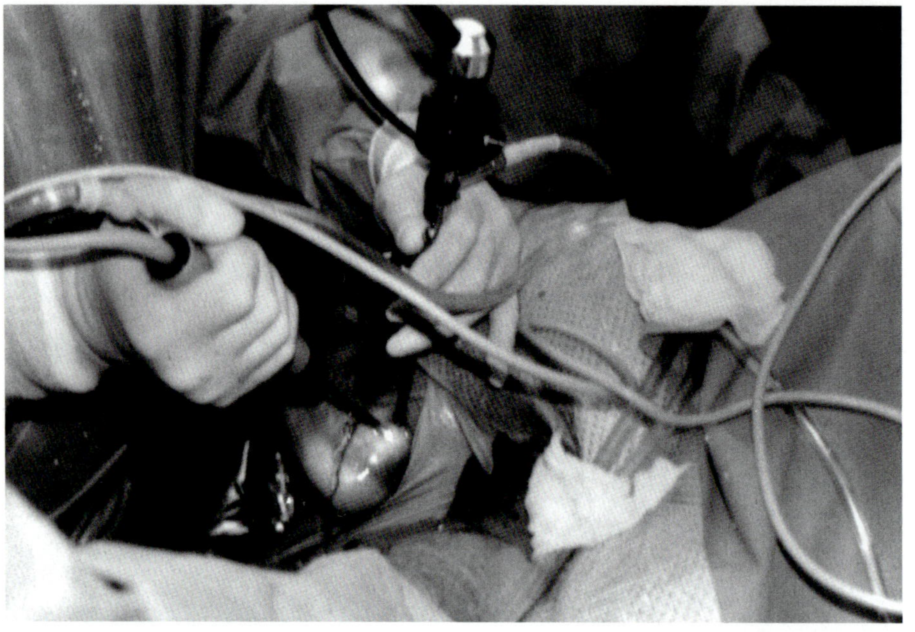

FIGURE 12.6. Two stacked portals are used for passing instruments during arthroscopic resection of an os trigonum.

arthroscopic cannula, and then placed in either portal. The inferior portal is usually used initially. It is now more difficult to palpate the posterior aspect of the joint to place the cannula. When the cannula is placed on the posterior aspect of the joint, the obturator is removed and the arthroscope inserted. Ingress of fluid is through tubing applied to the stopcock on the arthroscopic cannula with the aid of a powered infusion system. The irrigating system is turned on, and the force of the ingress fluid is used to "distend" the soft tissue at the posterior aspect of the joint, allowing the capsule to be visualized. Once seen, a shaver is used to make a rent in the capsule, thereby allowing visualization of the cartilage or joint surfaces of the posterior aspect of the posterior facet of the subtalar joint.

Upon initial entry into the joint, identification of the posterior capsule is aided by the typical reddish appearance of the hypertrophic synovium in the underlying joint pouch. Because the capsule is thin in this area, the brownish-red tint of the synovium is visible, aiding the orientation of the arthroscopist as to the proper placement of the arthroscope (Fig. 12.7).

Once the rent has been made in the capsule, a portion of the facet should be visible. The shaver is further used to perform a capsulotomy, which allows full visualization of the anatomic structures in the area. The position of the subtalar joint, again, must be confirmed by observing motion when inverting and everting the foot, verifying correct placement. Once verified, the capsulotomy is continued until all necessary anatomic structures are seen. In most cases the surface of the talus medial to the lateral process must be identified first and then followed anteriorly, looking for the separation or the fibrous synchondrosis between the talar body and the os trigonum.

Resection of the Trigonal Process

An os trigonum that is free and fully mobilized is easily pushed aside by the shaver, making direct visualization difficult. When the posterior talar facet can be identified, the shaver is used to free all soft tissue behind it, allowing the os trigonum to be visualized. When freed, the posterior talocalcaneal ligament and fibers attached to the fibrous tunnel

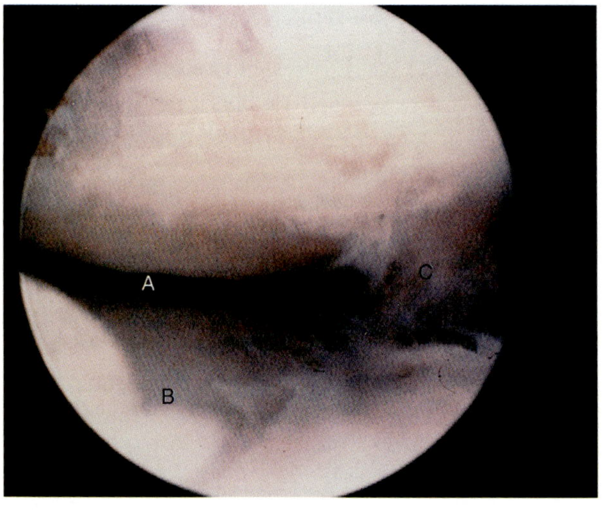

FIGURE 12.7. Posterior talar facet. A, posterior talar joint line; B, calcaneal facet; C, chronic hypertrophic synovitis.

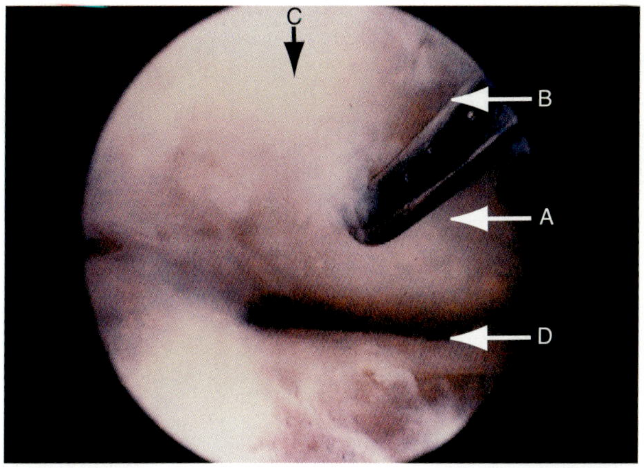

FIGURE 12.8. Note the os trigonum (A), synchondrosis (B) with probe inserted, fibers of the posterior talofibular ligament (C), and the calcaneal facet (D).

around the flexor hallucis longus tendon are still attached and must be released prior to resection. This can be done with an arthroscopic knife ("banana blade") or by securing the loose process with a grasper and rotating it in a circular motion to force avulsion of the soft tissue holding the ossicle.

A nonfree os trigonum is treated differently. A synchondrosis identifies the trigonal process (Fig. 12.8). Once identified and freed of soft tissue, a curved banana blade is inserted into an adjacent portal, and the posterior infracalcaneal facet is incised. Once free, the blade is removed from the portal, and a small Lambotte osteotome is inserted and brought into vision at the level of the synchondrosis. Because of the orientation of the talus on the calcaneus, a lateral portal, placed as described behind the peroneal tendons, forms a plane perpendicular to the axis of the lateral talar process, allowing accurate resection from the talar body (Fig. 12.9). After an osteotome is brought to the level of the synchondrosis, care must be exercised to ensure that it is oriented vertical to the plane of the joint line of the posterior facet. This allows flush resection of the ossicle from the posterior surface of the talus. It can be done by orienting the point of the osteotome in a plane perpendicular to the cartilaginous surface of the talar component of the posterior facet. A mallet is then used to drive the osteotome across the synchondrosis, freeing it from the talus. The fragment is still attached to the posterior tibiotalar ligament and the fibrous tunnel of the long flexor tendon to the hallux. These structures are released by sectioning with a knife or are avulsed by blunt dissection. If the ossicle breaks into pieces, care must be taken to remove all fragments. In these instances the shaver should be used to débride the surgical site further to visualize any remaining fragments.

Stieda's processes are resected similar to the nonfree os trigonum, in which a synchondrosis is present. In these cases the curved posterior portion of the trigonal process is identified at the level of the talar body. It is the same level at which the synchondrosis occurs and is directly in front of the talar attachment of the posterior talofibular ligament (Fig. 12.10) and behind the posterior talocalcaneal ligament. In place of the synchondrosis is the posteriorly curved portion (Fig. 12.11) of the trigonal process coursing away from the talar body. It is at the start of this curved portion that the osteotome is inserted and the process excised from the talus (Fig. 12.12). The posterior talocalcaneal ligament should first be incised and the fragments removed as described for the free os trigonum.

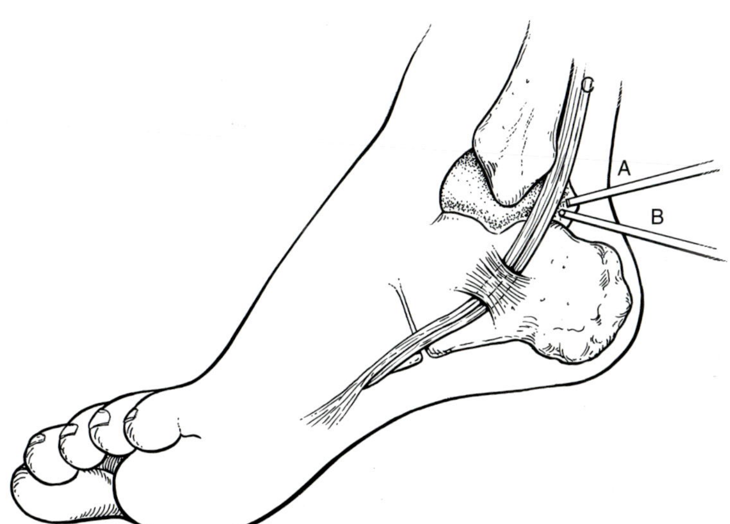

FIGURE 12.9. Lateral aspect of the foot showing the osteotome in the superior portal (A) and the os trigonum in the inferior portal (B) directly behind the peroneal tendons (C).

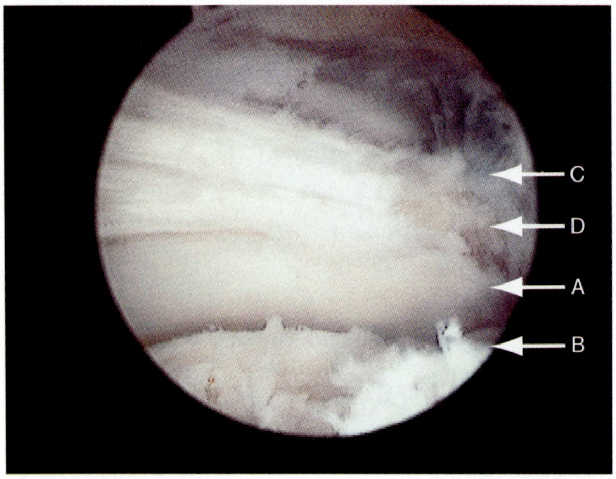

FIGURE 12.10. Note the talar facet (A), calcaneal facet (B), posterior talofibular ligament (C), and start of the posterior talar process (D).

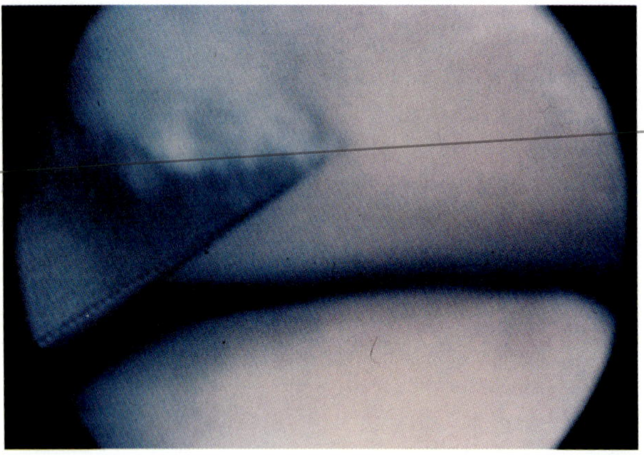

FIGURE 12.11. Osteotome placed perpendicular to the talar facet at the slant of the posterior talar process of the calcaneal facet.

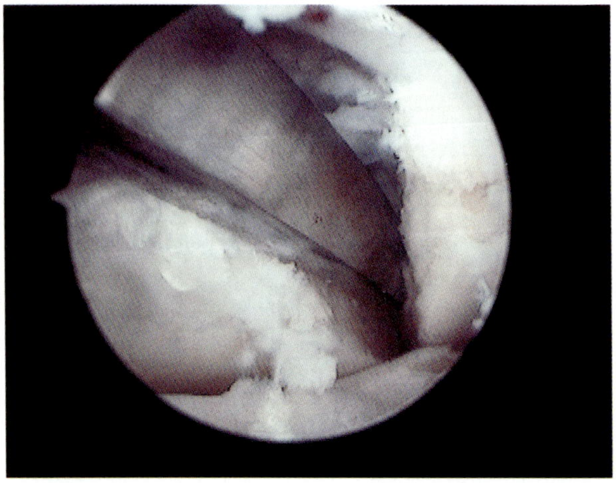

FIGURE 12.12. Note the fibers of the posterior talofibular ligament, osteotomized Stieda's process, osteotome, and calcaneal facet.

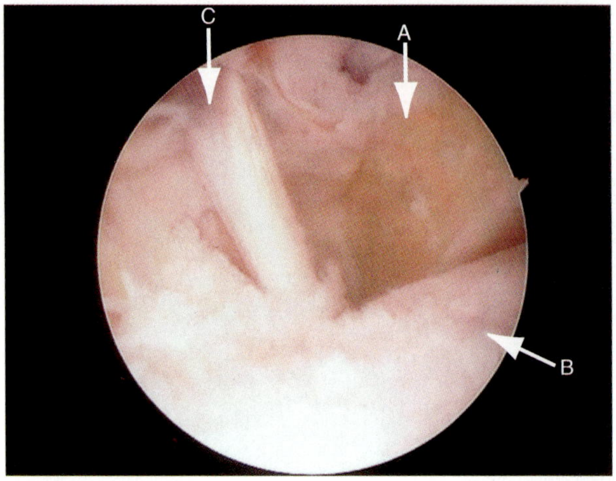

FIGURE 12.13. Resected posterior talar process exposing the talus (A), calcaneal facet (B), and flexor hallucis longus tendon (C).

Once the ossicle has been removed, the flexor hallucis longus tendon should be visible (Fig. 12.13). The tendon can be inspected for synovitis or other changes. Finally, the posterior aspect of the talus should be checked to make sure the process has been resected flush from the talus without leaving any remains. The joint is inspected for any further bony fragments or debris, after which the arthroscopic equipment is removed from the portals.

The incisions are closed with simple sutures of 5-0 nylon, and a mild compression dressing is applied. Prior to wound closure, the surgical site is infiltrated with 10 cc of a combination of 8 cc bupivacaine and 2 cc dexamethasone phosphate.

Postoperative Care

An above-the-ankle compression dressing is used on all patients. Most patients are placed in a cast brace and allowed to ambulate after the first 48 hours, bearing full weight on the operated foot. The patient is seen weekly. On the first postoperative visit, radiographs are obtained to verify excision of the os trigonum, and a compression dressing is reapplied. Sutures are removed on the second postoperative visit, and the compression dressing is reapplied. At the third postoperative week, if there is no pain on ambulation and minimal swelling an elastic wrap can be applied and the patient allowed to ambulate in the cast brace. If swelling persists, a compression dressing is continued until it subsides.

On approximately the fourth week following surgery, ambulation is allowed in a soft, oversized shoe using the cast brace as needed and increasing the amount and extent of walking. Physical therapy is used postoperatively at the discretion of the surgeon, usually following the clinical pathways for an acute ankle sprain.

ARTHROSCOPIC RESECTION OF THE OS TRIGONUM

Clinical Results

With continued utilization of the arthroscope for excising the trigonal process, the advantages over the open method are becoming increasingly more evident. A retrospective review of nine of my patients who underwent arthroscopic resection of the trigonal process further supports the advantages over the open method. The patient population consisted of five females and four males, with the procedure performed between 1993 and 1998. The average age of the patients was 29.8 years (range 13–71 years). Evidence of the presence of symptomatic os trigonum was confirmed clinically and radiographically. Conservative care, including rest, ice, elevation, application of a compression dressing, and local injection, did not significantly relieve the symptoms in these patients. Because of this lack of relief, I performed arthroscopic resection of the symptomatic trigonal process. A review of the postoperative course reveals that the average return to regular shoe wear was 28 days (range 26–54 days), and the average discharge time after surgery was 52.25 days (range 36–70 days).

Martin[8] reported on the postoperative course after using an open repair method, which included 2 weeks of no weight-bearing below the knee cast followed by a weight-bearing cast for another 2 weeks. Subsequent physical therapy was initiated after range of motion became pain-free. They emphasized the fact that complete recovery may take up to 6 months. When comparing this to the arthroscopic method, it is clearly evident that a much quicker recovery period, including earlier return to wearing shoes and an earlier discharge time, is achieved when utilizing the arthroscopic method.

Complications

Arthroscopic resection of the os trigonum can result in complications similar to those seen with traditional open procedures. The greatest risk is entrapment of the sural nerve due to inadvertent portal placement. To avoid this problem, the portal must be placed directly behind the peroneal tendons and a mosquito hemostat used to retract soft tissue structures under the skin incision. Also, do not use a trocar instead of the arthroscopic obturator. The obturator is sharp enough to place the cannula without inflicting inadvertent nerve or articular damage.

The peroneal tendons can be damaged if they are traumatized arthroscopically. To avoid this, place the arthroscopic cannula behind them and, when cleared, direct it anteriorly and inferiorly toward the posterior facet.

The flexor hallucis longus tendon can be damaged by overzealous shaving of the adjacent soft tissue structures or by using the osteotome or grasper. Watch for concurrent plantar flexion of the hallux to indicate contact with this structure.

Bony fragments can remain when removing the os trigonum in pieces. Inadequate resection of the trigonal process can result if it is not fully visualized or if the osteotome is used to resect it at an inadvertent angle, leaving portions of the lateral process. When there is no separation of the os trigonum from the talus, it is best to err on the side of too little resection of the process rather than osteotomize the talar body.

Arthroscopic resection of the os trigonum is an advanced procedure that requires an experienced arthroscopist. One of the most difficult tasks when performing arthroscopic resection of the os trigonum is the demand on the surgeon not to be one-hand dominant. Right-handed surgeons have an easier time on left ankles. Right ankles require the surgeon to watch the monitor backward for proper orientation.

BIBLIOGRAPHY

1. DuVries HC. *Surgery of the foot*, 2nd ed. St. Louis: Mosby, 1965;517–518.
2. Quirk T. Talar compression syndrome in dancers. *Foot Ankle* 1982;3:65–68.
3. Wredmare T, Carlstedt CA, Bauer H, Saartuk T. Os trigonum syndrome: a clinical entity in ballet dancers. *Foot Ankle* 1991;11:404–406.
4. Hedrick MR, McBride AM. Posterior ankle impingement. *Foot Ankle* 1994;15:2–8.
5. Johnson RP, Collier DB, Carrera GF. The os trigonum syndrome: use of bone scan in the diagnosis. *J Trauma* 1984;24:761–764.
6. Paulos LE, Johnson CL, Noyes FR. Posterior compartment fractures of the ankle. *Am J Sports Med* 1983;11:439–477.
7. Ecker ML, Ritter MA, Jacobs BS. The symptomatic os trigonum. *JAMA* 1967;201:882–884.
8. Martin BF. Posterior triangle pain: the os trigonum. *J Foot Surg* 1989; 28:312–318.

CHAPTER 13

Endoscopy for Excision of Haglund's Deformity and Retrocalcaneal Bursitis

Richard O. Lundeen

Pain at the posterosuperior aspect of the heel at or near the insertion of the Achilles tendon has been labeled with various terms, such as a "pump bump," Haglund's disease or deformity, achillobursitis, achillodynia, retrocalcaneal bursitis, retrocalcaneal bursitis, and bursitis retrocalcaneus.

Variations in the surgical treatment of Haglund's disease involve exostectomy of the posterosuperior aspect of the calcaneus with or without calcaneal osteotomy; the differences are mainly concerned with the incisional approach used. Approaches include a caudally based semielliptical incision across the posterior aspect of the heel,[1] a lateral linear incision parallel to the Achilles tendon,[2] or a medial linear incision along the Achilles tendon curving laterally across its insertion.[3] Remodeling of the posterosuperior aspect of the calcaneus varies among patients. Removal of too little bone might not cure the condition, and removal of too much bone could weaken the attachment of the Achilles tendon, possibly leading to rupture.[4]

ARTHROSCOPY OF THE POSTERIOR HEEL

The first presentation of a case where an arthroscope was used to assess the retrocalcaneal recess was by Nagai in 1985. He reported a 1979 case wherein he identified the Achilles tendon and an avulsed portion of its insertion from the calcaneus.[5] Arthroscopy of the retrocalcaneal bursae was reported by Zimmer and Meyers,[6] and Frey[7] forecast endoscopic evaluation of Haglund's deformity and Achilles tendinitis. Arthroscopic resection of the retrocalcaneal bursae and Haglund's deformity along with a description of the entry portals and the surgical technique appeared in 1997.[8]

INDICATIONS

Haglund's disease is verified by pain on palpation of the retrocalcaneal area in front of the Achilles tendon above its insertion. Radiographs show a prominence of the posterosuperior aspect of the calcaneus. Initial attempts at treatment may include changes or modifications of footwear, addition of a heel lift, and use of antiinflammatory medications. Often injection of a small amount of lidocaine and dexamethasone phosphate into the retrocalcaneal bursal area is helpful, but excessive injections or injection into the Achilles tendon can predispose to rupture of the tendon; therefore discretion must be exercised. Control of the function of the foot is important, and often various foot strappings and orthotic devices are employed. Cases that do not respond with aggressive conservative care are candidates for arthroscopic resection of the retrocalcaneal bursa and Haglund's deformity.

Several pathologic conditions can appear in the same area, which must be differentiated for correct treatment to resolve the particular problem. The differential diagnosis includes rheumatic disorders (usually bilateral and not responsive to mechanical therapy), traction exostosis (visible spurring in the middle one-third of the posterior calcaneus), bursitis (superficial or deep) of the Achilles tendon at or above its insertion, a prominent superior surface of the calcaneus, and biomechanical or functional abnormalities. A prominent posterosuperior surface of the calcaneus is generally referred to as Haglund's deformity when it is in the sagittal plane. Frontal plane abnormalities place the posterosuperior surface of the calcaneus laterally and are commonly referred to as a posterosuperior lateral retrocalcaneal exostosis, or "pump bump."

Biomechanical conditions are important because in a supinated or cavus foot the posterosuperior surface of the calcaneus is prominent laterally, leading to irritation by the counter of a shoe. This foot type also tends to have a tight Achilles tendon, which can lead to pain or insertional tendinitis. The adult pronated foot often presents with a tight heel cord that can also lead to insertional tendinitis or irritation of the bursa between the Achilles tendon and the superior calcaneal surface.

Arthroscopic treatment for Haglund's deformity is useful only for resecting the posterosuperior surface of the calcaneus and the bursa and soft tissue interposed between it and the Achilles tendon.

SURGICAL TECHNIQUE

The anatomy of the posterosuperior aspect of the calcaneus is straightforward and uncomplicated (Fig. 13.1). It is rounded with its superior surface coursing inferior to the attachment of the Achilles tendon (Fig. 13.2). The surface of the calcaneus is often covered with cartilaginous-appearing hyalinized tissue, thickened periosteum, or both. Often bursal tissue can be identified that consists of reddish synovium-like tissue or there are synovial villi, which can be acute (evidenced by a central injected vessel) or chronic (evidenced by the presence of fibrous tissue). Considerable amounts of fat are in this area as well. The Achilles tendon arises from the middle one-third of the posterior aspect of the calcaneus and courses superiorly, with its linear opaque fibers producing its characteristic appearance. With degeneration, the tendon becomes opaque and can become frayed or covered with fibrous tissue. Similarly, the posterosuperior aspect of the calcaneus can become fibrous and lose its normal glossy translucent appearance.

The instruments required for arthroscopic resection of Haglund's deformity and retrocalcaneal bursitis are those used for standard ankle arthroscopy, including a 4.0 mm or 2.7 mm 30 degree oblique arthroscope and accompanying obturators, trocars, cannulas, light source, light guide, and shaver. A 4.0 mm full-radius blade for the shaver is also needed, along with small probes, curettes, bell rasp, Lambotte osteotomes, and a nylon-headed mallet. The usual graspers or curved mosquito hemostats are also required.

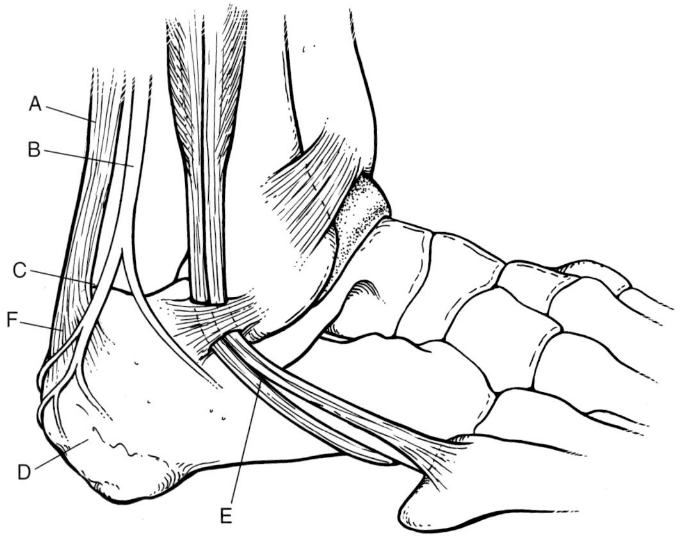

FIGURE 13.1. Anatomy of the posterior heel. A, Achilles tendon; B, sural nerve; C, retrocalcaneal recess; D, calcaneus; E, peroneal tendons; F, insertion of Achilles tendon in the posterior one-third of the calcaneus.

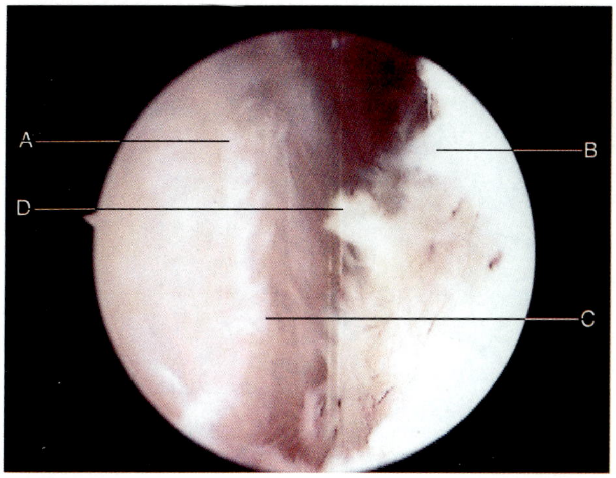

FIGURE 13.2. Note the retrocalcaneal recess, Achilles tendon (A), posterosuperior surface of the calcaneus (B), inflamed tendon tissue (C), hypertrophic inflammatory tissue (D).

The patient is placed in a prone position without a leg holder. The leg is elevated for exsanguination, and a thigh tourniquet is inflated. The foot can then be prepared and draped in the usual manner (Fig. 13.3).

The anatomic landmarks at the posterior aspect of the heel are identified. The junction of the posterosuperior surface of the calcaneus and the Achilles tendon is palpated medially and laterally; it is here that the portals are placed. A small cutdown incision is made on the medial and lateral aspects of the heel at the junction of the superior surface of the calcaneus and the Achilles tendon both medially and laterally. An incision is made perpendicular to the heel cord, and a curved mosquito hemostat is used to retract any vital structures under the incision. The obturator used to place the arthroscopic cannula is then used to create a channel between the medial and lateral portals and the space between the heel cord and the calcaneus. The obturator can also be used to palpate the anatomic areas including the insertion of the Achilles tendon and the smooth pseudocartilaginous surface of the superior aspect of the calcaneus for orientation at the anatomic site. Haglund's deformity should be probed in its entirety, emphasizing the extent of the deformity superiorly and anteriorly toward the superior surface of the calcaneus and talus.

The Achilles tendon expands laterally and medially around the back of the heel. Medial expansion is thicker and larger than lateral expansion. With large Haglund's deformities, the posterior surface of the calcaneus is significantly above the insertion of the Achilles tendon. Once these prominences have been resected, the portal is relatively higher, above the insertion of the heel cord. Therefore portals for large Haglund's deformities should be placed below the bony junction with the tendon. This prevents greater obliquity of the view of the retrocalcaneal area, which can make bone resection more difficult.

Vital structures other than the Achilles tendon include the sural nerve and saphenous veins anterior to the lateral portal. Medially, the neurovascular bundle lies anterior to the medial portal, with the medial calcaneal branch of the posterior tibial nerve at the most risk.

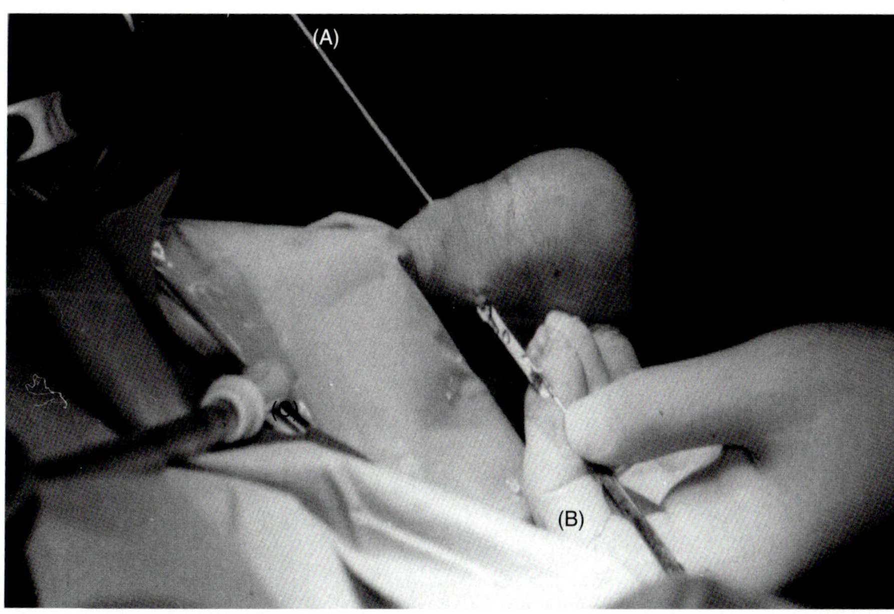

FIGURE 13.3. Arthroscopic setup for resection of Haglund's deformity. The arthroscope is placed laterally (A), and an osteotome is placed medially (B).

Once the area has been probed and a channel made into the space between the Achilles tendon and the calcaneus, the arthroscope is placed into either portal in the usual manner. Ingress is achieved by use of a powered infusion system through the cannula, and the retrocalcaneal area is inspected. Synovial tissue can be identified by the presence of injected vessels and hypertrophic synovial villi. A distinct bursal sac in this area is not usually identified. In addition to the synovial tissue, the area is laden with fat cells, and at times thickened periosteum can be seen along with fibrous tissue on the calcaneus or Achilles tendon.

The shaver is placed in the opposite portal and brought into view of the arthroscope (Fig. 13.4). The retrocalcaneal bursa and other soft tissue structures on or in front of the Achilles tendon are next resected. Once the retrocalcaneal area has been cleared of all soft tissue and the shaver is removed, a small osteotome is inserted into the opposite portal and brought into visualization. The upper portion of Haglund's deformity is resected initially, and then the deformity is gradually resected down to the level of insertion of the Achilles tendon in the middle one-third of the calcaneus. Care must be exercised that this surface of the calcaneus is resected at an approximately 45 degree angle to the plantar aspect of the foot, making sure not to leave a bony spicule at the superior aspect of the calcaneus (Fig. 13.5). It can be checked by palpating the superior surface of the calcaneus with a probe, osteotome, or shaver to ensure that no step-down defect exists. Following careful resection of the posterosuperior aspect of the calcaneus with the osteotome, the fragments are removed using a small grasper or a mosquito hemostat. Once the resection is complete, the superior surface of the calcaneus should be resected from the insertion of the Achilles tendon posteriorly and anteriorly at an approximately 45 degree angle onto the superior surface of the calcaneus (Fig. 13.6). To assist this move, a small bell rasp can be inserted into the retrocalcaneal space and the calcaneal surface

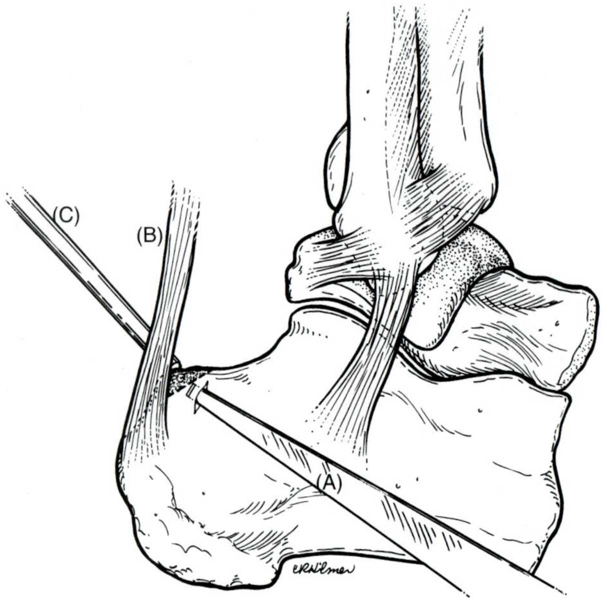

FIGURE 13.5. Orientation of the plane of the osteotome (A) relative to Achilles tendon (B) and the arthroscope (C).

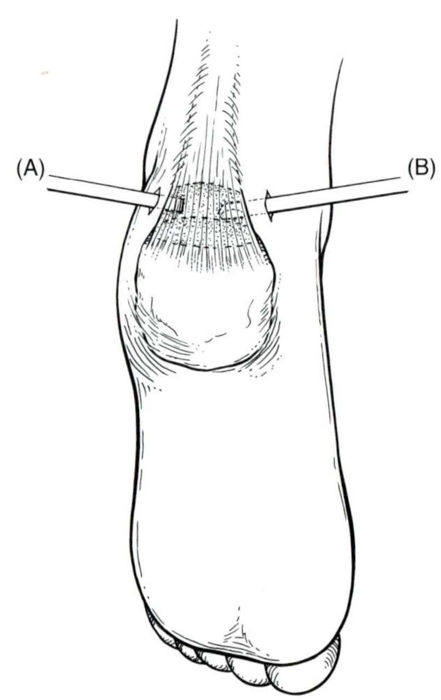

FIGURE 13.4. Proper placement of the arthroscope (A) and shaver (B) relative to Haglund's deformity.

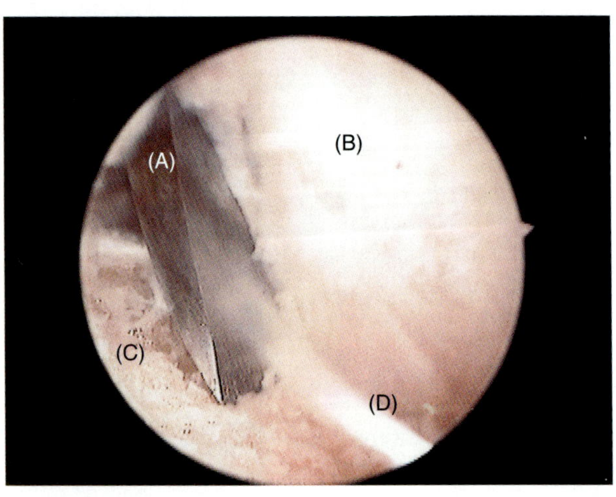

FIGURE 13.6. Plane of the osteotome (A) needs to be 45 degrees from the Achilles tendon (B) for proper resection of the calcaneus (C), as it is carefully resected from the tendon's uppermost insertion (D).

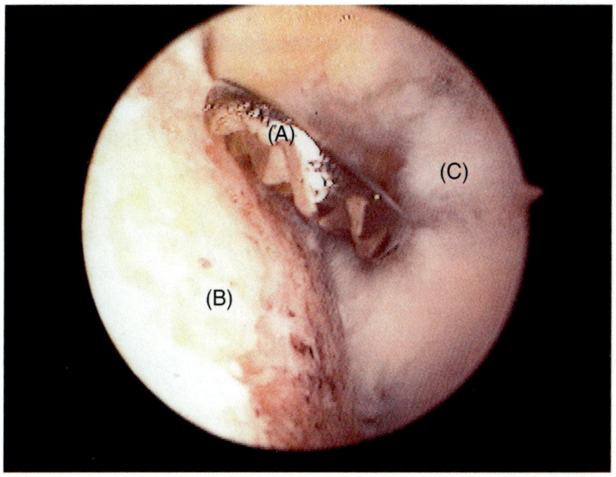

FIGURE 13.7. Small bell rasp (A) is useful for smoothing the resected calcaneus (B) away from the Achilles tendon (C).

gently remodeled to ensure that a smooth transition exists (Fig. 13.7). Once smoothed, the shaver is again inserted to remove any bony fragment or fibrous tissue that remains at the surgical site (Fig. 13.8).

The arthroscope should then be placed in the opposite portal and that area checked for any osseous defects or particulate matter, which is then treated appropriately. A particular concern is any bony irregularity at the opposite portal left by inadequate resection of the calcaneus directly under the point at which the arthroscope had been placed. Again the surgical site can be smoothed with the bell rasp. The full-radius shaver is used for final débridement of

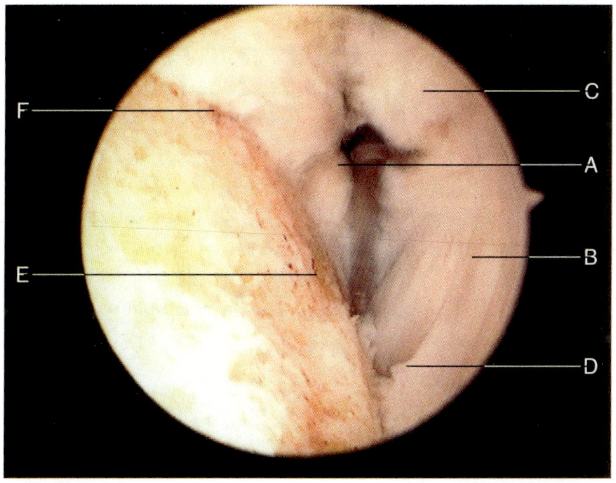

FIGURE 13.8. A 3.5 mm full-radius shaver (A) is used for final débridement of the retrocalcaneal recess including the Achilles tendon (B), whose fibers now appear normal following resection of fibrous tissue (C). The tendon's insertion (D) should be free of debris, the resected calcaneus smooth (E), and its superior portion rounded (F).

the area. When the procedure is finished, the arthroscopic equipment is removed from the portals and the incisions closed with a simple suture of 5-0 nylon. A mild compression dressing is applied, and the tourniquet is released.

After applying the mild compression wrap, a surgical shoe or a cast brace is applied, if warranted. Radiographs are obtained during the first postoperative visit, and the foot and ankle are covered again in a compression dressing. This compression dressing is changed weekly for 3–4 weeks, after which time the patient is allowed to increase ambulation in a soft shoe. If the swelling persists, an elastic wrap is utilized; or if pain persists after surgery, a cast brace is recommended. Physical therapy can be instituted at the discretion of the surgeon or can be performed on an at-home basis by the patient.

COMPLICATIONS

Complications of arthroscopic Haglund's resection are similar to those of open techniques and include medial calcaneal or sural nerve entrapment by inadvertent anterior lateral portal placement, injury to the Achilles tendon by overaggressive shaving, inadvertent under- or overresection of bone, or residual bony fragments in the surgical site.

Small bony fragments in the soft tissue around the surgical site may be seen on postoperative radiographs. They are of no consequence and should not present later problems. Incisional sloughing has not occurred even when resecting large deformities.

Technically, the procedure is somewhat demanding; but because of the subcutaneous nature of the deformity and easy palpation of the surgical site with instrumentation, most experienced arthroscopic surgeons are able to perform it. Because the operative site is subcutaneous, falling out of the incision is common during the procedure, and a steady hand is needed.

Nerve entrapment is a rare complication because of the portal placement. Moreover, owing to the nonaggressive nature of the full-radius shaver, inadvertent trauma to the Achilles tendon should not occur. Inadvertently leaving a dorsal spicule should not present a problem because of the frequent probing of the superior aspect of the resected portion of the calcaneus. Perhaps the least common complication is overzealous resection of the posterosuperior aspect of the calcaneus, or "chasing the bump," as is common with the open procedures. By directly

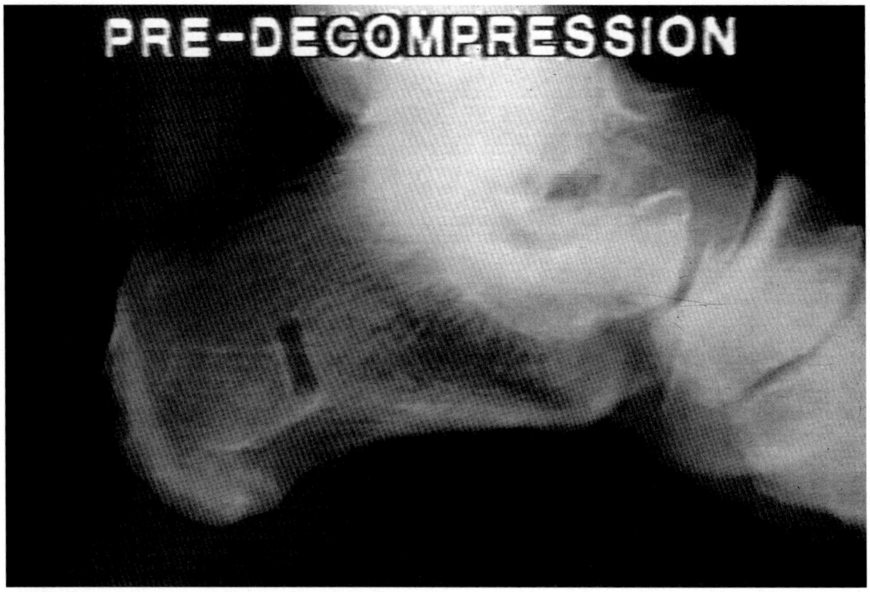

FIGURE 13.9. Preoperative lateral radiograph of a patient with symptomatic retrocalcaneal bursitis and a prominent posterosuperior calcaneal tuberosity. (Courtesy of T. Zimmer.)

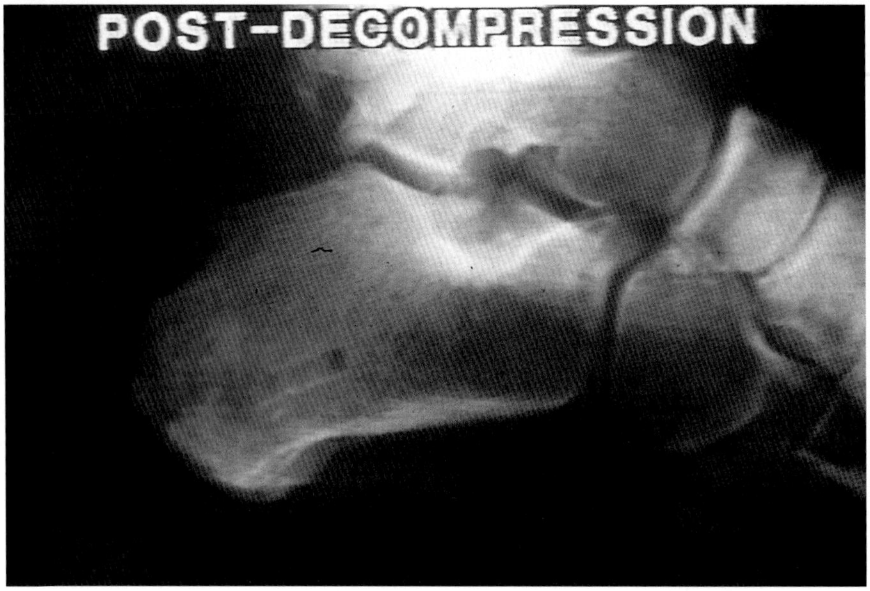

FIGURE 13.10. Postoperative radiograph of the patient in Figure 13.9. (Courtesy of T. Zimmer.)

visualizing the retrocalcaneal area, one can determine that an adequate amount of calcaneus has been resected and, under direct visualization, ensure that the insertion of the Achilles tendon has not been compromised (Figs. 13.9, 13.10).

BIBLIOGRAPHY

1. Keck SW, Kelly PJ. Bursitis of the posterior part of the heel. *J Bone Joint Surg Am* 1965;47:267–273.
2. DuVries HL. *Surgery of the foot*, 2nd ed. St. Louis, Mosby, 1965.
3. Arckinson DM, Loutts MB, et al. Tendo Achillis bursitis. *J Bone Joint Surg Am* 1966;48:77.
4. Nissen KI. Remodeling of the posterior tuberosity of the calcaneus. In: Rob C, Smith R (eds). *Operative surgery*, vol 5. London: Butterworth, 1957;317.
5. Nagai H. Tunnel endoscopy. In: Watanabi M (ed) *Arthroscopy of small joints*. New York: Igaku-Shoin, 1985;163–164.
6. Zimmer TJ, Meyers FF. Arthroscopic retrocalcaneal decompression. Presented at the AAOS annual summer meeting, 1989.
7. Frey C. Arthroscoping the foot and ankle practice. In: Guhl JF (ed) *Foot and ankle arthroscopy*, 2nd ed. Thorofare, NJ: Slack, 1993.
8. Lundeen RO. Arthroscopic resection of Haglund's deformity and retrocalcaneal bursae. Presented at the ASFAS annual meeting, Palm Springs, 1997.

CHAPTER 14

Arthroscopy of the First Metatarsophalangeal Joint

C.N. van Dijk

The development of small instruments has made arthroscopy in small joints possible. Arthroscopy of the elbow and wrist have become routine procedures.[1] Arthroscopy in small joints was first described by Burman (New York), who performed six wrist and three ankle arthroscopies on autopsy specimens.[2] In 1939 Tagaki described arthroscopy of the ankle joint in patients using an arthroscope with a diameter of 2.7 mm.[3] Watanabe et al. described the first arthroscopy of the first metatarsophalangeal (MTP) joint in 1985.[4] "The articulation between hallux and its metatarsal is entered at the point either lateral or medial to the extensor tendon. As this joint is extremely difficult to open with manual traction, a 2.7 mm outside diameter sheath must be used." Bartlett reported a case in 1988 in which successful arthroscopic débridement was performed on an osteochondral defect.[5]

A series of 20 patients with arthrosis of the first MTP joint was reported in which diagnostic arthroscopy was performed. Shaving gave some promising results. However, it was not the osteoarthritis that made us decide to perform arthroscopy on the first MTP joint. Members of our national ballet and other ballet groups often confronted us with pain problems and painful limitation of dorsiflexion in the first MTP joint. As with the anterior impingement syndrome of the ankle joint, the most likely cause is repetitive microtrauma on the dorsal aspect of the joint with secondary spur formation. Extension osteotomy of the first phalanx was our original approach to the problem. Because we were not always able to relieve the pain and because arthroscopic treatments of the anterior impingement syndrome of the ankle joint is highly successful, we tried the same procedure in the first MTP joint. The arthroscopic procedure has the advantage of less morbidity, outpatient treatment, and reduced risk of range of motion limitations that may be produced by the scarring that results from classic arthrotomy. Another advantage is faster return to sports and work. These advantages hold for every patient; therefore we looked for other indications as well.

INDICATIONS

Impingement Syndrome

Dorsal impingement on the big toe is the result of repetitive microtrauma on the dorsal aspect of the joint. It results from repetitive forced dorsiflexion movement, as occurs with ballet dancing.[6] This results in damage to the cartilage rim on the dorsal aspect of the distal phalanx and metatarsal head. An inflammatory reaction, synovitis, scar tissue formation, calcifications, and finally spur formation can be the final result.

Clinically, there is pain on the dorsal and dorsolateral aspect of the joint, especially during or after forced dorsiflexion. In more severe situations, limitation of dorsiflexion evolves.

On examination, there is pain on the dorsal aspect of the first MTP joint, where a rim can be palpated. Typically, it is located at the dorsolateral aspect of the metatarsal head. Dorsiflexion demonstrates slight limitation. On radiography, there are no degenerative changes on the anteroposterior (AP) or lateral views. On the lateral view, a spur beginning on the dorsal aspect at the junction of the metatarsal head and the shaft can be seen. The condition is comparable to the anterior impingement syndrome of the ankle joint. Here, we find the same painful limitation due to scar tissue and sometimes spur formation, usually without generalized arthrosis.[7]

Osteochondritis Dissecans

Osteochondritis dissecans in the first MTP joint is known pathology.[8] We regard osteochondritis dis-

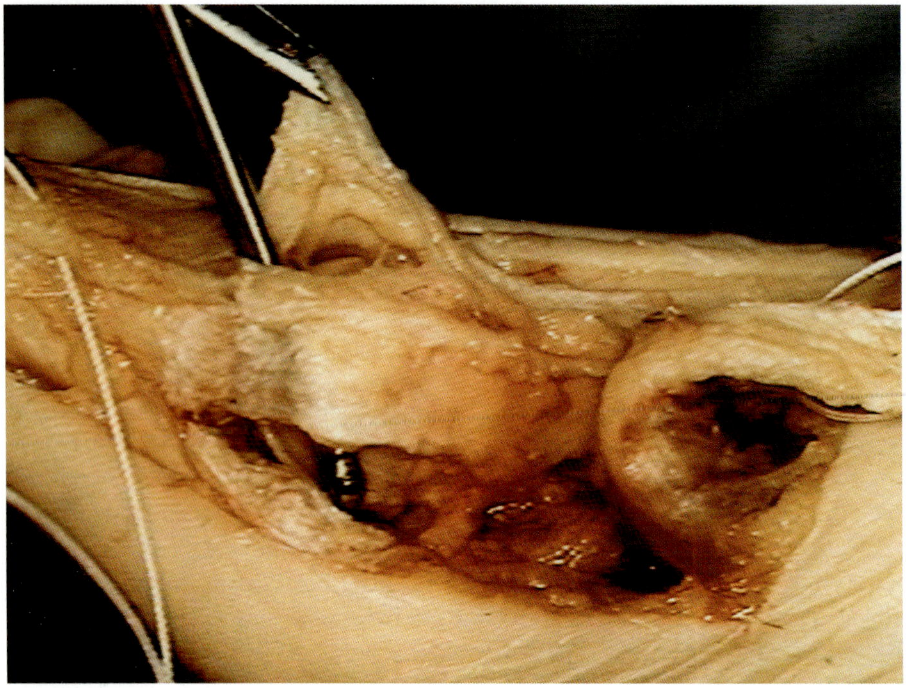

A

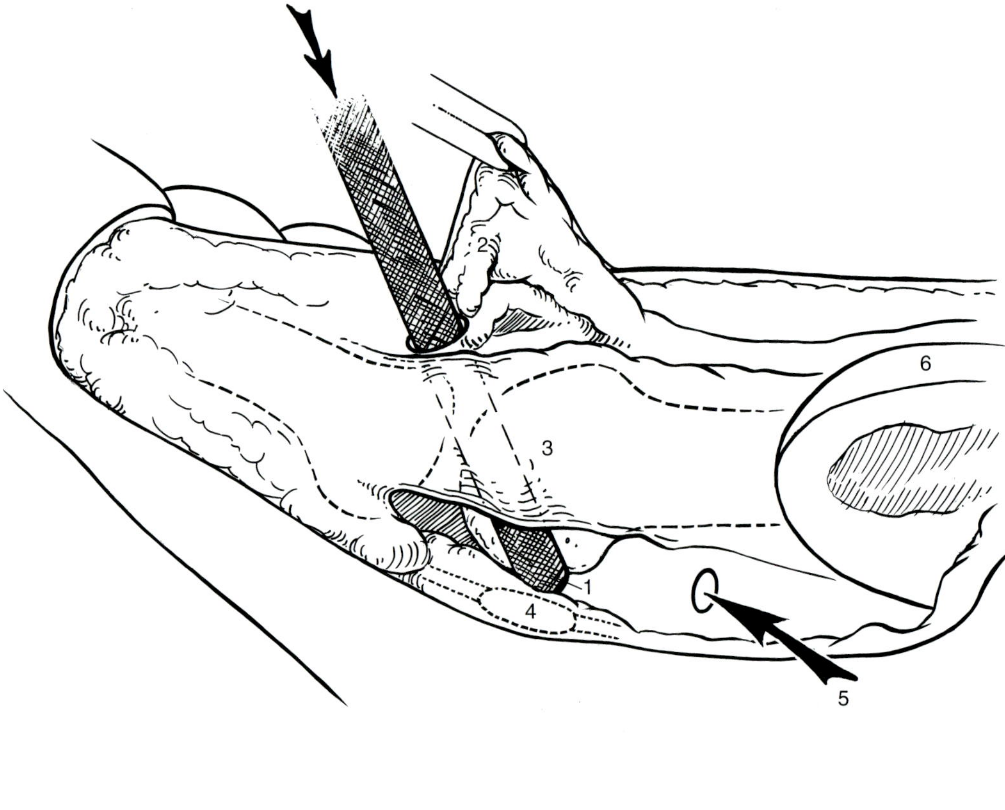

B

FIGURE 14.1. Dorsal capsula (2) is elevated. Metatarsal head (3). Arthroscope (1) has been introduced through the anteromedial portal directed downward toward the sesamoid bones (4). The abductor muscle (6) is reflected backward. Arrow indicates the additional proximal portal (5) for instrumentation of sesamoid pathology.

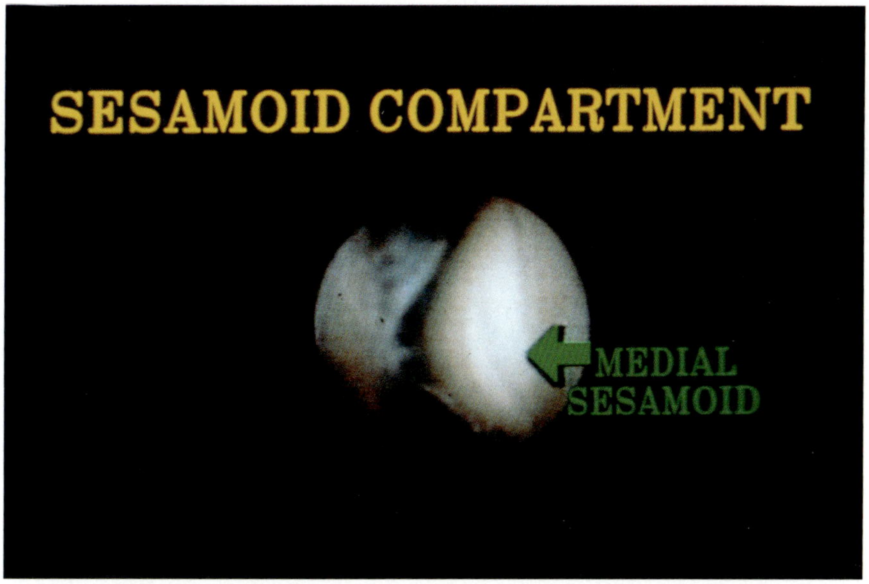

FIGURE 14.2. Arthroscopic view of the medial sesamoid bone.

secans to be a first step toward a hallux rigidus deformity. The symptoms and therapy are no different from osteochondritis dissecans in other joints such as the ankle or knee joints.

Sesamoiditis

The sesamoid bones are incorporated in the short flexors of the big toe and articulate with the plantar surface of the head of the metatarsal. A normal sesamoid bone can consist of multiple fragments.[9] Differentiation between a multifragmented sesamoid bone or a fracture/nonunion can be made by bone scans. A fracture may be the result of trauma, but more often complaints in this region are the result of repetitive microtrauma. A fatigue fracture may be the ultimate result. The pain, located on the plantar side of the head of the first metatarsal, is present during or after activity. It can be elicited by forced dorsiflexion of the big toe. There is local pressure and pain but usually no swelling. AP and lateral views can show the irregular, sometimes dislocated fragments. The axial view can demonstrate an irregular joint line between the sesamoid bone and the metatarsal head. A bone scan differentiates between active pathology and normal anatomy. Conservative treatment consists of a special inlay, anti-inflammatory drugs, plaster casting for a minimum of 6 weeks, and infiltration. Operative treatment

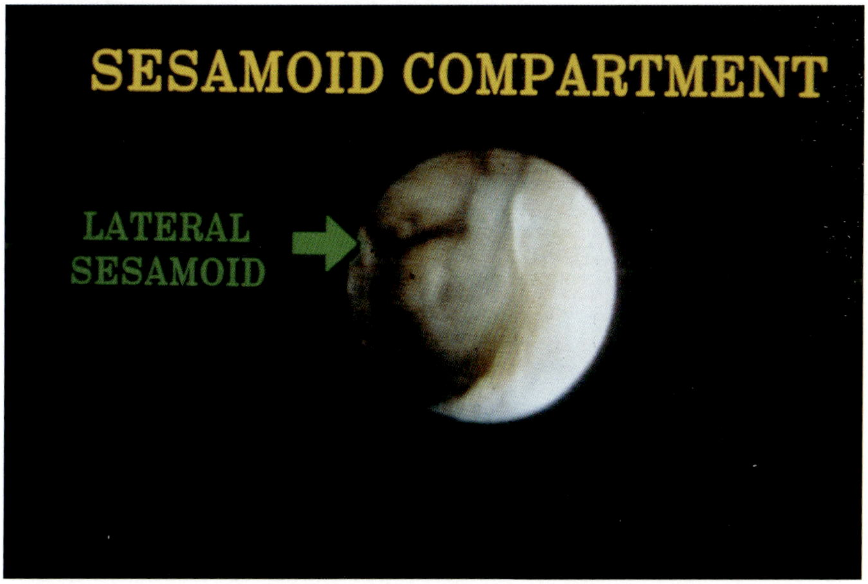

FIGURE 14.3. Arthroscopic view of the lateral sesamoid bone.

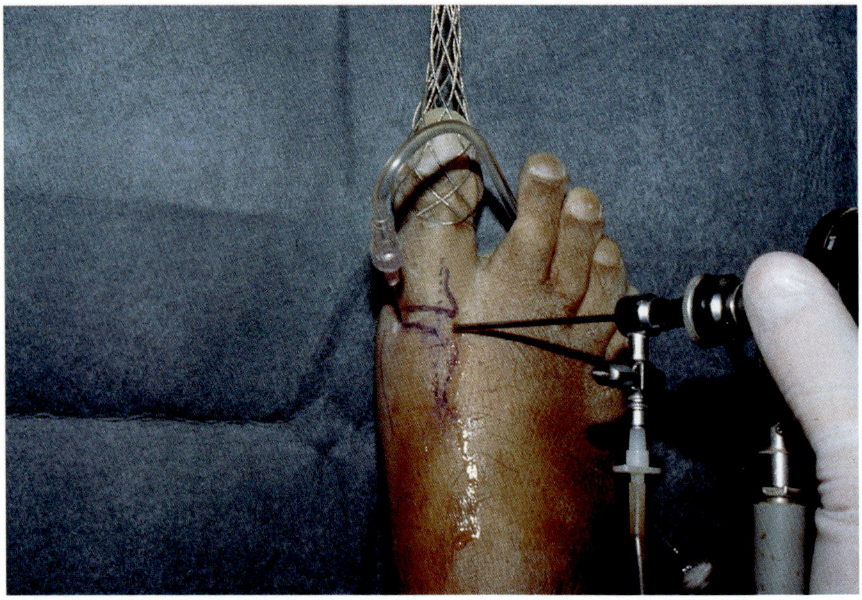

FIGURE 14.4. First metatarsophalangeal (MTP) joint in traction with arthroscope in the anterolateral portal.

(Figs. 14.1–14.3) with removal of the deformed sesamoid bone gives inconsistent results.

Hallux Rigidus

Davies-Colley (1887) was the first to describe hallux rigidus. Its possible etiologic factors are arthrosis deformans, repetitive microtrauma during sports activities,[10] macrotrauma, aseptic necrosis, osteochondritis dissecans,[11,15,16] and limited range of motion whereby dorsiflexion, especially, is progressively diminished. Progressive pain finally makes normal walking impossible. Radiography during the first stage may show no deformity. At a later stage, however, joint space narrowing and osteophytes become apparent. Operative options are resection of osteophytes, partial resection of the proximal one-third of the first phalanx,[12] arthrodesis, and silicon interposition arthroplasty.[13,17,19]

OPERATIVE TECHNIQUE

An autopsy study was first performed to verify portal anatomy (Figs. 14.4–14.7). Four main portals were developed, which allowed a complete overview of the first metatarsal joint. The two main portals

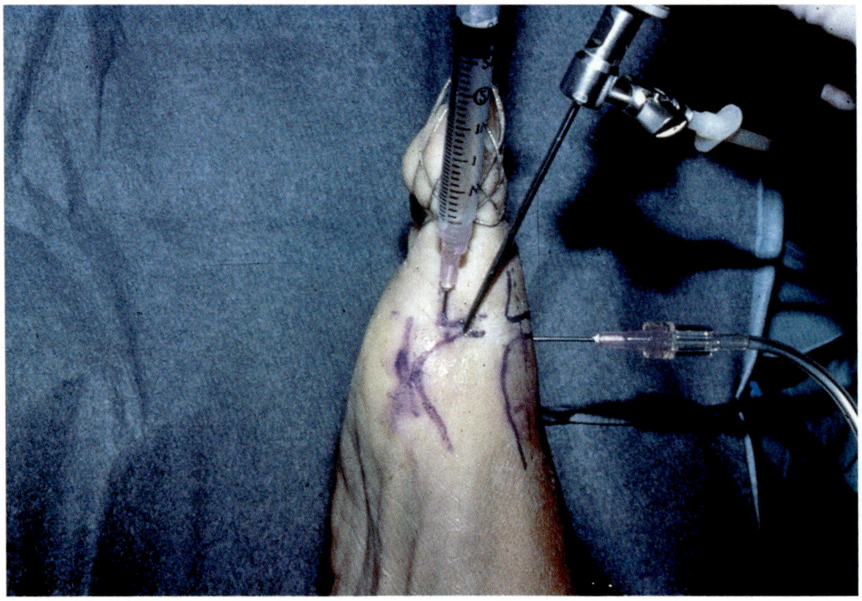

FIGURE 14.5. Lateral view. Arthroscope is in the anteromedial portal. Syringe and needle are below the arthroscope in the joint.

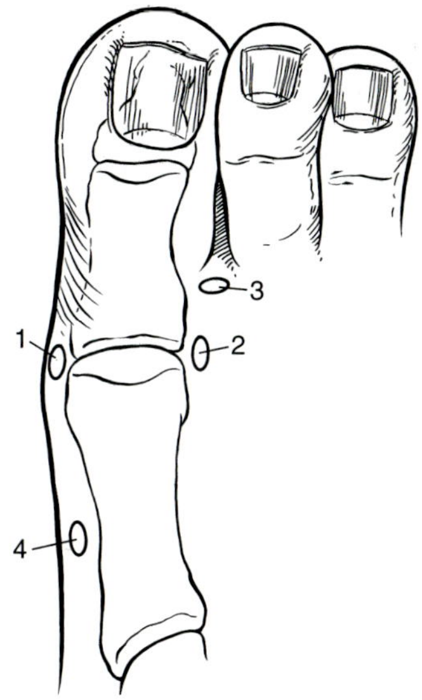

FIGURE 14.6. Anteromedial (1) and anterolateral (2) portals are the two main portals. Two additional portals were made to visualize the plantar side of the joint including the sesamoid bones. One is located in the web space between the first and second toes (3). The second one was made 4 cm proximal to the joint line between the abductor and short flexor muscle (4).

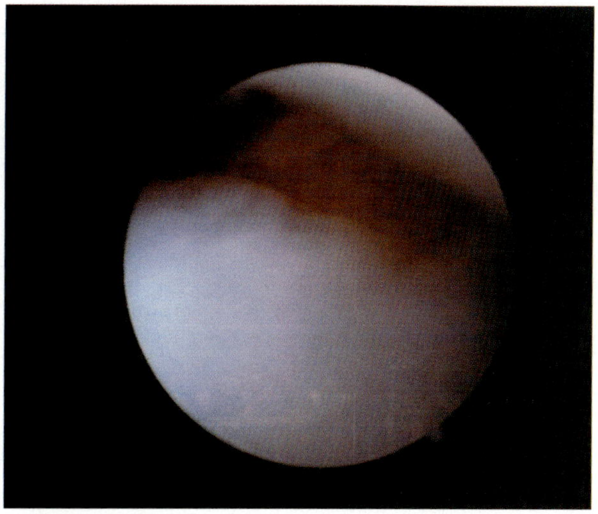

FIGURE 14.7. Arthroscopic view of the first MTP joint. Note the softening of the chondral surface of the head plus the irregularity. Some synovitis is seen.

are the anteromedial and anterolateral ones. They are located medially and laterally from the extensor hallucis longus tendon.[14] An incision is made through the skin only, and the joint is penetrated by blunt dissection. For visualizing the plantar side of the joint, including the sesamoid bones, two additional portals are needed. One is located in the web space between the first and second toes. The second is made 4 cm proximal to the joint line on the medial side of the joint between the abductor and short flexor muscles. A 2.7 mm arthroscope with an inclination angle of 30 degrees is introduced through the anteromedial portal. The instruments are introduced through the anterolateral portal. When the joint is filled with saline and placed in dorsiflexion, the dorsal aspect of the joint can be visualized. When synovitis is present, a shaver or whisker is used for removal, and osteophytes are resected by the abrader or small acromionizer (Figs. 14.8, 14.9). Manual distraction is usually sufficient to visualize the head of the metatarsal and base of the first pha-

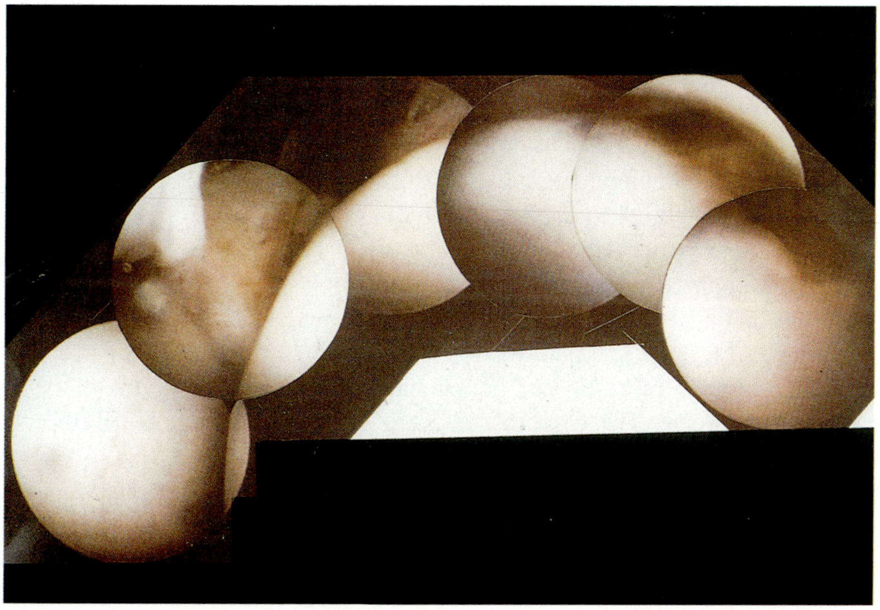

FIGURE 14.8. Arthroscopic view of the metatarsal head and the cartilage of the phalanx. The dorsal aspect of the cartilage of the metatarsal head is irregular and soft. Proximal to this cartilage rim the synovial reflection on the metatarsal bone can be seen.

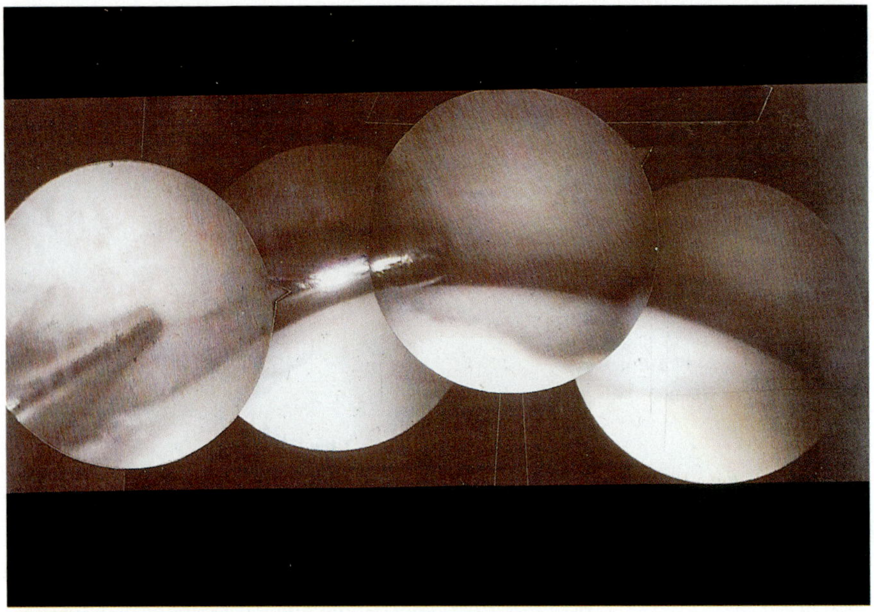

FIGURE 14.9. Arthroscopic view of the same patient as in Figure 14.8. Metatarsal head shows a cartilage defect with smooth edges. Note the obduration.

lanx. The arthroscope can be brought through the anteromedial portal to the plantar side of the joint as necessary to visualize and treat pathology in the lateral sesamoid bone (Figs. 14.1–14.5). The operation is performed as an outpatient procedure under general or regional anesthesia.

RESULTS

Altogether, 27 arthroscopies were performed in 26 patients.[19] There were 18 females and 8 males with an average of 33.6 years (range 16–61 years). In 15 cases the right joint was involved and in 12 patients the left joint. The indications were impingement syndrome (12 patients), nonunion of the sesamoid bone (5 patients), hallux rigidus (5 patients), and osteochondritis dissecans (4 patients). One patient was treated arthroscopically for bacterial arthritis of the first MTP joint.

There were no complications apart from a transient loss of sensibility in one patient on the medial side and in one patient on the lateral side of the big toe. In the impingement group at the 1-year follow-up, three patients had the same level of pain and swelling as they did preoperatively. All others improved, although three still had occasional pain after heavy exercise. The final results were already apparent at the 4-month follow-up. Eight patients had been unable to work preoperatively because of their deformity. At the 1-year follow-up only two patients had not resumed work. Resumption of sports participation was possible in nine patients. Any increased range of motion of more than 5 degrees was found in six patients, with an average increase of 13 degrees (7–20 degrees). There was a subjective good or excellent result in seven patients. In the sesamoid group, there were two patients in whom the lateral sesamoid was removed arthroscopically, whereas in the other three patients the medial sesamoid showed cartilage damage or fragmentation. Arthroscopic removal using a small burr was unsuccessful for the medial sesamoid. In all cases, the medial sesamoid was removed through a small, separate incision. There were two poor results and one fair result. The two patients who underwent arthroscopic excision of the lateral sesamoid had a good result, although they occasionally experienced pain during or after activity. In the hallux rigidus group, two patients showed no improvement, whereas the other three exhibited slight improvement.

In the osteochondritis dissecans group, treatment consisted of débridement and drilling or removal of loose bodies. Three of the four patients had a good or excellent result at the 1-year follow-up (Fig. 14.10).

DISCUSSION

Using the four portals described makes it possible to visualize the entire first MTP joint. The standard anteromedial and anterolateral portals provide ac-

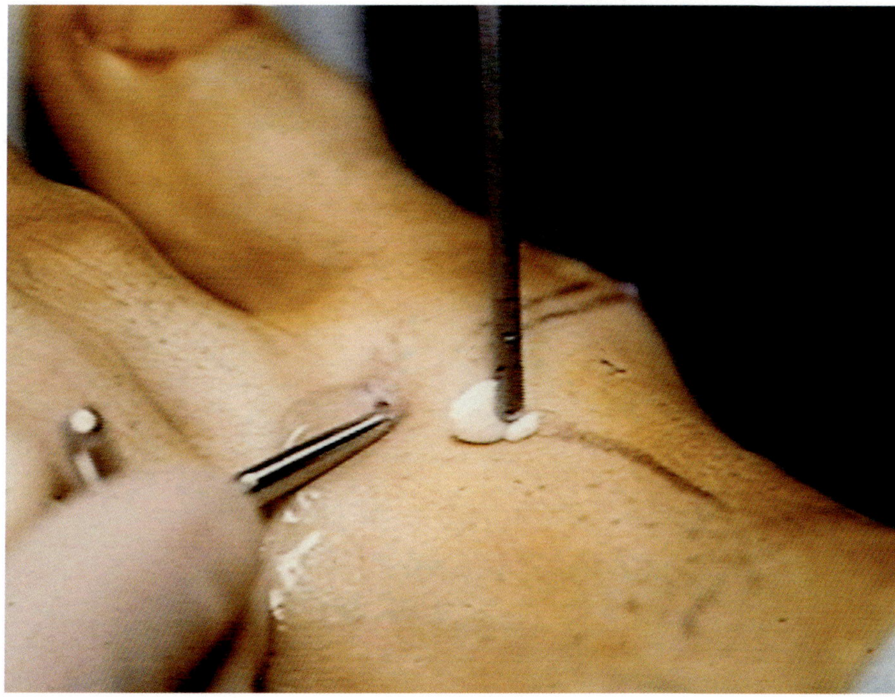

FIGURE 14.10. Arthroscopic loose body removal from the MTP joint of the right foot. The size of the loose body can be appreciated.

cess to the dorsal joint compartment. Osteophytes and synovitis can be removed by slight dorsiflexion of the joint. An osteochondral defect can be treated by applying traction to the big toe manually, making use of the same portals. For visualizing and treating pathology in the plantar compartment, the anteromedial portal should be combined with the two described additional portals in the web space and the proximal medial portal.

Five types of pathology were recognized preoperatively: impingement syndrome, nonunion of the sesamoid bone, hallux rigidus, osteochondritis dissecans, and infectious arthritis. Analysis of our results showed that osteochondritis dissecans and infectious arthritis can be easily treated arthroscopically. The dorsal impingement syndrome, with pain on forced dorsiflexion and limited range of motion, gave promising results. Especially in professional athletes, arthroscopic removal of osteophytes seems to be beneficial owing to less fibrous scarring and quicker rehabilitation. Only three patients still experienced pain at the 1-year follow-up. A significant increase in dorsiflexion was present in only half of the cases. The hallux rigidus group is too small to be considered separately, but our results are not encouraging for this group. The same is true for the sesamoid pathology group. Arthroscopy makes it possible to visualize the joint between the sesamoid bone and the plantar side of the phalanx. If there is degeneration or fragmentation, it might be an indication for removal. The results of removing a sesamoid bone in our patients, however, did not differ from those reported for open surgery series.

BIBLIOGRAPHY

1. Whipple TL. The wrist. In: Whipple TL (ed) *Arthroscopic surgery*. Philadelphia: Lippincott, 1992;1–9.
2. Burman MS. Arthroscopy or direct visualization of joints. *J Bone Joint Surg* 13:669–695.
3. Tagaki K. The arthroscope. *J Jpn Orthop Assoc* 1939;14:359–384.
4. Watanabe M, Ito K, Fujii S. Equipment and procedures of small joint arthroscopy. In: Watanabe M (ed) *Arthroscopy of small joints*. New York: Igaku-Shoin, 1985;3–30.
5. Bartlett DH. Arthroscopic management of osteochondritis dissecans of the first metatarsal head. *Arthroscopy* 1988;4:51–54.
6. Biedert R. Anterior ankle pain in sports medicine: etiology and indications for arthroscopy. *Arthrosc Orthop Trauma Surg* 1991;110:293–297.
7. Van Dijk CN, Lim LSL, Portmann A., et al. Degenerative joint disease in female ballet dancers. *Am J Sportsmed* 1995;3:295–301.
8. Carell B, Childress HM. Osteochondritis dissecans of a metatarsal head. *J Bone Joint Surg* 1940;22:442–443.
9. Kilokuim H. *Hallux valgus, allied deformities of the forefoot*. Philadelphia: Saunders, 1965;337–351.

10. Waterman H. Die arthritis deformans des Grosszehengrundgelankes. *Orthop Chir* 1927;48:236.
11. Kingreen O. Zur aetiologie de Hallux flexus. *Zentralbl Chir* 1933;60:2116–2118.
12. Brandes M. Zur operativen therapie des Hallus valgus. *Zentralblf. Chir* 1929;56:2434–2440.
13. Weirgart M, Klems H. Wert der Silikon-Interpositions arthroplastic am Gross-Zekegrundgelank am Grossehengrundgelenk. *Ortop Praxis* 1976;12:510.
14. Van Dijk CN. Arthroscopy of the MPTJ joint. *Acta Orthop Scand* 1993;64(suppl 253):11.
15. Goodfellow J. Etiology of Hallux rigidus. *Proc R Soc Med* 1966;59:821–824.
16. Hackenbroch M. Hallux rigidus. *Verh Dtsch Ortop* 1927;22:169.
17. Hohlmann D. *Fuss and Bein*, 5th ed. Munich: Bergmann, 1956.
18. Nilsoone H. Hallux rigidus and its treatment. *Acta Orthop Scand* 1930;1:295.
19. Dijk Van CN, Veenstra KM, Neusch B. Arthroscopic surgery of the MTP-I joint. *Arthroscopy* 1998;14: 851–855.

CHAPTER 15

Calcaneocuboid Joint Arthroscopy

Lawrence Oloff and Gary Fanton

The application of standard large-joint arthroscopic techniques to small joints has been a natural evolution primarily dependent on the development of appropriately small instrumentation. The 2.3 mm arthroscope and small shaver systems utilized and proven proficient for wrist arthroscopy have now been applied to the smaller joints of the foot. We have found arthroscopy quite useful for examining the calcaneocuboid joint and have reported our experience with several cases in 1996. The minishaver seems to have some limitations in terms of fully accessing the peculiar anatomy and confined calcaneocuboid articulation, which is a saddle-shaped joint. These anatomic space limitations of the calcaneocuboid joint in the past restricted the usefulness of arthroscopy to being mainly a diagnostic tool at this site. With the advent of the holmium laser and small radiofrequency devices, however, arthroscopy of the calcaneocuboid joint has proven to be as therapeutically rewarding as traditional arthroscopy of larger joints. Combined with new mechanical instrumentation, these devices may soon lead to more universal acceptance of arthroscopic procedures to small joints of the foot.[1,2]

INDICATIONS

Pathology of the calcaneocuboid joint is often poorly understood. It is not that midfoot complaints are uncommon but, rather, that they are not easily diagnosed and are often overlooked. Most calcaneocuboid complaints fall under the category of mechanically induced pain. Chronic synovitis and impingement syndromes identified in this area of the foot often result from hypermobility, arthritic erosions, and spur formation. The term cuboid syndrome (CS) has been used to describe these related conditions collectively. All of the aforementioned conditions are common indications for arthroscopy of the calcaneocuboid joint.[3,4]

The diagnostic workup for patients with CS is sometimes extensive. Diagnostic imaging techniques may be useful for arriving at a diagnosis before arthroscopy is considered. Magnetic resonance imaging (MRI) may be employed to rule out stress injuries and injuries to the contiguous peroneal tendons and then to identify soft tissue masses. Osteochondral lesions, osteophytic bone, and osseous neoplasia may be evaluated by computed tomography (CT). Even sophisticated imaging techniques may fail to establish the diagnosis. Furthermore, the diagnosis of CS is often unclear because of many secondary complaints, such as plantar fasciitis. Nonoperative care usually uncovers the secondary complaints, revealing focused pain in the calcaneocuboid joint. It is the refractory pain of the calcaneocuboid joint that best characterizes CS. If any doubt remains that the calcaneocuboid joint remains the primary source of pain, selective diagnostic blocks may be applied to this joint. Contrast dye is combined with local anesthetic to ensure that the injection enters the joint space. Only after the location of the pain is confirmed and nonoperative care fails to resolve the patient's complaints in a reasonable time should arthroscopy of this joint be considered. Nonoperative care options to try first are steroid injections, physical therapy, antiinflammatory drugs, orthotics, and immobilization.

Many patients have undergone calcaneocuboid joint arthroscopy for CS without a clear-cut diagnosis. In such cases, several pathologic conditions may be encountered and so should be considered. The differential diagnosis should include disorders considered for any chronically painful joint, including systemic diagnoses, such as the synovium-based rheumatic diseases as well as the more commonly encountered local conditions. Posttraumatic disorders are encountered as with any joint, such as the lateral impingement syndromes that result from fractures in this region, loose bodies, chronic synovitis, and osteochondral injuries.[3] We have also noted fibrotic synovial bands and plicas in this region. A previously undescribed anomaly of this joint—synovial hypertrophy of the dorsal joint margin—appears to correlate with rupture and repair of the dorsal capsule. When one becomes clinically astute as to the causes of pathology in this region, many potentially treatable cases should be identified. Arthroscopic intervention has proven useful in such cases and offers a less morbid approach than arthrodesis for chronic pain in this joint.

CONTRAINDICATIONS

There are relatively few contraindications to arthroscopy of the calcaneocuboid joint. The suitability of the patient for elective surgery is a consideration, as with any surgical procedure. The procedure is typically carried out with regional or general anesthesia. Any contraindications to these methods of anesthesia should be considered. The condition of the integument may be a consideration, especially in posttraumatic cases where the skin and underlying structures may have been previously violated. As the procedure is often facilitated by use of a tourniquet, vascular assessment of the lower extremity is important. Sometimes scarring of the area compromises access and visualization, such as with arthrofibrosis, and may prove to be a relative contraindication. When limitation of motion is noted, the patient should be forewarned that arthrotomy may be necessary.

The most significant complications and failures related to calcaneocuboid joint arthroscopy are the result of misdiagnosis. The key is to ensure that one is not dealing with an extraarticular phenomenon. Diagnostic blocks can prove useful for confirming the calcaneocuboid joint as the origin of the patient's complaints. It is important to confirm that what is thought to be calcaneocuboid joint pain is not in reality peroneal tendon pain. MRI and tenography can help rule out such pathology.[4,5]

SURGICAL TECHNIQUE

The procedure is usually carried out under regional or general anesthesia. The patient is positioned in the supine or lateral position, the preference often dictated by the need to do any additional procedures. A tourniquet is often required to facilitate visualization and can be placed at the ankle level. An attempt is first made to distend the joint by infusing saline with a 23-gauge needle and small syringe. The calcaneocuboid joint does not have much capacity for distension.

Mapping out the anatomy is important. The procedure is carried out by placing two closely approximated portals (Fig. 15.1). The more medial portal is made approximately at the level of the anterior process of the calcaneus. The intermediate dorsal cutaneous nerve thus lies just medial to this portal and must be mapped out. The more lateral portal is made 2 to 3 cm below the medial portal, near the joint line. This inferior portal is placed to avoid the peroneus brevis tendon and sural nerve. Both structures are just plantar to the portal. Because of neighboring subcutaneous structures, it is important to make the incision through the skin only and to proceed more deeply, utilizing blunt dissection with a small "mosquito" clamp. This helps prevent unnecessary trauma to underlying vascular and neurologic structures.

Standard arthroscopic small-joint instrumentation is employed (Fig. 15.2). An arthroscopic cannula and blunt obturator is inserted through one portal, and the joint is inspected. A 2.3 mm 30 degree arthroscopic lens is employed. Others have suggested use of a 4.0 mm lens, but it is difficult to introduce without damaging the joint. An 18-gauge needle is placed at the lateral portal or more inferiorly for initial distension and egress. A 2.5 mm mini-shaver may be utilized and provides adequate outflow, allowing the surgeon eventually to discard the 18-gauge needle. The portals may be used interchangeably to facilitate visualization and access. A switching rod is advised to maintain instrument position during the exchange, as position is easily lost. Although the mini-shaver is the mainstay débriding instrument, there are limitations with its use in some instances because of the joint shape and

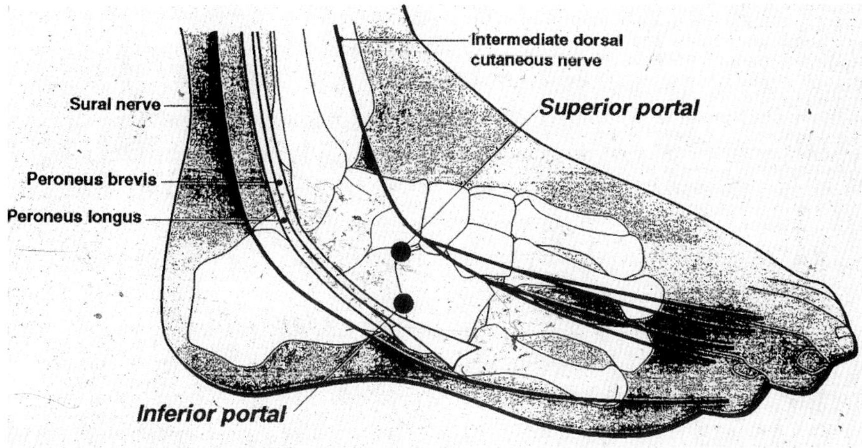

FIGURE 15.1. Calcaneocuboid joint anatomy and portal placement.

angle of approach. The 1.7 mm holmium-YAG laser has proven most useful for débriding the joint. The 30- and 70-degree handpieces may be employed. Recently, we started to use a smaller laser instrument designed for wrist arthroscopy. Although it is a straight handpiece, the smaller size makes it ideally suited for the confines of this small joint.

A small radiofrequency (RF) thermal probe (Oratec Interventions, Menlo Park, CA) has been utilized as well. The main advantage of the RF device is that it is much less likely to damage healthy cartilage inadvertently. Its smooth metallic tip and temperature-regulated energy output provide safer navigation and treatment than the laser devices. It ablates and sculpts unhealthy cartilage that is fibrillated in areas of chondromalacia. It is also useful for performing synovectomy and coagulation when necessary. The probes utilize a 1.5 mm shaft that can be bent at the time of surgery to facilitate access.

RESULTS AND COMPLICATIONS

Arthroscopy of the calcaneocuboid joint is relatively new. The indications and instrumentation to perform this procedure effectively are evolving. We have treated 12 such cases over the past 3 years. Two of the twelve patients were converted to open arthrotomy because of poor visualization. These two patients shared a traumatic etiology for their complaints and resultant arthrofibrosis that hampered instrumentation and visualization. Of the remaining ten cases, the results have been overwhelmingly favorable, and only one patient did not report significant improvement in his symptoms postoperatively. That patient went on to successful surgical fusion of the calcaneocuboid joint.

There were no complications encountered. However, there was an interesting side effect that occurred in this patient population postoperatively: 40% of the patients developed temporary peroneus

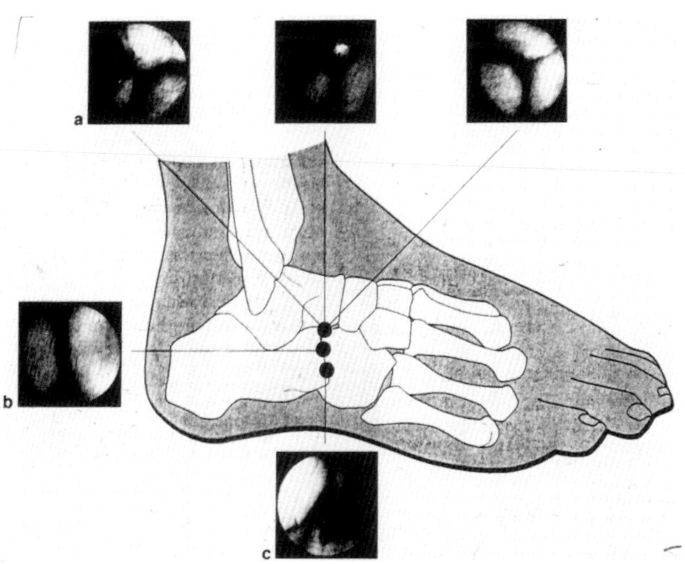

FIGURE 15.2. Another version of Figure 15.1 with three portals.

brevis tendonitis. The exact mechanism for this inflammatory response is unclear. We can only postulate that the mechanism observed may be analogous to what is seen with subtalar joint irritation, where peroneal spasm can limit motion in the hindfoot. In the case of calcaneocuboid joint arthroscopy, the peroneal symptoms were transient and dissipated after a few weeks with organized physical therapy and antiinflammatory medications.

Most of our patients had a diagnosis of CS. In some of them the onset of pain resulted from a traumatic episode. Various pathologies were discovered in this group, including osteochondral lesions, impingement lesions, posttraumatic arthritis, and loose bodies. Although diagnostic imaging was universally carried out, the pathology was not appreciated in all of the cases by such means. Chondral lesions in particular were appreciated only on direct arthroscopic visualization of the joint. Most of the CS patients had no antecedent traumatic event, and in such cases the cause was suspected to be related to poor foot mechanics. One arthroscopic procedure was performed in a patient with CS that seemingly originated as a result of complete plantar fascial release for chronic heel pain. Overloading of the lateral column is a recognized sequela after plantar fascial release, and the chronic synovitis that ensues may potentially be treated by arthroscopy.

The postoperative program in patients who have undergone calcaneocuboid joint arthroscopy is evolving as well. Our protocol has been to keep the patients non-weight-bearing for 3 weeks but to initiate motion via a continuous passive motion apparatus on the second postoperative day. Although this approach may seem conservative, the overall rate of recovery has been faster than that of the initial study patients who ambulated early.

An arthroscopic approach to a variety of pathologies of the calcaneocuboid joint is clearly feasible at this time. Disorders of this joint are not uncommon, and arthroscopy effectively expands the surgeon's armamentarium of techniques for treating chronic, painful disorders of this joint. Admittedly, the learning curve of this procedure is rather steep and is probably best reserved for the more experienced arthroscopist.

BIBLIOGRAPHY

1. Frey C, Glasser S, Feder K. Arthroscopy of the subtalar joint. *Foot Ankle Int* 1994;15:424–428.
2. Nagle DJ, Benson LS. Wrist arthroscopy: indications and results. *Arthroscopy* 1992;8:198–203.
3. Oloff L, Schulhofer SD, Fanton GS, Dillingham MD. Arthroscopy of the calcaneocuboid and talonavicular joints. *J Foot Ankle Surg* 1996;35:101–108.
4. Parisien JS, Vangsness T. Arthroscopy of the subtalar joint: an experimental approach. *Arthroscopy* 1992;8:198–203.
5. Scranton PE Jr, Ferkel RD, Hamilton WG, et al. Symposium: arthroscopy of the ankle and foot. *Contemp Orthop* 1993;26:67–93.

CHAPTER 16

Hindfoot Endoscopy for Posterior Ankle Pain

C.N. van Dijk

During the past decades arthroscopy has become a major tool for diagnosing and treating articular lesions. The role of arthroscopy has been established for indications such as impingement syndromes, synovitis, osteochondral lesions, loose bodies, and arthrosis. Extraarticular pathology demands open surgery, which requires postoperative plaster immobilization to prevent equinus malformation and to stimulate wound healing.[1,2]

A variety of soft tissue pathology can be present around the ankle joint. In the absence of intraarticular damage, posteromedial ankle complaints most often are caused by disorders of the posterior tibial tendon.[3] In the event of failure of conservative treatment, posterior tibial tendon disorders can be treated by open surgery.[1]

Posteromedial overuse and posttraumatic injuries in ballet dancers and soccer players most often are caused by tenosynovitis of the flexor hallucis longus tendon, a posterior impingement syndrome, or both. Posterolateral ankle complaints most often are caused by disorders of the peroneal tendons such as tenosynovitis, partial rupture, and tendon subluxation.

Endoscopic surgery offers the advantage of less morbidity, reduced postoperative pain, and outpatient treatment.[4] We performed a cadaver study as well as a subsequent prospective study in which 240 diagnostic and therapeutic endoscopic procedures were performed in 229 consecutive patients.

POSTERIOR ANKLE IMPINGEMENT

Posterior ankle syndrome is a pain syndrome. The patient experiences posterior ankle pain mainly present on forced plantar flexion. Forced dorsiflexion is also painful in some patients. In this hyperdorsiflexion position, traction is applied to the posterior joint capsule and posterior talar fibular ligament, both of which attach to the posterior talar process. Posterior ankle impingement is caused by overuse or trauma. Distinction between these two disorders seems important because posterior impingement through overuse has a better prognosis.[5] A posterior ankle impingement syndrome through overuse is found mainly in ballet dancers and runners.[6–8] Running that involves forced plantar flexion (e.g., downhill running) can put repetitive stress on the posterior aspect of the ankle joint.[8] In ballet dancers, forceful plantar flexion during the en pointe or demi-pointe position produces compression at the posterior aspect of the ankle joint. Joint mobility and range of motion gradually increase through exercise. In the presence of a prominent posterior talar process or an os trigonum, this can lead to compression of these structures.

In 1995 we reported on a group of 19 retired dancers and examined their ankle and subtalar joints.[6] The mean length of ballet dancers' professional career was 37 years. All of the dancers had been dancing en pointe. None of these dancers had suffered a posterior ankle impingement syndrome. A hypertrophic posterior talar process or an os trigonum was present in 18 of the 38 investigated ankle joints. The presence of an os trigonum itself therefore does not seem to be relevant. This anatomic anomaly must be combined with a traumatic event such as supination trauma, dancing on hard surfaces, or pushing beyond anatomic limits. The pain is caused by an abnormal movement between the os trigonum and talus or compression of a thickened joint capsule/scar tissue between the os trigonum and the posterior tibial rim.

A diagnosis can be made on the basis of the history, physical examination, and radiographs. During examination there is pain at palpation of the posterior aspect of the talus. The posterior talar process can be palpated posterolaterally between peroneal tendons and the Achilles tendon. On the posteromedial side, the neurovascular bundle and flexor tendons cover the talus. Posteromedial pain on palpation therefore does not automatically indicate impingement pain. The passive forced plantar flexion test is most important. With this test the examiner performs repetitive quick passive forced plantar hyperflexion movements. The test can be repeated in slight exorotation or slight endorotation of the foot relative to the tibia. The investigator should apply this rotation movement on the point of maximal plantar flexion, thereby "grinding" the posterior talar process/os trigonum between the posterior tibial rim and the calcaneus. A negative test rules out a posterior impingement syndrome. A positive test in combination with pain on posterolateral palpation can be followed by a diagnostic infiltration. The infiltration is performed from the posterolateral position, whereby the capsule between the prominent posterior talar process and the posterior edge of the tibia is infiltrated with lidocaine (Xylocaine). If the pain disappears on forced plantar flexion, the diagnosis is confirmed. A lateral radiograph is obtained if an os trigonum is suspected.

Flexor hallucis longus tendinitis is often present in patients with posterior ankle impingement syndrome, with the pain located posteromedially. The flexor hallucis longus tendon can be palpated behind the medial malleolus. By asking the patient to flex the toes repetitively with the ankle in 10°–20° plantar flexion, the flexor hallucis longus tendon can be palpated in its gliding channel behind the medial malleolus. The tendon glides up and down under the palpating finger of the examiner. In a case of stenosing tendinitis or chronic inflammation, there may be crepitus and recognizable pain. Sometimes a nodule in the tendon can be moved up and down under the palpating finger.

Nonoperative treatment of posterior ankle impingement syndrome and flexor hallucis longus tendinitis involves modifications of activities, physical therapy (massage stretching and muscle strengthening), and steroid injections. The steroids are injected posterolaterally into the posterior joint capsule between the prominent posterior talar process and the posterior tibial edge. Physicians who are not familiar with this type of infiltration are advised to perform the infiltration under fluoroscopic control.

ACHILLES TENDINITIS

Overuse injuries of the Achilles tendon can be divided into insertional and noninsertional tendinitis.[9] Because there is no evidence of inflammation in patients with "tendinitis," the term tendinosis has been proposed.[10]

Noninsertional tendinitis can be divided into three subgroups: paratendinitis, paratendinitis + tendinosis, and tendinosis. Paratendinitis is characterized by inflammation of only the lining of the tendon. With acute paratendinitis there is diffuse swelling around the tendon. Most cases of isolated paratendinitis respond well to conservative treatment.

In patients with paratendinitis + tendinosis there is localized swelling, most often 4–7 cm above the insertion of the Achilles tendon. On examination there is pain, particularly when the tendon is squeezed. Most often the pain is localized predominantly on the medial side. Magnetic resonance imaging (MRI) demonstrates marked thickening of the tendon.

In patients with Achilles tendinosis, fields of local degeneration in the tendon are present. With advanced tendinosis, as a result of chronic degeneration the tendon elongates and is no longer in functional continuity. There is often an increase in passive range of dorsiflexion. Insertional tendinitis can be classified as retrocalcaneal bursitis, retrocalcaneal bursitis + insertional tendinosis, and insertional tendinosis.

Chronic retrocalcaneal bursitis is accompanied by deep pain and swelling of the posterior soft tissue just in front of the Achilles tendon. The prominent bursa can be palpated medially and laterally from the tendon at its insertion. The lateral radiograph demonstrates the characteristic prominent superior calcaneal deformity. Operative treatment involves removal of the bursa and resection of the lateral and medial posterosuperior aspect of the calcaneus. Postoperative treatment involves use of a below-knee weight-bearing cast for 4 weeks.[9] Retrocalcaneal bursitis is often accompanied by midportion insertional tendinosis. Often a partial rupture of the midportion of the tendon is present at its insertion. When operative treatment for retrocalcaneal bursitis is indicated, débridement of the midportion of the Achilles insertion should be considered in case of a partial rupture.

In the case of insertional tendinosis, there is pain at the bone–tendon junction that worsens after exercise. The tenderness is specifically located directly posterior to the junction. Radiographic signs of ossification at the most distal extent of the insertion of the tendon (bone spur) are typical signs of insertional Achilles tendinosis. Most patients can be managed with nonoperative means, such as widening and deepening of the heel counter of the shoe. When operative treatment is indicated, the pathological ossifications and spurs can best be approached by a central heel-splitting incision.

Heavy-load eccentric calf muscle training has been demonstrated to be effective treatment for chronic Achilles tendinosis + paratendinitis.[11] For operative treatment of paratendinitis, the diseased and thickened paratenon is excised. Operative treatment of chronic tendinosis consists of débridement of the paratenon and removal of degenerative necrotic tissue. The thickened degenerative portion of the tendon is excised, and the defect is closed primarily.

Revascularization is stimulated by making multiple longitudinal incisions into the tendon.[9] Open surgery produces a guarded prognosis. In fact, Maffulli recently reported poor results in more than 60% of patients.[12]

Open surgery for insertional tendinitis with removal of the chronic inflamed bursa and the posterosuperior prominence of the calcaneus can be associated with a poor outcome. Open surgical treatment requires plaster immobilization to prevent equinus malformation and to stimulate wound healing.[1,2] Angermann reported a cure rate of only 50% after open surgery for chronic retrocalcaneal bursitis.[13] Endoscopic treatment offers the advantage of less morbidity, reduced postoperative pain, and outpatient treatment.[4]

POSTERIOR TIBIAL TENDON PATHOLOGY

On the posteromedial side of the ankle joint, intraarticular lesions such as posteromedial impingement syndrome, calcifications in the dorsal capsule of the ankle joint, subtalar pathology, loose body, or osteochondral defect must be excluded. The most common extraarticular disorders are tenosynovitis of the posterior tibial tendon, disorders of the flexor hallucis longus tendon, and the tarsal tunnel syndrome.

Postsurgery and postfracture adhesions and irregularity of the posterior aspect of the tibia (posterial tibial sliding channel) can be responsible for symptoms in this region (Fig. 16.1). The posterior tibial tendon plays an important role in normal hindfoot function.[14] Several investigators have described the development of posterior tibial dysfunction as the disease progresses from peritendinitis to elongation, degeneration, and rupture.[2,3,15–17]

Tenosynovitis is often seen in association with flat feet and with psoriatic and rheumatic arthritis. In the early stage of posterior tibial dysfunction, tenosynovitis is the main symptom. Tenosynovectomy can be performed if conservative treatment fails.[18]

Entrapment of the posterior tibial nerve in the tarsal canal is commonly known as a tarsal tunnel syndrome.[19] Clinical examination should be sufficient to differentiate these disorders from an isolated posterior tibial disorder.

PERONEAL TENDON DISORDERS

Tenosynovitis of the peroneal tendons, dislocation, rupture, and snapping of one of the peroneal tendons account for most of the symptoms at the posterolateral side of the ankle joint.[20,21] This disorder must be differentiated from (fatigue) fractures of the fibula, lesions of the lateral ligament complex, and posterolateral impingement (os trigonum syndrome).

Peroneal tendon disorders are often associated and secondary to chronic lateral ankle instability. Because the peroneal muscles act as lateral ankle stabilizers, more strain is placed on their tendons in the presence of chronic lateral instability, resulting in hypertrophic tendinopathy, tenosynovitis, and ultimately in (partial) tendon tears.[2,3,22] The diagnosis may be difficult in a patient with lateral ankle pain. Peroneal tendon dislocation and tenosynovitis can be established by clinical examination. In the case of subtotal tears of the peroneus brevis or longus tendon, supplemental investigations might be helpful for establishing the diagnosis.[22] Postsurgery and postfracture adhesions and irregularities in the posterior aspect of the fibula (i.e., ten-

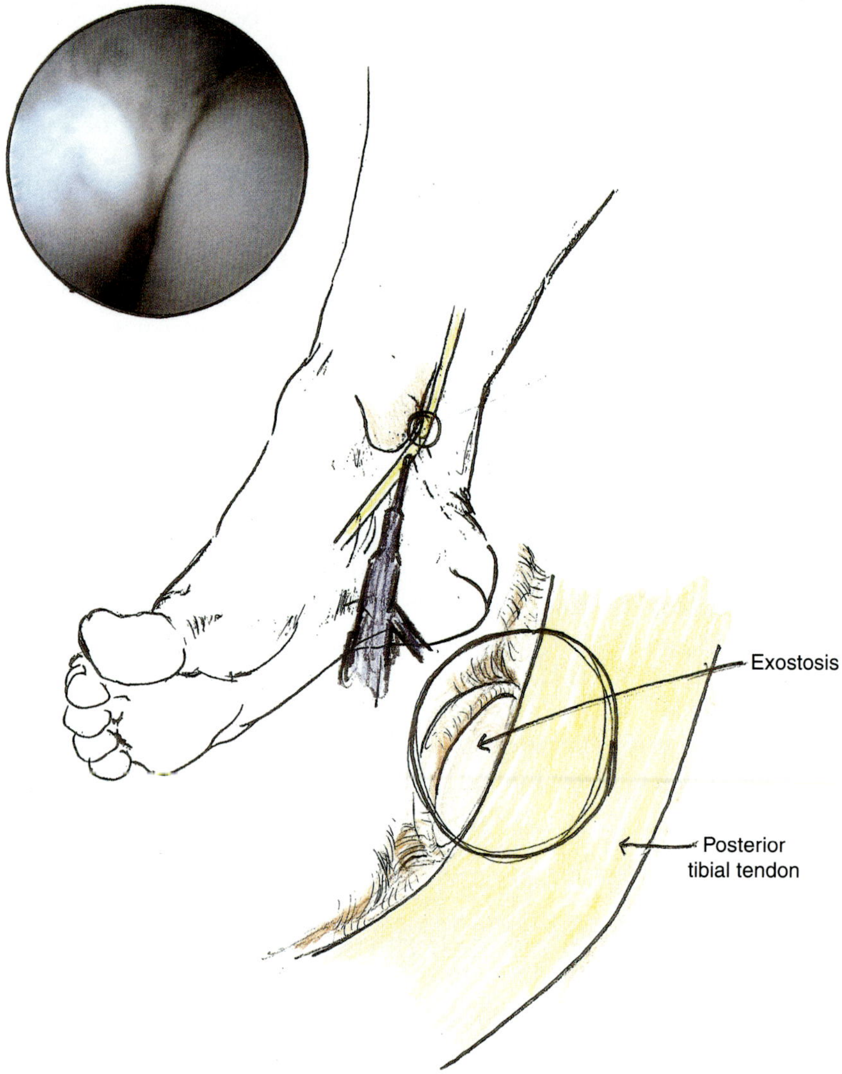

FIGURE 16.1. Exostosis of the medial malleolus compressing on the posterior tibial tendon in a right ankle.

dons sliding channel) can be responsible for symptoms in this region.

OPERATIVE TECHNIQUE

Access to the tendons can be obtained anywhere along the tendons. The two main portals for posterior tibial and peroneal tendoscopy are located directly over the involved tendon 1.5–2.0 cm distal and 1.5–2.0 cm proximal to the posterior edge of the malleolus. The distal portal is made first, with an incision through the skin. The tendon sheath is penetrated by the arthroscope shaft with a blunt trocar. A 2.7 mm arthroscope with an inclination angle of 30° is introduced. After introducing a spinal needle under direct vision, an incision is made through the skin into the tendon sheath to create a proximal portal. Instruments such as probes, a disposable cutting knife, scissors, or a shaver system are introduced. Through the distal portal on the medial side, a complete overview can be obtained of the posterior tibial tendon, from its insertion (navicular bone) to some 6 cm above the level of the tip of the medial malleolus. The complete tendon sheath can be inspected by rotating the scope over the tendon (Fig. 16.2). Through the distal portal on the lateral side, a complete overview can be obtained of both peroneal tendons. The inspection starts some 6 cm proximal from the posterior tip of the lateral malleolus, where a thin membrane splits the tendon compartment into two chambers (Fig. 16.3). More distally, both tendons lie in one compartment (Fig. 16.4). The complete compartment can be inspected by rotating the endoscope over and between the two tendons (Figs. 16.5, 16.6).

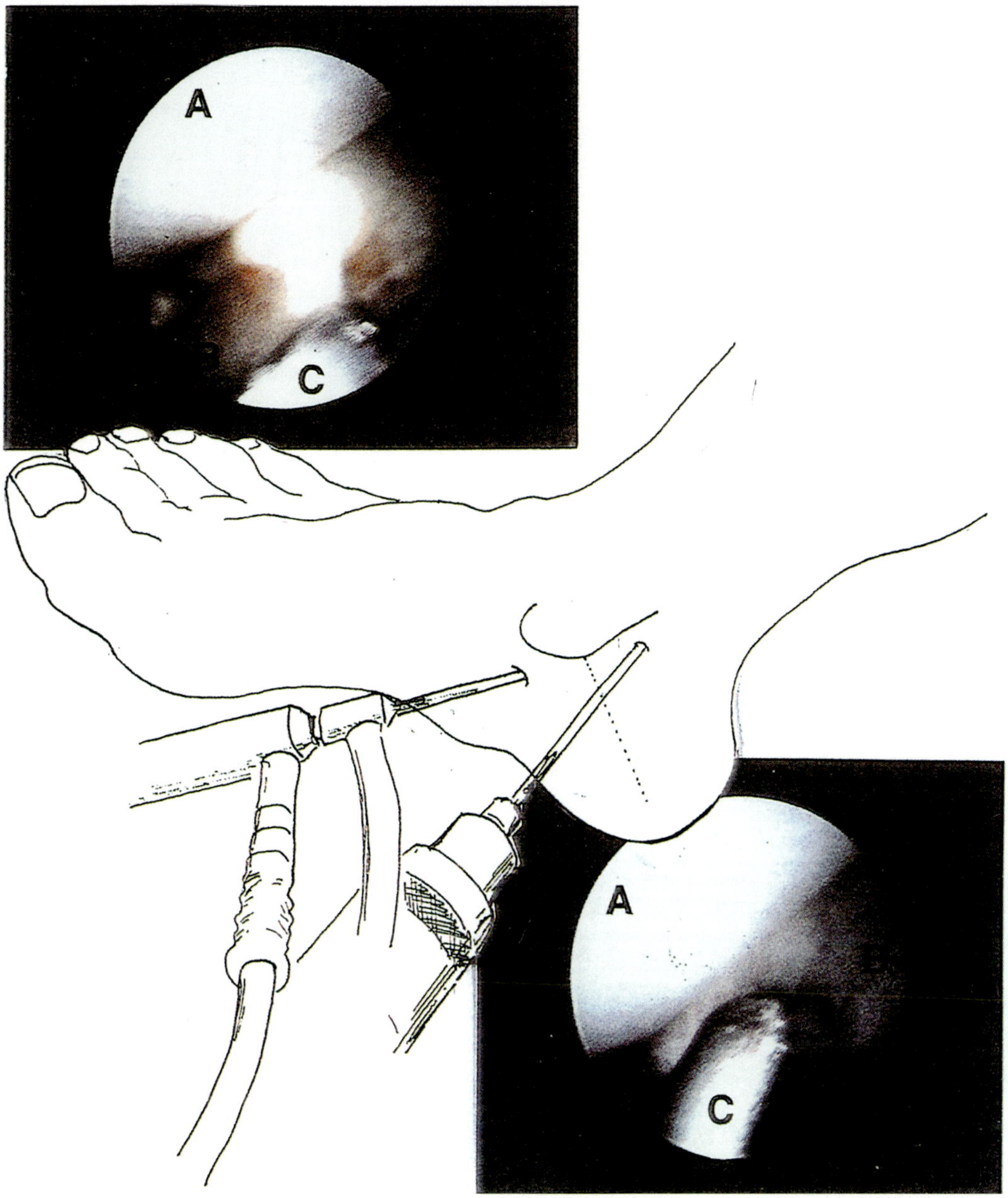

FIGURE 16.2. Posterior tibial tendoscopy of the right ankle. The portals are located directly over the tendon 1.5–2.0 cm distal and 1.2–2.0 cm proximal to the posterior edge of the medial malleolus. Synovectomy is performed with the shaver (here introduced through the proximal portal). A, posterior tibial tendon; B, inflamed synovium; C, tip of shaver.

Achillotendoscopy for retrocalcaneal bursitis is performed in the prone position. Two portals are created, medial and lateral to the Achilles tendon, at the level of the superior border of the os calcis. A 4 mm arthroscope with a inclination angle of 30 degrees is introduced through the posterolateral portal. A probe and subsequently a 5 mm full-radius resector are introduced through the posteromedial portal. After removing the bursa and inflamed soft tissue, the calcaneal prominence is removed using a full-radius resector and small acromionizer (Figs. 16.7, 16.8).

For peritendinitis of the Achilles tendon, the portals are created 2 cm proximal and 2 cm distal of the lesion. The distal portal is made first: An incision is made through the skin only. The crural fascia is penetrated by the arthroscope shaft with a blunt trocar, and a 2.7 mm arthroscope with an inclination angle of 30 degrees is introduced. After introducing a spinal needle under direct vision, an incision is made at the location of the proximal portal. An instrument such as a probe or a small shaver is introduced. The pathologic paratenon is removed by

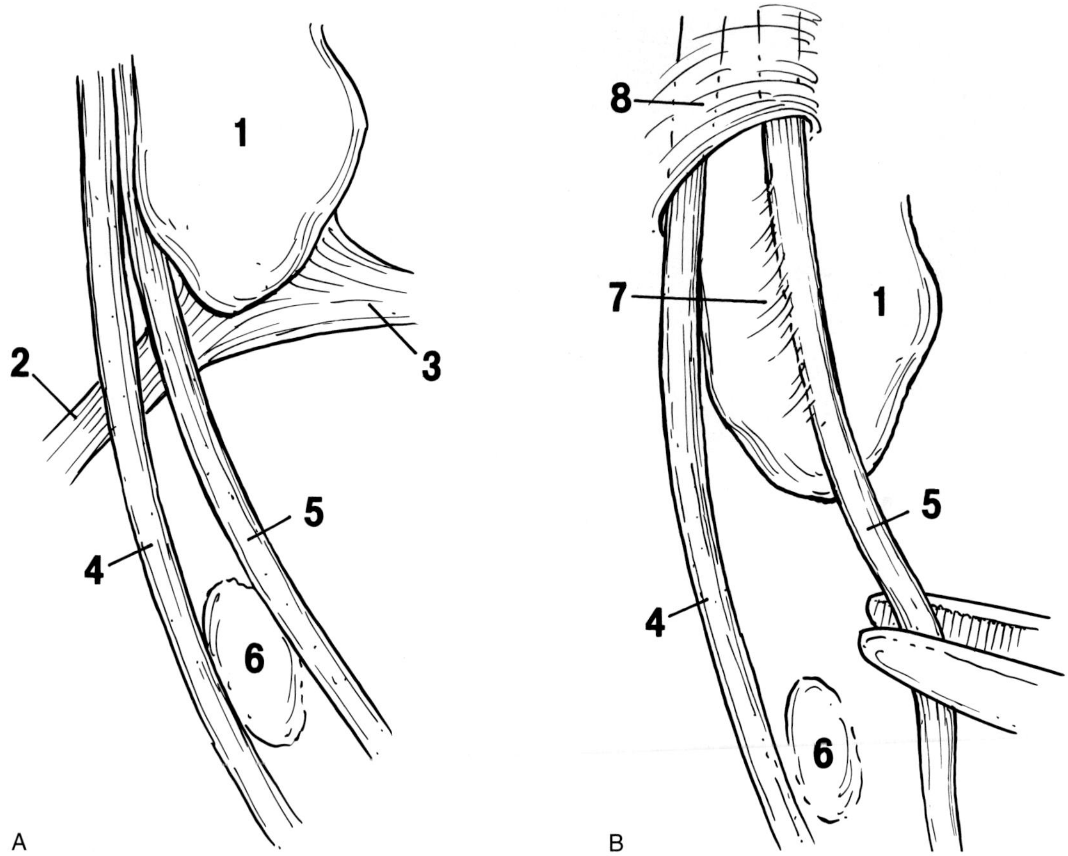

FIGURE 16.3. **A:** Right ankle. Peroneal brevis and peroneal longus tendons are separated by the peroneal tubercle. 1, tip of fibula; 2, fibulocalcaneal ligament; 3, anterior talofibular ligament; 4, peroneal longus tendon; 5, peroneal brevis tendon; 6, peroneal tubercle. **B:** Right ankle. Anterior dislocated peroneal longus tendon is separated by the peroneal tubercle. 1, Tip of fibula; 4, peroneal longus tendon; 5, peroneal brevis tendon; 6, peroneal tubercle; 7, vinculum (stretched); 8, intact tendon sheath.

shaver. The Achilles tendon can be inspected by rotating the scope over the tendon. The plantaris tendon can be recognized and released or resected when indicated.

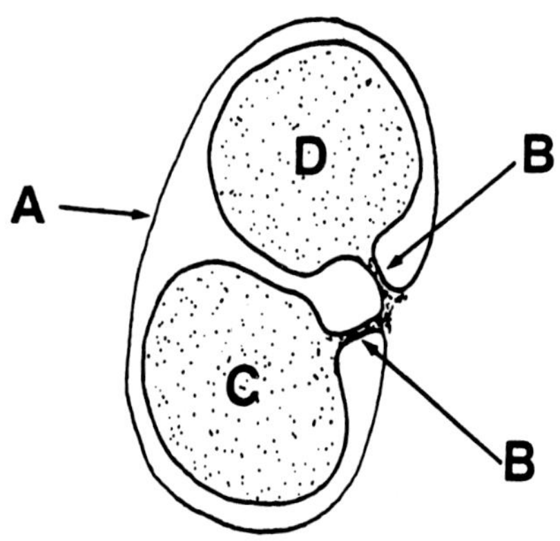

FIGURE 16.4. Peroneal tendons with their tendon sheath and vincula (cross section). A, tendon sheath; B, vinculum; C, peroneal longus tendon; D, peroneal brevis tendon.

Posterolateral and posteromedial portals are used for approaching the flexor hallucis longus tendon. These same two portals are used to gain access to the posterior aspect of the ankle joint and subtalar joint.[23] The patient is placed in the prone position. The posterolateral portal is made at the level of or slightly above the tip of the lateral malleolus, just lateral to the Achilles tendon. After making a vertical skin incision, the subcutaneus layer is split by a mosquito clamp. The mosquito clamp is directed toward the interdigital web space between the first and second toes. The mosquito clamp is exchanged for the 4 mm arthroscope shaft with a blunt trocar, pointing in the same direction. Subsequently, the posteromedial portal is made just medial to the Achilles tendon; in the horizontal plane it is located at the same level as the posterolateral portal. After making a skin incision, the mosquito clamp is directed toward the arthroscope shaft (which has been placed through the posterolateral portal). When the

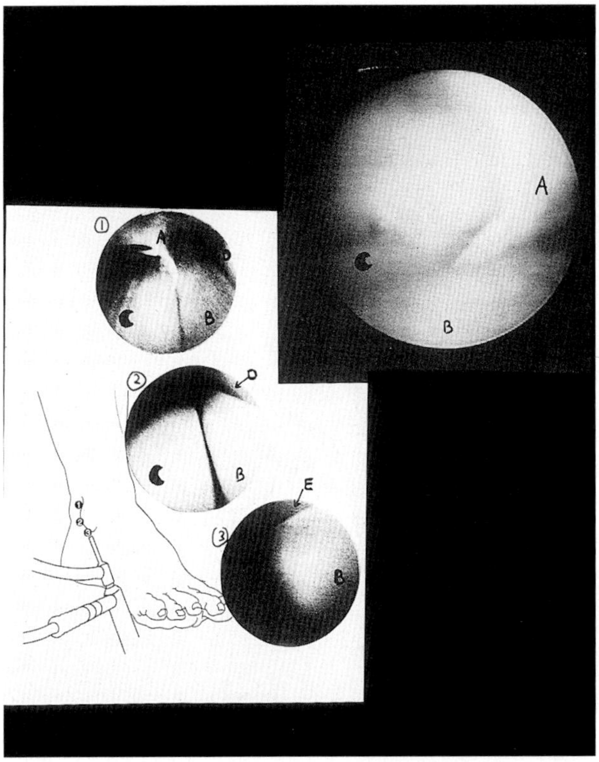

FIGURE 16.5. Normal arthroscopic appearance of the anterior aspect of both peroneal tendons of the right ankle. **1:** Proximal view. The vinculum, which attaches the tendons to each other and to the tendon sheath, arises from the posterior surface of both tendons (not visible here). More proximally, both tendons are separated by a membrane. Above this level both tendons have their own tendon sheath. **2:** Middle view. Both tendons are located in the same tendon sheath. The vinculum is posteriorly located and therefore not visible in this picture. **3:** Distal view. More distally, both peroneal tendons curve around the tip of the lateral malleolus in the sliding channel. A, free edge of the tendon sheath membrane; B, peroneal brevis tendon; C, peroneal longus tendon; D, lateral malleolus; E, tip of the lateral malleolus.

mosquito clamp touches the arthroscope shaft, the shaft is used as a guide to "travel" in the direction of the ankle joint. The arthroscope shaft is subsequently pulled slightly backward until the tip of the mosquito clamp is visualized. The mosquito clamp is used to spread the soft tissue just in front of the tip of the arthroscope. The mosquito clamp is exchanged for a 5 mm full-radius resector to resect the fatty tissue lateral to the flexor hallucis longus tendon. The ankle and subtalar joint can easily be entered by opening the extremely thin joint capsule.

The operation is performed as an outpatient procedure under general regional or local anesthesia. Local anesthesia has the advantage of allowing a possible dynamic investigation. Before the anesthe-

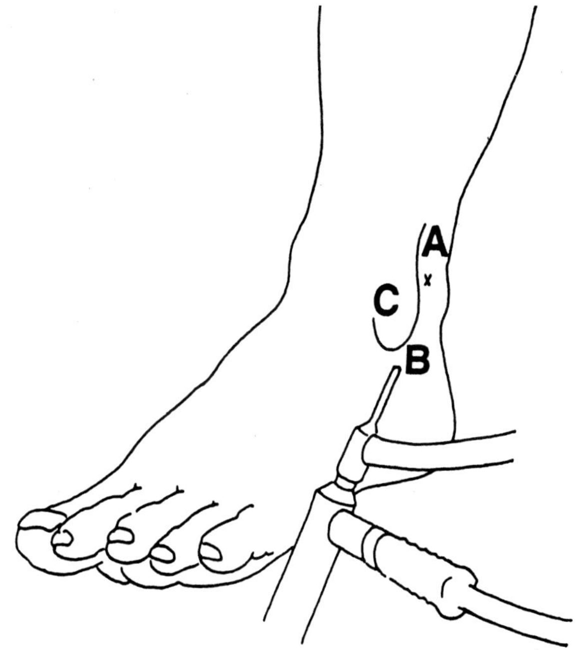

FIGURE 16.6. Peroneal tendoscopy of the left ankle. The two main portals are located 2.0–2.5 cm proximal and 1.5–2.0 cm distal to the posterior edge of the lateral malleolus. A, proximal portal; B, distal portal; C, lateral malleolus.

sia is administered the patient is asked to actively evert (for peroneal tendoscopy), invert (for posterior tibial tendoscopy), or dorsiflex (for anterior tibial tendoscopy) his or her foot. The tendon than can be palpated, and the sites of the portals are drawn on the skin. When using local anesthesia, the anesthetic is administered around the portals and into the tendon sheath. When total synovectomy of the tendon sheath is to be performed, it is advisable to create a third portal more distal or more proximal to the previously described portals. To prevent sinus formation, the portals are closed by monofilament sutures. Postoperative treatment consists of a pressure bandage and partial weight-bearing for 2–3 days. Active range of motion exercise is advised immediately after operation.

PATIENTS

Since 1994 at the Academic Medical Center in Amsterdam, 240 endoscopic soft tissue procedures were performed in 229 consecutive patients. The main indication for an endoscopic hindfoot procedure was a posterior ankle impingement syndrome. In 52 patients a bony impediment such as an os trigonum or hypertrophic posterior talar process was removed.

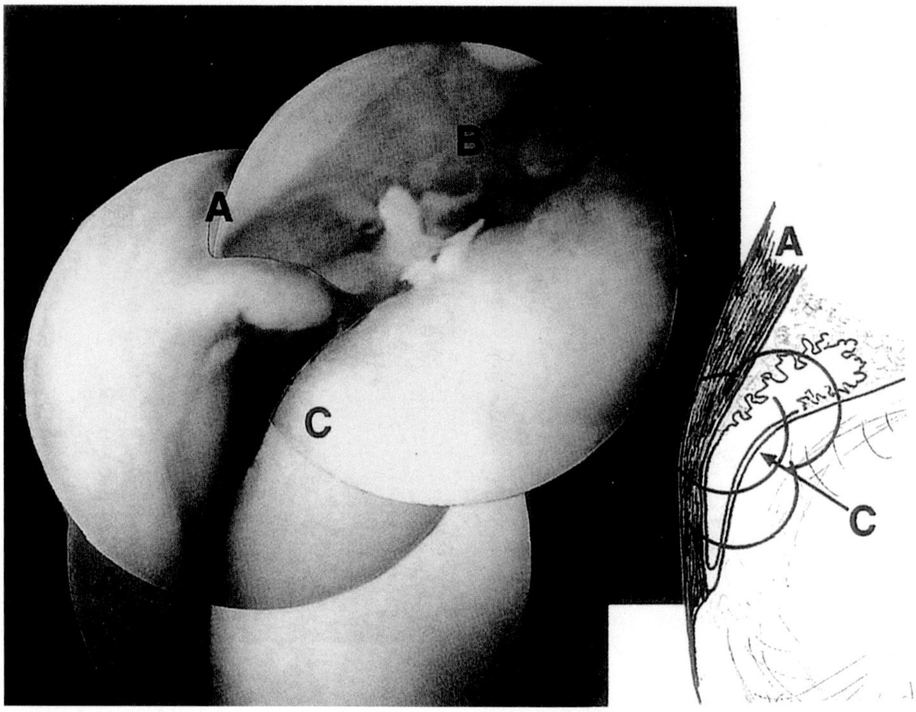

FIGURE 16.7. Achillotendoscopic view of an inflamed retrocalcaneal bursa. Treatment consisted of removing all bursal tissue (with a 4 mm synovator) and the posterosuperior calcaneal rim (5.5 mm burr or acromionizer). A, Achilles tendon; B, inflamed bursal tissue; C, posterosuperior calcaneal rim.

In 28 patients the posterior ankle impingement syndrome was combined with flexor hallucis longus tendinitis. In these patients, in addition to removing the bony impediment, the flexor hallucis longus was released (Table 16.1). In 8 of the 60 patients the cause of the posterior ankle impingement syndrome was a soft tissue impediment, which was removed by a shaver system. In total, 44 patients had flexor hallucis longus tendinitis. There was isolated flexor hallucis longus tendinitis in only 7 patients, whereas in the other patients the flexor hallucis longus tendinitis was combined with a bony impingement syndrome (28 patients), an avulsion fracture of the posteromedial tibial rim, or an ossicle near the flexor hallucis longus tendon (4 patients). In 5 patients the flexor hallucis longus tendinitis was combined with a posteromedial talar osteochondral defect.

The main indications for endoscopic treatment of Achilles tendon pathology were retrocalcaneal bursitis (39 patients) (Fig. 16.9) and peritendinitis (23 patients). The indication for endoscopic calcaneoplasty was failure of 6 months of conservative treatment. The indication for endoscopic release of chronic paratendinitis was failure of conservative treatment for at least 1 year in a patient with localized symptoms and a mechanically intact tendon. The diagnosis of paratendinitis was confirmed on MRI in all cases. Degenerative changes in the Achilles tendon should not exceed more than 30% of its diameter. Conservative treatment consisted of modifying the patient's activity level and shoe wear, stretching, ice application, and eccentric calf muscle training.[11]

Tendoscopy of the posterior tibial tendon was performed in 31 patients (Table 16.2). For the peroneal tendons the main indication was detection of a longitudinal rupture in the peroneal brevis tendon (Fig. 16.10). All patients had a history of an acute lateral ankle ligament rupture. Five of these eight patients presented with pain and swelling over the posterior aspect of the lateral malleolus, and three patients presented with a snapping sensation at the level of the lateral malleolus. Seven patients had chronic tenosynovitis after operative treatment of a lateral malleolar fracture or lateral ankle ligament reconstruction (Table 16.1).

Hindfoot endoscopy for treatment of posterior ankle joint pathology was performed in 36 patients (Table 16.3). In 13 patients a localized osteochondral defect was débrided and drilled. In seven patients the osteochondral defect was located at the

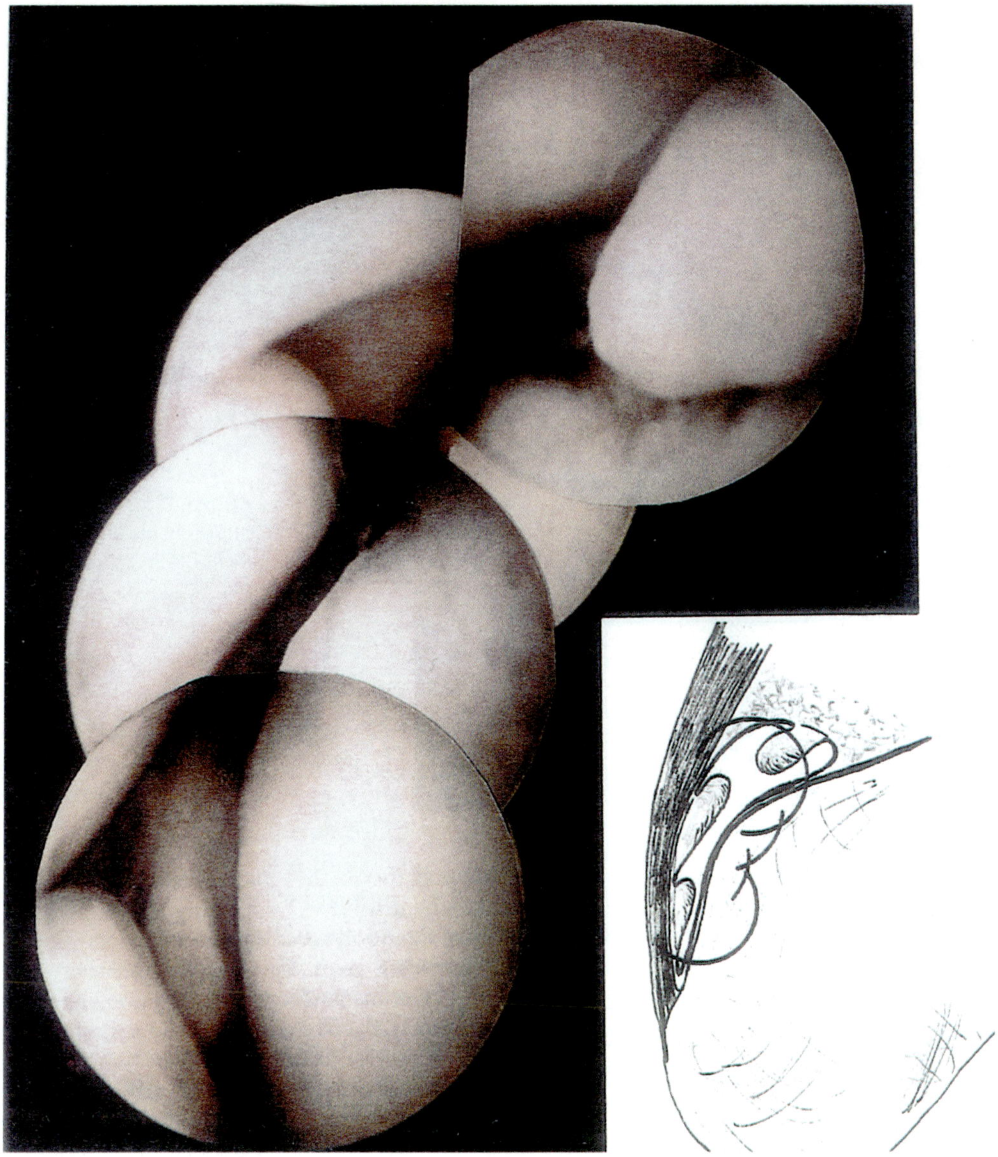

FIGURE 16.8. Achillotendoscopic view of a chronically inflamed retrocalcaneal bursa. Treatment consisted of removing bursal tissue and part of the calcaneus.

TABLE 16.1. *Endoscopy for periarticular hindfoot pathology (n = 78): indications and procedures*

Patients (no.)	*Diagnosis*	*Treatment*
8	Soft tissue impingement	Resect soft tissue impediment
24	Bony impingement	Resect os trigonum
28	BI + FHL tendinitis	Resect OT + release FHL
7	FHL tendinitis	Release FHL
4	FHL tendinitis + ossicle	Release FHL + remove ossicle
5	FHL tendinitis + OD	Release FHL + drill OD
2	Tarsal tunnel syndrome	Release tarsal tunnel

BI, bony impingement; OT, os trigonum; FHL, flexor hallucis longus, OD, osteochondral defect.

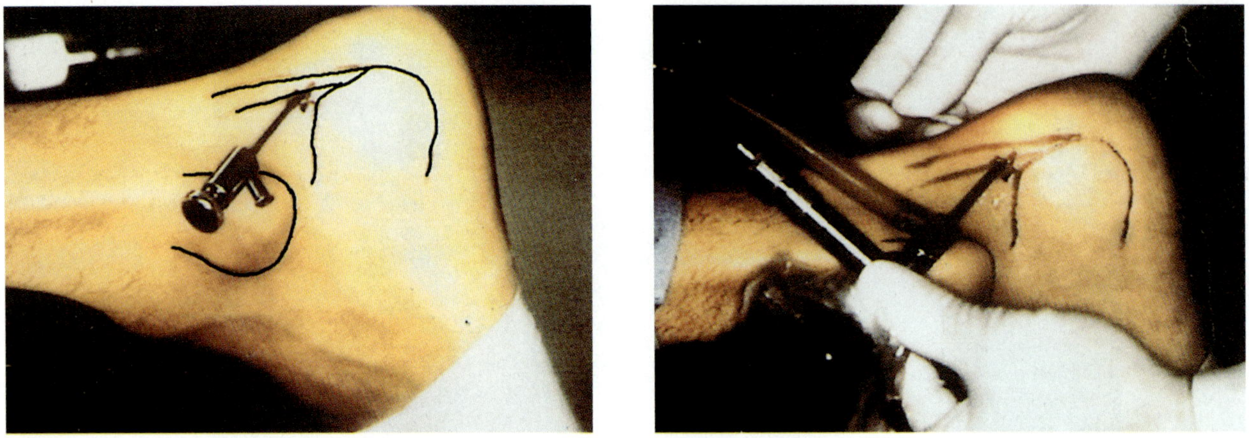

A B

FIGURE 16.9. A: Achillotendoscopy for chronic retrocalcaneal bursitis. The arthroscope shaft (2.7 mm) with blunt trocar is introduced into the bursa after making a skin incision just proximal to the laterosuperior border of the os calcis. **B:** Achillotendoscopy. Medial portal is made under direct vision by introducing a spinal needle just proximal to the mediosuperior border of the os calcis.

posteromedial talar dome, in four patients in the tibial plafond, and in two patients in the posterolateral talar dome. Posttraumatic calcifications in the posteromedial capsule or the posteromedial deltoid ligament were present in five patients. Two patients had a Cedell fracture (avulsion flexor retinaculum). All calcifications were removed endoscopically.

Total synovectomy was performed in nine patients. The procedure started with a two-portal posterior approach in the prone position. When the posterior synovectomy was complete, the knee was flexed, and an anterior synovectomy was subsequently performed by means of the standard anterolateral and anteromedial approach. The indications were chondromatosis ($n = 2$), pigmented villonodular synovitis ($n = 3$), rheumatoid arthritis ($n = 2$), and crystal synovitis ($n = 2$). Two-portal hindfoot endoscopy for subtalar pathology was performed for degenerative articular changes ($n = 10$) or removal of a loose body ($n = 1$), and a large talar intraosseous ganglion was treated in three patients. These multicystic lesions originated from the subtalar joint. The chondral defect (origin of the ganglion) was identified in the subtalar joint by means of the two-portal hindfoot approach. The ganglion then was drilled through the posterior talar process. The drill hole was enlarged to 4.5 mm to make introduction of a curette possible. After curetting and drilling, the cystic defect was filled with cancellous bone from the iliac crest.

TABLE 16.2. *Tendoscopy of the posterior tibial tendon (n = 31): indications and procedures*

Patients (no.)	*Diagnosis*	*Treatment*
8	Tenosynovitis	Tenosynovectomy
1	Medial malleolar fracture	Remove screw
1	Exostosis sliding channel	Remove exostosis
21	Tenosynovitis *e.c.i.*	Various[a]

[a]In this diagnostic group four patients had a pathologic thickened vincula, which was resected; six patients had a longitudinal rupture, which was sutured by means of a mini open approach; four patients had degenerative tendon changes, which were débrided; four patients had adhesions, which were removed; three patients had synovitis that required synovectomy.

RESULTS

Complications were seen in only three patients, who experienced a small area of diminished sensation over the posterior aspect of the hindfoot. Tenosynovectomy, screw removal, and exostosis removal were performed successfully by means of posterior tibial tendoscopy and peroneal tendoscopy.[4,24] When a longitudinal rupture was detected, a small incision was made and the rupture was sutured. A pathologic thickened posterior tibial vincula was successfully removed in four patients (Tables 16.2, 16.4). Removal of an inflamed retrocalcaneal bursa together with the prominent posterosuperior part of the calcaneus (endoscopic calcaneoplasty) was as-

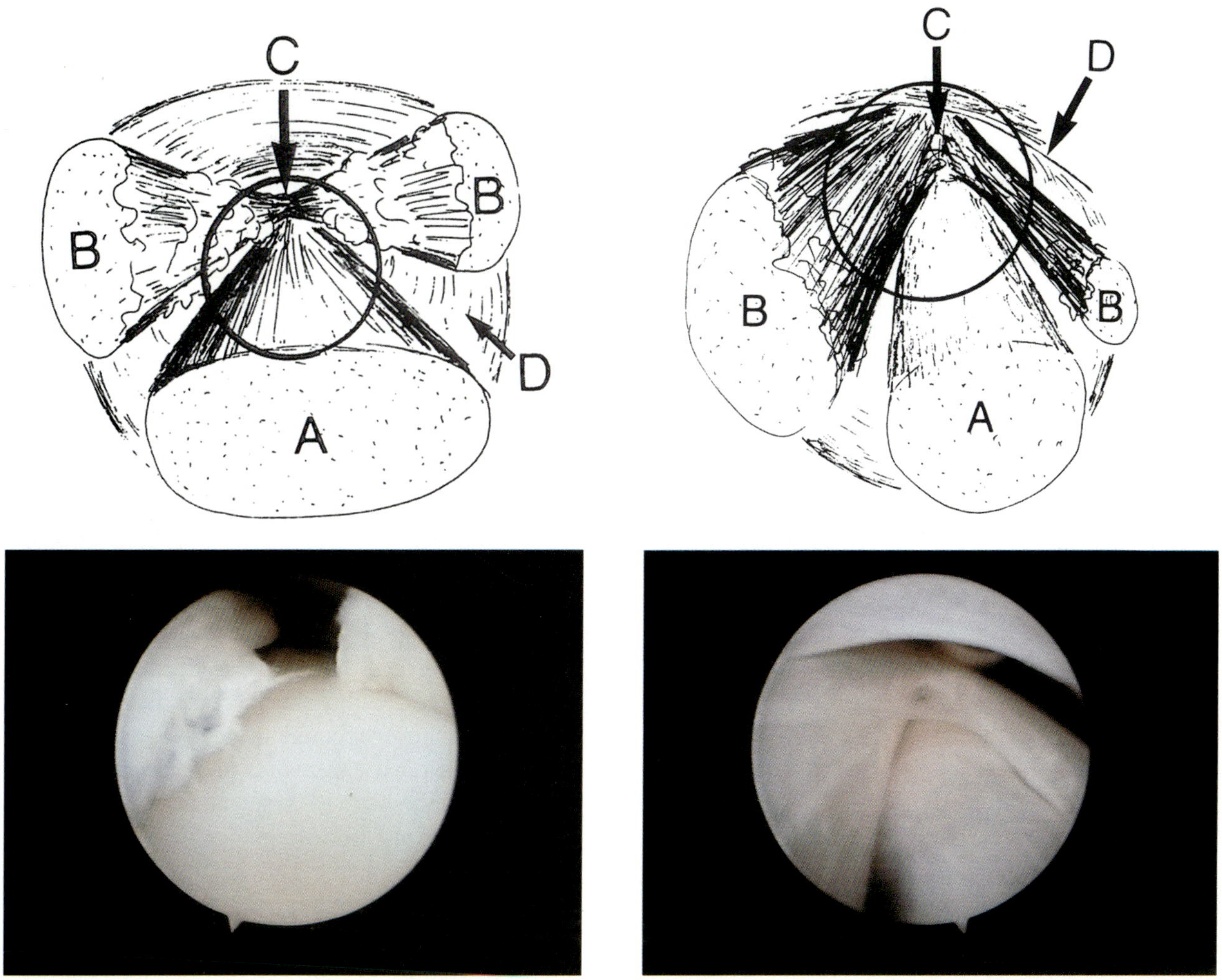

A B

FIGURE 16.10. A: Longitudinal rupture of the peroneal brevis tendon of the right ankle. The view is from distal to proximal (see drawing). Below is the intact peroneal longus tendon. Above left and right are the split legs of the ruptured peroneal brevis tendon. The two legs meet more proximally where the rupture ends (not visible in the picture). A, peroneal longus tendon; B, split legs of the ruptured peroneal brevis tendon; C, ending of the peroneal brevis tendon rupture; D, inside of the tendon sheath. **B:** When moving the arthroscope more proximally, the ending of the longitudinal rupture of the peroneal brevis is visible. A, peroneal longus tendon; B, split legs of the peroneal brevis tendon; C, ending of the peroneal brevis tendon rupture; D, tendon sheath.

sociated with a good or excellent result in 80% of our patients[25] (Fig. 16.11). Resection of an inflamed peritendinium in the case of localized Achilles tendinitis gave promising early results (Table 16.5). Removal of a pathologic os trigonum or a painful posterior soft tissue impediment did not cause any technical problems and was successful in most patients (Table 16.1, Fig. 16.12). In patients in whom

TABLE 16.3. *Hindfoot endoscopy for posterior ankle joint pathology (n = 36): indications and procedures*

Patients (no.)	*Diagnosis*	*Treatment*
13	Osteochondral defect	Débridement + drill
5	Loose body	Remove loose body
7	Calcification/avulsion	Remove ossicles
2	Osteophyte posterior tibial rim	Resect osteophytes
2	Chondromatosis	Anterior + posterior removal
7	Chronic synovitis	Anterior + posterior synovectomy

TABLE 16.4. *Tendoscopy of the peroneal tendon (n = 13): indications and procedures*

Patients (no.)	*Diagnosis*	*Treatment*
5	Snapping tendon	Suture length rupture (*n* = 3)[a]
1	Calcaneal exostosis	Remove exostosis
7	Posttraumatic tenosynovitis	Suture longitudinal rupture (*n* = 5)[a]

[a]When a longitudinal rupture of the peroneus brevis tendon was detected, an open repair was performed by means of a small incision.

a total synovectomy was performed there was no recurrence of the synovitis. All loose bodies were successfully removed. Of the 13 débrided/drilled osteochondral defects, 9 had a good or excellent result (Table 16.3). The three patients with treatment of an intraosseous talar ganglion were without symptoms at the last follow-up. All of the patients treated for degenerative changes in the subtalar joint experienced clear alleviation of their symptoms. None of these patients had deterioration of their results over time (Table 16.6).

DISCUSSION

The balance between peroneal tendons and posterior tibial tendons plays an important role in normal hindfoot function. Posttraumatic posterior tibial tendon dysfunction can lead to peritendinitis. Tenosynovitis is often associated with flat foot deformity. When conservative measures fail at an early stage, tenosynovectomy can be performed. Postoperative treatment consists of plaster immobilization for several weeks. Endoscopic release in combination with synovectomy has demonstrated several advantages, such as less pain, outpatient treatment, functional after-treatment, and rapid resumption of work and sport activities. Posttraumatic and postsurgery complaints regarding the posterior margin of the lateral and medial malleolus often pose difficult diagnostic and therapeutic problems. Adhesions between the tendon and tendon sheath or an irregularity of the tendon sliding channel can give rise to pain. Open tendon release demands postoperative plaster immobilization with a subsequent chance of new adhesion formation. Endoscopic release has the advantage of a diagnostic and therapeutic procedure that can be performed under local anesthesia and is associated with functional postoperative care.

A new finding in our cadaver specimens as well

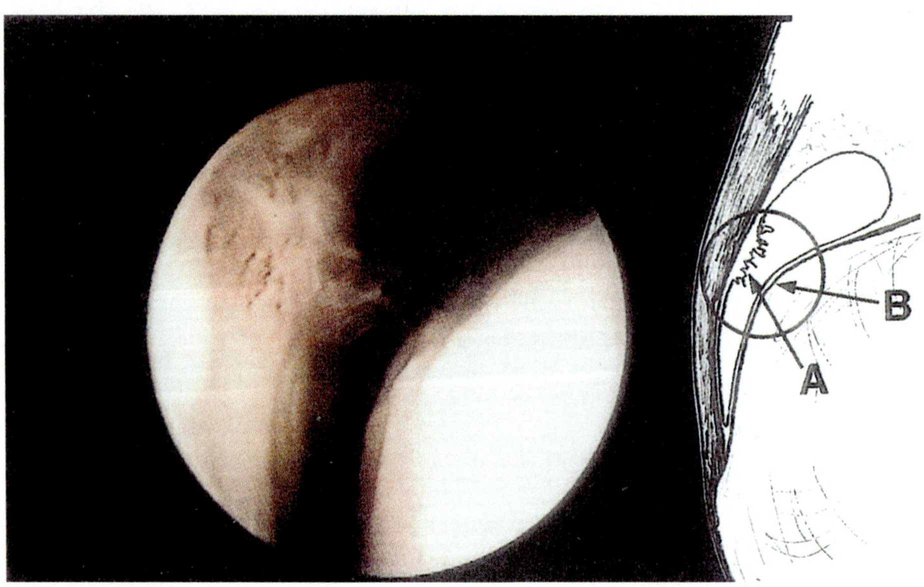

FIGURE 16.11. Achillotendoscopy for chronic retrocalcaneal bursitis. Typically in these quadrants inflammation of bursal tissue overlies the Achilles tendon (A) seen opposite the posterosuperior calcaneal rim (B). This is the area where impingement is seen between a proximal calcaneal rim and the Achilles tendon.

TABLE 16.5 *Endoscopic treatment for Achilles tendon pathology (n = 62): indications and procedures*

Patients (no.)	*Diagnosis*	*Treatment*
39	Retrocalcaneal bursitis	Endoscopic calcaneoplasty
23	Peritendinitis (+ tendinosis)	Resect peritendineum

as during all endoscopic procedures of the posterior tibial tendon was the posterior tibial vincula (Fig. 16.13). Posttraumatic or postsurgical damage to this vincula can cause thickening and scarring of its distal free edge. This thickened vincula can be palpated at the posterior edge of the distal tibia, 3–5 cm above the posterior tip of the medial malleolus. Active movement of the tendon and hyperdorsiflexion causes pain due to traction by the shortened, thickened vincula on its attachment. Endoscopic resection was successful in these patients.

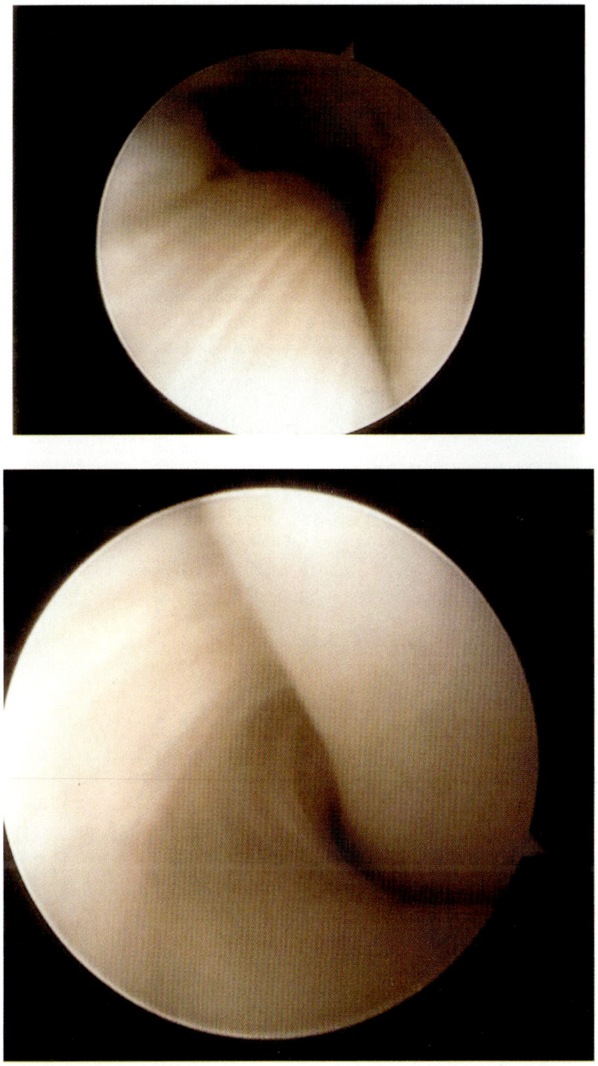

FIGURE 16.12. Original prints of the flexor hallucis longus tendon and its sheath.

An important cause of posterior ankle pain in athletes—especially ballet dancers and soccer players—is chronic tenosynovitis of the flexor hallucis longus tendon. Open surgery involves opening the tendon sheath, débriding the tendon, and resecting the flexor retinaculum. Postoperative treatment is associated with plaster immobilization. The patient is advised to expect up to 6 months for a full recovery. Endoscopic release is associated with a significant reduction in recovery time. Another advantage is that the procedure is performed on an outpatient basis.

The reported results of open treatment for chronic retrocalcaneal bursitis has not been favorable. Nesse and Finsen[26] reported persisting symptoms and complications in 22 of 35 patients, and Angermann and Hovgaard[27] reported a 50% failure rate. Myersen and McGarvey[9] reported more favorable results. Despite these figures, endoscopic calcaneoplasty offers a good alternative to open resection. Surgeons who were used to performing arthroscopy have found this endoscopic technique a more rewarding experience. Advantages of the endoscopic technique are related to the small incisions. Complications such as wound dehiscence, painful and ugly scars, and nerve entrapment in the scar are minimized. Endoscopic surgery allows excellent visualization from both medial and lateral sides. Thus the Achilles tendon, its insertion, and the calcaneus can be inspected and subsequently treated. This minimizes the chance of removing and disturbing the Achilles attachment. Because of functional postoperative treatment, late complications such as stiffness and pain are avoided. We have reported 80% good to excellent results in our patients with this technique.

The reported results for conventional operative treatment of chronic paratendinitis have been favorable. The percentage of good to excellent results vary between 78% and 96%.[28–32] This same positive outcome has been experienced by means of endoscopic treatment. The advantage is that the endoscopic treatment is well received by our patients.

TABLE 16.6. *Hindfoot endoscopy for posterior subtalar joint pathology (n = 13): indications and procedures*

Patients (no.)	*Diagnosis*	*Treatment*
10	Degenerative changes	Remove + débride osteophyte
1	Loose body	Remove
2	Intraosseus talar ganglion	Drill, curette + graft

A

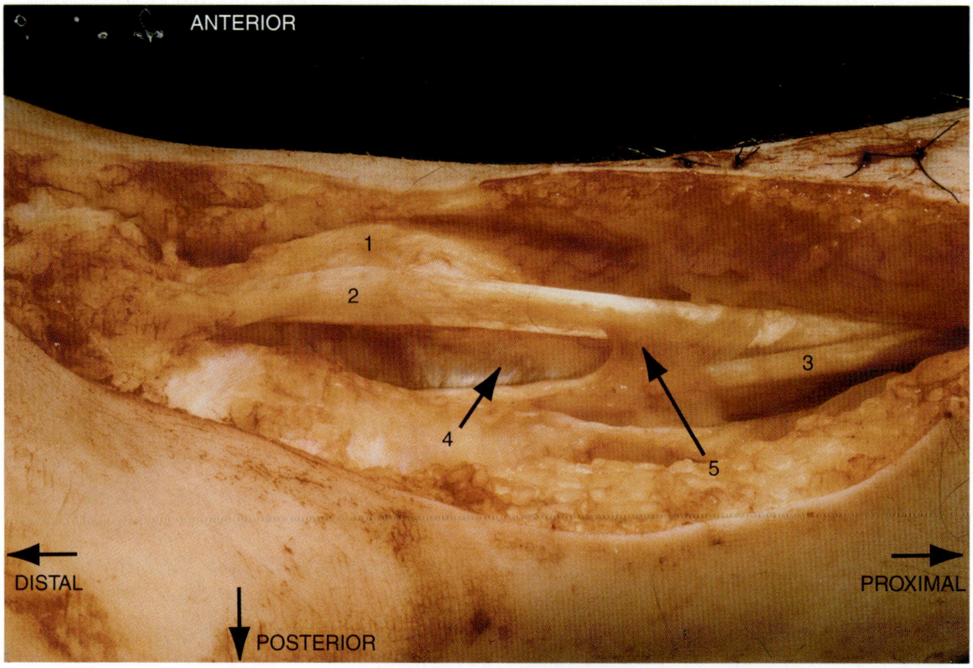

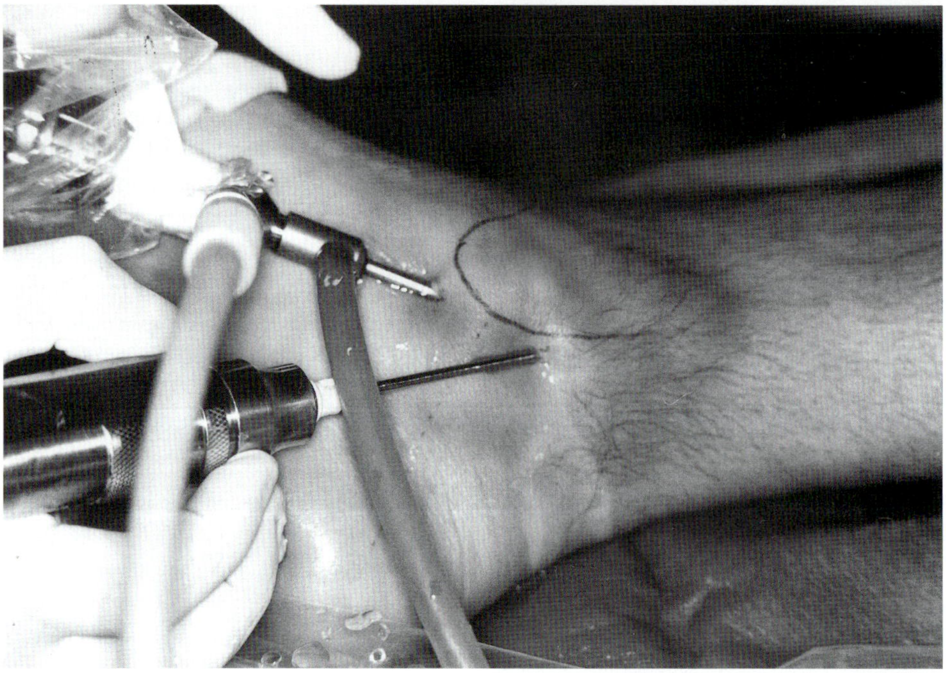

B

FIGURE 16.13. A: Gross anatomy shows medial malleolus and anterior displaced posterior tibial tendon. 1, medial malleolus; 2, posterior tibial tendon; 3, flexor digitorum longus; 4, sliding channel for posterior tibial tendon; 5, vinculum (posterior tibial tendon). **B:** Arthroscope is in the distal portal, and the shaver/abrader is located proximally and anteriorly to shave the exostosis (medial malleolus) for relieving pressure on the medial malleolus. The vinculum may be cut if necessary.

TABLE 16.7. *Etiology of Achilles tendon pathology*

Overuse
Age
Errors in training: shoe, malalignment, strength imbalance
Compression/friction
Inactivity
Rheumatoid arthritis
Drugs
Endocrine disorders

Tolerance to this type of outpatient surgery with minimal scarring is favorable. In selected cases the procedure can be performed under local anesthesia.

The two-portal posterior endoscopic ankle approach with the patient in the prone position offers excellent access to the posterior compartment of the ankle joint, the posterior subtalar joint, and the flexor hallucis longus tendon and os trigonum. When combined with anterior ankle arthroscopy, most surgeons regard the posteromedial portal to be contraindicated in all but the most extreme situations because of the potential for serious complications. The posterolateral portal, however, is advocated as a routine portal by most authors. When the arthroscopic shaft is placed through this posterolateral portal, the instruments through the posteromedial portal must be directed toward the arthroscopic shaft. This shaft subsequently is used as a guide for the medially introduced instruments to travel in the direction of the joint. The neurovascular bundle is thus passed without problem. Since 1994 we have created a posteromedial portal during 127 consecutive procedures without relevant complications. When performed in the above-described manner, posterior ankle arthroscopy is a safe, reliable, exciting method for diagnosing and treating a variety of posterior ankle problems. It is recommended that the procedure be performed by an experienced arthroscopist who has studied the local anatomy in a cadaver setting.

The various causes of Achilles tendon pathology are listed in Table 16.7.

BIBLIOGRAPHY

1. Lapidus PW, Seidenstein H. Chronic non-specific tenosynovitis with a fusion about the ankle. *J Bone Joint Surg* 1950;32:175–179.
2. Richardson EG. Disorders of tendons. In: Grenshaw AH (ed). *Campbell's Operative Orthopaedics*. St. Louis: Mosby, 1992;2851–2873.
3. Myerson M. Tendons and ligaments. In: Myerson, M. (ed.) *Current therapy in foot and ankle surgery*. St. Louis: Mosby, 1992:123–187.
4. Van Dijk CN, Scholten PE, Kort NP. Tendoscopy (tendon sheath endoscopy) for overuse tendon injuries. *Operative Techniques Sports Med* 1997;5:170–178.
5. Stibbe AB, van Dijk CN, Marti RK. The os trigonum syndrome. *Acta Orthop Scand Suppl* 262 1994;XX: 59–60.
6. Van Dijk CN, Lim LSL, Poortman A, et al. Degenerative joint disease in female ballet dancers. *Am J Sports Med* 1995;23:295–300.
7. Hamilton WG, Geppert MJ, Thompson FM. Pain in the posterior aspect of the ankle in dancers. *J Bone Joint Surg Am* 1996;87:1491–1500.
8. Hedrick MR, McBryde AM. Posterior ankle impingement. *Foot Ankle Int* 1994;15:2–8.
9. Myerson MS, McGarvey W. Disorders of the insertion of the Achilles tendon and Achilles tendinitis. *J Bone Joint Surgery Am* 1998;80:1814–1824.
10. Puddu G, Ippolito E, Postacchini F. A classification of Achilles tendon disease. *Am J Sports Med* 1976; 4:145–150.
11. Alfredson H, Pietila T, Jonsson P, Lorentzon R. Heavy-load eccentric calf muscle training for the treatment of chronic Achilles tendinosis. *Am J Sports Med* 1998;26:360–366.
12. Maffulli N, Binfield PM, Moore D, King JB. Surgical decompression of chronic central correlations of Achilles tendon. *Am J Sports Med* 1999;27:747–752.
13. Angermann P. Chronic retrocalcaneal bursitis treated by resection on the calcaneus. *Foot Ankle* 1990;10: 285–287.
14. Funk DA, Cass JR, Johnson KA. Acquired adult flatfoot secondary to posterior tibial tendon pathology. *J Bone Joint Surg Am* 1986;68:95–102.
15. Cosen L. Posterior tibial tenosynivitis secondary to foot strain. *Clin Orthop* 1965;42:101–102.
16. Johnson KA, Strom DE. Tibialis posterior tendon dysfunction. *Clin Orthop* 1989;239:196–206.
17. Williams R. Chronic non-specific tendovaginitis of tibialis posterior. *J Bone Joint Surg Br* 1963;45:542.
18. Trevino S, Gould N, Korson R. Surgical treatment of stenosing tenosynovitis at the ankle. *Foot Ankle* 1981;2:37.
19. Coughlin MJ, Mann RA. Tarsal tunnel syndrome. In: *Surgery of the Foot and Ankle*. 6th ed, vol 1. St. Louis: Mosby, 1993; chap 11.
20. Roggatz J, Urban A. The calcareous peritendinitis of the long peroneal tendon. *Arch Orthop Trauma Surg* 1980;96:161–164.
21. Schweitzer GJ. Stenosing peroneal tenovaginitis. case reports. *S Afr Med J* 1982;4:521–523.
22. Yao L, Tong JF, Cracchiolo A, Seeger LL. MR findings in peroneal tendinopathy. *J Comput Assist Tomogr* 1995;19:460–464.

23. Van Dijk CN. Ankle joint arthroscopy. In: Duparc J, Wülker N (eds) *Surgical techniques in orthopaedics and traumatology*. Paris: Editions Scientifiques et Medicales Elsevier SAS, 2001 (55-630-A-10).
24. Van Dijk CN, Kort N, Scholten P. Tendoscopy of the posterior tibial tendon. *Arthroscopy* 1997;6:692–698.
25. Van Dijk CN, van Dyk E, Scholten P, Kort NP. Tendoscopic calcaneoplasty. *Am J Sports Med* 2001; 29(2):185–189.
26. Nesse E, Finsen V. Poor results after resection for Haglund's heel: analysis of 35 heels in 23 patients after 3 years. *Acta Orthop Scand* 1994;65: 107–109.
27. Angermann P, Hovgaard D. Chronic Achilles tendinopathy in athletic individuals: results of non-surgical treatment. *Foot Ankle Int* 1999;20:304–306.
28. Kvist H, Kvist M. The operative treatment of chronic calcaneal paratendonitis. *J Bone Joint Surg Br* 1980; 62:353–357.
29. Leach RE, Schepsis AA, Takai H. Long-term results of surgical management of Achilles tendinitis in runners. *Clin Orthop* 1992;282:208–212.
30. Nelen G, Martens M, Burssens A. Surgical treatment of chronic Achilles tendinitis. *Am J Sports Med* 1989;17:754–759.
31. Schepsis AA, Leach RE. Surgical management of Achilles tendinitis. *J Sports Med* 1987;15:308–315.
32. Williams JGP. Achilles tendon lesions in sport. *Sports Med* 1986;3:112–135.

CHAPTER 17

Endoscopic Plantar Fasciotomy

Stephen L. Barrett

Heel pain is one of the most common foot complaints. Plantar fasciitis is a common cause of heel pain, although there are many other causes as well, including stress fracture, nerve entrapment syndromes, Achilles tendonitis, and posterior ankle pathology. About 80–90% of plantar fasciitis resolves with currently available nonoperative treatments, including stretching exercises, rest, intrinsic muscle strengthening, and cortisone. For the 10–20% of patients who do not respond to nonoperative treatment, plantar fascia release may alleviate the symptoms. Endoscopic plantar fasciotomy has been performed more than 500,000 times in the U.S. and throughout the world.

ENDOSCOPIC PLANTAR FASCIOTOMY

Indications

Endoscopic plantar fasciotomy (EPF) is a minimally invasive endoscopic approach to the management of intractable plantar fasciitis/heel spur syndrome. This procedure is indicated only in situations where exhaustive nonoperative care has been performed and the patient's symptoms have not resolved. EPF is indicated for the surgical intervention of mechanical heel pain and does not have any indications when nerve pathology exists or when there is some other etiology contributing to the patient's heel pain. Hence EPF is indicated only in patients for whom the surgeon would consider performing an open fasciotomy/fasciectomy.

Contraindications

Endoscopic plantar fasciotomy should not be performed in any patients who would otherwise not be considered good surgical candidates. Patients who have unrealistic expectations about the technique are usually not good candidates for any procedure. EPF is contraindicated in any patient who has not had a prolonged, complete course of nonoperative care, including physical therapy, orthotics, and even injections.

Surgical Techniques

Since the mid-1990s the EPF technique has evolved into a simple, precise procedure. It is stressed, though, that the surgeon must complete adequate training, including time in a cadaveric hands-on skills laboratory, to ensure efficacious, safe treatment with this technique. The surgeon is also encouraged to perform the first few cases with an experienced mentor to aid in patient safety and quality of care.

The EPF procedure can be performed with a general or local anesthetic, depending on the patient's needs. We have found this technique to be easily completed with a local anesthetic and monitored anesthesia care. If using a local anesthetic block, it is recommended that the surgeon perform both a sural and posterior tibial nerve block, with additional infiltration of the anesthetic in the area of the medial and lateral calcaneal nerve branches. The surgeon is cautioned to avoid infiltrating the local anesthetic in the area of cannula placement, as it would decrease visualization during the technique. Usually, less than 14 cc of local anesthetic is needed.

The patient is placed on the operating room table in a supine position, with the feet hanging off the end of the table. This positioning is important because it allows freer movement with the camera and endoscope by the surgical assistant. An ankle tourniquet is preferred to a thigh cuff. Hemostasis is essential for this technique to be performed correctly.

The foot should be exsanguinated with an Esmark bandage, in preference to simply elevating the extremity to ensure better hemostasis. The foot is then abducted, which allows easier medial portal incisional placement. Portal placement is critical. There are two ways to ensure proper placement of the instrumentation. One method is to calculate the location for cannula placement from a non-weight-bearing lateral projection radiograph (Fig. 17.1). The cannula should be placed 1–2 mm anterior of the medial calcaneal tubercle, or inferior calcaneal exostosis if present, at the inferior level of the plantar fascial shadow. An x and y coordinate can then

A

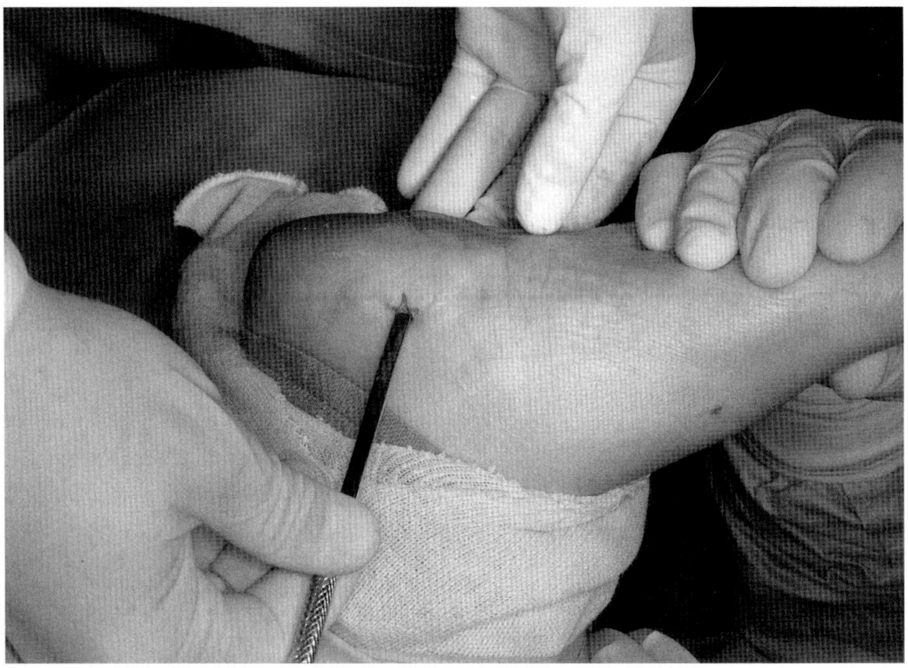

B

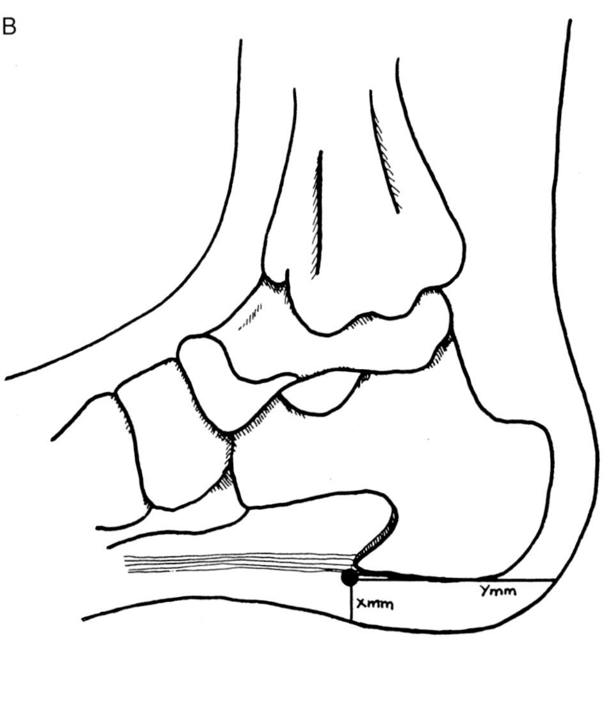

FIGURE 17.1. Ideal cannula placement should be 1–2 mm anterior or distal to the medial calcaneal tubercle (or inferior calcaneal exostosis if present) at the level of the inferior aspect of the plantar fascia.

be measured from the plantar and posterior aspects of the heel, respectively. These measurements can be transposed to the patient intraoperatively. Another method that can be used intraoperatively is placement by palpation (Fig. 17.2). This method is sometimes alluded to as the "rule of thumb." The surgeon should take the right thumb if a right foot is being operated on (use the left thumb if it is a left foot) and place the thumb on the plantar aspect of the heel, over the medial calcaneal tubercle. Rocking the thumb anteriorly, the surgeon should be able to feel a "drop-off" from osseous tissue to soft tissue. This drop-off corresponds to the inclination of the calcaneus. When the drop-off is palpated, it is the level of the thumbnail that the surgeon uses for the anterior-to-posterior positioning of the cannula. The inferior-to-superior measurement is then used from the radiograph. This measurement is frequently in the area of 17 mm. This inferior-to-superior measurement should never exceed 20 mm, even in large-boned men.

This is the essence of the technique, and affording time for proper planning preoperatively ensures ease of technique for the surgeon once the procedure begins. The medial incision is a 6- to 7-mm vertical incision. Care is taken to keep the incision superficial and to avoid a "stab"-type incision. The main medial calcaneal nerve branch is usually posterior to this incisional placement and with good technique it is not endangered. Once through the dermis, simple blunt dissection with some small tenotomy scissors is performed through the subcutaneous adipose tissue down to the level of the plantar fascia. The fascial elevator is introduced from a superomedial to inferior (more than plantar) position. The surgeon should grip this instrument in pencil fashion, and there should be minimal resistance felt if the surgeon is in the proper tissue plane. Once the tip of the elevator "palpates" the plantar fascia, the surgeon can feel the elevator drop down along the fascia as it courses inferiorly around the abductor hallucis muscle. Once this "drop-off" is felt by the surgeon, the elevator is then brought into a transverse position, which allows the instrument to course closely underneath the plantar fascia as it is moved laterally. When the surgeon is able to palpate the tip of the elevator on the lateral aspect of the heel, the surgeon can then check the position of the elevator laterally. With gentle dorsal pressure, the instrument is moved retrogradely out of the medial portal incision, allowing the surgeon to feel the bottom of the plantar fascia. Medially, the surgeon feels this elevator fall back up the drop-off as the instrument exits the foot. Such psychomotor skills are important for the surgeon to develop, as these simple techniques ensure proper cannula placement and avoid perforating the plantar fascia.

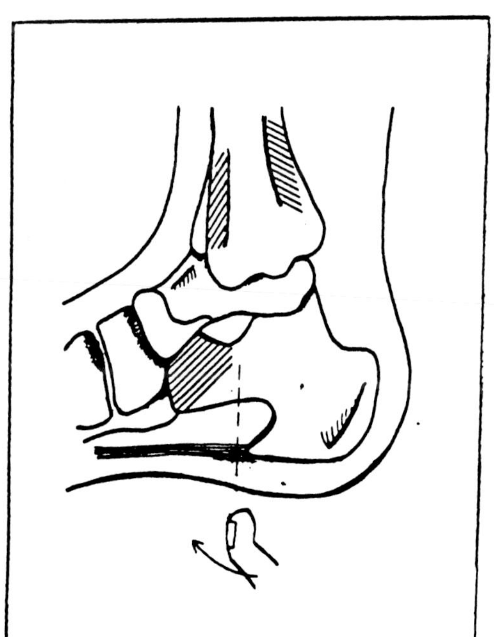

FIGURE 17.2. "Rule of thumb" method of palpation to locate the anterior to posterior positioning of the cannula.

The obturator/cannula is now placed in the heel in a manner similar to that described for the plantar fascial elevator. It is important to stress again that the surgeon must initially approach the medial portal in a superomedial, more plantar than lateral fashion, until the drop-off is felt. The instrumentation can then be brought into a transverse position. The surgical assistant can now make a small 5 mm vertical incision over the tip of the obturator when it is palpated laterally, allowing the instrumentation to exit the lateral portal. The obturator is removed from the cannula, leaving the cannula in proper position.

The cannula should be cleaned with several cotton-tipped applicators from a medial to lateral direction to remove any adipose tissue from the area (Figs. 17.1–17.6). The cannula is marked internally so the surgeon has some starting reference points. The goal of the procedure is to release the medial one-third of the plantar fascia completely. With the improved instrumentation, the surgeon's eyes never have to leave the video monitor. There is a set of double markings 9 and 11 mm from the medial portal and a single marking 13.5 mm lateral from the midpoint of the double marks. Beginning the fas-

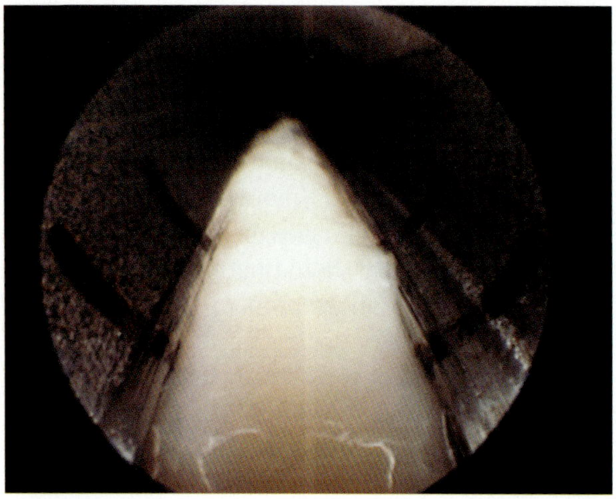

FIGURE 17.3. View from the medial portal. Double marks indicate the approximate location of the medial investment, at which point the surgeon begins the fasciotomy.

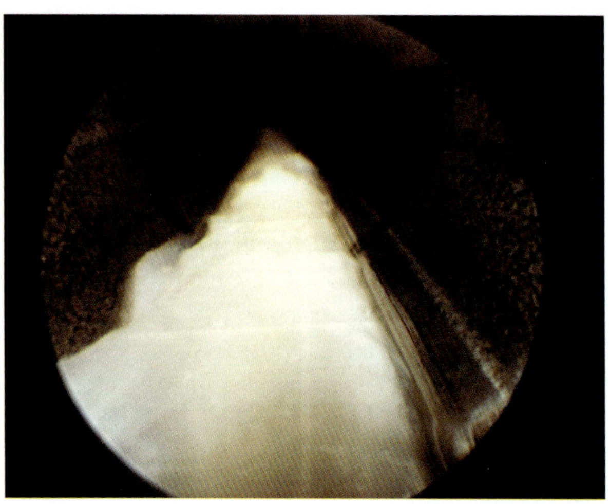

FIGURE 17.4. Single mark indicates approximate stopping point for a medial one-third fasciotomy. Note that the single mark is 13.5 mm lateral to the central part of the double marks.

ciotomy at the point between the double marks and stopping laterally at the single mark helps the surgeon perform a medial one-third fasciotomy. Anatomic studies have shown that the width of the medial band, on average, is 13.48 mm.[1] It must be cautioned that these marks are only anatomic guides, and the surgeon must still recognize anatomically how much fascia is being cut. One excellent anatomic reference point is the first intermuscular septum, which separates the abductor hallucis from the flexor digitorum brevis. It correlates with a medial one-third release. The surgeon should always be able to identify this landmark during an EPF.

It takes several passes with the hook blade to cut completely through the fascia. Use of the hook blade prevents damage to the intrinsic musculature. The triangle knife should be used only to release the intermuscular septum and the medial investment. Once the fascia is cut, the surgeon must be able to identify two well-demarcated edges of plantar fascia, with the muscle belly between them. These edges should separate further with dorsiflexion of the foot. Once this is achieved, the surgeon intro-

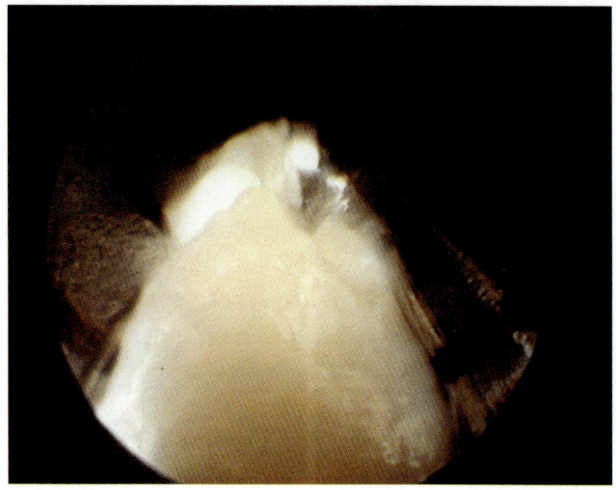

FIGURE 17.5. Medial portal view. Note the reflection from the hook knife starting the fasciotomy in the center of the photograph.

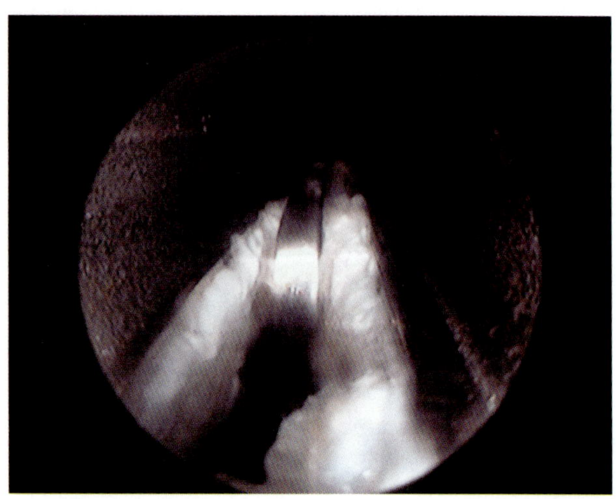

FIGURE 17.6. Medial portal view showing a medial one-third fasciotomy with the fasciotomy stopping at the single mark.

duces the camera through the lateral portal, identifies the medial investment, and then releases it with the triangle knife. The EPF is now complete.

The cannula is irrigated with several bulb syringes of sterile water or saline and then can be removed once the obturator is reintroduced. Closure of the incisions is easily attained with a couple of simple interrupted sutures. The area is then infiltrated with local anesthetic and a water-soluble corticosteroid before placing a light gauze dressing on the patient.

Postoperative management is essential with this technique to ensure efficacy and avoid complications. Patients are advised to be fully weightbearing immediately after surgery but are also advised to avoid excessive ambulation. On the third postoperative day, the dressings are removed and replaced with sterile cloth adhesive bandages. The patient is then allowed to wear a regular shoe.[2]

RESULTS AND COMPLICATIONS

Although endoscopic plantar fasciotomy is not a panacea, and I have never proposed it as such, the technique is highly efficacious and effective in trained hands. I have reported a 97% success rate in a multisurgeon study of 652 cases.[3] This rate of success is comparable to success rates in the literature for open plantar fasciotomy.[4] Several other important studies have shown EPF to be associated with an earlier return to work in one study by up to 55 days,[5] when compared to open heel spur surgery. Kinley et al.[6] showed a decreased complication rate for EPF when compared to traditional heel spur surgery. Stone and Davies'[7] study showed that there is high patient satisfaction with the technique. An article by Palumbo et al.[8] stated that cadaveric training is mandatory.

As with any surgery, EPF has complications. Some are more inherent to this procedure than those associated with traditional forms of open surgery for heel spur syndrome/plantar fasciitis. I believe that this is simply due to the fact that the patient is much more ambulatory during the initial postoperative phase after EPF than after some of the more invasive forms of surgery, such as open fasciotomy.

Complications associated with EPF have been classified into three categories.[3] The first group of complications can be categorized as medial column problems, the second as lateral column destabilization problems, and finally a group as simply "other." Medial column complications include arch fatigue and cramping of the muscles on the plantar aspect of the foot. These problems usually occur during the immediate postoperative period because of too much ambulating by the patient. When the surgeon understands the biomechanical structural significance of the plantar fascia to the human foot, it is easy to understand the development of these complications after severing the medial one-third of the plantar fascia. In fact, they should be expected if the patient ambulates too much before the fascia has reattached, usually about 6–8 weeks after surgery.

Lateral column sequelae are the most serious complications a surgeon can expect from this type of surgery. Such problems include pain at the calcaneocuboidal joint, peroneal tenosynovitis, sinus tarsitis, and pain at the level of the fourth to fifth metatarsal cuboid articulation. Some patients have complained of pain in the sub-fifth metatarsal head and occasionally of a decrease in sensation along the course of the lateral plantar nerve. Other complications sometimes encountered with EPF are infection, painful scar formation, wound dehiscence, and any other complication associated with surgery.

With proper training and judicious postoperative management, endoscopic plantar fasciotomy is a highly successful, minimally invasive surgical technique that can be performed with few complications. In fact, modification of postoperative management has cut the complication rate associated with lateral column destabilization problems by half.

BIBLIOGRAPHY

1. Barrett SL, Day SV, et al. Endoscopic heel anatomy: analysis of 200 fresh frozen specimens. *J Foot Surg* 1995;34:51–56.
2. Barrett SL, Day SV. Endoscopic plantar fasciotomy: two portal endoscopic surgical techniques—clinical results of 65 procedures. *J Foot Ankle Surg* 1993;32: 248–256.
3. Barrett SL, Day SV, et al. Endoscopic plantar fasciotomy: a multi-surgeon prospective analysis of 652 cases. *J Foot Surg* 1995;34:400–406.
4. Anderson RB, Foster MD. Operative treatment of subcalcaneal pain. *Foot Ankle* 1989;9:317–323.
5. Tomczak RL, Haverstock BD. A retrospective comparison of endoscopic plantar fasciotomy to open

plantar fasciotomy with heel spur resection for chronic plantar fasciitis/heel spur surgery. *J Foot Surg* 1995; 34:305–311.
6. Kinley S, Frascone S, et al. Endoscopic plantar fasciotomy versus traditional heel spur surgery: a prospective study. *J Foot Surg* 1993;32:595–603.
7. Stone PA, Davies JL. Retrospective review of endoscopic plantar fasciotomy 1992–1994. *J Am Podiatr Med Assoc* 1996;86:414–420.
8. Palumbo RC, et al. Endoscopic plantar fasciotomy: indications, techniques and complications. *Sports Med Arth Rev* 1994;2:317–322.

CHAPTER 18

Endoscopic Tarsal Tunnel Release

Frederick N. Day III

Tarsal tunnel syndrome (TTS) is an entrapment neuropathy involving the posterior tibial nerve in the tarsal canal or one of its branches leaving the canal.[1] The surgical objective is to release the entrapped nerve. In the classic technique, a long J-shaped incision is made along the medial aspect of the ankle. This approach provides excellent exposure to the tarsal canal and vital structures. If the pathology is caused by compression of the posterior tibial nerve by the laciniate ligament, a different approach may be utilized that offers a smaller scar and faster recovery.

Endoscopic tarsal tunnel release (ETTR) is an example of endoscopic surgery replacing an open technique. Endoscopy offers the surgeon an alternative procedure that results in less patient trauma and faster recovery time. As with any emerging procedure, modifications have been made in the procedure to help simplify the process and improve the end result. Caution must be used by the surgeon when performing this technique. If the surgeon is not skilled enough to perform an open release, the endoscopic approach should not be attempted. I highly recommend cadaveric experimentation to the skilled surgeon prior to implementation. I believe that ETTR is an excellent alternative procedure to the classic open technique for the skilled surgeon.

The classic open surgical approach to decompression of the posterior tibial nerve is a 10 cm curved incision along the tarsal canal. The laciniate ligament is divided and the posterior tibial nerve mobilized. The incision is usually then closed using only skin sutures. TTS may recur if a hypertrophic scar should form over the nerve secondary to skin healing, but ETTR can prevent this problem.

The tarsal canal is located behind the medial malleolus; it becomes the tarsal canal when the flexor retinaculum or laciniate ligament passes over the structures. The laciniate ligament is a thickened band of deep fascia that attaches to the medial malleolus and medial process of the calcaneus. As the retinaculum passes toward and into the plantar aspect of the foot, it helps provide an origin for the abductor hallucis muscle, which lies deep to the ligament and then becomes continuous with the plantar aponeurosis. The posterior tibial artery, vein, and nerve pass deep to the ligament and lie within a fascial canal in the neurovascular bundle.[2]

INDICATIONS

The etiologies of tarsal tunnel syndrome are multiple; they have soft tissue, neoplastic, metabolic, congenital, biomechanical, traumatic, and idiopathic origins. Bony masses may also be responsible. Included in the soft tissue impingements are accessory muscles, varicosities, ganglions, abductor hallucis hypertrophy, tenosynovial cysts, hypertrophy of the laciniate ligament, and tumors such as lipoma, neurilemoma, hemangioma, and other neoplasms. Swelling due to metabolic disorders can also cause symptoms. Congenital deformities such as residual clubfoot, Charcot-Marie-Tooth disease, Down syndrome, and cerebral palsy can produce TTS. Hyperpronation and bony exostosis near the tarsal canal or coalitions may cause symptoms. Trauma to the ankle joint, including sprains, fractures, previous surgery, or other injuries resulting in inflammation or scarring of the tarsal canal, may cause TTS.[3]

The diagnosis of TTS is made after a complete, detailed history and physical examination. A varied history of pain in the foot (whether shooting, burning, or electric) while walking, at night, all the time, or intermittently (and in any combination) can be found in the history. I have found that the underlying common denominator in all patients is unrelieved pain.

A complete neurologic and biomechanical examination are performed, and muscle weakness and sensory loss are documented. Percussion of the posterior tibial nerve may elicit Tinel's sign (distal radiation of pain into the foot and toes) or a Valleix sign (radiation of pain proximally up the leg).[3] Gait patterns are observed to rule out hyperpronation. Radiographic and laboratory studies may be indicated to rule out bony etiologies and metabolic disorders such as diabetes mellitus, rheumatoid arthritis, or seronegative arthritis.

Nerve conduction velocity (NCV) studies and electromyography can be performed to evaluate nerve latency, amplitude, and velocity and the polyphasic intrinsic foot muscle potentials. These tests are specific but not sensitive. A negative result does not rule out the possibility of TTS. Patients with negative NCV studies can still have pathology. Pfeiffer and Cracchiolo demonstrated that not all patients with TTS had positive nerve conduction velocities. There were 18% of the patients with a normal NCV who had tarsal tunnel release, and the authors found no clinical correlation between clinical outcome and the results of the study.[4]

Once the proper diagnosis has been made, a treatment protocol is chosen. If a space-occupying lesion is present, it should be excised using an open technique. Conservative treatment is initially instituted. Injection therapy, nonsteroidal antiinflammatory drugs, physical therapy, and orthotics are possible modalities. If conservative management fails, surgical intervention should be considered.

CONTRAINDICATIONS

There are contraindications for ETTR. Tarsal tunnel syndrome that recurs after an initial release cannot be treated endoscopically, as there is no ligament to ligate. The open technique is then indicated to release the hypertrophic scar that has formed. If the instrumentation does not slide up the neurovascular canal, the surgeon must reevaluate the instrument's position. Consideration should be given to the tarsal canal that adheres to the underlying neurovascular structures or if the passage is blocked by tissue such as fat, soft tissue, muscle, or tumor. Abundant varicosities around the ankle joint may be inadvertently cut or may be the cause of the TTS; in such cases I recommend the open technique. This technique is not recommended for an orthopedic deformity that inhibits full utilization of the instrumentation, such as a severe rear foot varus or clubfoot deformity.

SURGICAL TECHNIQUE

Endoscopic tarsal tunnel release uses instrumentation from the Smith & Nephew Dyonics ECTRA system. The retrograde cutting knife, probe, obturator, and cannulated sleeve are used during the procedure. A 30 degree 4.0 mm Smith & Nephew Dyonics endoscope and standard viewing equipment are also utilized.

Anatomic landmarks are identified. The medial malleolus, abductor hallucis, and proximal portion of the laciniate ligament are marked. The ligament is palpated via eversion and dorsiflexion of the foot followed by palpation of the neutral triangle behind the ankle joint. A tight band of tissue is felt between the most prominent part of the medial malleolus and the Achilles tendon. A 1 cm mark is made transversely over the superior aspect of the ligament. The superior aspect of the abductor hallucis muscle is then palpated where the neurovascular bundle penetrates deep into the foot. The soft and supple area is easily found. A 2- to 3-cm elliptical mark is then made immediately superior to the muscle belly.

After a thigh cuff is inflated, the proximal incision is placed; and dissection is carried through subcutaneous fat to the ligament with sharp and then blunt dissection. The ligament is left at this point, and attention is directed distally.

An elliptical incision is made, and a skin flap is created over the superior aspect of the abductor hallucis muscle, which is reflected plantarly. Vessels encountered along the way are identified and cauterized. Dissection is meticulously performed to the tarsal canal. The ligament is gently teased away at the intersection of the laciniate ligament and abductor hallucis muscle, exposing the neurovascular bundle, tarsal canal, and porta pedis (Fig. 18.1). The obturator is fitted into the cannulated sleeve, and the

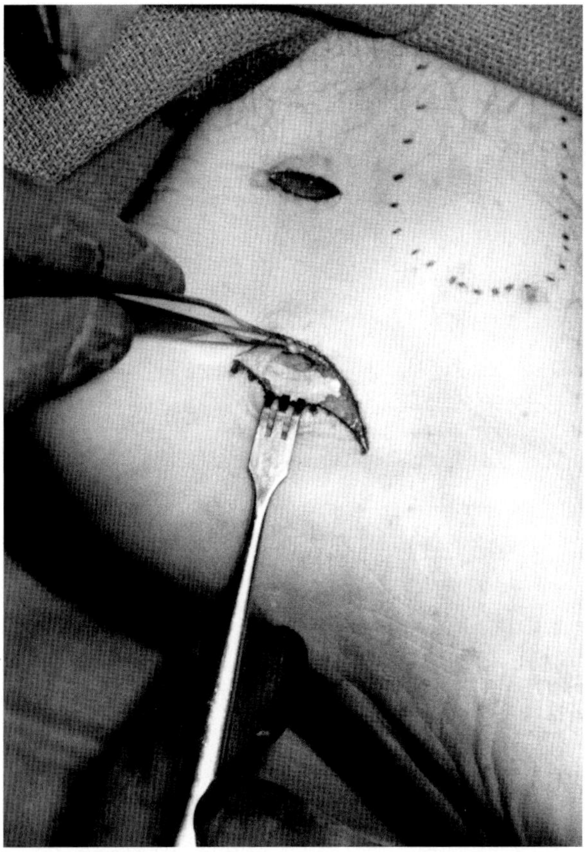

FIGURE 18.1. Dissection demonstrating the tarsal canal. (From Day FN, Naples JJ. Endoscopic tarsal tunnel release: update 96. *J Foot Ankle Surg* 1996;3:225–229, with permission from Elsevier.)

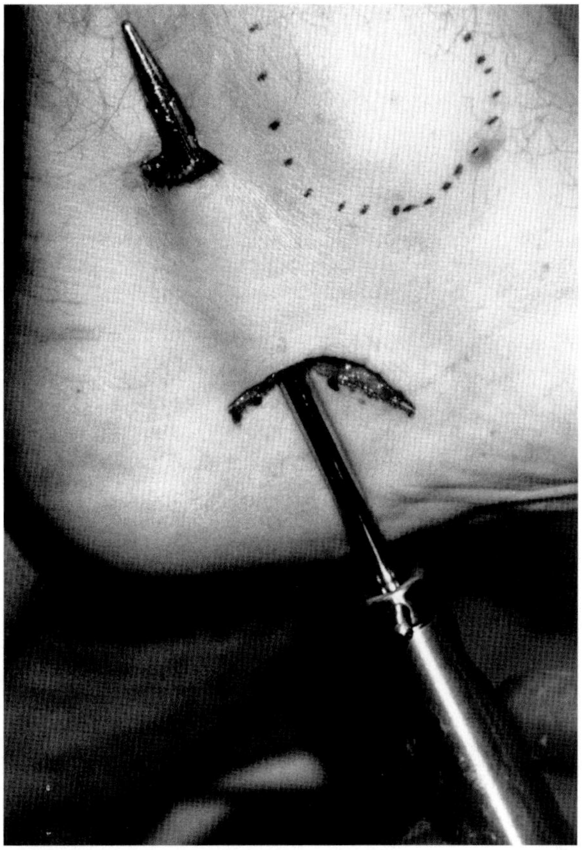

FIGURE 18.2. Obturator and cannula within the tarsal canal. (From Day FN, Naples JJ. Endoscopic tarsal tunnel release: update 96. *J Foot Ankle Surg* 1996;3:225–229, with permission from Elsevier.)

assembly is then placed in the tarsal canal from distal to proximal. Care is taken not to force the instrumentation into the canal. Slow advancement with a clockwise–counterclockwise motion of the assembly is all that is needed. If the instrumentation is unable to enter the canal, the surgeon should attempt to reposition the instrument and check the dissection. The surgeon must be able to stop this procedure if unable to maneuver the instrument up the canal, proceeding then with the open technique. The tip of the obturator is now penetrating the proximal incision; if not, carefully using a knife a small incision is made, allowing the assembly to pass through and out into the surgical field (Fig. 18.2). The laciniate ligament may be continuous with the deep fascia of the leg (seen in about 30% of cases by the author). The obturator is then removed, and the endoscope is placed in the cannula from the proximal end; the probe is placed in the distal end.

The transverse fibers of the laciniate ligament should now be visualized (Fig. 18.3A). Superficial veins may appear as purple streaks in the fibers, and care is taken to avoid them during cutting. The probe is used to remove any fat from the area and test the integrity and extent of the ligament. The probe is removed, and the retrograde cutting knife is inserted (Fig. 18.3B). The ligament is then divided from proximal to distal under endoscopic visualization (Fig. 18.3C,D). A retrograde force toward the cannula while cutting pulls the ligament away from the superficial veins and helps avoid inadvertent laceration. The instruments do not need to be reversed. After removing the knife and endoscope the obturator is reinserted into the cannula, and the entire assembly is gently removed. Attention is now directed to the porta pedis dissection.

The aponeurosis that surrounds the abductor hallucis muscle may need to be freed to enter the porta pedis if visualization of the nerves is obstructed. Care is taken not to "buttonhole" the aponeurosis, which may result in muscle herniation. As the posterior tibial nerve divides, it passes the abductor hallucis muscle and enters the plantar aspect of the foot. The septa that form individual compartments for the

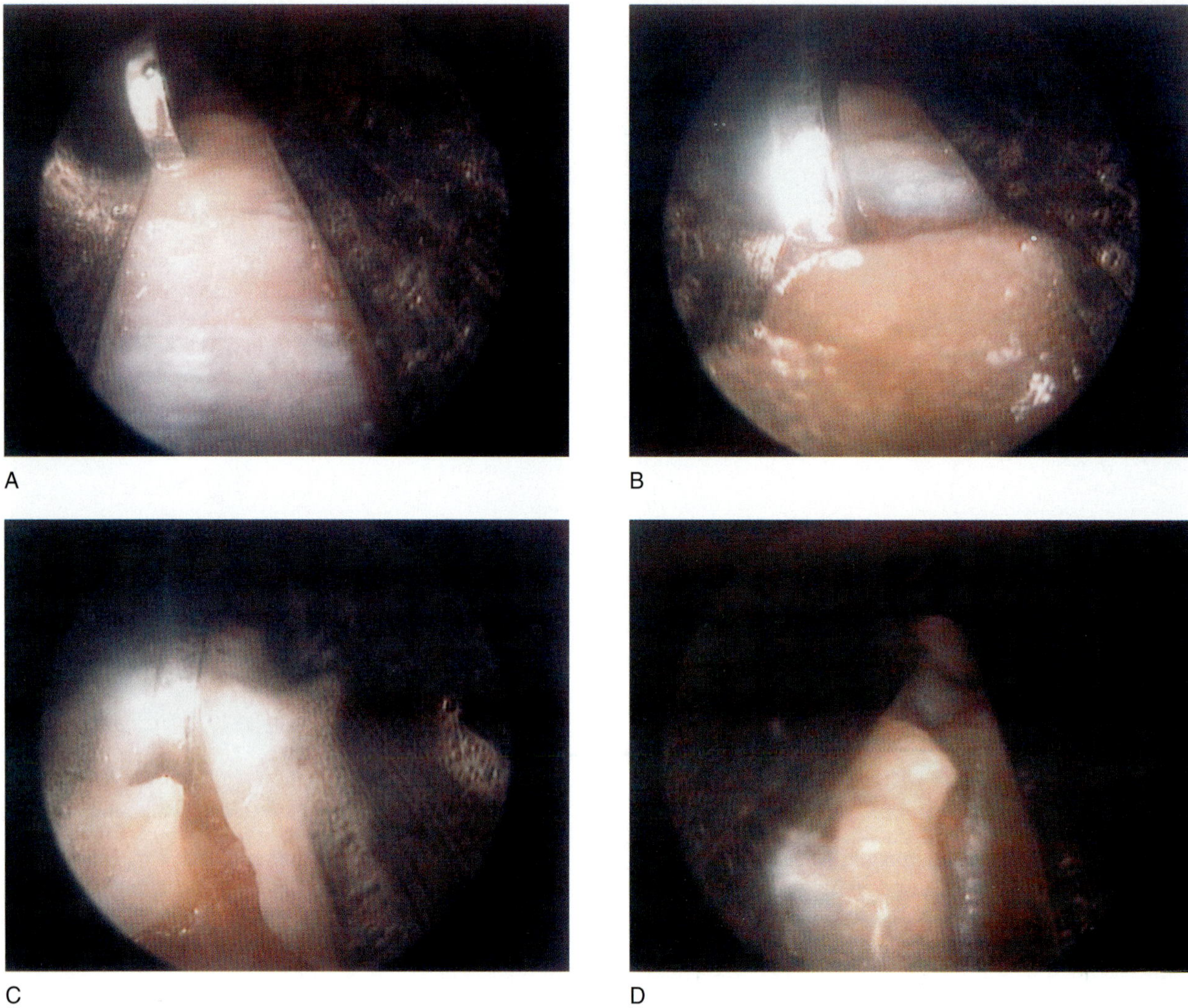

FIGURE 18.3. Endoscopic visualization of laciniate ligament ligation. (From Day FN, Naples JJ. Endoscopic tarsal tunnel release: update 96. *J Foot Ankle Surg* 1996;3:225–229, with permission from Elsevier.)

medial and lateral branches of the posterior tibial nerve must be dissected. Also, because the laciniate ligament may be continuous with the deep fascia of the leg proximally, the surgeon may need to cut the fascia to ensure no constriction on the posterior tibial nerve. The thigh cuff is then released to check for bleeding. Dexamethasone phosphate (0.5–1.0 cc) is placed in the surgical site, and the skin is closed with simple nonabsorbable suture. The patient should remain non-weight-bearing for 1 week, partial weight-bearing during the second week (with active range of motion of the ankle joint), and fully weight-bearing by the end of the third week. Sutures are removed at the end of the third week. The foot and ankle must remain clean, dry, and bandaged for the 3-week period.

RESULTS AND COMPLICATIONS

Two studies were performed by the author on a total of 15 patients. A multisurgeon sample included 22 patients, 7 of whom were lost to follow-up. In the first study of 10 patients, a three-incision approach was used.[5] This procedure was then modified to the present two-incision approach, and the second study was conducted with five patients.[6] A 90% success rate was found in the first study and a 100% success rate in the second study. To date, more than 100 procedures have been performed by various surgeons at Doctors Hospital using the two-incision approach previously described. No recurrence of TTS has been reported. One patient had no relief after surgery in the first study, which was attributed to extensive polyneuropathy. The only complication encountered was inadvertent ligation of superficial veins. Electrocautery or compression was used through the distal incision to stop any bleeding. The posterior tibial artery, vein, or nerve has never been compromised.

BIBLIOGRAPHY

1. Coughlin MJ, Mann RA. Tarsal tunnel syndrome. In: *Surgery of the foot and ankle*, 6th ed, vol 1. St. Louis: Mosby-Year Book, 1993;554.
2. Draves DJ. *Anatomy of the lower extremity.* Baltimore: Williams & Wilkins, 1986;153–154.
3. Pfeiffer WH, Cracchiolo A. Clinical results after tarsal tunnel decompression. *J Bone Joint Surg Am* 1994;76: 1222–1230.
4. Mahan KT, Rock JJ, Hillstrom HJ. Tarsal tunnel syndrome a retrospective study. *J Am Podiatr Med Assoc* 1996;2:81–91.
5. Day FN, Naples JJ. Tarsal tunnel syndrome: an endoscopic approach with 4–28 month follow-up. *J Foot Ankle Surg* 1994;3:224–228.
6. Day FN, Naples JJ. Endoscopic tarsal tunnel release: update 96. *J Foot Ankle Surg* 1996;3:225–229.

CHAPTER 19

Use of Laser and Radiofrequency for Foot and Ankle Arthroscopy

Marc A. Samson, Michael F. Dillingham, Gary S. Fanton, and George Thabit III

Many arthroscopists have found the laser to be a user-friendly device that speeds the operating time and lessens morbidity. The holmium:YAG (yttrium-aluminum-garnet) laser has supplanted the carbon dioxide (CO_2) laser as the primary laser for arthroscopic surgery. Other laser systems are either too impractical or too expensive for widespread use. Furthermore, a new radiofrequency device (Oratec, Menlo Park, CA) has been developed that shows promise as a tissue shrinker and coagulator, with the benefit of more refined ability to transfer energy to the tissue.

There are numerous advantages of the laser as a tool for ankle arthroscopy compared to traditional instruments. The small size of the laser probe facilitates arthroscopy in the small, tight recesses and spaces of the joints in the foot and ankle. In addition to the laser's ability to cut tissue and cauterize bleeders, as with traditional Bovie cautery, it is uniquely able to ablate and vaporize tissue, shrink collagen, and weld tissue. Furthermore, it is an excellent coagulator and produces approximately half as much tissue reaction as electrocautery, with necrosis varying from 5 to 50 μm (T. Vangsness, personal communication, 1998).

The CO_2 laser was the first laser used in arthroscopic surgery, although several of its aspects hindered its popularization. The requirement of an articulated arm for laser delivery, the need for a gas environment with its requirement for nonstandard technique, and a significant tendency for major complications made CO_2 lasers less than attractive.[1–10] In time it became obvious that most of these problems could be avoided by using a wavelength that could be transmitted fiberoptically and through a fluid medium. Lasers with these characteristics include the neodymium:YAG (Nd:YAG), holmium:YAG (Ho:YAG), KTP, excimer, and possibly the erbium:YAG (Er:YAG).[11–15] Use of the Ho:YAG laser began during the mid-1980s. It is a mid-infrared wavelength laser with fiberoptic transmission capacity (Fig. 19.1). Holmium is a rare earth element that when doped into a YAG crystal can emit a photon energy beam at 2.1 μg wavelength. It is well absorbed by water and is transmissible through readily available quartz fibers. Typically, 15–20 watts of energy are used with a pulse rate varying from 1 to 20 Hz and a pulse energy of 0.5–2.0 joules per minute. Machines are able to produce up to 80 watts of energy. The holmium laser delivery device is typically a plastic-sheathed, 400 μm fiberoptic cable with a metal handpiece. Various-diameter handpieces are available with different delivery angles and several specialized handpieces (Figs. 19.2–19.5). The laser is used in a contact or near-contact mode, permitting cutting and manipulation of the target tissue with a single instrument. Because the amount of laser energy delivered to a surface can be varied by defocusing the laser (moving and varying the intensity of the energy as one would with a

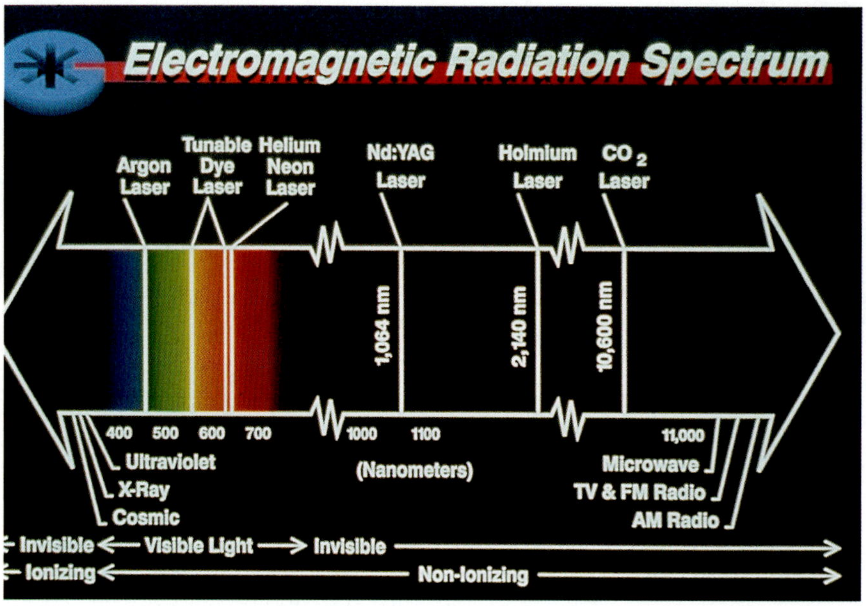

FIGURE 19.1. Electromagnetic laser spectrum.

magnifying glass), congealing or contouring the articular or meniscal cartilage is possible. With the holmium laser the thermal effect ensures excellent coagulation, and the dissipation of heat is sufficient to avoid charring and carbonization (Fig. 19.6).

The holmium laser works in a free beam mode (near-contact) rather than contact mode (hot tip). The laser beam therefore interacts directly with the tissue. This is the same manner by which the CO_2 laser works. When the beam enters the tissue, it is reflected, absorbed and then converted to heat, scattered within the tissue, or transmitted.[16,17] Absorption results in heat, which boils the tissue. Lasers that are not safe to use in a free beam mode must be used in a contact mode by way of a hot tip that acts as a heat sink. With this mode the laser energy is used only indirectly, and only cutting is possible.

In addition to its free beam use, the holmium laser also enjoys the advantage of having a short absorption length. Lasers with long absorption length, such as the Nd:YAG laser, travel deep into tissue and produce significant surrounding thermal effects that may be dangerously uncontrolled. A laser with a short absorption length is safer and more precise, producing minimal deep tissue heating and damage. The holmium laser, along with the CO_2, erbium, and excimer lasers, has a short absorption length and thus significant precision when cutting and abrading tissue.

Neither the erbium laser, which is not easily transmitted through glass fibers,[18] nor the xenon chloride excimer laser, which is a slow, poorly coagulating tool, has been used successfully in orthopedics. The neodymium:YAG laser also has a limited role in orthopedic surgery. Because its wavelength is longer (1.06 μm), it penetrates deeper into

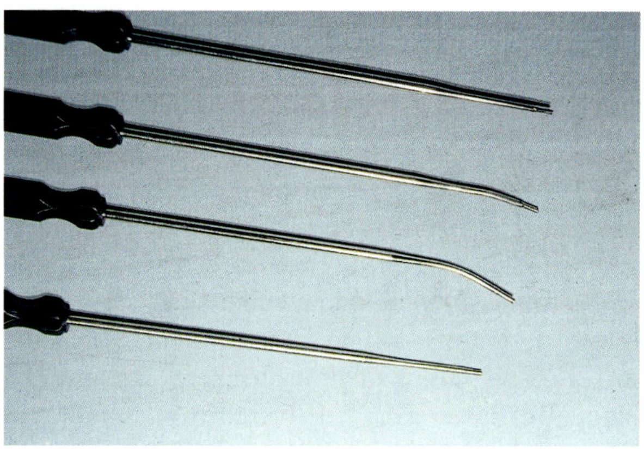

FIGURE 19.2. Various curved probes.

FIGURE 19.3. End firing probe.

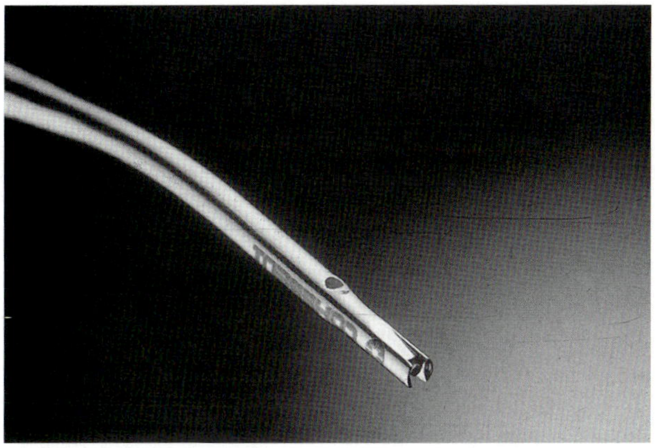

FIGURE 19.4. Later model, end firing probe, curved.

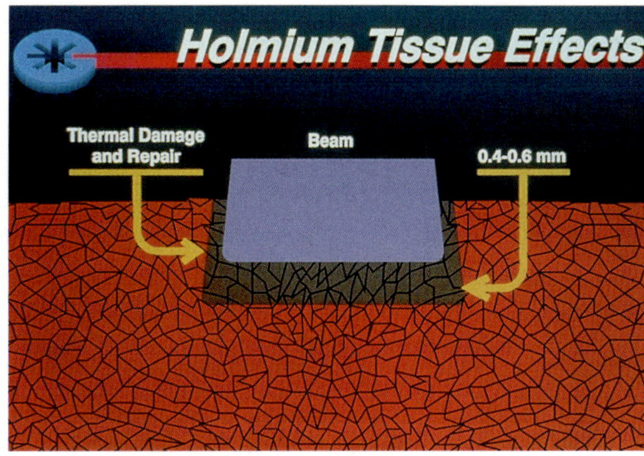

FIGURE 19.6. Holmium tissue effects.

tissue and causes significant, uncontrolled collateral damage. It creates a wide zone of necrosis and thick area of carbonization, with thermal effects up to 5 mm from the beam entrance. Furthermore, it must be used as a hot-tip device, and energy delivery is slow. As a result, the Nd:YAG laser is no longer marketed in the United States for orthopedic use.

The holmium laser is a pulsed laser with a 2.1 μm wavelength. This wavelength is between that of the neodymium:YAG and CO_2 lasers and incorporates the advantages of both (Fig. 19.1). Its thermal effect is well controlled, and thermal damage in the meniscus does not exceed 550 μm[19–25] (Figs. 19.7, 19.8). The zone of thermal necrosis is limited to approximately 80 μm. Because it can be used in a fluid environment through a small fiberoptic handpiece, it offers precision and speed. Regarding absorption characteristics, it offers excellent ablation and produces slight to moderate thermal damage, which is much more predictable and precise than electrocautery, free beam Nd:YAG, or contact probe systems. Because it is truly a pulsed laser, heat conduction is minimized between pulses, during which time the arthroscopic fluid cools the target tissue.[26–29] This is a significant advantage over hot tip contact devices or continuous-wave lasers. Given the intermittent and dependable cooling of the fluid environment, high energy can be delivered and the rate of ablation varied by changing the pulse frequency. A Ho:YAG laser can be used in a near contact mode and defocused to create a large spot, allowing effective meniscal ablation, synovial reduction, and coagulation.

The holmium:YAG laser has distinct advantages when compared to electrocautery. Cautery works best in nonphysiologic fluid such as sterile water.[30] Its zone of necrosis is poorly controlled, generally involving the path of greatest conduction or least resistance. Collateral necrosis may reach several millimeters into surrounding tissue. Laser photocoagulation is more accurate and better controlled.

We have studied the clinical applications of the holmium:YAG laser since 1988 and found it to be

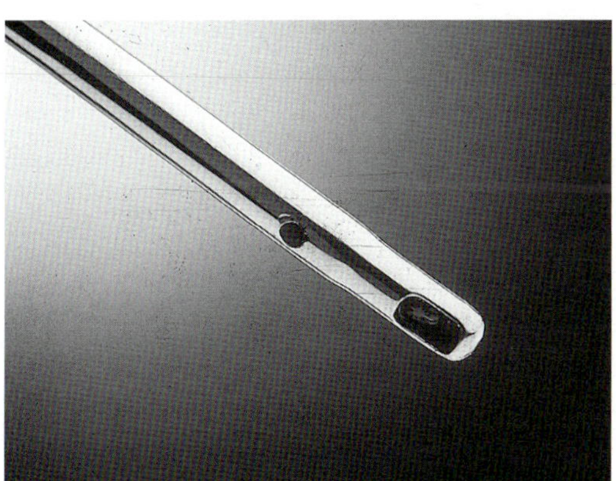

FIGURE 19.5. Ninety degree right angle firing probe.

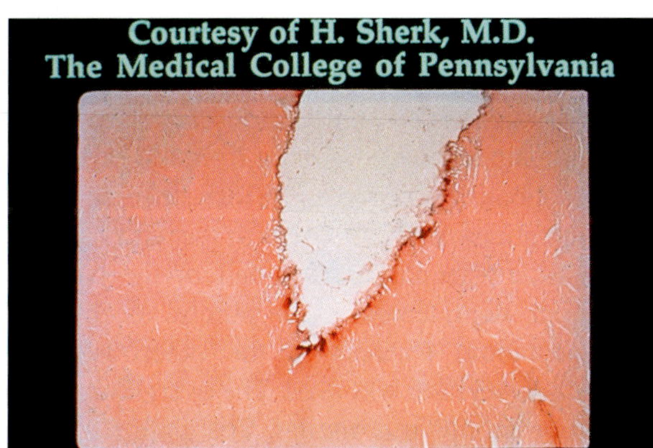

FIGURE 19.7. Thin zone of necrosis with holmium:YAG laser. (Courtesy of H. Sherk.)

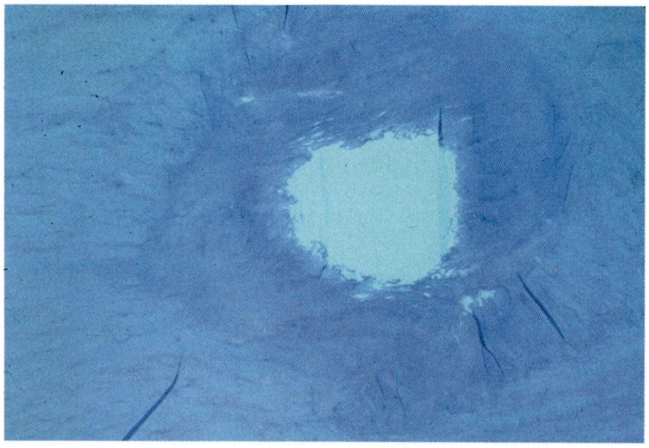

FIGURE 19.8. Same effect as seen in Figure 19.7.

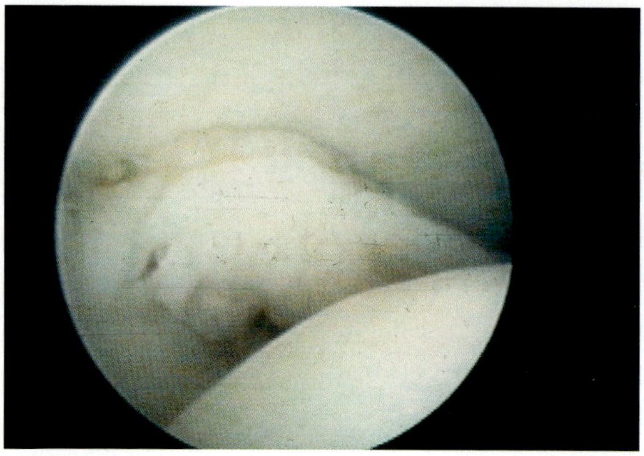

FIGURE 19.9. Lateral soft tissue impingement (L/STI) prior to laser treatment.

safe and effective. The fiberoptic instrumentation allows easy and increased joint accessibility, which minimizes joint trauma compared to conventional instrumentation. Postoperative bleeding, hemarthrosis, inflammation, and pain were substantially reduced in the laser-treated patients compared to the conventional instrumentation group.[16] We believe that the hemostatic capability of the laser is one of its greatest advantages. The contact or near-contact delivery technique allows safe application of energy to the target tissue with a tactile feedback that is helpful during tissue manipulation. With a single instrument, the surgeon is able to cut, contour, resect, ablate, and coagulate. Furthermore, there is reduced operating time because of the decreased need for instrument swapping, and there is no need to change the arthroscopic fluid environment. We have used the laser successfully in a variety of settings. In the knee, it has proved valuable for plica resection, synovectomy, and lateral retinacular release; and has proven to be dependable in its capacity to prevent bleeding postoperatively. Since its early development, application of the laser has now been extended to the shoulder, elbow, and ankle.

Zangger and Gerber looked at a series of 16 patients who underwent ankle arthroscopy for mostly posttraumatic disorders, ranging from impingement to osteochondritis dissecans. Most suffered from posttraumatic synovitis and scar tissue with or without anterior osteophytes. One-half of the patients underwent débridement with purely mechanical instrumentation, whereas in the other half the holmium:YAG laser was used. The overall outcome of the two groups was similar. The authors found, however, that using the laser had improved the analgesic effects, permitted easier approach to the tight recesses of the joint, and allowed contouring of convex surfaces, which cannot be performed as easily with standard instruments.[31]

For the reasons that have been discussed, the holmium laser offers significant advantages during surgery of confined joints such as the ankle and the subtalar joints. The curved handpieces or side-firing handpieces allow access to the entire anterior ankle joint, the medial and lateral gutter areas, and almost all talus and tibial articular surfaces via a routine anterior portal. Fibrillated or degenerative areas of articular surfaces can be smoothed, contoured, and débrided. Areas of posttraumatic fibrosis such as Wolin's lesion in the anterior lateral ankle or posttraumatic fibrosis after fracture or osteoarthritic fibrosis can be safely cut and its volume reduced. Chronic synovitis and adhesions can be treated quickly and effectively. Furthermore, the laser appears to be beneficial when treating soft tissue impingement lesions (Fig. 19.9–19.11), fibroarthrosis and capsulitis because it causes less

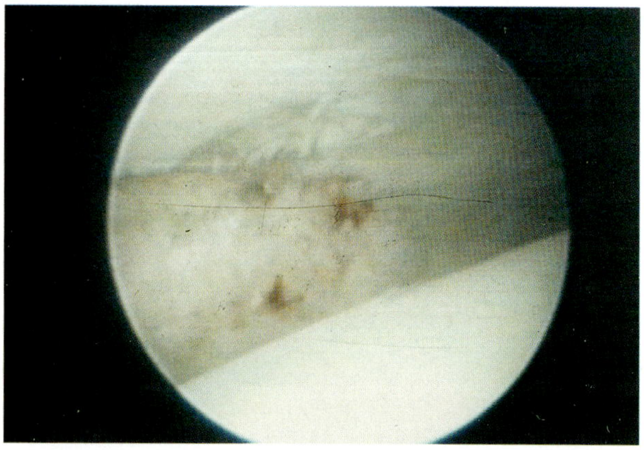

FIGURE 19.10. Same ankle as in Figure 19.9 after laser ablation.

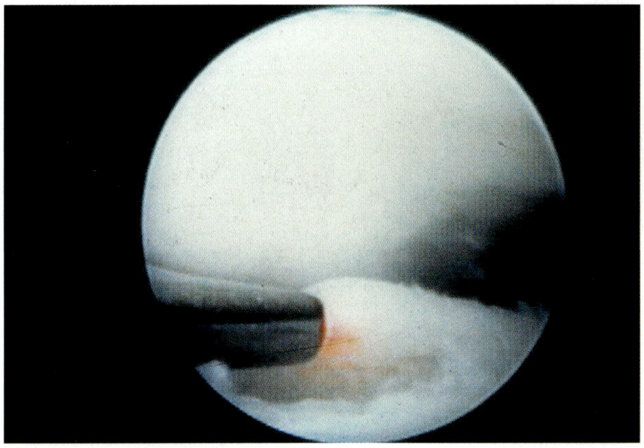

FIGURE 19.11. Laser beam used to trim chondral defect. In our experience this seems to reduce or prevent further peeling of the cartilage layer.

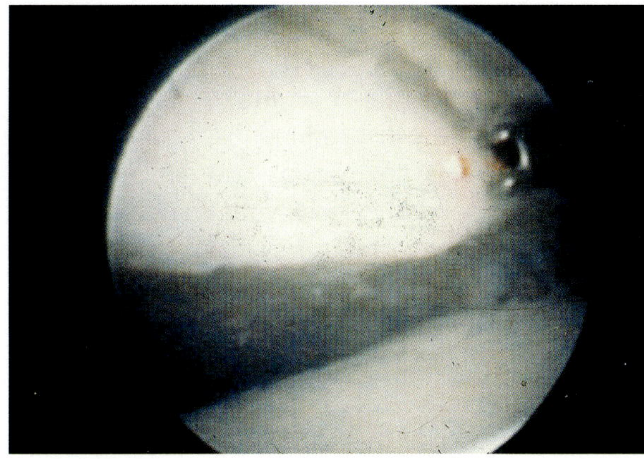

FIGURE 19.13. Laser is used here to trim an osteophyte.

chondral damage, less bleeding, a lower recurrence rate, and quicker rehabilitation.

Osteochondritic lesions or chondral lesions of the talar dome or tibial plafond can be easily débrided using the laser. Curettes and abraders are best for removing articular cartilage down to bleeding bone. Laser or radiofrequency probes might be beneficial in débriding recesses or "tight" areas. There have been at least two cases of osteonecrosis reported when this tool was used extensively. As with other joints, the laser is also useful for removing ossicles or entrapped loose bodies (Fig. 19.12). The laser can be used to either ablate the loose body directly or to shrink or pulverize the loose body to a more manageable size. Osteophytes (Figs. 19.13, 19.14) can be significantly reduced directly with high-power laser application; alternatively, once mechanical instrumentation has removed the osteophyte, the residual bone base can be photocoagulated. In this case, the laser results in less instrument crowding, better proprioception, greater accuracy, less postoperative bleeding, and greater speed. For treatment of chronic nonunions, the laser can help débride a pseudoarthrosis and contour and sculpt articular cartilage in chondral defects and chondromalacia.

Pathology of the posterior recess, such as spurs and soft tissue entities, is amenable to arthroscopic laser surgery. Here the combined posterolateral approach or accessory posterolateral approach should be employed. Furthermore, subtalar joint pathology (synovitis, adhesions, fibroarthrosis, chondromalacia, chondral defects) is more easily approached with a laser than with conventional mechanical instrumentation because of the confined space. In addition, it is conceivable that plantar fasciitis can be transected by a laser in less traumatic fashion, similar to the use of the laser in carpal tunnel release, although this has not been reported. In this case, no fluid pump or electrocautery would be required to

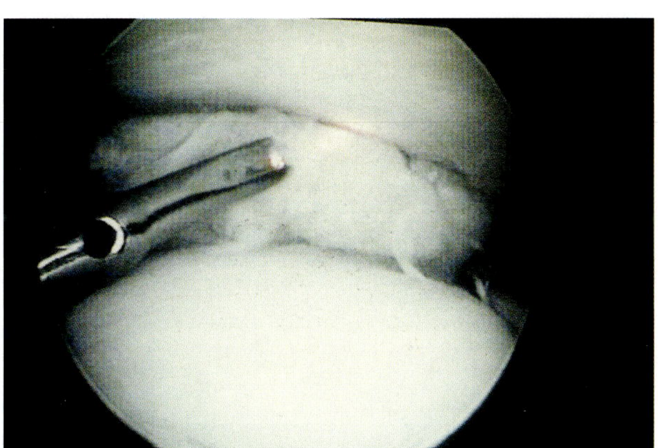

FIGURE 19.12. Laser is used here to ablate an entrapped loose body in the posterior recess (P/OCI).

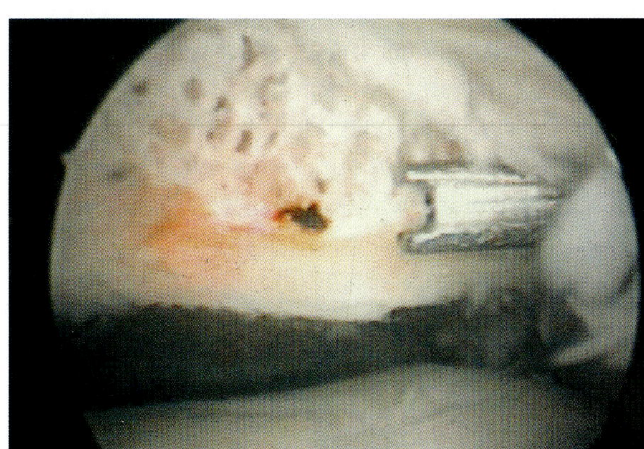

FIGURE 19.14. Osteophyte after removal via holmium: YAG laser.

maintain hemostasis. The laser may also be useful for treating retrocalcaneal bursitis.

We have used the laser on multiple occasions in the foot and ankle. Most commonly, it has been used for coagulation, synovectomy, trimming the margins only of chondral or osteochondral defects, and cutting and ablating fibrous tissue. One of the more promising laser surgery techniques is in the area of tissue welding and collagen shrinkage. Extrapolating the techniques used for laser-assisted capsular shrinkage and collagen shrinkage used in shoulder instability (see Radiofrequency Applications section for more information); the laser can be used to shrink lax ligamentous tissue in the ankle and foot as well. We have successfully treated chronic ankle instability by thermal stabilization of the lateral ligamentous complex arthroscopically. Short-term results have been promising.

In all, there have been no complications in these cases attributable to the laser, and in fact in many of these of these cases access, maneuverability, speed, and visibility were substantially improved by using the laser device. For instance, synovectomy in the medial and lateral gutters of the ankle utilizing a 70 degree laser probe for tissue ablation and coagulation cannot be done as easily using mechanical instrumentation and cautery. Additionally, the 1.5 mm laser probe can be placed much farther back into the gutters and tibiotalar joint than can be done with traditional instrumentation.

RADIOFREQUENCY APPLICATIONS

A device has been developed that applies radiofrequency technology to surgical techniques originally created for the laser. The Oratec device (Oratec Systems, Menlo Park, CA) (Fig. 19.15) and other radiofrequency systems by other manufacturers can be used for tissue contouring, collagen shrinkage, chondroplasty, and coagulation or in the power mode for cutting, scraping, and coagulation.

Thermal techniques such as laser-assisted capsular shrinkage, thermal-assisted capsular shrinkage, and collagen shrinkage utilize the intrinsic biochemical properties of the collagen molecule to enable tissue shrinkage. Type I collagen is the most abundant protein in the human body[32] (Fig. 19.16), comprising approximately 90% of all ligaments and tendons.[34] The molecules themselves are usually oriented longitudinally in the direction of stress and are held in extended configuration under tension.[34,35] Collagen is comprised of a triple helix molecule with an organized crystalline structure, it contains heat-sensitive bonds that are crosslinked with hydrogen bonds for greater strength[34,35] (Fig. 19.17).

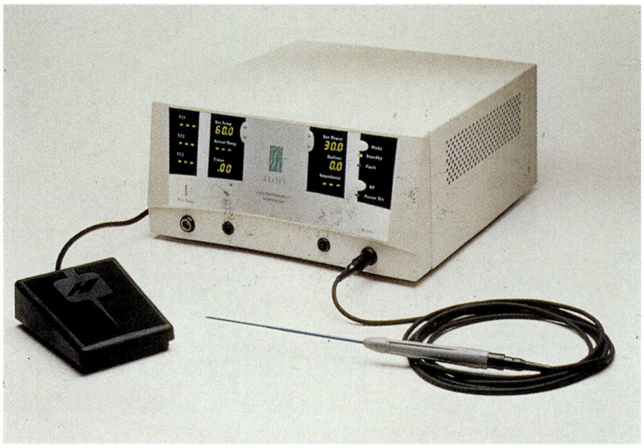

FIGURE 19.15. Power source of Oratec radiofrequency application.

The structural basis underlying the shrinkage of collagenous tissue is a conformational change from the crystalline, extended state to the random coil, contracted state.[34–36] When heat higher than 60°C is applied to the collagen molecule, the heat-sensitive (primarily hydrogen) bonds break[35] and the crystalline extended structure begins to uncoil and shrink; as the molecule contracts, its diameter increases,[34–36] which causes the collagen molecule to "denature" or exist in the random coil state. Over time, fibroblasts invade and grow over the shortened, denatured collagen scaffolding, creating new but shorter collagen molecules.[37]

It has been shown that contraction of the collagen molecule is both time- and temperature-depen-

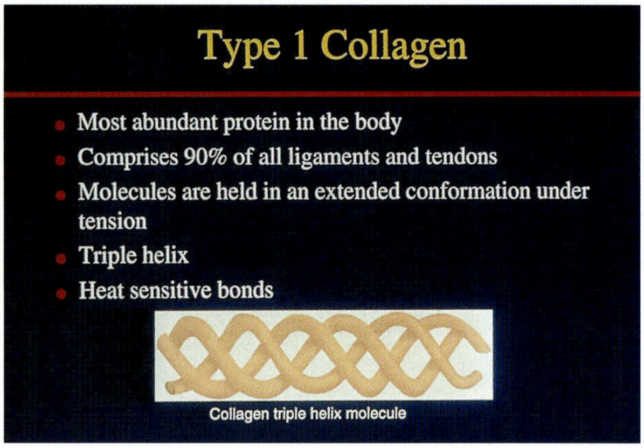

FIGURE 19.16. Type I collagen. Molecules are held in an extended conformation under tension.

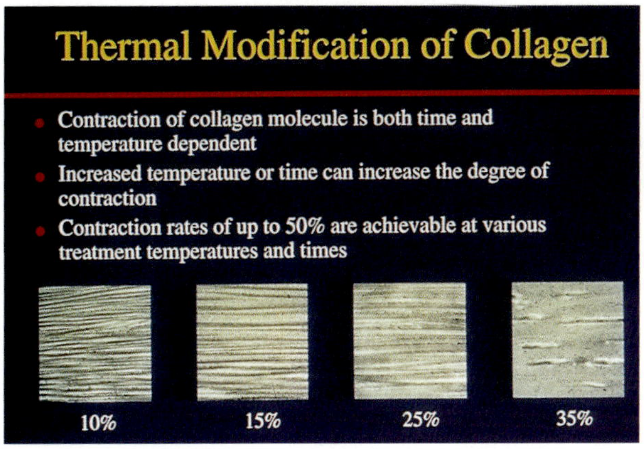

FIGURE 19.17. Thermal modification of collagen. Contraction of collagen molecule.

dent.[38,39] Increasing the temperature or the duration of application of the increased temperature can increase the degree of contraction. Contraction rates of up to 50% are achievable at various treatment temperatures and durations.[38,39] Animal laboratory studies have shown an inverse relation between treatment temperature and posttreatment mechanical properties. It has been shown that the reduction in mechanical properties is caused by increasing disassociation of the collagen as the tissue temperature increases. As the temperature increases above 60°C the normalized stiffness increases significantly, whereas the rate of shrinkage decreases.[38] Furthermore, increased shrinkage at temperatures above the "therapeutic range" may significantly alter mechanical properties (Figs. 19.18, 19.19).

These principles have been applied to the laser-assisted capsular shift technique utilizing the holmium:YAG laser. Our unpublished 4-year clinical data validate the arthroscopic thermal approach with more than 90% efficacy and a high success rate. Furthermore, these procedures can be done as an outpatient procedure, whereas open stabilization has been an inpatient procedure.

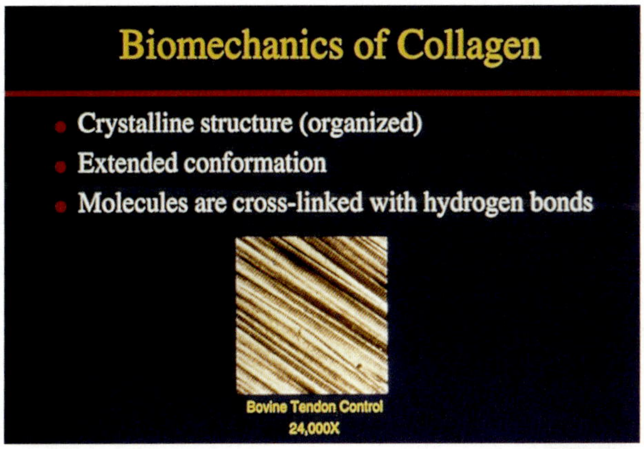

FIGURE 19.18. Biomechanics of collagen. Crystalline structure (organized). Molecules are crosslinked with hydrogen bonds.

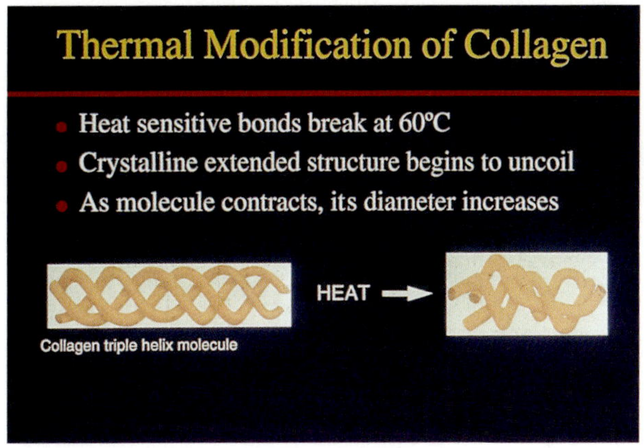

FIGURE 19.19. Thermal modification of collagen. Thermal shrinkage at increased temperature results in significant attentuation of mechanical properties.

Although this technique was originally developed for use with the low-energy laser, the laser itself perhaps is not the ideal energy delivery device. The laser, used in a hot-tip technique, is focal and applies only superficial energy and heat to the tissue. There is no temperature control, and the laser is costly. The radiofrequency device (Oratec Systems, Menlo Park, CA) attempts to improve on the energy delivery technique while offering a more cost-effective alternative to traditional laser use.

The Oratec device transmits radiofrequency energy into the soft tissue, thereby creating oscillation in intercellular electrolytes in host tissue. This molecular movement generates heat in the tissue, so the tissue itself (not the probe) generates heat. The transmission of radiofrequency energy provides consistent, predictable thermal effects that are more even than microwaves. Three temperature-controlled handpieces have been developed (TAC-S, TAC-C, Mini-TAC) that modulate the temperature in the tissue to preset levels (Fig. 19.20). It is the only device available with temperature feedback regulation. The probes themselves are highly versatile, low-profile devices that are designed for use with saline or lactated Ringer's solution. In addition, the temperature-controlled probes are malleable, which facilitates access to specific areas in a joint. Furthermore, they can be used either on the temperature setting for thermal modification of collagen or a power setting for coagulation. The laser transmits energy to only the first millimeter of tis-

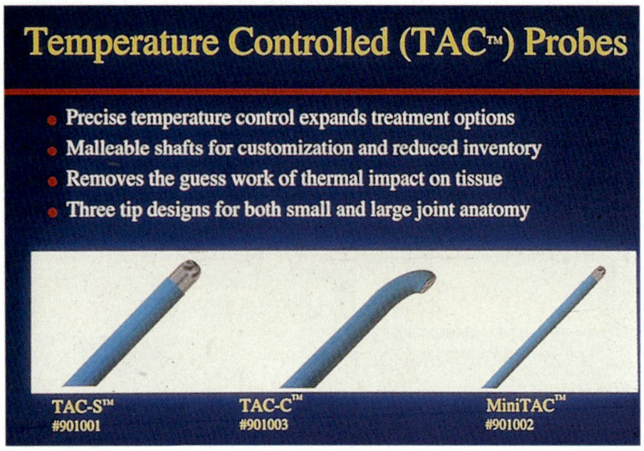

FIGURE 19.20. Three temperature controlled handpieces.

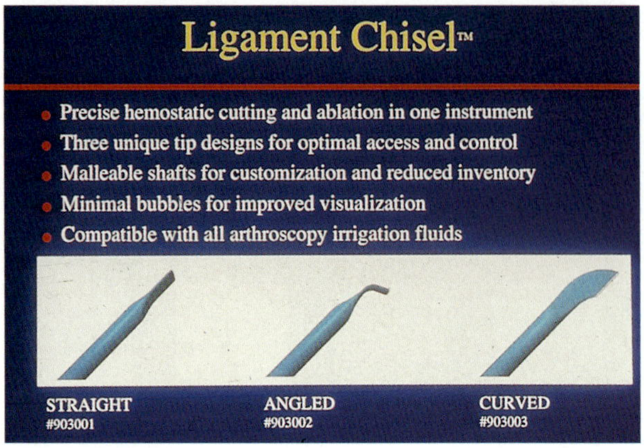

FIGURE 19.21. Three cutting and ablation handpieces.

sue, causing intense heat, whereas the bipolar device transmits energy via the path of least resistance in conductive irrigating solution and therefore creates a broad area of tissue destruction. In contrast, the Oratec monopolar probe induces current into the tissue, causing heat by molecular friction and conduction in a well-controlled area and under precise temperature control.

Our follow-up with the thermal-assisted capsular shift device has been extremely promising in the shoulder, with results at least equal to if not superior to those seen with other arthroscopic stabilization techniques. Our early results with the Oratec radiofrequency device in the shoulder have encouraged us to expand the application for such procedures. We have recently begun radiofrequency thermal stabilization of ankle ligaments and have used the thermal capacity of the Oratec to shrink lax anterior tibiofibular, anterior talofibular, and calcaneofibular ligaments entirely arthroscopically. Our preliminary results have been exciting. We have used this technique in more than 20 patients and have corrected ankle instability in nearly all of them, with no significant complications to date.

The technique involves a standard arthroscopic approach to the ankle. The TAC-S probe is then inserted via the anteromedial portal. With the generator set at 67°C and 40 watts on the temperature setting, the probe is delivered in a contact fashion along the lax ligament or tissue. The thermocouple in the probe tip measures tissue temperature through conduction, and thus accurate tissue temperature is best obtained by leaving the probe in direct contact with the tissue. The probe is then slowly swept back and forth along the tissue, creating a thermal response. As a result of the thermal energy, the lax ligaments slowly tighten as they shrink. Once the desired response is achieved, the arthroscopy is terminated and the ankle is immobilized. The patient is then protected with a cast or boot for 4–6 weeks (Fig. 19.22).

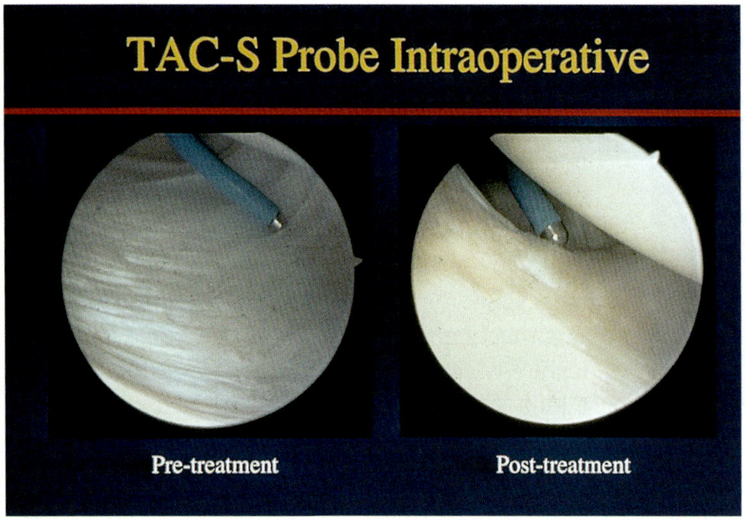

FIGURE 19.22. Pre- and post-treatment with thermal shrinkage of the shoulder capsule of the inferior axillary recess with a temperature controlled probe.

The second application of radiofrequency is more like that of traditional cautery. Several cost-effective probes with different tip configurations have been developed that can be used in a power mode. The desired effects on tissue can be modulated by varying the power setting (low power for coagulation, high power for cutting and ablating). The power probes (straight chisel, curved chisel, angled chisel) are highly effective coagulators and soft tissue ablators (Fig. 19.21). By modulating the power somewhere between pure cutting and pure coagulation, a cutting/coagulation ratio can be attained concurrently. Although these probes are as effective as the laser in terms of ablation of soft tissue and coagulation, they are not as effective as the laser for ablating bone and articular cartilage. Perhaps the most appealing aspect of the radiofrequency device is its cost. A typical radiofrequency system costs approximately 10% of a typical holmium:YAG laser system, and the handpieces are comparable if not less expensive than the laser handpieces.

CONCLUSIONS

The application of therapeutic heat, by either holmium laser or radiofrequency, provides a safe, effective arthroscopic alternative to mechanical instrumentation for peripheral joint surgery. Their small probe sizes and fluid medium transmissibility provide significant advantages over electrocautery and other laser systems developed for biomedical applications. Developing radiofrequency technology provides a more cost-effective alternative to laser systems in most applications with similar results. As the surgeon's ability and skill increase with time using these devices, the laser and radiofrequency devices should allow greater versatility and speed of use in the future.

BIBLIOGRAPHY

1. Philandrianos G. Carbon dioxide laser in arthroscopic surgery of the knee. *Presse Med* 1985;14: 2103–2104.
2. Smith JB, Nance TA. Arthroscopic laser surgery. Presented at the annual meeting of the Arthroscopy Association of North America, Coronado, CA, 1983.
3. Whipple TL, Caspari RB. Laser energy in arthroscopic meniscectomy. *Orthopedics* 1983;6:1165–1169.
4. Whipple TL, Caspari RB, Meyers JF. Arthroscopic laser meniscectomy in a gas medium. *Arthroscopy* 1985;1:2–7.
5. Whipple TL, Caspari RB, Meyers JF. Synovial response to laser induced carbon ash residue. *Lasers Surg Med* 1984;3:291–300.
6. Whipple TL, et al. Electron microscopy of CO_2 laser-induced effects in human fibrocartilage. *Lasers Surg Med* 1987;7:184–188.
7. Lane GJ, et al. CO_2 vs. holmium:YAG laser arthroscopic debridement [abstract]. In: *American Society for Laser Medicine and Surgery*, Suppl. 3, 1991.
8. Brillhart AT. Arthroscopic laser surgery: the CO_2 laser and its use. *Am J Arthroscopy* 1991;2:7–12.
9. Meller M, Black H, Sherk H: Wavelength selection in laser arthroscopy. Presented at the American Society for Laser Medicine and Surgery. San Diego, CA, April 1991.
10. Gruenwald JM. Fatal air embolism during arthroscopy. *J Bone Joint Surg Br* 1990;72:929.
11. Berns MW, Nelson JR. Laser applications in biomedicine. I. Biophysics, cell biology, and biostimulation. *J Laser Applications* 1988;1:34–39.
12. Fronck, J, Krakauer J, Clowell CW Jr. Effects of the Nd:YAG laser on the meniscus of the knee joint. *SPIE* 1990;1200:214–220.
13. Miller DV, et al. The use of contact Nd:YAG laser in arthroscopic surgery: effects on articular cartilage and meniscal tissue. *Arthroscopy* 1989;5:245–253.
14. O'Brien SJ, Miller DV. The contact neodymium yttrium-aluminum-garnet laser: a new approach to arthroscopic laser surgery. *Clin Orthop* 1990;252: 95–100.
15. Sherk HH, Killmer C. Arthroscopic surgery with a freebeam Nd:YAG laser. In: Sherk HH (ed) *Lasers in orthopedics*, Philadelphia: Lippincott, 1990;134–139.
16. Fanton GS, Dillingham MF. Arthroscopic meniscectomy using the holmium:YAG laser: a double-blind study. Presented at the Arthroscopy Association of North America annual meeting, Orlando, April 1990.
17. Fanton GS. Use of the holmium laser in arthroscopy: multiple joint applications. Presented at the Coherent Symposium on Advances in Laser Arthroscopy: New Techniques in Orthopedic Surgery, Anaheim, March 1991.
18. Rand JA, Gaffey TA. Effect of electrocautery on fresh human articular cartilage. *Arthroscopy* 1985;1: 242–246.
19. Nishioka NS, Damankevitz Y. Reflectance during pulsed holmium laser irradiation of tissue. *Lasers Surg Med* 1989;9:375–381.
20. Trauner K, Nishioka N, Patel D. Pulsed holmium yttrium-aluminum-garnet (Ho:YAG) laser ablation of fibrocartilage and articular cartilage. *Am J Sports Med* 1990;18:316–321.

21. VanLeeuwen TG, et al. Non-contact tissue ablation by holmium:YAG laser pulses in blood. *Lasers Surg Med* 1991;11:24–26.
22. Nishioka, et al. Ablation of rabbit liver, stomach and colon with pulsed holmium laser. *Gastroenterology* 1989;96:831–837.
23. Stein E, et al. Acute and chronic effects of bone ablation with a pulsed holmium laser. *Lasers Surg Med* 1990;10:384–388.
24. Vari SG, et al. Ablation study of the knee structure tissues with a Ho:YAG laser. Am Soc Laser Med Surg 1991 (Suppl 3) (abstr).
25. Lane GJ, Mooar PA. Holmium:YAG laser arthroscopic debridement [abstract]. In: *American Society for Laser Medicine and Surgery*. Suppl. 3, 1991.
26. Berns MW. Laser surgery. *Sci Am* 1991;264:85–90.
27. Decklebaum, et al. Reduction of laser-induced pathologic tissue injury using pulsed energy delivery. *Am J Cardiol* 1985;56:662–667.
28. Hobbs ER, et al. Superpulsed lasers: minimizing thermal damage with short duration, high irradiance pulses. *J Dermatol Surg Oncol* 1987;13:955–964.
29. Walsh JT Jr, et al. Pulsed CO_2 laser tissue ablation: effect of tissue type and pulse duration on thermal damage. *Laser Surg Med* 1988;8:108–118.
30. Reagan BF, McInerny VK, Treadwell BV, et al. Irrigation solutions for arthroscopy. *J Bone Joint Surg Am* 1983;65:624–631.
31. Zangger P, Gerber BE. Use of the laser in arthroscopy of the ankle: indications, method, first results. *Orthopade* 1996;25:73–78.
32. Tanzer ML. Cross-linking of collagen—endogenous aldehydes in collagen react in several ways to form a variety of unique covalent cross-links. *Science* 1973;180:561–566.
33. Birk DE, Silver FH, Trelstad RL. Matrix assembly. In: Hay ED (ed) *Cell biology of extracellular matrix*, 2nd ed. New York: Plenum, 1991;221.
34. Flory PL. Role of crystallization in polymers and proteins. *Science* 1956;124:53–60.
35. Gustavson KH. *The chemistry and reactivity of collagen*. San Diego: Academic, 1956.
36. Lennox FG. Shrinkage of collagen. *Biochim Biophys Acta* 1949;3:170–187.
37. Hayashi K, Nieckarz JA, Thabitt G III, et al. Effect of nonablative laser energy on the joint capsule: an in vivo rabbit study using a holmium:YAG laser. *Laser Surg Med* 1997;20:164–171.
38. Wall MS, et al. Thermal modification of collagen. *J Shoulder Elbow Surg* 1999;8:339–344.
39. Weir CE. Rate of shrinkage of tendon collagen—heat, entropy and free energy of activation of the shrinkage of untreated tendon; effect of acid salt, pickle, and tannage on the activation of tendon collagen. *J Am Leather Chem Assoc* 1949;44:108–138.

CHAPTER 20

Office Foot and Ankle Arthroscopy

Neal C. Small and Walter A. Del Gallo

Despite the fact that arthroscopy is one of many types of minimally invasive surgery, most arthroscopic procedures are still being performed in a hospital setting. The modern practice of foot and ankle surgery has largely evolved from trauma centers and children's hospitals that have traditionally been an integral part of orthopedic training. Orthopedic surgeons, throughout residency training and most fellowship programs, are trained in surgical techniques that are applied in the hospital setting. Therefore arthroscopic surgery, although minimally invasive, has evolved in a similar manner and has remained a hospital procedure.

In contrast with foot and ankle surgery, many other surgical specialties have removed minimally invasive surgery from the hospital or ambulatory surgery center to the office setting. Among these specialties are ear-nose-throat, ophthalmology, plastic surgery, obstetrics-gynecology, colorectal procedures, and general surgery. Gastroenterologists and rheumatologists have also significantly increased the number of procedures performed in the office environment.

For years, oral surgeons and podiatrists were unable to acquire full hospital privileges in many states, so these practitioners developed protocols and anesthesia techniques for office procedures performed under local anesthesia. In many instances, intravenous sedation was used as well. Despite the fact that hospital privileges are now available for these practitioners, many still choose to perform minimally invasive procedures and other, more extensive procedures in the office setting for reasons of convenience, cost-effectiveness, and patient preference.

INDICATIONS

The indications for office foot and ankle arthroscopy are listed in Table 20.1. The indications are similar to those for ankle arthroscopy performed in the hospital under general or regional anesthesia. However, procedures requiring major bony work, such as arthroscopic ankle arthrodesis, cannot be performed with local anesthesia and sedation.

CONTRAINDICATIONS

The surgical contraindications to office foot and ankle arthroscopy (Table 20.2) are identical to those for ankle arthroscopy performed in the hospital. Patient selection for local anesthesia with sedation in the office setting is extremely important and is discussed later.

PATIENT SELECTION

Medical screening is done prior to scheduling a patient for office surgery. At that time it is determined whether a particular patient is a candidate for office operative foot and ankle arthroscopy. The patient is asked to fill out a questionnaire concerning previous medical and surgical diagnoses, allergies, and medications. This allows identification of patients who require other medical consultations or who would be better treated in a hospital setting. Laboratory tests, electrocardiography (ECG), and chest radiography are not performed on patients scheduled for office operative arthroscopy. Patients who

TABLE 20.1. *Indications for office ankle and foot arthroscopy*

Soft tissue impingement (anterolateral synovial impingement)
Osteochondral or chondral lesions
Bony impingement (osetophytes, tibiotalar spurs)
Synovitis (posttraumatic, inflammatory)
Loose bodies
Arthrofibrosis
Instability (open modified Brostrom combined with arthroscopic synovectomy and débridement)
Undiagnosed foot and ankle symptomatology (diagnostic foot and ankle arthroscopy)

have surgery in the office are basically healthy. The yield from such studies is extremely small in this age group. The tests are expensive, so eliminating them serves to keep the overall costs of the procedure more reasonable.

The psychological makeup and personality of the patient is an important factor. If the patient becomes concerned by the sight of blood or a needle, the surgery should not be performed under local anesthesia in the office setting. If the nurse reports that the patient is too nervous for office operative arthroscopy, the surgeon should listen.

Once the patient has been identified as a candidate for office surgery, the date and time are set for the procedure. The next step is preauthorization by the third-party payer. Occasionally, a second surgical opinion is mandated by the payer, but this practice has become less frequent.

Patients between the ages of 16 and 65 years of age are selected. Patients under the age of 16 may not have the emotional maturity to cooperate during a 30- to 45-minute procedure under local anesthesia. Patients over the age of 65 were thought to have a potentially higher risk of medical problems that would be better treated in a hospital environment should the need arise. Patients in American Society of Anesthesiologists (ASA) categories I and II are selected.

TABLE 20.2. *Contraindications to foot and ankle arthroscopy*

Local soft tissue infection
Severe arthritis with deformity
Poor vascular status
Severe edema
Acutely injured ankle with ruptured ligaments and capsule

Most mature, stable patients are pleased that they will not be subjected to a general anesthetic for their arthroscopic procedure in the office. Those who have had a previous general anesthetic are well aware of the sometimes unpleasant sensation as the anesthesia wears off. Many of these patients are also eager to view the procedure on the video monitor.

FACILITY

The facility may vary from an operating room (OR) with minimal approval requirements to the state-of-the-art facility shown in Figure 20.1. For office operative arthroscopy, the minimum size for a functional office OR is 16 × 12 feet. This space is necessary to allow free movement of the surgeon and assistants. A few extra square feet is welcomed by the surgeon and staff. The patient is prepared for surgery in an examination room prior to entering the office OR. No presurgery holding area is necessary. The office OR must have room to accommodate video equipment, monitoring equipment, a crash cart with cardiopulmonary resuscitation (CPR) equipment, and an OR table with a leg holder, soft tissue ankle distractor, or both, as well as an autoclave, Cidex basin, nitrogen and oxygen tanks, and suction equipment (Fig. 20.2).

The layout of the office OR is an important factor in maximizing the available space. The nurse-anesthetist, physician's assistant, or anesthesiologist who is monitoring the patient is at the head of the table. The table is situated so it allows access to the patient from either side. A floor drain is present in the OR and is situated in the center of the room. The OR table is placed so the patient's lower extremity is directly over the floor drain after positioning.

A formal surgical scrub sink is not necessary but is desirable. The surgeon and the surgical assistant use hexachlorophene (Septisol) foam solution for 2 minutes at the beginning of the surgical day and for 1 minute prior to each additional operation.

Recovery room facilities are not necessary for office arthroscopy. At completion of the procedure, the patient walks from the OR to the adjacent examination room (Fig. 20.3). The patient stays in this room until ready to go home. Because the sedation is light, no postanesthesia recovery room monitoring is necessary. The infection rate associated with arthroscopy is low (approximately 1 per 500 procedures), so no special ventilation or air-exchange equipment is necessary for arthroscopic surgery in the office.

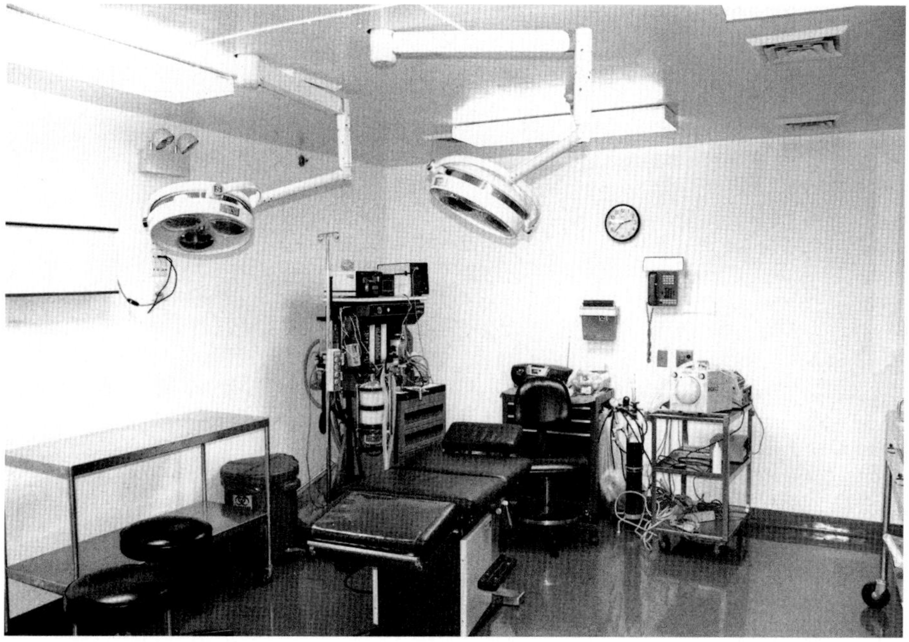

FIGURE 20.1. Operating room, showing the overhead lights, video setup, and light support system (center). The latter includes the Dynamap, pulse oximeter, and defibrillator.

If the office OR is to be constructed as a completely new facility rather than as a modification of existing space, certain considerations would create a more ideal situation, including ceiling supports for overhead lights (Fig. 20.1). Floor drains also are helpful for office arthroscopy and are relatively inexpensive to install. Ideally, the floor should slope directly toward the drain. Two floor drains with slopes for drainage at both the foot of the table (knee, foot, and ankle arthroscopy) and the head of the table (shoulder and elbow arthroscopy) would be ideal. In addition, a cabinet or closet for nitrogen and oxygen tanks would eliminate some of the clutter in the room.

If the clinic wishes to construct a licensed, Medicare-certified ambulatory surgery center (ASC), the state guidelines for development and construction must be used. Having a licensed, Medicare-certified ASC opens the facility to many payers who would not reimburse facility charges in a nonlicensed facility. The licensed facility also allows general anesthesia to be administered, which

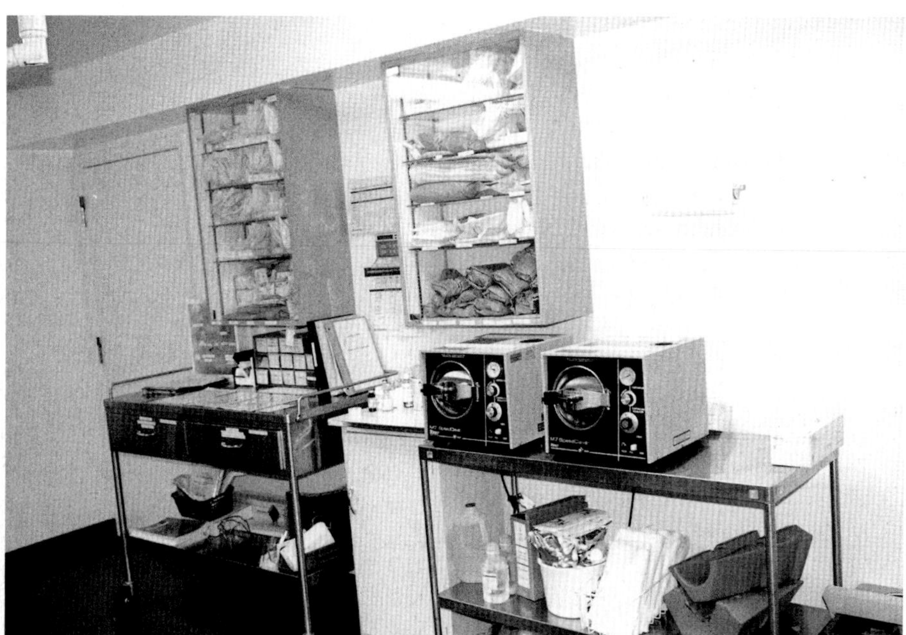

FIGURE 20.2. Along the opposite wall of the operating room shown in Figure 20.1 are the "flash" autoclave, shelves for storing the sterile-wrapped operative instruments, and a cart for needles and dressing material.

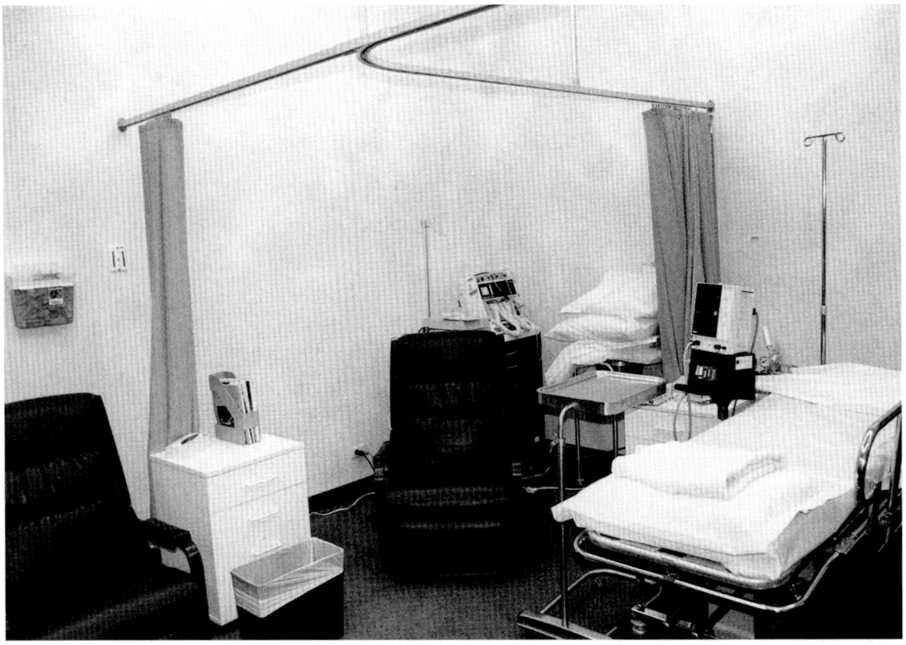

FIGURE 20.3. Recovery area immediately adjacent to the office operating room. Tool gurneys with rails are shown where patients spend the next few hours for immediate recovery. They then proceed (walk) to the recliner to await discharge.

in turn allows virtually all arthroscopic procedures on the foot and ankle to be performed in the office environment.

EQUIPMENT

The OR table used for office ankle arthroscopy requires a few basic elements. The table should raise and lower electronically, as it saves time and minimizes the physical effort required by the nurse or whoever is monitoring the patient at the head of the table. The table should also allow lowering and raising the foot section.

Because space in the office OR is at a premium, a compact camera and video system is essential. Many of the newer camera and video systems include an integrated light source. The integrated camera with light source and the video system are on a movable cart on the contralateral side of the OR table. This cart is placed at the patient's mid-trunk level. The video monitor is rotated toward the surgeon but not enough to prevent the patient from observing the video image.

A printer is helpful for providing a convenient photograph of the operative findings and the appearance following the corrective arthroscopic procedure. These images, which are reviewed with the patient and family following the procedure, are made part of the patient's permanent medical record.

The arthroscopes used for office arthroscopy are 2.7, 3.0, or 4.0 mm in diameter. These arthroscopes are available with 30 and 70 degree angled optics.

The back table is set against one wall. It contains the contents of the disposable office arthroscopy pack including draping equipment, tubing, and bandage equipment used during the procedure. A Mayo stand is necessary to hold the instruments used during the procedure. This movable Mayo stand is usually placed where the surgeon and assistant can easily reach the necessary instruments. By positioning the back table and Mayo stand in this fashion, the surgeon can reach virtually everything needed during the procedure. A scrub technician is usually not required for foot or ankle arthroscopy.

ANESTHESIA

Office arthroscopy is a new area of orthopedic surgery that offers the patient quality care and greater convenience at less cost. The procedures performed offer varied challenges to the anesthesia care provider. First, discomfort must be reduced to acceptable levels; second, provisions must be made for a quick return to a functional state. Last, all of this must occur within established guidelines that provide high margins of safety.

Every anesthesia care provider must have detailed knowledge of the anesthetic agents available to them to make competent, individualized selections. This knowledge must include safe dosage levels, effects, interactions with other drugs, and potential adverse reactions. This, in combination with adequate evaluation of the patient, allows correct anesthetic management. Once an anesthetic plan is formulated, safe delivery must be ensured. Adequate monitoring of the patient from the initial administration of the anesthetic agent until such time as the patient is no longer at risk is mandatory. Monitoring should include, but not be limited to, constant monitoring of the blood pressure, ECG, and oxygen saturation via pulse oximetry. Additionally, preparedness for known consequences of anesthetic administration, as well as unforeseen problems, is a given. Most problems arising in this setting involve airway management and, to a lesser extent, hypotension, brachycardia, or both. Having said this, there is no reason why a qualified, alert, well-prepared anesthesia care provider cannot provide excellent, reproducible results with a high degree of safety.

Monitored anesthesia care (MAC) is the most commonly employed technique for office anesthesia when foot and ankle arthroscopy is performed. In conjunction with local and intraarticular injection, MAC provides a safe, effective anesthetic technique for foot and ankle arthroscopy. When using MAC, reversible or short-acting intravenous agents (or both) are preferred. The most common drugs used in this setting are midazolam (Versed) and fentanyl (Sublimaze).

Anesthesia for office arthroscopy of the foot and ankle includes intraarticular injection, portal site injections, and light intravenous sedation. The intraarticular injection consists of 0.25% bupivacaine (Marcaine) with epinephrine. It is important to wait at least 10 minutes after this intraarticular injection for synovial absorption prior to starting the arthroscopy. The portal sites are injected at the same time with a second syringe containing a mixture of 0.25% bupivacaine with epinephrine and lidocaine (Xylocaine) 1% plain. Usually, potential portal sites are injected. The usual sites include the anterolateral, anteromedial, and posterolateral portal sites. Other portal sites are injected during the procedure as needed.

Attention has been given in recent years to the toxic levels of bupivacaine. The dosage used for office arthroscopy, even with supplemental portal site injections during the procedure, is far below the reported toxic levels for bupivacaine. The 1% lidocaine used during the procedure is far below the reported toxic levels for that drug as well.

Light intravenous sedation, which is administered by the surgeon just prior to the arthroscopic procedure itself, includes midazolam HCl 0.025–0.05 mg/kg and fentanyl 2 μg/kg. These agents are administered consecutively over an approximately 2- to 3-minute period. The patient is monitored during administration of this intravenous sedation. Naloxone (Narcan) 1 mg/cc is available on the anesthesia cart, as is flumazenil (Mazicon) 0.1 mg/cc. Although rarely utilized, these agents are necessary to reverse the effects of fentanyl and midazolam, respectively, if reversal should become necessary.

MONITORING EQUIPMENT

The monitoring equipment necessary when intravenous sedation is used during the procedure includes a pulse oximeter, ECG monitor, and a blood pressure monitor with printout. The printouts become part of the patient's office record. The presence of a registered nurse (RN), certified physician's assistant (PA-C), certified registered nurse-anesthetist (CRNA), or physician familiar with these monitoring devices is mandatory. Oxygen is administered during each procedure if intravenous sedation is used. A nasal cannula or mask is utilized. Oxygen is administered at 6 L/min.

Equipment for CPR must be available in the OR. Care should be taken to ensure that this resuscitative equipment is in good working order. Basic CPR equipment includes a defibrillator, CPR board, ambu bag, endotracheal tubes, laryngoscope with several blades, and oxygen. The crash cart should include the appropriate medications for CPR.

In addition to the equipment necessary for action in case of a cardiopulmonary event, a working knowledge of CPR by the OR team is mandatory. Basic CPR certification by the entire team is recommended. Consideration should be given to taking an advanced life support (ACLS) course.

Arrangements should be made with a nearby hospital for transfer of patients in case of an emergency. A local ambulance service should be available for patient transfer if necessary. The above precautionary measures are recommended if intravenous sedation is to be used in the office OR. No oversedation or cardiovascular incidents occurred during the first 100 knee arthroscopy procedures in our office.[1] Being prepared for such an occurrence is the responsibility of the surgeon.

STAFF

The staff necessary to perform smooth office foot and ankle arthroscopy comprises three team members in addition to the surgeon. A registered nurse, a PA-C, or a nurse-anesthetist is necessary to monitor the patient after the surgeon has administered the intravenous sedation. Some surgeons prefer that the sedation be administered by an anesthesiologist. When the patient is taken from the office OR to the examination room at the completion of the procedure, the individual who has been monitoring the patient throughout the procedure accompanies him or her.

A circulating nurse is necessary to ensure that the proper instruments, sutures, dressings, and other equipment related to office arthroscopy are available during the procedure. The circulating nurse is responsible for cleaning and turning over the room between cases, in addition to helping the surgeon during the procedure.

A surgical assistant is necessary during the procedure to assist the surgeon and in certain cases to hold the arthroscopy instruments or the arthroscope itself. The assistant usually stands on the contralateral side of the lower extremity from the surgeon. The surgical assistant can be another physician or any individual who is trained and competent as an arthroscopy assistant.

If the arthroscopy assistant is another physician, a PA-C, or an RN, he or she can start the intravenous infusion in the next patient and inject the joints of the ankle and portal sites. The surgeon is therefore free to talk to the previous patient and patient's family, dictate the notes on the case, return phone calls, and even see patients.

PREOPERATIVE MANAGEMENT

Several items require attention on the day before the procedure, well before the patient's arrival. Charts and radiographs must be reviewed. Consent forms must be completed and awaiting the patient's signature. An intravenous tray and pole should be set up in the examination room or preoperative area. The OR, of course, must be ready to go. The efficiency for the surgeon is greatly increased if these steps are accomplished. A checklist of all items necessary for surgery is reviewed the day prior to the procedure.

If the surgeon and staff are prepared, the patient has the correct impression that the surgical routine has been performed many times before in the office setting. This preparation goes a long way toward providing a more positive experience for the patient and the patient's family. The patient arrives 20–30 minutes prior to the procedure. Once checked in at the front desk, the patient is taken back to the examination room or preoperative area. The chart is reviewed with the patient, and the involved extremity is reexamined. The patient marks and initials the operative extremity with an indelible marker. The patient's diagnosis and planned procedure are discussed. Questions are answered, and the consent form is signed. Any family members who are with the patient are sent to the waiting room prior to injecting the local anesthesia. The patient is given a pair of examination shorts and a surgical gown. Shoe covers are placed over the patient's bare feet. An intravenous infusion is started with 5% dextrose/Ringer's lactate and adjusted to a slow drip.

The foot and ankle are shaved and cleaned with a betadine alcohol preparatory solution (DuraPrep). Local anesthetic intraarticular and portal injections are then performed as described earlier in the Anesthesia section.

EQUIPMENT

Standard arthroscopy equipment is required for ankle arthroscopy as described above. A 4.0, 3.0, or 2.7 mm arthroscope may be used. The 2.7 mm arthroscope is easier to manipulate in the small space of the foot and ankle joint. Likewise, standard size or small joint (2.0 or 2.7 mm) motorized suction shavers may be used. Again, small joint shavers are easier to manipulate in the small space of the foot and ankle joint. These small shavers, however, are much less aggressive and slower for débridement. Standard-size shavers (3.5–5.5 mm) are more aggressive but are more likely to cause chondral scuffing of the talar dome and tibial plafond when being swept between the tibiotalar articulation and other joints of the foot. They are, however, easily introduced into the medial and lateral recesses through anteromedial and anterolateral portals, respectively. Therefore the availability of both size shavers is ideal. Small-joint arthroscopic probes, burrs, punches, and graspers are also useful. Skeletal ankle distraction cannot be performed in the office under local anesthesia with sedation and is not necessary. Noninvasive distraction is well tolerated with local anesthesia and sedation. Again, familiarity with ankle arthroscopy, with its minimization of operative time (and therefore distraction time), is important. Commercially available distractors may be used.

PATIENT POSITIONING

The patient is placed supine on the operating table. The ankle distractor is placed in the appropriate position prior to preparation and draping. The surgeon and first assistant then perform a surgical scrub with hexachlorophene (Septisol) foam solution for 2 minutes if the procedure is the first of the day. A Septisol foam scrub for 1 minute is adequate for subsequent procedures that same operating day. A surgical scrub sink is not necessary.

The patient is prepared with an iodophor and isopropyl alcohol (DuraPrep) solution for 2 minutes. The extremity is then draped using the specially designed office arthroscopy draping pack. The surgical procedure is then performed.

SURGICAL TECHNIQUE

After preparation and draping, the foot of the operating table is flexed approximately 30 degrees. Surface anatomic landmarks may be marked on the ankle prior to local anesthesia or at this time. Such landmarks include the dorsalis pedis, superficial peroneal nerve, tibialis anterior, peroneus tertius, medial and lateral malleoli, ankle mortise, and Achilles tendon. Appropriate landmarks for other joints of the foot should also be marked in a similar fashion. The sterile straps of the ankle distractor are wrapped over the anterior aspect of the midfoot and posterior aspect of the heel, and distraction of the ankle joint is then applied by an assistant.

POSTOPERATIVE MANAGEMENT

At the conclusion of the procedure, dressings are applied and the patient is placed in a solid ankle foot orthosis (short leg walking boot). The patient is given an injection of ketorolac tromethamine (Toradol) 60 mg IM or 30 mg IV.

The patient is then asked to exit the OR with assistance and is allowed to walk back to the examining room accompanied by the person who monitored him or her during the procedure. Upon entering the examining room, the patient sits in a chair with the operated extremity elevated. A compressive ice wrap is applied to the operated extremity. Crutches are provided if needed. Simple crutch training can be given by the nursing staff or a physical therapist if available.

The arthroscopy findings and the surgical procedure are then discussed with the patient and the patient's family. The patient is given comprehensive postoperative instructions, both verbal and printed, as well as appropriate prescriptions. He or she is then allowed to dress and leave the office. The patient is not allowed to drive home independently.

When leaving the office, the intraarticular and portal site anesthesia is still in effect. The patient is given prescriptions for hydrocodone and cephalexin upon leaving the office. At home the patient should elevate the extremity as much as possible during the next 48 hours. The patient should avoid taking aspirin or other medications that might alter platelet functioning and clotting. Foot and ankle range of motion exercise is encouraged immediately upon arrival home to enhance venous drainage from the extremity. The patient is allowed to become increasingly active during the next 2–3 days prior to the start of the home exercise program or physical therapy.

Frequently, patients experience an acceleration of postsurgical discomfort when the bupivacaine portion of the intraarticular injection wears off after surgery, about 4–8 hours following the surgical procedure. The patients are warned of this possibility and are asked to take the oral hydrocodone.

The patient returns to the office approximately 2–3 days after the surgery, at which time the ankle is inspected, dressings are changed, and Band-Aids are applied. The patient begins rehabilitation at a time dictated by the procedure performed.

The turnover time between cases in the OR is typically 10–15 minutes, although surgeons just starting an arthroscopy program should allow as long as an hour. There is a learning curve, especially for the staff, that shortens the turnover time as experience is gained. Scheduling patient arrival times varies accordingly.

BIBLIOGRAPHY

1. Small NC, Glogau AI, Berezin MA, Farless BL. Office arthroscopy of the knee: technical considerations and preliminary analysis of the first one hundred patients. *Arthroscopy* 1994;10:534–539.

CHAPTER 21

Regional Anesthesia for Ankle Arthroscopy

Thomas J. Guhl

Several methods can be used to provide anesthesia for ankle arthroscopy. This chapter deals mainly with the use of regional techniques to accomplish this goal. These methods can be used in conjunction with sedative/hypnotic medications to attain the optimum comfort for the patient provided the procedurist is skilled at giving these medications. Otherwise, I recommend that a trained provider of anesthesia be present to ensure the safety and comfort of the patient, allowing the surgeon to concentrate on the procedure at hand.

LOCAL ANESTHETICS

No text on regional techniques is complete without a brief discussion of the drugs used to obtain anesthesia. This section discusses the local anesthetic agents that are generally used and reviews important information to allow the practitioner to choose the appropriate one. It is necessary to understand the basic characteristics of local anesthetics to use them effectively. The simple physicochemical properties become more complex when applied to the individual patient, especially those who have moderate to severe medical conditions that compromise their function and reserves.

Structure

There are essentially two classes of local anesthetics, grouped according to their basic chemical structure. They are divided into the "ester" and "amide" compounds, with the difference lying in the linkage between the common aromatic, hydrophilic portion and the amino group. The importance of this division lies mainly in their metabolism. The "ester" compounds are metabolized by plasma cholinesterase, producing paraaminobenzoic acid, a common allergen. The "amide" compounds are metabolized by the liver, and the potential for allergic reactions is minimal.

The main physicochemical properties that are of importance include the following: Lipid solubility correlates with potency in that the more lipid-soluble the agent the greater is its potency. Protein binding of the anesthetic agents influences the duration of action, whereby increased protein binding leads to decreased release of the substance for metabolism, increasing the duration of action. Finally, the pH or pKa of the drug, which determines its ionization, affects the speed of onset of the drug action. The nonionized form crosses the neural membrane readily, whereas the ionized form is chiefly responsible for the drug's effect. When the pKa of the drug is close to the physiologic pH of the body, the onset of action is more rapid.

Function

In simplistic terms, the function of local anesthetics is to block the sodium channels of the neuron, which in turn inhibit propagation of the nerve impulse along the axon. Nerve propagation begins when the threshold potential of a neuron is exceeded, causing an increase in membrane permeability for Na^+. This sudden influx of Na^+ causes depolarization of the nerve membrane, which is conducted down the length of the nerve. As the nerve impulse travels down the nerve, Na^+ influx decreases and K^+ outflow reaches its peak. The ion pump then exchanges Na^+ and K^+, returning the membrane to its resting potential.

This action of local anesthetics is to penetrate the lipid membrane via its nonionized state. Once inside the cell, the local anesthetic dissociates into its charged form, which then binds to the intracellular side of the sodium channel, blocking the movement of Na^+ ions and so blocking the action potential from developing and inhibiting nerve transmission.

FACTORS AFFECTING LOCAL ANESTHETIC FUNCTION

Vasoconstrictors

The addition of vasoconstrictors such as epinephrine allows an increase in the duration and intensity of neural blockade by causing an increase in the length of time the nerve tissue is being penetrated. It also has the effect of decreasing toxicity by slowing absorption into the bloodstream.

Bicarbonate

Some have recommended adding bicarbonate to produce a faster onset of the nerve block. This practice increases the pH and pKa, thereby allowing more unchanged local anesthetic to penetrate the nerve membrane faster. Local anesthetics are usually supplied at a low pH to prolong storage.

Dosage

The onset, quality, and duration of the blockade is determined essentially by the total dose of the anesthetic used. Varying the concentration does not matter if one uses the same total amount of drug in milligrams. Volume usually does not affect these factors with peripheral nerve blockade.

Combinations

Combinations of local anesthetics have been used to combine the favorable characteristic of each agent, such as rapid onset and duration of action. This practice has met with mixed results, as other factors (e.g., pH) may be altered, thereby changing the characteristics and sometimes negating the advantage sought.

Toxicity

The toxicity of local anesthetics is usually due to direct intravascular injection of the medication and only rarely to the cumulative dosage. Central nervous system (CNS) toxicity is usually most apparent. As blood levels increase, patients may begin to experience such things as perioral paresthesias, tinnitus, lightheadedness or dizziness that can progress to confusion, slurred speech, or other unusual mental status changes. Eventually, if left unchecked, the endpoint is grand mal seizures. Methods to prevent such toxicity are to inject a small dose (i.e., 1–2 ml) of local anesthetic and monitor the patient for signs and symptoms before proceeding with larger doses. Intravascular injection may be detected early when the local anesthetic has epinephrine added, as the epinephrine may cause tachycardia and hypertension. Nonetheless, safe administration, continuous monitoring, and vigilance are the best methods for preventing adverse outcomes.

Cardiovascular toxicity is due to local anesthetic action on the heart and vasculature. Usually hypotension is an early sign and is due to myocardial depression combined with peripheral vasodilation. It worsens progressively with increasing blood levels; later signs are decreases in heart rate and conduction. These alterations can lead to cardiac arrest if they go unnoted. Bupivacaine, specifically, and the other, more potent anesthetics are most likely to cause this problem.

SPECIFIC AGENTS

Esters

Procaine (Novacaine) was one of the first local anesthetics in use, but its slow onset, short duration, and low potency have limited its use, as has its allergic potential. *Tetracaine* (Pontocaine) is used mainly for its potency and long duration of action. Its drawbacks are high toxicity and poor tissue diffusion, rendering it essentially useless for peripheral nerve blockades.

"Amides"

Lidocaine (Xylocaine) is the most commonly used local anesthetic because it has a fairly rapid onset, moderate duration of action, and moderate potency. Moreover, it is relatively safe to use when administered with care. *Bupivacaine* (Nesacaine, Sensorcaine) is an excellent agent for peripheral nerve blockade because of its ability to produce differential blockade: sensory fibers are blocked more intensely and for a longer duration than motor fibers. This provides an earlier return of function before the anesthesia and analgesia effects dissipate. Its disadvantages include greater toxicity and a slower onset of action compared to lidocaine. *Mepivacaine* (Carbocaine) has a profile similar to that of lidocaine, with a slightly longer duration of action. *Prilocaine* (Citanest) is less toxic than other "amides" owing to its rapid metabolism, but its propensity to cause methemoglobinemia and cyanosis is a major drawback. Otherwise, it has a rapid onset, high potency, and moderate duration of action. *Ropivacaine* (Naropin) is similar to bupivacaine except it has the advantage of being less cardiotoxic and creating a greater differential blockade (sensory more than motor blockade). *Etidocaine* (Duranest) has a rapid onset and long duration of action but is more toxic than lidocaine and can produce stronger motor than sensory blockade, making it less desirable.

EQUIPMENT

The essential pieces of equipment necessary are essentially those that deliver the medication and those that provide resuscitation for adverse events.

1. *Syringe*. I recommend the use of a 10 cc control syringe, one with eyelets for the thumb, index, and middle finger. This allows proper administration of medication during the block yet leaves one hand free to palpate landmarks. The 10 cc is adequate to deliver appropriate amounts of medication without frequently refilling the syringe. Also, the force of aspiration with the smaller syringe size allows one to be able to detect intravascular injections more readily. An alternative to the control syringe is to have a needle with extension tubing attached to a syringe. This requires two people; the person performing the block and an assistant who aspirates and injects the syringe's material under the practitioner's guidance.

2. *Needles*. The optimum needle for peripheral nerve blockade is a short, blunt, beveled, or "B" beveled, needle. The blunt bevel produces less trauma to nerve tissue and allows greater perception of tissue planes. The smaller needle gauge provides less trauma but does not allow adequate aspiration of blood. Therefore, a 22 or 23 gauge needle is the best compromise.

3. *Resuscitative equipment*. This must include all appropriate materials required to provide advanced cardiac life support, as recommended by the American Heart Association. It should include materials to intubate, ventilate, defibrillate, and medicate the patient should an adverse event occur. Before any regional procedure, this equipment must be available with trained personnel present.

TECHNIQUES

Informed consent must be obtained, after a complete discussion of all the alternatives to ensure the patient's comfort and optimize the success of the procedure. Intravenous access is recommended for the purpose of administering sedative agents as well as resuscitative medication as needed. Once everything is in place, one can proceed with the anesthetic.

The one caveat when choosing peripheral nerve blockade at the ankle or foot is that the injection sites must be above the portal sites for ankle (and foot) arthroscopy (Fig. 21.1). Ankle blockade is a simple, relatively safe procedure that allows blockade of five peripheral nerves. Use of non-epinephrine-containing local anesthetic is recommended.

1. *Deep Peroneal Nerve*. The deep peroneal nerve lies lateral to the anterior tibial artery and the tendon of the extensor hallucis longus muscle, approximately 2–3 cm above the level of the malleolus. Palpate the artery or ask the patient to point the great toe upward. After a skin wheal is placed just lateral to these landmarks, advance the needle to contact the tibia, withdraw a few millimeters, and inject 3–5 ml of the local anesthetic. This anesthetizes the web space of the first and second digits.

2. *Superficial peroneal nerve*. The superficial peroneal nerve supplies the dorsum of the foot and toes except for the area supplied by the deep peroneal nerve. The nerve can be blocked by subcutaneous infiltration of local anesthetics (5–10 ml) from the anterior tibia to the lateral malleolus above the portal sites in an intradermal or subcutaneous fashion.

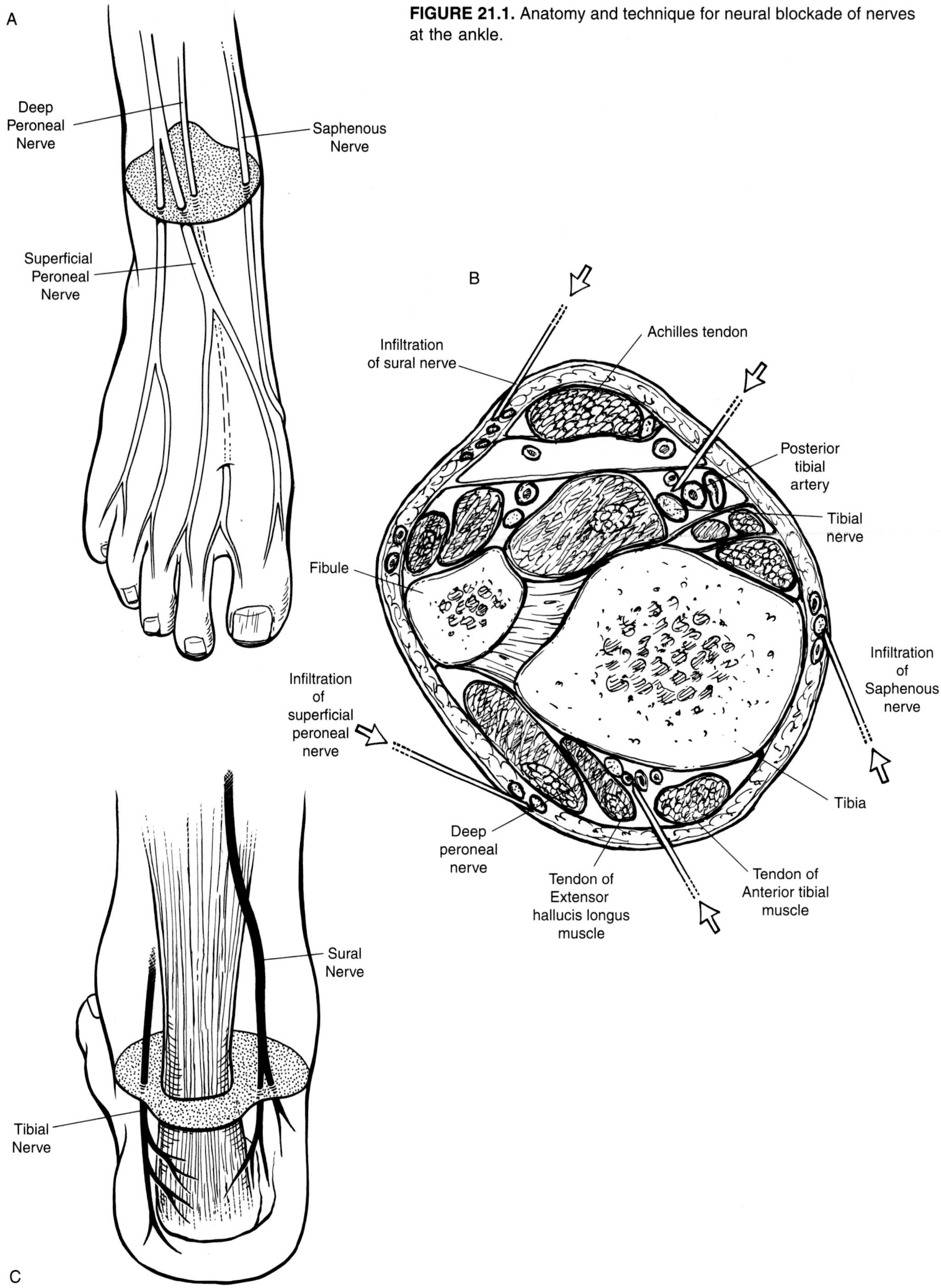

FIGURE 21.1. Anatomy and technique for neural blockade of nerves at the ankle.

3. *Sural nerve*. The sural nerve supplies the lateral side of the foot and lateral portion of the fifth toe. To block it, insert the needle lateral to the Achilles tendon and infiltrate with 3–5 ml to the lateral malleolus's superior outer border in a fanwise distribution.

4. *Saphenous nerve*. The saphenous nerve supplies the medial portion of the foot to the metatarsophalangeal joint. It can be blocked by subcutaneous infiltration of 3–5 ml of local anesthetic, proceeding medially from the superior aspect of the medial malleolus to the anterior tibia.

5. *Posterior tibial nerve*. The posterior tibial nerve supplies the medial side of the foot and plantar surface of the toes. The block is performed by rotating the ankle externally, palpating the posterior tibial artery, and placing the needle lateral to this point. One can attempt to elicit a parethesia by advancing the needle perpendicular to the posterior aspect of the tibia. If paresthesias are not elicited, advance the needle until the tibial surface is contacted; then withdraw 1 cm and inject 5–8 ml of the local anesthetic.

OTHER ANESTHETIC TECHNIQUES

Nerve blocks at the knee should be used when ankle block is not feasible, as during prolonged tourniquet application. It requires the patient to be prone during blockade of the tibial and common peroneal nerves. Otherwise, its safety and efficiency nearly rivals that of the ankle block. It is recommended that it be performed by a trained specialist.

Also known as an IV or Bier block, *intravenous regional anesthesia* is used when a tourniquet is applied to the extremity where exsanguination and occlusion of the dorsal limb can be obtained. A large volume of dilute local anesthetic, usually lidocaine, is then injected. The advantage is rapid anesthesia with a bloodless field. The disadvantage is that once the tourniquet is released the anesthetic dissipates and does not provide any postoperative pain relief. This technique should be performed by personnel familiar with it.

CONCLUSIONS

This chapter has concentrated on the regional techniques needed to provide anesthesia for ankle arthroscopy. They can be used in an outpatient setting when the required equipment and personnel are present. Intravenous sedation used as an adjunct to regional anesthesia can provide optimal conditions for the patient, especially when administered by trained personnel. It provides the added benefit of patient safety. Obviously, general anesthesia is a viable alternative.

CHAPTER 22

Rehabilitation after Ankle Arthroscopy

Lars Konradsen and Per F.A.H. Renstrom

The goals of rehabilitation after most ankle arthroscopies are to restore (1) range of motion, (2) muscle strength, (3) proprioception, and (4) coordination of movement to a preinjury level. This chapter discusses the normal requirements for each of these functions and the causes of their restrictions or deficits. The function of the foot/ankle complex during gait and the kinematics during running are presented. Also discussed are the scientific basis behind relevant rehabilitation modalities and programs for acute postoperative and long-term ankle rehabilitation.

NORMAL REQUIREMENTS

Range of Motion

To be able to perform a movement with ease, the movement must lie within the range of passive motion of the foot/ankle complex. An inability to participate in various activities can occur with decreased passive motion. For example, a slight loss of ankle plantar flexion would be considered a handicap by professional dancers, whereas it would not be of significance to most people in their everyday life. In contrast, an inability to dorsiflex the ankle at least 10 degrees beyond neutral would cause anyone to limp while walking, no matter how well the elements of strength, coordination, and proprioception were trained.

Anatomically, the foot/ankle complex is usually divided into the talocrural and the subtalar joints. The range of passive motion of the talotibial joint varies from one report to another, mostly owing to differences in methods of measurement. Maximal dorsiflexion ranges from 10 to 23 degrees and maximal plantar flexion from 23 to 48 degrees.[1,2] From maximal dorsiflexion to maximal plantar flexion, all of the articular surface of the talus at some point is contained under the tibial articular surface. The main restriction for passive dorsiflexion in the health subject is the Achilles tendon complex, whereas plantar flexion is stopped by tightened anterior tendon structures or by posterior bony impingement.

The subtalar joint (talocalcaneonavicular joint complex) rotates around an axis that continuously changes during movement.[3] The axis has a 42 degree inclination in the sagittal plane and 23 degrees of medial deviation in the horizontal plane.[4] The range of motion is variable, but 30 degrees of inversion and 10 degrees of eversion is a practical average in clinical settings.[5]

When considering the ankle for rehabilitation, it is important to consider the movement of the ankle/foot complex in a field of motion that mirrors a combination of talotibial and subtalar movements (Fig. 22.1).[6] This field is individual and can decrease with age. Injury can affect large or small areas of the field. If the arthroscopic procedure has removed the cause of a decreased field, rehabilitation must try to restore it to what was normal for the individual.

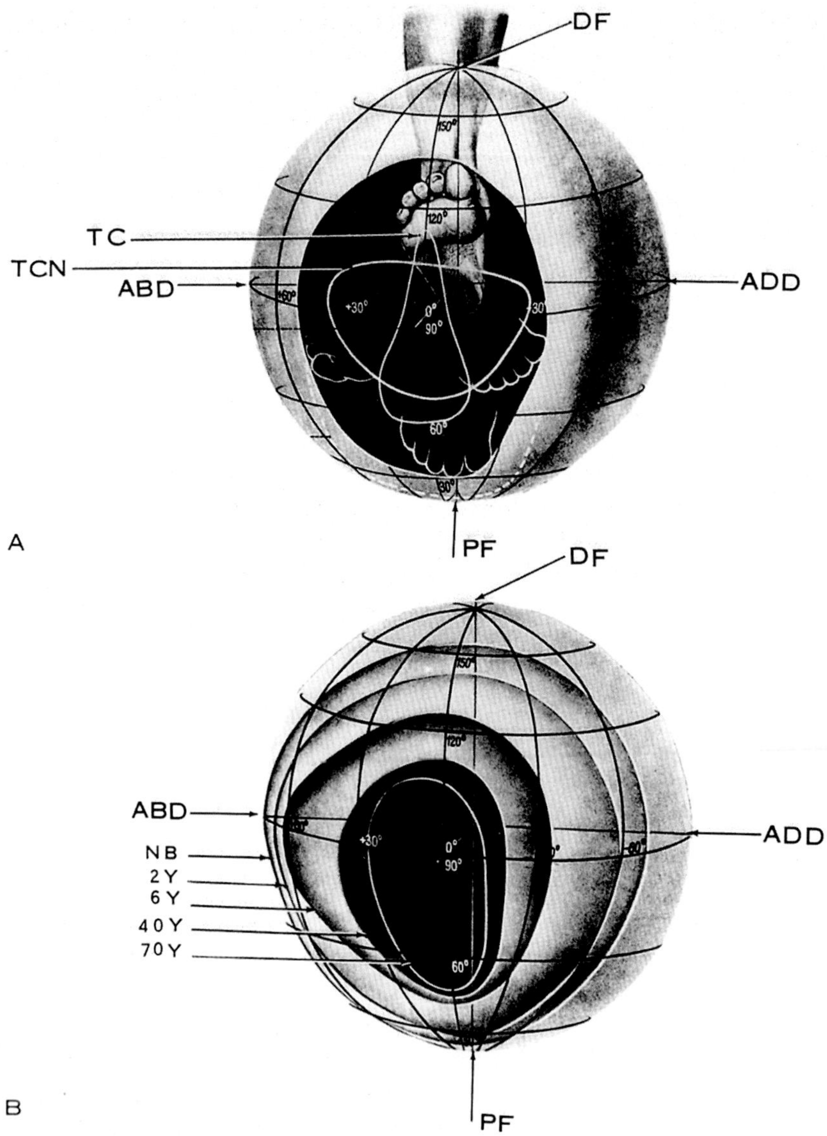

FIGURE 22.1. Range of motion of the foot/ankle complex. **A:** Oval contour of the field of motion. TC, contribution of the talocrural joint; TCN, contribution of the talocalcaneonavicular joint; DF, dorsiflexion; PF, plantar flexion; ABD, abduction; ADD, adduction. **B:** Field of motion in various age groups. NB, newborn; 2Y, 2 years old [and so forth.] (From Sarrafian SK. *Anatomy of the Foot and Ankle.* Philadelphia: Lippincott, 1993;476, with permission.)

A reduced field of motion can be caused by both mechanical and dynamic restrictions. Mechanical restrictions include bony restraints, capsular contracture, and increased passive muscle/tendon resistance. Bony spurs and synovitis in the anterior compartment of the talocrural joint have been mentioned in previous chapters as a cause of reduced dorsiflexion. The arthroscopic procedure usually addresses these changes. In the presence of decreased dorsiflexion, contracture of the soleus complex may occur, adding to the problem, reducing the immediate effect of an anterior decompression procedure. Dynamic restrictions may be involuntary or voluntary. Increased muscle tone due to spinal or central nervous system (CNS) disease may involuntarily restrict ankle movement, whereas other CNS or general diseases or local tendon or nerve affections may make it impossible for the subject to utilize part of the field of motion open to her or him. Voluntary restrictions to range of motion may be induced if pain elicited from the joint or from periarticular structures causes the subject to avoid movements in an area of the field that would elicit pain. For example, a subject may decide to avoid eversion movements and choose to walk with increased inversion during the stance phase to avoid loading a chondral lesion on the lateral talus.

MUSCLE STRENGTH

There are 32 muscles—13 extrinsic and 19 intrinsic—that control the actions of the foot. The extrinsic muscles of the calf are responsible for the major torque generation of the talotibial and subtalar joints. They can be categorized into antagonistic groups responsible for (1) dorsal/plantar flexion or (2) inversion/eversion, but due to the oblique placement of the subtalar axis dorsal/plantar flexors have an element of inversion/eversion action and vice versa (Fig. 22.2).[4] Even the soleus muscle with its Achilles tendon attachment on the calcaneus medial to the subtalar axis acts with an inversion component. The gastrocnemius and the soleus complex have a primary propulsive function as the strongest plantar flexors of the talotibial joint. Their function is mediated through the subtalar joint, however, which requires that many of the other muscles work in combination to secure the stability of the foot and ankle complex.

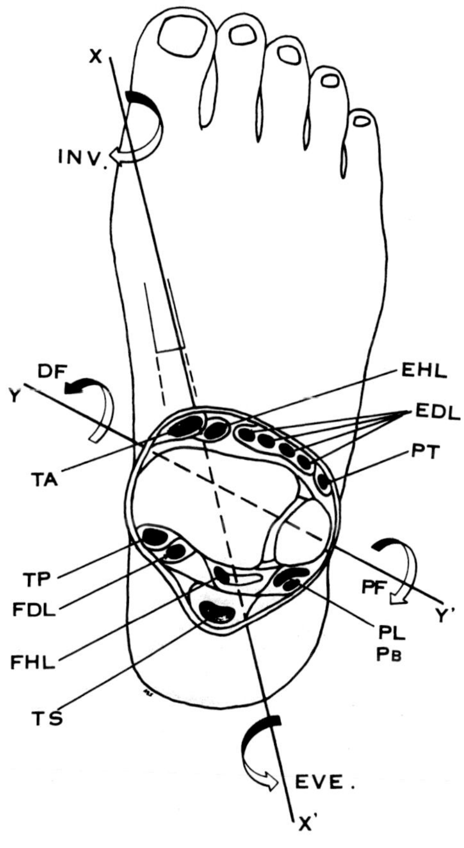

FIGURE 22.2. Motors of the ankle and the talocalcaneonavicular joint. X–X′, axis of the TCN joint; Y–Y′, axis of the talocrural joint; INV, inversion; EVE, eversion; DF, dorsiflexion; PL, plantar flexion. Invertors: TA, tibialis anterior; TP, tibialis posterior; FDL, flexor digitorum longus; FHL, flexor hallucis longus; TS, triceps surae. Evertors: PL, peroneus longus; PB, peroneus brevis; EHL, extensor hallucis longus; EDL, extensor digitorum longus; TA, tibialis anterior; PT, peroneus tertius. Plantar flexors: TP, FDL, FHL, TS, PL, PB. Dorsiflexors: TA, EHL, EDL, PT. (From Sarrafian SK. *Anatomy of the Foot and Ankle.* Philadelphia: Lippincott, 1993;551, with permission.)

It is not possible to define required levels of strength for each of the crural muscles. Activities of daily living do require a substantial degree of force generation from the muscles working against gravity. Various components of muscle strength must be considered. Peak or maximal muscle strength in both isometric and isokinetic setups is often used as a measurement of functional muscle ability, especially in rehabilitation situations. Maximal muscle strength, however, indicates only if it is within the ability of the individual to perform a specific task. If a muscle is too weak to do a necessary task, other muscles that can create a similar torque must be recruited, as is seen for the tibialis posterior in the presence of Achilles tendon deficiency, or another pattern of motion must be sought, as in cases of peroneal nerve palsy. In either case other structures are at risk of being injured because of overload.

Often maximal strength seems to be sufficient but muscle endurance is reduced, rendering the muscle too weak for the task after a number of repetitions. Finally, the balance between antagonistic muscles may have been disturbed, rendering one of the seemingly strong muscle groups too weak (compared to the antagonists) to be able to provide functional balance. Thus excessive ankle inversion strength compared to ankle eversion strength seems to predispose to repeated lateral ankle ligament injuries.[7]

Injury, immobilization, and reduced muscle activation result in muscle wasting as early as 1–2 weeks after the onset. The degree of muscle atrophy depends on the duration of immobilization (the longer the immobilization, the greater the atrophy) and the position of immobilization (tissue under tension atrophies significantly less than when placed in a relaxed position).[8] Persistent reduction in muscle strength continues for years after the primary injury. In healthy individuals the peak force and muscle cross-sectional area correlate well, but after injury the reduction in maximal peak force is greater than suggested by the reduction in the cross-sectional area. Neural factors are responsible for this discrepancy. In the injured or immobilized state, full activation might not be possible because of an unspecific effect of disuse by the lack of optimal nerve drive or it may be due to reflex inhibition.[9] Inhibition of muscle activation may be present even though there is no pain or discomfort. A mild joint effusion causes a significant reduction in muscle activation ability.[9] Pain impedes muscle activation as well.

PROPRIOCEPTION

There are numerous receptors for motion and position sense in the capsule and ligaments of the ankle joint.[10] These receptors are complemented by muscle/tendon receptors and cutaneous receptors in the surrounding skin and subcutaneous tissue.[11] Afferent information from these receptors, collected and processed in cortical centers, constitutes proprioception: the sensation of limb position and limb and joint movement.[12] The ability to sense limb position and movement is extremely accurate. Slow movements of about 1 degree are detectable, and reproduction of joint angles can be done within 2 degrees of accuracy.[13,14]

Ankle proprioception is primarily governed by input from the ankle area. It is not only receptors in ankle ligaments and capsule that supply the necessary information, however, as local anesthetic injections in these areas did not affect movement threshold detection or postural stability.[15] Totally stopping afferent information from the ankle/foot area by an ankle block results in decreased ankle angle reproduction abilities.[16] If the crural muscles are allowed to be active, however, mechanoreceptors here are able to supply the input that quite accurately judges ankle position.

Loss or gross deterioration of proprioception as seen with degenerative neuropathic diseases can cause destruction of the joints, as with Charcot feet. However, acute injury to the ankle (e.g., ankle sprains) may also result in a proprioceptive deficit.[17–19] In subjects with repeated inversion injuries, a proprioceptive defect can be measured as impaired postural control,[20] as an increased reaction time for the peroneal muscles in response to sudden inversion,[21] as increased detection threshold to ankle movement,[22] and as an increased error in ankle angle reproduction.[14]

MOTION PATTERNS

When repeating known sequences of movement (e.g., walking, running, balancing), we usually rely on preprogrammed patterns.[23–25] Each pattern can then again be altered or modified based on afferent input.[23] New tasks often are approached using patterns that have proven successful from previous experience in similar situations combined with markedly increased activity of all of the muscles that may be needed for the task. With increased experience, fewer and fewer muscles are recruited, and the muscles that are involved show decreasing activity, resulting in less fatigue.[26] In cases of functional impairment of the ankle joint due to altered mechanics or painful conditions, a new gait pattern may be chosen by the subject. With time, a crossover effect is seen, affecting the pattern of the normal limb as well. Relieving the initial mechanical or pain problem by surgery often does not change the pattern of movement to normal; this must be relearned, often in the beginning with the overrecruitment of muscle activity, as is seen when learning new tasks.

LOCOMOTION: GAIT CYCLE

Walking requires constant maintenance of body equilibrium while achieving forward propulsion. For the body to stay in equilibrium, the gravitational force acting in the center of gravity should pass through the supporting surface of the foot or through the support base, which is defined by both feet joined anteriorly and posteriorly by a double tangent.[27] Walking requires the coordinated movement of all major parts of the body, and displacements occur in three planes of space, which must be considered for adequate rehabilitation. The pelvis and lower extremities move in phase, whereas the upper back, shoulders, and upper extremities move out of phase relative to the lower segments. The support phase of walking accounts for approximately 60% of the cycle and the swing phase 40% (Fig. 22.3).

Rotational Movements

The pelvis, femur, and tibia rotate inward from heel-strike to 20% during the walking cycle and then rotate externally from this point until toe-off (Fig. 22.3). The average total ranges of rotational motion are as follows: pelvis, 8 degrees; femur, 15 degrees; tibia, 19 degrees. Distally, transverse rotation is transmitted to and absorbed by the ankle/foot complex. Because of the obliquity of the talocrural joint axis, a limited degree of transverse rotation can be absorbed by concomitant dorsiplantar flexion. The major transmission of tibial rotation occurs at the level of the subtalar joint. At heel-strike, the subtalar joint is slightly inverted, followed by eversion, which peaks at foot-flat and is maintained during the major portion of the stance phase. Just prior to heel-off the subtalar joint is inverted followed by eversion close to a neutral position during the swing

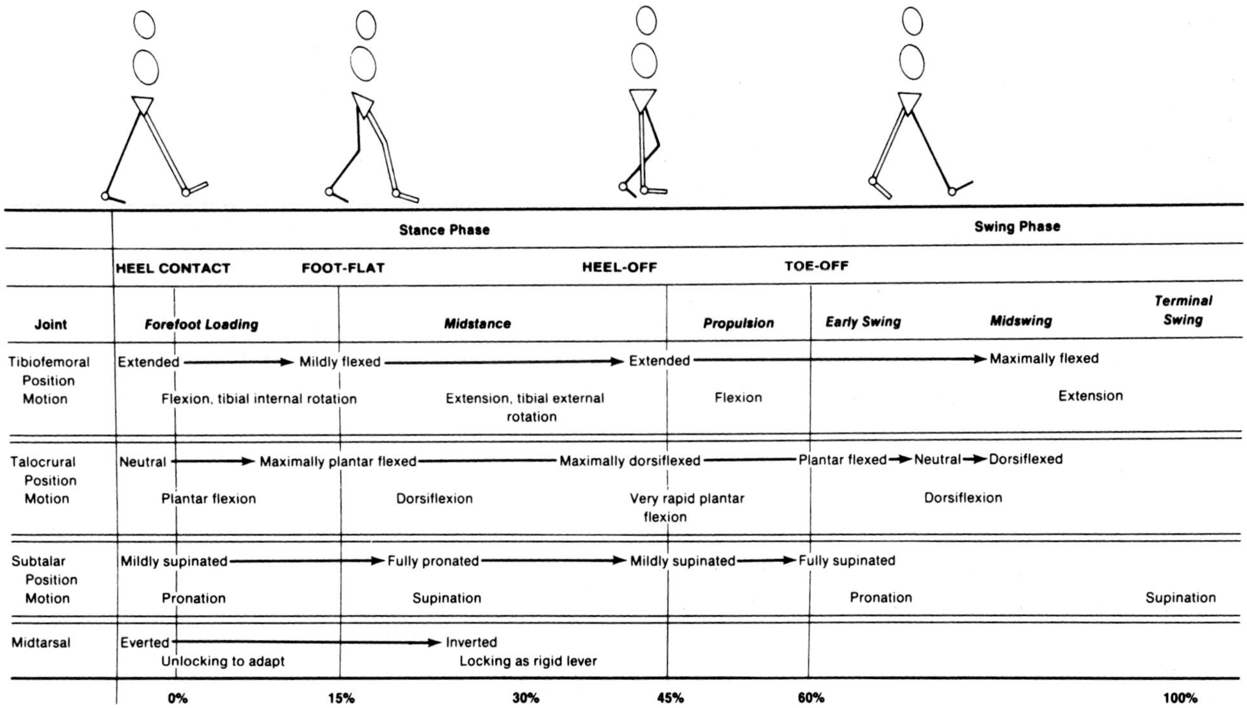

FIGURE 22.3. Normal gait cycle. (From Mulligan E. Lower leg, ankle, and foot rehabilitation. In: Andrews JR, Harrelson GL (eds) *Physical Rehabilitation of the Injured Athlete.* Philadelphia: Saunders, 1991;217, with permission.)

phase. The motion of the subtalar joint during the stance phase averages approximately 6 degrees.[28] According to Mann, the internal rotation of the lower extremity is initiated distally through subtalar eversion during weight-bearing and is transmitted to the proximal joints.[29] The external rotation of the weight-bearing extremity is initiated proximally through the swinging opposite lower extremity, producing external rotation of the pelvis for the stance leg. This external rotation is transmitted distally and is further enhanced by the obligatory external rotation of the leg through its anterior flexion during the stance phase. Additional external rotation of the leg occurs through the metatarsal break along the oblique axis oriented posterolaterally at the time of heel-rise.[29]

Regarding the sagittal plane motion, during the stance phase the ankle goes from a 10 degree dorsiflexed position to a 25 degree plantar-flexed position.[4] During the swing phase the ankle is initially plantar-flexed, followed by dorsiflexion to neutral to clear the toes of the ground.

Stability of the Foot During Gait

At heel-strike the heel is minimally inverted. From heel-strike and 20% into the cycle the tibia rotates internally, the os calcis is everted at the subtalar joint, and the forefoot is relatively supinated. As a result, the foot is in a low-arched, closely packed stable position acting as an efficient structure to support the body weight. The stretching of the plantar ligaments helps them store elastic strain energy, which can be returned during the latter part of the stance phase during toe-off.[28] The following external rotation of the tibia during the progression of the stance phase induces high-arched remodeling with inversion of the os calcis and relative pronation of the forefoot. The tension of the plantar soft tissue structures is now maintained through anterior flexion of the leg or relative dorsiflexion of the foot. Thus the continuum of remodeling ensures stability during locomotion from foot-flat to toe-off.

Forces on the Ankle During Gait

Forces are imparted to the ground by the body in motion through the contact surface of the foot. At the beginning of the stance phase, at heel strike, the decelerating foot comes down and the heel cushion strikes the ground with an initial shock wave, which travels in the lower extremity with impulses up to 100 Hz.[30] The initial vertical spike force is approximately 80% of the body weight. A second force peak occurs at the middle of the cycle, surpassing the body weight by 10%. The magnitude of the force varies with the speed of the gait. Slow walk diminishes peak forces, and rapid walk increases them.

Electromyographic Activity During Gait

Some muscles (e.g., soleus complex and anterior tibial muscle) show highly consistent cyclic patterns that seem to express primarily preprogrammed strategies. In contrast, other muscles (e.g., tibialis posterior and the peroneal muscle group) show variable activity, suggesting a pattern that relies more on afferent input registering immediate foot/ankle balance.

KINEMATICS OF RUNNING

Compared to walking, the floating noncontact phase is 20% of the cycle time for jogging and 40% for running.[27] The support portion of the running stride is generally categorized into the impact phase, mid-stance phase, and push-off phase. The initial impact usually begins at the lateral aspect of the heel with the foot in slight inversion. In mid-stance, defined as the time during which the entire foot is on the ground, the subtalar joint passes from an inverted to an everted position. Eversion continues to about 85% of the support phase, with maximum values ranging from 5 to 25 degrees depending on various factors including footwear. Seen in the sagittal plane following initial footfall, the leg rotates forward, resulting in about 20 degrees of ankle dorsiflexion. In mid-stance the ankle begins to plantar-flex, reaching a maximum of 20 degrees shortly after toe-off.

REHABILITATION MODALITIES AND SCIENCE

Improving Range of Motion and Flexibility

Stretching

The effectiveness of stretching techniques has been attributed to neurophysiologic and mechanical factors.[31,32] The neurophysiologic foundation of muscle/tendon stretching is neural inhibition of the muscle undergoing stretch. Decreased reflex activity results in reduced resistance to stretch, which results in further gain of range of motion.[32] The biomechanical aspect relates to the viscoelastic properties of the connective tissue. The viscoelastic properties can be defined as two components of stretch.[33,34] The elastic component allows elastic temporary stretching, and the viscous component allows plastic stretching with more permanent tissue elongation after the load is removed. The various stretching techniques can be categorized as ballistic stretching, static stretching, contraction with relaxing stretching, and relaxing agonist contraction.[32,35–37] The latter two are commonly referred to as proprioceptive neuromuscular facilitation (PNF) stretch techniques. A single stretch cycle has been shown to reduce passive torque at a given joint angle by about 20%.[38] A plateau in torque decline is reached after about 45 seconds of stretching. Using a PNF technique, an improvement in joint range of motion compared to a static stretch can be accomplished.[39,40] No measurable stretch effect remains 1 hour after a single stretch cycle. Repeated stretches are necessary to produce an effect that can last more than 1 hour.[38] Taylor et al.[31] found that four stretch cycles seemed to be the threshold for producing maximal effect, but there is no scientific support for their findings. We propose that stretching should be repeated regularly (e.g., every 6–8 hours) for a lasting effect.

When stretching, it remains important to remember that it is the movement sphere that must be restored, not just movements in the usually defined anteroposterior and lateral planes (see Figure 22.1).

Joint Mobilization

Joint mobilization addresses the accessory motions of a joint (called "roll and glide") using joint distraction and oscillations of varying amplitude. Mechanical effects include stretching capsular restrictions and breaking adhesions, distracting impacted tissue, providing movement of articular surfaces, and maintaining fiber distance for an orderly alignment or remodeling of collagen tissue.[41]

Friction Massage

Friction massage is performed over an area of soft tissue adhesions perpendicular to the direction of the fibers. The technique is believed to encourage longitudinal orientation of the scar tissue instead of allowing a disorganized connective tissue healing pattern.[42] It increases the strength of the tendon or ligament involved and improves the extensibility of the tissues.[41] Friction produces significant hyperemia in the target area and may stress newly injured tissue to the degree of reinjury.[41] The application of friction massage to acute injuries cannot be advised.

Improving Muscle Strength

The principal measures to consider when choosing a postoperative treatment program are the avoidance of reflex inhibition and an increase in neural activation over the first 2–4 weeks after surgery. Reflex inhibition is prevented primarily by preventing both short-term and long-term postoperative pain.[43] As mentioned, a moderate degree of joint swelling without pain can induce reflex inhibition,[9] so preventing effusion also becomes important throughout the rehabilitation period.

Increased neural activation is achieved by functional and dynamometer training.[44] For functional training the patient is required to activate his or her musculature in normally occurring activities. Dynamic stability, including proprioceptive information, motor control, and appropriate muscle force development, is enforced by the training. Schedules may start with walking and two-leg jumping and progress to different levels of balancing, jumping, jogging, and running. Strength, as measured with a dynamometer, has been found to improve with this functional approach.

During the early phases of dynamometer training with isokinctic or variable resistance modalities the increased neural activation plays a dominant role. Here it seems that training at high speeds increases high-speed maximal activation while not affecting low-speed maximal activation, and vice versa.[45]

If reflex inhibition is avoided or overcome, a major effect of training on muscle structure (muscle hypertrophy) can be expected over the following weeks. It does not seem important whether dynamometric training is done isokinetically or with variable resistance.

Summary

Three postinjury/postsurgical periods can be identified.[46] The first phase, with immobilization, requires prevention of reflex inhibition and maintenance of muscle structure. This period usually lasts from day 0 to 1 week after surgery.

During the second phase, with activation, emphasis is placed on neutral activation through functional training, and several training principles may be employed. Dynamometer training during this phase allows training of maximal effort with a stabilized joint but should never be more important than functional training. This period usually lasts from week 2 to week 4.

During the third phase, with adaptation to function, the specific needs of the patient must be considered. The training regimen should include activities similar to the activities of daily living or sport-specific functions of the patient. The need for muscle strength and muscle endurance should be kept in mind (Table 22.1). The third phase usually starts after 4–6 weeks.

IMPROVING PROPRIOCEPTION AND MOTION COORDINATION

Treatment of a proprioceptive ankle deficit consists of a progressive series of coordination exercises to reeducate the ankle. Although the idea of rehabilitating proprioception seems well established, little research has been done to establish the effect of training on ankle-specific proprioceptive functions. Tropp found significantly improved balance during single-limb stance in functionally unstable ankles after 10 weeks of balance-board exercises.[20] The same group reported a decrease in the frequency of inversion injuries and ankle "giving way" feelings when compared to an untrained, unstable ankle control group. Tropp also found that the subjects in question showed a change in their strategy of single-limb stance, going from a broken chain strategy before training to the normal inverted pendulum strategy after training was completed.[20] It may be that proprioceptive rehabilitation is as much a relearning program as it is physical recovery after surgery.[13] Often the subjects themselves have a clear feeling of a perception/proprioception deficit in the ankle joint area; they cannot "feel" the ankle as they used to. When this "feeling" returns it seems to co-coincide with complete rehabilitation. Leandersson et al. found that return of single-limb balance to normal values coincided with a subjective feeling of full rehabilitation in dancers.[17] It can be argued, however, that in this group balance during single-limb stance was as much a specific functional test as a nonspecific test for ankle proprioception.

Proprioceptive function is gained through coordination exercises using unilateral balance boards, uniaxial and multiaxial teeter boards, and jumping ropes. Restitution of normal function relies primarily on the individual's subjective feeling of return

TABLE 22.1. *Treatment modalities for muscle weakness*

Treatment	*Main indications*	*Advantages*	*Disadvantages/limitations*
Isometric exercise	Limited joint mobility or pain-free range of motion	Easy to implement; choice of specific angles	No training of full range of motion; nonfunctional except at certain positions
Dynamic exercise			
Constant resistance	Basic at home training programs	Concentric and eccentric training exercise; simple equipment	Inefficient matching of muscle and load torque; does not accommodate to pain
Variable resistance	Neurogen and muscle volume training	Exercise through full range of motion; accommodate and eccentric exercise	Eccentric exercise cannot be avoided; does not accommodate to pain
Isokinetic concentric	Specific effects at high and low speed; muscle volume training	Voluntary maximum load through range of motion; accommodates to pain; reduced joint compression force at high speed with maintained motor unit recruitment	No load at the end of movement
Isokinetic eccentric	Muscle volume training at relatively good muscle strength	High force development	Muscle soreness when unaccustomed; difficult to accommodate to pain

From Grimby G. Clinical aspects of strength and power training. In: Komi PV (ed) *Strength and Power in Sports*, Oxford: Blackwell Scientific, 1992, with permission.

to normal sensation, with the major effect of training seeming to be achieved within 6–10 weeks.

CONCOMITANT MODALITIES

External Compression

External compression using inflatable splints reduces blood flow and edema in the compressed area.[47,48] If the external pressure of an elastic bandage can reach approximately 80 mm Hg, the oozing of blood in the acutely injured tissues is markedly diminished.[49]

Cryotherapy

Cryotherapy consists of cold being delivered to the target tissue by conduction. The primary objective is to reduce hemorrhage, inflammation, edema, and pain. Physiologically, the reduced temperature results in arteriolar vasoconstriction, slowing the local inflammatory process and increasing the pain threshold.[50] There is an optimum temperature in terms of vasoconstriction, as excessive cryotherapy causes vasodilatation.[51,52] With appropriate cooling, blood flow is reduced by two-thirds after 10–15 minutes.

The cryotherapy method is important. Ice chips are superior to frozen gel packs, chemical ice, or cool sprays.[53] Maximal contact can be achieved with cooling systems such as the Cryocuff, which is used by many professionals during the postoperative and rehabilitation phases. Although it achieves beneficial short-term effects, cold therapy does not seem to alter the outcome of tissue regeneration.[50]

Superficial Heat Application

Like cold, heat is transmitted to the body by conduction. When superficial heat is applied to the skin, internal temperatures rise slowly, not exceeding 40°C, and the duration of the peak temperature is relatively short.[54] The heat-induced increase in blood flow primarily occurs in vessels of the skin and subcutaneous tissues, whereas deeper tissues seem to be unaffected.[55] The vasodilatory effect causes increased vessel permeability with concomitant intercellular fluid outflow and edema. Although the neurologic mechanism by which it occurs is unknown, it seems well established that superficial heating agents relieve pain.[55,56] Heat application also decreases connective tissue stiffness.[57] In conclusion, topical application of heat is indicated when more rapid healing, a mild increase in blood flow, partial relief of pain, muscle relaxation, and decreased joint stiffness are desired.

Ultrasonography

Ultrasonography is thought to have thermal, nonthermal, and neural effects. The thermal effect is caused by absorption of energy by the given tissue. Depending on the frequency, ultrasound can penetrate 5–10 cm into tissue and cause a 5°–6°C temperature increase in bone after just 2–20 seconds of application.[58] Nonthermal effects include the ability to drive large externally applied molecules deep into the tissue. Topically applied medications have thus been found at a tissue depth of up to 10 cm after 5 minutes of ultrasound treatment.[59] Vibration of gas bubbles in the tissues and changes in cell permeability, thereby inducing alterations in sodium, potassium, and calcium diffusion, are other nonthermal effects.[58] The neural effect is primarily an analgesic effect that has been reported in numerous clinical reports, although the mechanism of the pain relief is not clear.[59]

During rehabilitation, the ability of ultrasound to heat deep structures remains the prime indication. The sessions should not last more than 5–7 minutes, with constant movement of the ultrasound transducer to avoid overheating.[60]

PRACTICAL REHABILITATION

After Arthroscopic Surgery with Expected Return to Normal Function

A graded rehabilitation program after ankle arthroscopy is suggested in Table 22.2. Compared to arthroscopic meniscal surgery of the knee, for example, reduced weight-bearing may be advised for a longer period of time after simple ankle arthroscopic procedures owing to an increased tendency to effusion. Practical ways to apply the excises and modalities in the program are presented below.

Range of Motion

Active range of motion exercises are started after a few days. Traditional "alphabet exercises"—drawing the letters of the alphabet with the foot—encourage movements in all planes. Progressing at a pace at which swelling and pain are not provoked, stretching can be achieved with extra force using a towel sling (Fig. 22.4). As motion in the joint improves, gentle Achilles tendon and ankle dorsiflexion stretches are allowed (Fig. 22.5). If possible, stretches should be done with prewarmed muscles. Based on the research mentioned previously, the stretch must be held for as long as 45 seconds and be repeated at least four times every 6–8 hours. Joint mobilization using manual distraction and anteroposterior glides can also be started during this phase, progressing to a full program if the patient is pain-free.

Strength Training

If pain-free, strengthening exercises can be initiated early. Isometric exercises can usually be started fairly quickly in the dorsiplantar flexion direction, primarily as toe raises with an increasing amount of body weight. As with range of motion exercises, strength exercises should be performed in the combined planes of motion. These exercises are performed with elastic tubing (Fig. 22.6). Weights and machines that utilize weights are often difficult to control for the ankle and should be used for the final phases of a rehabilitation program. Soleus pumps, full arch isokinetics, and heel raise progression also belong at the end of the program. The last phase of the strengthening program should be established to recreate the functional demands of the patient (fast versus slow, eccentric versus concentric, endurance versus high load).

Proprioception and Coordination

Proprioceptive exercises usually begin as simple standing and balancing on one leg, followed by exercises using some type of balance board (Fig. 22.7). Improvement has been seen in chronically unstable ankles using the balance board 10 minutes a day five times a week for 2.5 months.[20] A reduction in sprains is seen using the balance board only 2 minutes twice a day.[61] Usually, however, the patients themselves have a definitive feeling of when they have regained full proprioceptive function. During the final phase

TABLE 22.2. *Rehabilitation after ankle arthroscopic surgery or injury*

Parameter	*Acute immobilization phase*	*Subacute postimmobilization phase*	*Terminal phase*	*Return to activity phase*
Goals	Protect joint integrity. Control inflammation. Control pain, edema and spasm	Maintain and increase soft tissue and adjacent joint mobility	Functional progression of closed chain activities. Proprioceptive retraining. Correct and control abnormal biomechanics	Preparation for return to ADL requirements
Weight-bearing status	Non-weight-bearing to touch weight-bearing	Crutch partial weight-bearing progressing toward full weight-bearing	Full weight-bearing	Full weight-bearing
Modalities	Ice; compression; elevation	Ice—ROM—ice—ROM, for example	Ice—ROM—ice—ROM, for example. Manipulative treatment	Ice after functional stress
External support	Orthosis/splint	ROM orthosis	ROM orthosis	Support if necessary
ROM flexibility	Early pain-free mobilization	Manipulative joint mobilization	Achilles tendon stretching	Muscle stretching
Open kinetic chain exercises	Pain-free isometrics	Alphabet ROM. Toe curls; marble pickups. Surgical tubing exercises in all planes	Full arch isokinetics	Ensure normal inversion/eversion strength ratios
Closed kinetic chain exercises		Low-weight-bearing heel raises. Soleus pumps. Body weight transfers	Heel raise progression. Body weight transfers with elastic tubing resistance	Body weight transfers in inversion/eversion with tubing resistance
Proprioception, agility, balance drills	Low-weight bearing tilt board	Partial weight-bearing. Tilt board. Stork stands	Full weight-bearing on tilt board. Jumping rope	Tilt board with weight-bearing overload. Hopping. Functional programs
Alternative exercises	Gluteus medius strengthening	Stationary cycling	Minitramp; stationary cycling	Stair climber and lateral step-ups

Adapted from Mulligan E. Lower leg, ankle, and foot rehabilitation. In: Andrews JR, Harrelson GL (eds) *Physical rehabilitation of the injured athlete.* Philadelphia: Saunders, 1991, with permission.
ADL, activities of daily living; ROM, range of motion.

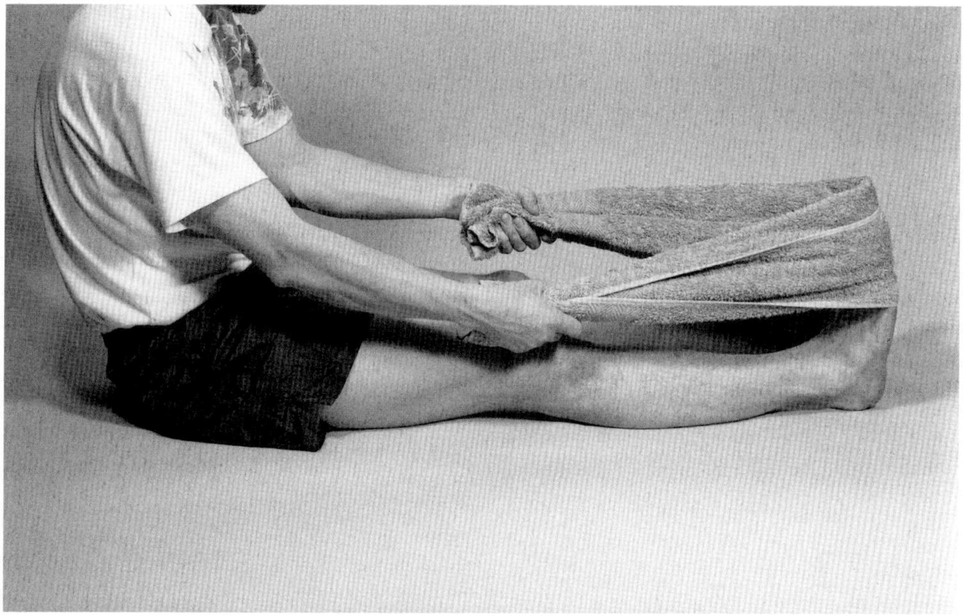

FIGURE 22.4. Training with a towel sling to improve passive and active range of motion.

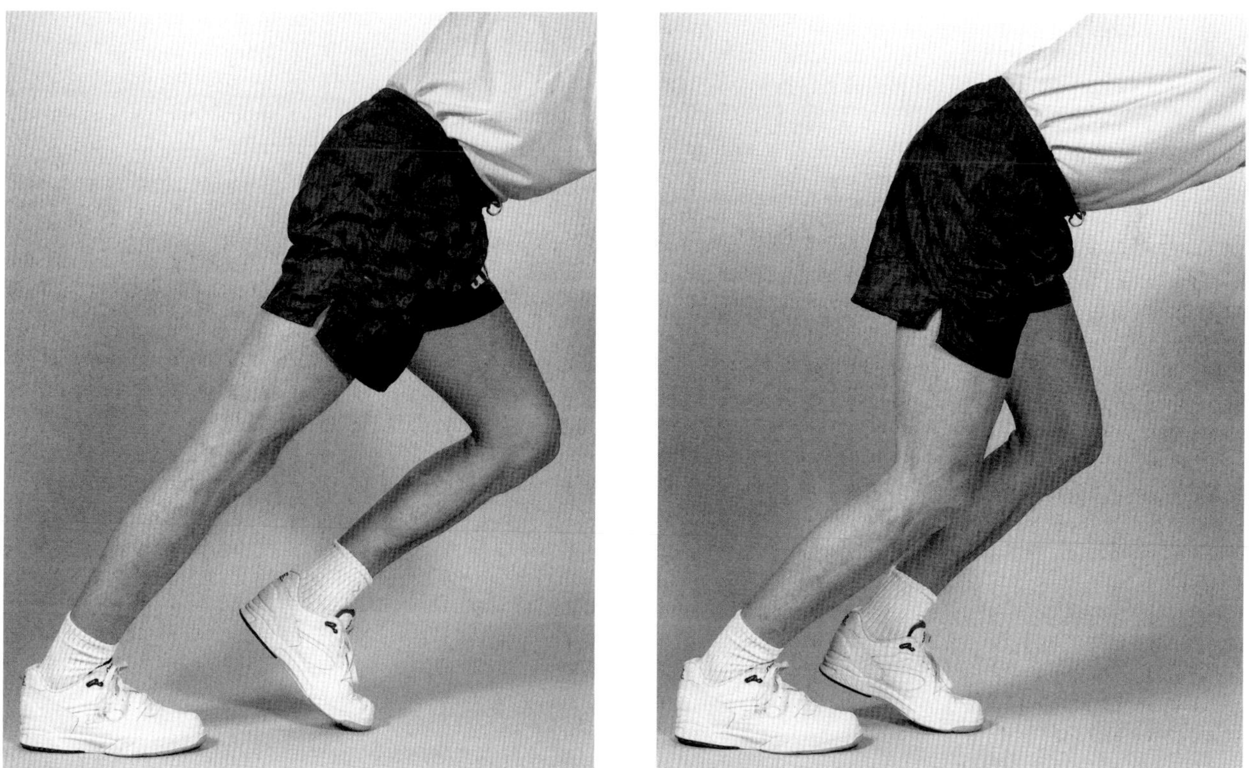

A B

FIGURE 22.5. Stretching the peripheral (**A**) and deeper parts (**B**) of the triceps surae.

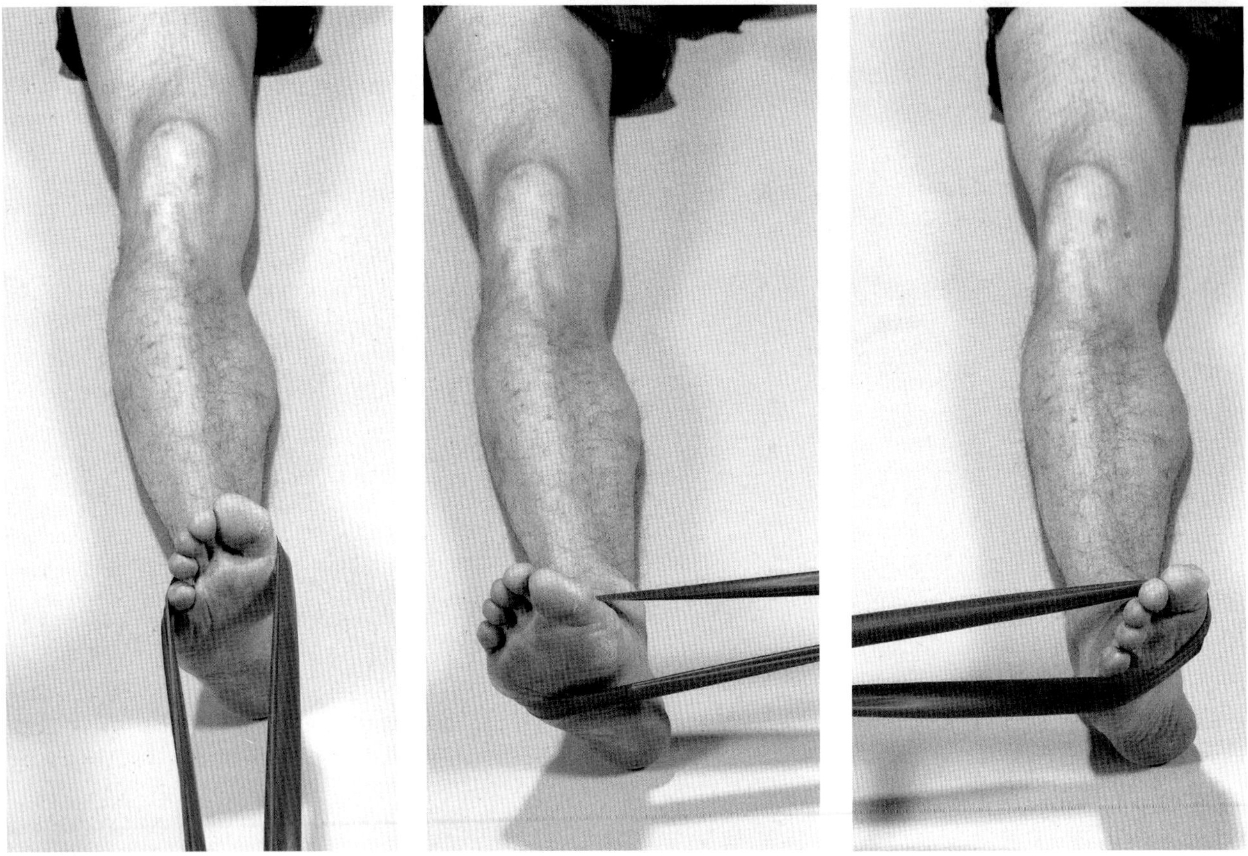

A B C

FIGURE 22.6. Rubber tubing exercises promoting strength and endurance. **A:** Dorsiflexor muscles. **B:** Everting muscles. **C:** Inverting muscles.

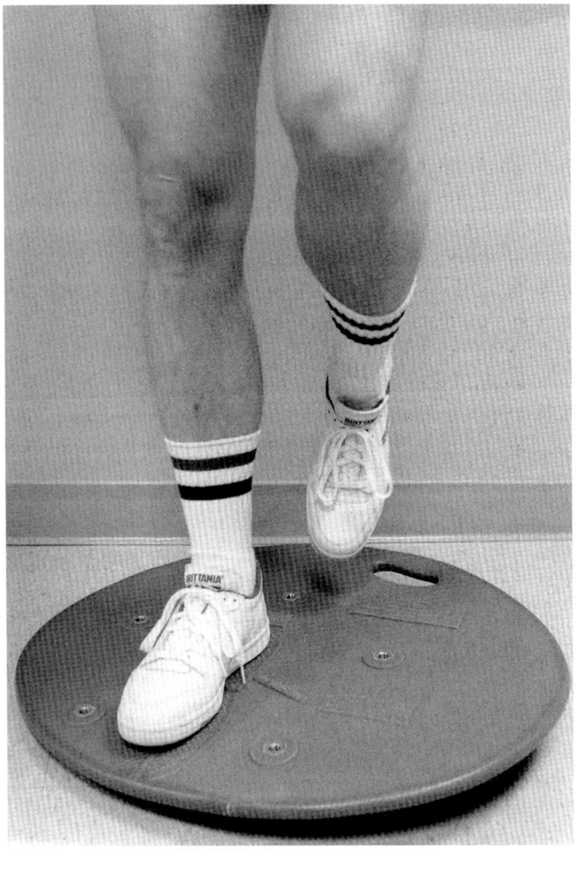

FIGURE 22.7. Balance board training.

of rehabilitation, functional progression is instituted to restore agility and confidence. If the patient is an athlete, functional exercises must be sports-specific. Having the subject run in tight figures-of-eight often helps determine the level of proprioceptive capability and allows the subject to determine whether he or she feels properly rehabilitated.

After Arthroscopic Ankle Arthrodesis

The goal following arthrodesis of the ankle is to achieve bony fusion by securing total immobilization of the talocrural joint while preserving motion in the surrounding joints and strength and mobility in the musculotendinous structures. The position of choice for ankle arthrodesis is in neutral dorsiflexion, 5–10 degrees of external rotation, and 5 degrees of valgus.[62,63] Although tibiotalar motion is lost, plantar flexion of up to 20 degrees can be achieved owing to motion in Chopart's and Lisfranc's joints. Dorsal flexion is restricted to the neutral position.[63] Muscle atrophy has been reported following ankle arthrodesis.[64,65] Walking speed is decreased owing to a shortened stride,[65] but two-thirds of the patients appear to have a normal gait.[63]

Depending on the choice of fixation device, the period of non-weight-bearing and partial weight-bearing may vary. As soon as ankle fusion is present, range of motion exercises of the subtalar joint and of Lisfranc's and Chopart's joints can commence coupled with proprioceptive training of balance. Walking is aided by a rocker bottom sole and increased heel cushioning. Quite early in the rehabilitation fitness maintenance can begin with stationary biking. Swimming can also be started.

BIBLIOGRAPHY

1. American Academy of Orthopedic Surgeons. *Joint motion: method of measuring and recording*, Chicago: AAOS, 1965;69–85.
2. Sammarco GJ, Burstein AH, Frankel VH. Biomechanics of the ankle: a kinematic study. *Orthop Clin North Am* 1973;4:75–96.
3. Van Langelaan EJ. A kinematical analysis of the tarsal joints: an x-ray photogrammetric study. *Acta Orthop Scand* Suppl 204 1983;54:147–269.
4. Inman VT. *The joints of the ankle*. Baltimore: Williams & Wilkins, 1976;37.
5. Sarrafian SK. *Anatomy of the foot and ankle*, 2nd ed. Philadelphia: Lippincott, 1993;508–513.
6. Lang J, Wachsmuth W. *Paktische anatomie: ein Lehr und Hilfsbuch der anatomischen gundlagen firtzlichen handelns*, vol 1, Part 4: *Bein und Statik*. Berlin: Springer, 1972;370.
7. Baumhauer JF, Alosa DM, Renstrom PA, et al. A prospective study of ankle injury risk factors. *Am J Sports Med* 1995;23:564–570.
8. Kannus P, Jozsa L, Renstrom P, et al. The effects of training, immobilization and remobilization on musculoskeletal tissue. 2. Remobilization and prevention of immobilization atrophy. *Scand J Med Sci Sports* 1992;2:164–176.
9. Stokes M, Young A. The contribution of reflex inhibition to arthrogenous muscle weakness. *Clin Sci* 1984;67:7–14.
10. Michelson JD, Hutchins C. Mechanoreceptors in human ankle ligaments. *J Bone Joint Surg Br* 1995;77: 219–224.
11. McCloskey DI. Kinesthetic sensibility. *Physiol Rev* 1978;58:763–820.
12. Sherrington CS. On the proprioceptive system, especially in its reflex aspects. *Brain* 1906;29:467–472.
13. Glencross D, Thornton E. Position sense following joint injury. *J Sports Med* 1981;21:23–27.
14. Jerosch J, Hoffstetter I, Bork H, Bischof M. The influence of orthoses on the proprioception of the ankle joint. *Knee Surg Sports Trauma Arthroscopy* 1995;3:39–46.
15. De Carlo MS, Talbot RW. Evaluation of ankle joint proprioception following injection of the anterior talofibular ligament. *J Orthop Sports Phys Ther* 1986;8:70–76.
16. Konradsen L, Ravn JB, Soerensen AI. Proprioception at the ankle: the effect of anaesthetic blockade of ligament receptors. *J Bone Joint Surg Br* 1993; 75:433–436.
17. Leandersson J, Eriksson E, Nilsson C, Wykman A. Proprioception in classical ballet dancers: a prospective study of the influence of an ankle sprain on proprioception in the ankle joint. *Am J Sports Med* 1996;24:370–374.
18. Kleinrensink GJ, Stoeckart IL, Meulstee J, et al. Lowered motor conduction velocity of the peroneal nerve after inversion trauma. *Med Sci Sports Exerc* 1994;26:877–883.
19. Konradsen L, Olesen S, Hansen HM. Ankle sensorimotor control and eversion strength after acute ankle inversion injuries. Am J Sports Med 1998; 26(1): 72–77.
20. Tropp H. Functional instability of the ankle joint. Thesis, Linkoping University Medical Dissertation no. 202, Linkoping, Sweden, 1985.
21. Karlsson J. Chronic lateral instability of the ankle joint: a clinical, radiological and experimental study. Thesis, Gothenburg University Hospital, Gothenburg, Sweden, 1989.
22. Gain SN, Newton RA. Kinesthetic awareness in sub-

jects with multiple ankle sprains. *Phys Ther* 1988;68: 1667–1671.
23. Dietz V. Human neuronal control of automatic functional movements: interaction between central programs and afferent input. *Physiol Rev* 1992;72:33–69.
24. Mann RA, Moran GT, Dougherty SE. Comparative electromyography of the lower extremity in jogging, running, and sprinting. *Am J Sports Med* 1986; 14:501–510.
25. Shiavi R, Bugle HJ, Limbird T. Electromyographic gait assessment. Part 1. Adult EMG profiles and walking speed. *J Rehabil Res Dev* 1987;24:13–23.
26. Dietz V, Quintera J, Sillem M. Stumbling reactions in man: significance of proprioceptive and preprogrammed mechanisms. *J Physiol (Lond)* 1987;386: 149–163.
27. Inman VT, Ralston HJ, Todd F. *Human walking*, Baltimore: Williams & Wilkins, 1981;22.
28. Wright DG, Desai SM, Henderson WH. Action of the subtalar and ankle joint complex during the stance phase of walking. *J Bone Joint Surg Am* 1964;46:361–365.
29. Mann RA. Overview of the foot and ankle biomechanics. In: Jahss MH (ed). *Disorders of the foot and ankle: medical and surgical management*, 2nd ed. Philadelphia: Saunders, 1991;385–408.
30. Folman Y, Wask J, Voloshin A, Liberty S. Cyclic impacts on heel strike: a possible biomechanical factor in the etiology of degenerative disease of the human locomotor system. *Arch Orthop Trauma Surg* 1986;104:363–365.
31. Taylor DC, Dalton JD Jr, Seaber AV, Garrett WEJ. Viscoelastic properties of muscle-tendon units: the biomechanical effects of stretching. *Am J Sports Med* 1990;18:300–309.
32. Hutton RS. Neuromuscular basis of stretching exercise. In: Komi PV (ed) *Strength and power in sports*. Oxford: Blackwell Scientific, 1993;29–38.
33. Kottke FJ, Pauley DL, Ptak KA. The rationale for prolonged stretching for correction of shortening of connective tissue. *Arch Phys Med Rehabil* 1966;47: 345–352.
34. Sapega AA, Quedenfeld TC, Moyer RA, Butler RA. Biophysical factors in range of motion exercise. *Physician Sportsmed* 1981;9:57–64.
35. Moore MA, Hutton RS. Electromyographic investigation of muscle stretching techniques. *Med Sci Sports Exerc* 1980;12:322–329.
36. Etnyre BR, Lee EJ. Comments on proprioceptive neuromuscular facilitation stretching techniques. *Res Q* 1987;58:184–188.
37. Magnusson SP, Simonsen EB, Aagaard P, et al. Mechanical and physiological responses to stretching with and without preisometric contraction in human skeletal muscle. *Arch Phys Med Rehabil* 1996;77:373–378.
38. Magnusson SP, Simonsen EB, Aagaard P, et al. Viscoelastic response to repeated static stretching in the human hamstring muscle. *Scand J Med Sci Sports* 1995;5:342–347.
39. Bohannon RW. Effect of repeated weight-minute muscle loading on the angle of straight-leg raising. *Phys Ther* 1984;64:491–497.
40. Godges JJ, MacRae H, Longdon C, et al. The effects of two stretching procedures on hip range of motion and gait economy. *J Orthop Sports Phys Ther* 1989; 11:350–357.
41. Hertling D, Kessler RN. *Management of common musculoskeletal disorders*, 2nd ed. Philadelphia: Lippincott, 1980.
42. Kessler RM. Friction massage. In: Kessler RM, Hertling D (eds) *Management of common musculoskeletal disorders*. Philadelphia: Harper & Row, 1983.
43. Arvidsson I, Eriksson E, Knutsson E, Arner S. Reduction of pain inhibition on voluntary muscle activation by epidural analgesia. *Orthopaedics* 1986;9: 1415–1419.
44. Grimby G. Clinical aspects of strength and power training. In: Komi PV (ed) *Strength and power in sports*. Oxford: Blackwell Scientific, 1992.
45. Thome R, Renstrom P, Grimby G, Peterson L. Slow or fast isokinetic training after knee ligament surgery. *J Orthop Sports Phys Ther* 1987;9:475–479.
46. Grimby G, Thomee R. Principles of rehabilitation after injuries. In: Knuttgen HG, Tittel K (eds) *Olympic book of sports medicine*, vol 1. Oxford: Blackwell Scientific, 1988;489–508.
47. Ashton H. The effect of increased tissue pressure on blood flow. *Clin Orthop* 1975;113:15–26.
48. Nielsen HV. External pressure-blood flow relations during limb compression in man. *Acta Physiol Scand* 1983;119:253–260.
49. Thorsson O. Muscle injuries in athletes. Dissertation, Lund University, Lund, Sweden, 1996.
50. Hurme T, Rantanen J, Kalimo H. Effects of early cryotherapy in experimental skeletal muscle injury. *Scand J Med Sci Sports* 1993;3:46–51.
51. Barcroft H, Edholm K. The effect of temperature on blood flow and deep temperature on the human forearm. *J Physiol (Lond)* 1943;102:5–20.
52. Kellett J. Acute soft tissue injuries: a review of the literature. *Med Sci Sports Exerc* 1986;18:489–500.
53. McMaster WC, Liddie S, Waught TR. Laboratory evaluation of various cold therapy modalities. *Am J Sports Med* 1978;6:291–294.
54. Lehmann JF. *Therapeutic heat and cold*, 3rd ed. Baltimore: Williams & Wilkins, 1982.
55. Michlovitz S. *Thermal agents in rehabilitation*. Philadelphia: Davis, 1986.
56. Licht S. *Therapeutic heat and cold*, 2nd ed. Baltimore: Waverly, 1965.
57. Wright V, Johns RJ. Physical factors concerned with

the stiffness of normal and diseased joints. *Bull Johns Hopkins Hosp* 1960;106:215–231.

58. Drez D. *Therapeutic modalities for sport injuries.* Chicago: Year Book, 1989.
59. Griffin JE, Karselis TC. *Physical agents for physical therapists*, 2nd ed. Springfield, IL: Charles C Thomas, 1982.
60. Rivenburgh DW. Physical modalities in the treatment of tendon injuries. *Clin Sports Med* 1992;11:645–660.
61. Rebman L. Suggestions from the clinic: ankle injuries: clinical observations. *J Orthop Sports Phys Ther* 1986;8:153–156.
62. Baker PL. SACH heel improves results of ankle fusion. *J Bone Joint Surg Am* 1970;52:1485–1486.
63. Ouzouian TJ, Kleiger B. Arthrodesis in the foot and ankle. In: Jahss MH (ed) *Disorders of the foot and ankle*, 2nd ed. vol 3. Philadelphia: Saunders, 1991.
64. Lynch AF, Bourne RB, Rorabeck CH. The long term results of ankle arthrodesis. *J Bone Joint Surg Br* 1988;70B:113–116.
65. Mazur JM, Schwartz E, Simon SR. Ankle arthrodesis, long term follow-up with gait analysis. *J Bone Joint Surg Am* 1979;61:964–975.

Index